Anne McNulty RN CCRN

clinical
MONITORING

CAROL L. LAKE, M.D.
Professor of Anesthesiology
University of Virginia Health Sciences Center
Charlottesville, Virginia

1990
W. B. SAUNDERS COMPANY
Harcourt Brace Jovanovich, Inc.

Philadelphia ■ London ■ Toronto ■ Montreal ■ Sydney ■ Tokyo

W. B. Saunders Company
Harcourt Brace Jovanovich, Inc.

The Curtis Center
Independence Square West
Philadelphia, PA 19106

Library of Congress Cataloging-in-Publication Data

Clinical monitoring.

  1. Patient monitoring. I. Lake, Carol L.
[DNLM: 1. Monitoring, Physiologic—methods.
WB 142 C641]
RC86.7.C53 1990   616.07′5   89-10171
ISBN 0-7216-2961-X

Editor: Lisette Bralow
Designer: Joan Owen
Production Manager: Bill Preston
Manuscript Editor: Mimi McGinnis
Illustration Coordinator: Brett MacNaughton
Indexer: Ella Shapiro

CLINICAL MONITORING   ISBN 0-7216-2961-X

Printed in the United States of America

Last digit is the print number: 9 8 7 6 5 4 3 2 1

Contributors

WILLIAM P. ARNOLD III, M.D.
Associate Professor of Anesthesiology, University of Virginia Health
Sciences Center, Charlottesville, Virginia
Perioperative Biochemical Monitors

JOHN L. ATLEE III, M.D.
Professor of Anesthesiology, Medical College of Wisconsin, Madison, Wisconsin
Electrocardiography: Monitoring for Arrhythmias

STEVEN J. BARKER, Ph.D., M.D.
Associate Professor and Vice-Chairman; Active Staff, University of California, Irvine Medical Center, Irvine, California
Monitoring of Oxygen

FIONA M. CLEMENTS, M.D.
Assistant Professor; Attending Anesthesiologist, Duke University Medical
Center, Durham, North Carolina
Electrocardiography: Monitoring for Ischemia

HARRY COMERCHERO, M.Sc.
Marketing Manager, EMTEK Health Care Systems, Inc., Tempe, Arizona
Patient Data Management Systems

D. RYAN COOK, M.D.
Professor of Anesthesiology and Pharmacology, University of Pittsburgh
School of Medicine; Director; Staff Anesthesiologist, Department of Anesthesiology, Children's Hospital of Pittsburgh, Pittsburgh, Pennsylvania
Monitoring the Neuromuscular Junction

NORBERT P. de BRUIJN, M.D.
Associate Professor of Anesthesiology; Assistant Professor of Surgery; Attending Anesthesiologist; Duke University Medical Center, Durham, North
Carolina
Electrocardiography: Monitoring for Ischemia

COSMO A. DiFAZIO, M.D., Ph.D.
Professor of Anesthesiology, University of Virginia Health Sciences Center, Charlottesville, Virginia
Maternal-Fetal Monitoring in Obstetrics

CHARLES G. DURBIN, Jr., M.D.
Associate Professor of Anesthesiology and Surgery, University of Virginia School of Medicine; Medical Director of Surgical Intensive Care Unit; Medical Director of Respiratory Therapy Department, University of Virginia Health Sciences Center, Charlottesville, Virginia
Monitoring Arterial Blood Gases and Acid-Base Balance

THOMAS J. GAL, M.D.
Professor of Anesthesiology, University of Virginia Health Sciences Center, Charlottesville, Virginia
Monitoring the Function of the Respiratory System

BERNICE R. HECKER, M.D.
Attending Anesthesiologist, Virginia Mason Medical Center; Clinical Assistant Professor of Anesthesiology, University of Washington, Seattle, Washington
Monitoring Anesthetic Gases

ZAHARIA HILLEL, M.D., Ph.D.
Assistant Professor of Anesthesiology, Mount Sinai School of Medicine, Mount Sinai Medical Center, New York, New York
Intraoperative Echocardiography

JOHN W. HOYT, M.D.
Clinical Professor of Anesthesiology and Critical Care Medicine, University of Pittsburgh School of Medicine; Medical Director, Medical/Surgical Intensive Care Unit, Saint Francis Medical Center, Pittsburgh, Pennsylvania
Patient Data Management Systems

GAVIN N. C. KENNY, B.Sc. (Hons.), M.B., Ch.B., M.D., F.F.A.R.C.S.
Senior Lecturer, University Department of Anaesthesia, Glasgow University; Honorary Consultant Anaesthetist, Royal Infirmary, Glasgow, Scotland
Computerized Monitoring in Anesthesia

KEITH D. KNOPES, M.D.
Staff Anesthesiologist, Virginia Mason Medical Center; Clinical Assistant Professor of Anesthesiology, University of Washington, Seattle, Washington
Monitoring Anesthetic Gases

STEVEN N. KONSTADT, M.D.
Assistant Professor of Anesthesiology; Director, Cardiovascular Anesthesiology, Loyola University Medical Center, Maywood, Illinois
Intraoperative Echocardiography

CAROL L. LAKE, M.D.
Professor of Anesthesiology, University of Virginia; Staff Anesthesiologist, University of Virginia Health Sciences Center, Charlottesville, Virginia
Introduction; Monitoring of Arterial Pressure; Monitoring of Ventricular Function; Stethoscopy, Thermometry, and Miscellaneous Monitors; Evoked Potentials

STUART C. LAW, M.D.
Assistant Professor, University of Pittsburgh; Staff Anesthesiologist, Presbyterian Hospital; Staff Anesthesiologist, Children's Hospital of Pittsburgh, Pittsburgh, Pennsylvania
Monitoring the Neuromuscular Junction

WARREN J. LEVY, M.D.
Associate Professor of Anesthesia, Hospital of the University of Pennsylvania, Philadelphia, Pennsylvania
Electroencephalography

ROBERT G. LOEB, M.D.
Assistant Professor, Department of Anesthesiology, University of California Davis School of Medicine, Davis; Anesthesiologist, University of California Davis Medical Center, Sacramento, California
Intravascular Pressure Monitoring Systems

WAYNE K. MARSHALL, M.D.
Associate Professor, Department of Anesthesia, M. S. Hershey Medical Center, Pennsylvania State University College of Medicine, Hershey, Pennsylvania
Intracranial Pressure

ROGER A. MOORE, M.D.
Associate Professor, University of Pennsylvania School of Medicine, Philadelphia, Pennsylvania; Co-Chairman, Department of Anesthesiology, Deborah Heart and Lung Center, Browns Mills, New Jersey
Intraoperative Evaluation of Hemostasis

ALAN W. MURRAY, M.B., Ch.B., F.F.A.R.C.S.
Research Fellow in Anaesthetics, University Department of Anaesthetics, Royal Infirmary, Glasgow, Scotland
Computerized Monitoring in Anesthesia

MARK J. RICE, M.D.
Assistant Professor of Anesthesiology, University of Wisconsin, Madison, Wisconsin
Electrocardiography: Monitoring for Arrhythmias

CONTRIBUTORS

WILLIAM T. ROSS, Jr., M.D.
Associate Professor of Anesthesiology; Medical Director, Virginia Ambulatory Surgery Center, University of Virginia Health Sciences Center; Anesthesiologist, University of Virginia Hospitals, Charlottesville, Virginia
Monitoring the Anesthesia Machine

KAREN J. SCHWENZER, M.D.
Assistant Professor of Anesthesiology; Associate Director, Surgical Intensive Care Unit, University of Virginia Health Sciences Center, Charlottesville, Virginia
Venous and Pulmonary Pressures

DANIEL M. THYS, M.D.
Associate Professor of Anesthesiology, Mount Sinai School of Medicine; Director, Cardiothoracic Anesthesiology, Mount Sinai Medical Center, New York, New York
Intraoperative Echocardiography

KEVIN K. TREMPER, Ph.D., M.D.
Associate Professor and Chairman; Active Staff, University of California, Irvine Medical Center, Irvine, California
Monitoring of Oxygen

ANDREW M. WOODS, M.D.
Associate Professor of Anesthesiology, University of Virginia Health Sciences Center, Charlottesville, Virginia
Maternal-Fetal Monitoring in Obstetrics

Preface

A monitor is a machine that repetitively performs a measurement of a physiologic parameter such as heart rate, systemic blood pressure, or cardiac output. The anesthesiologist, working in conjunction with many machines, spends almost 70–80% of her or his working time as a monitor of the cardiovascular, respiratory, central nervous, and biochemical systems of her or his patients. In addition, the anesthesiologist must monitor the function of the anesthetic administration system and its environment. In critical situations, the electromechanical or computer-based monitor performs independently of the anesthesiologist in an automated fashion, indicating alterations in variables from preset limits. Finally, the vast quantities of measured variables are acquired, analyzed, and stored.

This text describes both invasive and noninvasive monitoring devices as well as automated and nonautomated monitoring methods. The approach to monitoring in this book is in its role as a specific subspecialty of anesthesiology. The book is organized by devices designed to perform specific monitoring functions rather than by descriptions of monitors used for specific types of anesthetic and operative procedures. However, the clinical uses of each monitoring device are discussed, including a comprehensive review of the specialized monitoring required in cardiac anesthesia, neuroanesthesia, obstetric anesthesia, pediatric anesthesia, and intensive care. Chapters on special monitoring needs, such as the measurement of biochemical parameters including arterial blood gases, glucose, or electrolytes; the use of computers for patient data acquisition and management in the operating room; and intensive care are presented.

The book is intended for residents and fellows in anesthesiology and attending anesthesiologists with specific interests in the monitoring of patients receiving cardiac anesthesia, neuroanesthesia, obstetric anesthesia, and intensive care. However, the general anesthesiologist clinician will find the device- and method-oriented approach useful in daily practice. The multiauthor format overcomes the inability of a single author to be expert in all areas of monitoring. The goal of this text is to provide complete, authoritative information without the bias or inclusion of monitoring methods utilized or applicable only to research-oriented institutions.

Acknowledgments

The inspiration and support for writing and editing this text has come from many people. The editor extends sincere thanks to the many authors who contributed their time, experience, and expertise in the writing of the individual chapters in this text. A special debt of gratitude is owed to the families, friends, and colleagues of the chapter authors for their share in the hard work that made this text a reality.

Skillful preparation of the text and illustrations was performed by Mrs. Barbara Lane of Lane Business Services, Ms. Linda Hamme and Ms. Cindy Hiter of the Division of Biomedical Communications at the University of Virginia, and others in the institutions of the contributing authors. Numerous authors and publishers have kindly permitted us to reprint figures and tables from their work. Special thanks are due to Mr. Dana Dreibelbis, former medical editor at W.B. Saunders for his assistance is the early phases of planning of the book. The staff of W.B. Saunders and particularly Ms. Lisette Bralow were particularly helpful in the preparation of the manuscript and understanding about the inevitable and unavoidable delays. Finally, I am most grateful to the chairman, Dr. Robert M. Epstein, and the faculty of the Department of Anesthesiology at the University of Virginia for encouragement and guidance in the preparation of the manuscript.

Contents

Introduction

■ CAROL L. LAKE, M.D.

In perioperative patient care, monitoring can be defined as continuous or repeated observation and vigilance.[1] The best monitor is the totally aware anesthesiologist who is looking and listening and sensing significant changes in the patient. No electronic device can replace this function.

The goal of monitoring is to identify trends and to prevent untoward events. Repeated observations must be performed frequently, either intermittently, semicontinuously, or continuously to record trends. Machines make repetitive measurements at frequencies impossible for humans. The value of any specific monitor in the achievement of this goal is how likely a change in a particular monitored variable predicts poor outcome or contributes directly to it. Adequate warning time to change conditions and alter outcome is implicit in the definition of monitoring. For these reasons, use of a variable to establish a diagnosis is not monitoring. An example is the placement of an intra-arterial catheter in a critically ill patient. The direct measurement of arterial pressure allows identification of hypotension while there is time to reverse it rather than making the diagnosis of hypertension as blood pressure determination does in an outpatient. Another example is the oxygen analyzer which detects a condition of reduced oxygen delivery but fails to pinpoint the source of the problem. Although this monitor functions well to prevent injury, correct action (increased oxygen delivery) must be taken to assure a good outcome.[2]

More than 50% of the critical incidents occurring during anesthesia result from inadequate or incomplete monitoring of the patient, anesthesia machine, or patient-machine interface. Equipment failure is one of the recurrent causes of anesthesia-related injuries.[3] Problems with electrocardiograph, blood pressure equipment, or other monitoring devices, disconnections or incorrect connections in breathing circuits, and incorrect types or flows of gases or vapors are frequent causes of critical perioperative inci-

1

dents. Although the monitoring device itself may be the source of the incident, failure to use an adequate array of monitors, inadequate recognition of the changes displayed, or failure to respond to an undesirable monitored event constitutes most anesthetic management problems.

Human error continues to play a major role in anesthetic mishaps.[4] In this regard, inexperience and exchange of personnel are critical factors. Either the relief of one person by another or the return of the primary caretaker may permit detection and control of untoward events.[4]

However, the proliferation of new monitors and safety features has often occurred without regard for the ability of the human anesthesiologist to assimilate the additional information. There is a need to limit the complexity of control and information displays (increase their manageability or make them more "user friendly") so that adverse outcomes are prevented, not caused.[5] The vast array of monitors currently available for use in the perioperative period allows the anesthesiologist or critical care physician greater access to variables measured by machines but may actually reduce his or her direct personal observation of the patient. The British anesthetist Pask suggested in 1965 "that the best patient-monitoring device would be a tube of contact adhesive: Place a small dab of it over the patient's temporal artery, another small dab on one of the anesthetist's fingers and bring these two into contact so that they could not be readily separated."[6] Although times have changed, there is still much truth in these words.

HISTORY OF MONITORING

The monitoring technology of the twentieth century is best appreciated in the light of history. The earliest historical observations of the circulatory, respiratory, and central nervous systems concerned either their anatomy or their physiology.

Pulse

Herophilus around 300 BC used a water clock for counting the pulse, upon which he placed considerable importance as an index of health or disease.[7] Galen also contributed 16 volumes detailing the uses of the pulse and its role as a predictive variable.[7] Pulsus paradoxus and pulsus alternans, changes in the pulse volume, were described in 1873 and 1892, respectively.[8]

Stethoscopy

Clinical observations were restricted to external observations, palpation, percussion (introduced by Auenbrugger in 1761), or postmortem examination until the development of the stethoscope in 1816 by Laënnec.[8] It permitted judgment on the patient's internal conditions, specifically position of organs, presence of fluid, and location of lesions. Laënnec's original stethoscope was a wooden tube, 9 inches long and 1.5 inches in diameter. One version had a bell-shaped opening at one end that reduced to a small-diameter hole at the other; another had a single-diameter hole for its entire length.[9] Piorry improved the monaural stethoscope, introduced the trumpet chestpiece, and improved the earpieces. The binaural stethoscope was developed by Cammann in 1852. Microphonic amplification stethoscopy was used in 1878.[9] In 1909, Sprague invented the combined stethoscope with both bell and diaphragm chestpieces. Use of the precordial stethoscope in the operating room is attributed to Cushing.[10]

Blood Pressure

The first person to measure or monitor a physiologic function was Stephen Hale, who directly measured the blood pressure of a horse in 1733. Into the crural artery, Hale inserted a brass pipe to which was attached a 9-foot length of glass tubing. Release of the arterial ligature allowed blood to rise in the tube to a distance of 8 feet 3 inches above the heart. Hale also noted that the blood in the tube rose and fell different amounts with each pulse, with greater excursions of 12–14 inches alternating with lesser changes. During hemorrhage of the animal, Hale noted that the amount of blood loss failed to correlate with the decrease in pressure. However, it was more than 150 years later before the importance of measuring blood pressure was appreciated.

Sphygmomanometry

Over the years, attempts were made to measure blood pressure either by direct cannulation or with a sphygmograph. One of the links between direct arterial measurement and noninvasive methods was made by Poiseuille in 1828 when he used a U-shaped tube containing mercury (which counterbalanced the pressure of the blood) to replace the long glass tube into which blood flowed from a cannulated artery. Herisson invented an instrument that showed the beat of the pulse in a column of mercury, thus obviating the need for intra-arterial measurement of blood pressure. This instrument was later combined with a kymographion (a pen- and-drum recorder), creating the sphygmograph. The sphygmograph consisted of a series of levers that could be loaded until arterial pulsations were abolished. The levers also recorded the movements that the pulse imparted to a button, and the force necessary to impede the arterial pulse completely was measured in grams.

Basch in 1881 modified the sphygmograph by using a rubber ball, which communicated with a mercury manometer, to compress the artery. However, Basch's instrument was inaccurate. Other modifications included the securing of the ball in a bandage, the substitution of air for water as the medium to transmit the impulses, and finally the evolution of a device consisting of a measuring apparatus with a tube connecting to a compressing apparatus, which was a double ball secured to a metallic ring.

Riva Rocci stressed the importance of monitoring blood pressure and its variation. In his sphygmomanometer, blood pressure equaled the pressure in the inflated cuff, compressing the arm at the point where the pulse was felt during cuff deflation. Riva Rocci described the stress produced by the pressure on the arterial wall in 1896 in *A New Sphygmomanometer*. His sphygmomanometer was intended for rapidly repeatable measurement of radial artery pressure. However, in 1905 Korotkoff, using the stethoscope to monitor the pulse, discovered that the pulse sound disappeared as cuff pressure declined, at the point roughly corresponding to ventricular diastole, the diastolic pressure.[11]

Intraoperative Blood Pressure Measurement

Intraoperative recording of blood pressure was introduced by Cushing, who recognized that arterial pressure indicated the physiologic condition of a laboratory animal or human.[12] Crile also advocated blood pressure monitoring by use of the Gärtner tonometer, but neither his nor Cushing's recommendation for routine use of blood pressure measurement during surgery was widely accepted in the first decade of the twentieth century. However, by the time of publication of Gwathmey's book, *Anesthesia*, in 1914, a section on the intraoperative monitoring of blood pressure by McKeson was included.[13] Rovenstine in 1934 promoted systematic data collection for statistical purposes in anesthesia.[14] Collected observations of blood pressure, pulse, and respiration became the first anesthesia records.[15]

Intravascular Pressures

Intracardiac pressures were measured by Wiggers using a vertical glass fluid-filled cannula with one end covered by a distensible rubber membrane with a mirror attached to it that could be introduced directly into the heart.[16] A beam of light reflected from the oscillations of the mirror were recorded on a photographic plate. A thistle-shaped glass vessel, called a cardiometer, placed over the ventricle and connected to a piston recorder, was used to determine volume changes in the heart.

Both direct and indirect methods were used to measure venous pressure. The indirect method was the amount of external pressure required to collapse a small superficial vein or the pressure that prevented its refill. Venous pressure was measured directly by insertion of a needle connected by a rubber tube to a manometer into the median basilic vein. Pressure changes in the central venous system were measured in the jugular vein by placing a small metal cup over the vein and connecting it to a Marey tambour. Refinements in the measurement of pressure and flow in the heart were made by Cournand and Richards in the early 1940s.[11]

Electrocardiography

The electrocardiogram (ECG) was first described by Einthoven.[17] It consisted of a sensitive string galvanometer or iron oscillograph. In the Einthoven galvanometer, a fine silvered glass fiber is suspended in an electro-magnet. Minute oscillations occur when current passes through the fiber. The shadow of the oscillating fiber is magnified and projected onto a photographic plate. Adjustment of the tension of the fiber allowed a potential difference of 1 mV between the two ends of the fiber to cause a 1-cm deflection on the recording plate. Intracavitary electrograms using saline-filled catheters were described in 1949.[18] The development of closed chest cardiac resuscitation and defibrillation in the 1960s furthered the need to continuously monitor the ECG in coronary care units.

Cardiac Output

The Fick principle to measure cardiac output was theorized in 1870, but it was not in common use until the 1930s.[19] Collection of mixed venous blood from humans was difficult. The Fick principle forms the basis for dye dilution and thermodilution cardiac output determinations used in modern times.

Thermometry

Although the importance of body temperature was recognized by Hippocrates, the first thermometer was probably constructed by Galileo in 1592. However, his thermometer had no measurement scale, was influenced by atmospheric pressure, and gave only gross indications of temperature alteration.[11] Essential steps toward clinical measurements came with the development of fixed temperature scales by Christian Huygens (Celsius scale) and Gabriel Fahrenheit (Fahrenheit scale).[11] Boerhaave introduced the thermometer into clinical practice in the seventeenth and eighteenth centuries, but it did not become an integral part of medical monitoring until the nineteenth century with the publication of Carl Wunderlich's *The Temperature in Diseases* in 1868.[9, 11] Early thermometry was complex and cumbersome, which precluded its acceptance even though its significance was apparent. Anton deHaen, one of Boerhaave's students, recognized that movement of the temperature toward normal indicated improvement in the patient's condition. The shape and size of the clinical thermometer used today were designed in 1870 by Albutt.[11]

Respirometry

Hutchinson in his monograph, *On the Capacity of the Lungs, and on the Respiratory Functions, with a View of Establishing a Precise and Easy Method of Detecting Disease by the Spirometer*, defined five variables for measurement of respiratory performance. These were vital capacity (quantity expelled during greatest exhalation after deepest inspiration), residual air (amount of air remaining in lungs after deepest breathing), reserve air (amount of air left after gentle expiration), complemental air (amount beyond normal inspiration by deep breathing), and breathing air (normal inspiration and expiration).[9] Hutchinson's spirometer did not require skilled interpretation, and he verified the association between pulmonary disease and alterations in spirometric variables.[9]

Laboratory Medicine

Evaluation of the appearance and chemical properties of the blood and urine was initially done in the late eighteenth century. However, most of the determinations were for diagnosis of chronic conditions such as diabetes and renal disease. The importance of laboratory evaluation was demonstrated by the development of "ward labs," a precursor of the present-day "stat lab."

REASONS FOR MONITORING

Many reasons have been promulgated for perioperative monitoring of surgical patients. Two of the major reasons are physiologic monitoring and patient safety. Physiologic monitoring includes the ECG and devices that monitor intravascular pressures, intracranial pressures, neuromuscular function, cardiac output or ventricular function, and biochemical variables. Patient safety monitors include breathing circuit oxygen analyzers, breathing circuit disconnect alarms, and other monitors of the anesthesia delivery system as well as devices such as capnographs or pulse oximeters that monitor the patient–anesthesia machine interface. Whitcher and colleagues suggest that a minimally acceptable monitoring configuration should permit positive identification of all major pathways of patient injury.[20] They further suggest that the expected savings in the prevention of injuries outweighs the costs of sophisticated monitors.[20] The emphasis is on *preventable* injuries such as disconnection of the anesthetic circuit, esophageal intubation, hyperthermia, and the like.

ESSENTIAL MONITORING

Establishment of minimal monitoring standards has been difficult, although the goals of such standards are clear. Monitors may be essential for the conduct of the anesthetic (e.g., respirometers, oxygen analyzers, breathing circuit alarms, volatile anesthetic vapor analysis), for the conduct of perioperative care for a specific procedure (pulmonary artery and intra-arterial catheters, intracranial cannulas), or for general perioperative management (blood pressure, pulse, ECG, temperature measurement, pulse oximetry, capnography).[21] Eichhorn and associates suggest that standards for

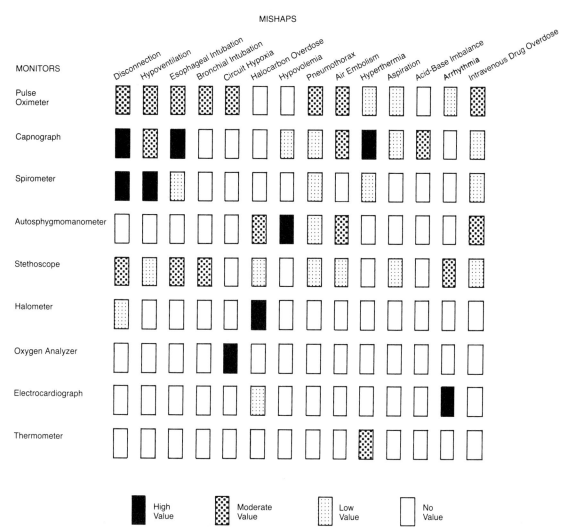

MISHAPS

MONITORS

Figure I–1. A matrix of the type of monitoring device versus its value in the prevention of accidents. (From Whitcher C, Ream AK, Parsons D, et al: Anesthetic mishaps and the cost of monitoring: A proposed standard for monitoring equipment. J Clin Monit 1988; 4:11. With permission.)

monitoring codify accepted practices, provide the means for objective evaluation of individual practice, reduce patient injury from anesthesia accidents (and possibly eventually liability insurance premiums), and apply collective experience to rare events (occurring one or two times in the career of an individual anesthesia practitioner).[22] The reduction in insurance premiums (based on paid claims) may amount to $27,000/operating room/year.[20]

The essential monitors proposed by Whitcher and colleagues include automatic sphygmomanometer, pulse oximeter, capnograph, spirometer, halometer, breathing circuit oxygen analyzer, stethoscope, electrocardiograph, and thermometer.[20] Most essential monitors provide continuous, as opposed to intermittent, information. The value of these devices to prevent

Mishap

Monitor	Disconnection	Hypoventilation	Esophageal Intubation	Bronchial Intubation	Circuit Hypoxia	Halocarbon Overdose	Hypovolemia	Pneumothorax	Air Embolism	Hyperthermia	Aspiration	Acid Base Imbalance	Arrhythmia	Intravenous Drug Overdose	Hypotension	Hypoxia	Cerebral Ischemia	Airway Obstruction	Circuit Valve Malfunction	Anesthetic Agent Error	Pulmonary Edema	Inadequate Cardiac Output	Inadequate Peripheral Perfusion	Residual Neuromuscular Blockade	Hypothermia
Pulse Oximeter	1	2	1	1	1	1	1	1	1	1	1	0	2	1	2	3	0	1	1	0	2	3	3	0	0
Capnograph	3	3	3	2	0	0	2	2	2	3	1	2	0	1	2	1	0	3	3	0	1	2	1	2	2
Spirometer	3	3	1	0	0	0	0	1	0	1	0	0	0	1	0	0	0	3	2	0	1	0	0	1	0
Autosphygmomanometer	0	0	0	0	0	2	2	1	1	0	0	0	0	2	3	0	0	0	0	0	1	2	2	0	0
Stethoscope	2	1	2	2	0	1	0	1	1	0	1	0	1	0	1	0	0	2	0	0	2	1	0	0	0
Halometer	1	0	0	0	0	3	0	0	0	0	0	0	0	0	0	0	0	1	0	1	0	0	0	0	0
Oxygen Analyzer	1	0	0	0	3	0	0	0	0	1	0	0	0	0	0	0	0	0	0	0	0	0	0	0	0
Electrocardiograph	0	0	0	0	0	1	0	0	0	2	0	0	3	0	0	1	0	0	0	0	1	0	0	0	0
Thermometer	0	0	0	0	0	0	0	0	0	1	0	0	0	0	0	0	0	0	0	0	0	0	0	0	3
Electroencephalograph	0	1	0	0	1	3	1	0	2	0	0	2	0	3	2	3	3	0	0	1	0	3	3	0	1
Evoked Potentials	0	0	0	0	0	2	1	0	1	0	0	1	0	0	2	2	2	0	0	1	0	2	1	0	1
Airway Pressure	3	1	1	2	0	0	0	2	1	0	1	0	0	0	0	0	0	3	1	0	2	0	0	0	0
Agent-specific Halometer	1	0	0	0	3	0	0	0	0	0	0	0	0	0	0	0	0	1	0	3	0	0	0	0	0
Nitrogen Analyzer	1	0	0	0	1	0	0	0	3	0	0	0	0	0	0	0	0	0	0	0	0	0	0	0	0
Cardiac Output	0	0	0	0	0	2	2	1	2	0	0	0	1	2	2	1	0	0	0	1	2	3	2	0	1
Two-Dimensional Echocardiograph	0	0	0	0	0	2	3	0	3	0	0	0	2	2	1	0	0	0	0	1	1	2	1	0	0
Continuous Blood Pressure	0	0	0	0	0	2	3	1	2	0	0	0	2	3	0	0	0	0	0	1	2	2	2	0	1
Pulse Plethysmograph	0	0	0	0	0	2	3	2	2	0	0	0	2	2	2	0	0	0	0	2	3	3	3	0	2
Transcutaneous Po_2	1	1	1	3	2	1	2	3	2	1	3	1	0	1	2	3	0	1	1	0	3	3	3	0	1
Transcutaneous Pco_2	1	3	1	1	1	1	2	1	2	3	1	2	0	0	2	2	0	1	1	0	2	1	1	0	0
Neuromuscular Twitch	0	0	0	0	0	0	0	0	0	0	0	0	0	0	0	0	0	0	0	0	0	0	0	3	0

Figure I–2. Capability of different monitors to detect critical events during administration of anesthesia. 3 = high value, 2 = moderate value, 1 = low value, 0 = no value. (From Block FE: A proposed standard for monitoring equipment: What equipment should be included? J Clin Monit 1988; 4:1–4, with permission.)

or limit mishaps is detailed in Fig. I–1. However, the use of monitors must be realistic and easily attainable for the average anesthesiologist. Cost-benefit ratios must be considered in detailing standards. Costs to equip one operating room with essential or enhanced monitoring arrays vary from $22,000 to $82,000.[20, 23]

Other authors have suggested different values for the monitors proposed by Whitcher for the detection of various critical events and recommended different essential arrays (Fig. I–2).[5, 20, 23] Block suggests that the essential monitors are pulse oximeter, capnograph with waveform display, automatic sphygmomanometer, electrocardiograph, thermometer, electroencephalograph, transcutaneous oxygen and carbon dioxide tension monitor, and neuromuscular function monitor.[23] However, he highly recommends the addition of a continuous blood pressure measurement, such as the Peñaz method, and use of a noninvasive monitor of cardiac output, such as the thoracic impedance or transesophageal Doppler devices, to this monitoring array.[23]

Philip and coworkers noted other factors—such as predictability (freedom from aberrant output or malfunction), specificity (few false-positive results), sensitivity (few false-negative results), simplicity of use, distraction of caregiver, cost, and availability—that must be considered when recommendations for equipment or guidelines for monitoring are regarded as standards. The optimal monitoring array must be effective, noninvasive, manageable, and economical.[5]

An automated anesthesia record has also been suggested as an essential monitor.[21] This suggestion results from the diagnostic information derived from trend plots, which form patterns of great clinical importance (see Chapter 11). However, acceptance of automated records may require improvement in the current input of much artifactual information.

Table I–1. THE HARVARD MEDICAL SCHOOL STANDARDS FOR ANESTHESIA MONITORING PRACTICE

These standards apply for any administration of anesthesia involving department of anesthesia personnel and are specifically referable to preplanned anesthetics administered in designated anesthetizing locations (specific exclusion: administration of epidural analgesia for labor or pain management). In emergency circumstances in any location, immediate life support measures of whatever appropriate nature come first, with attention turning to the measures described in these standards as soon as possible and practical. These are minimal standards that may be exceeded at any time based on the judgment of the involved anesthesia personnel. These standards encourage high-quality patient care, but observing them cannot guarantee any specific patient outcome. These standards are subject to revision from time to time, as warranted by the evolution of technology and practice.

Anesthesiologist's or Nurse Anesthetist's Presence in Operation Room
For all anesthetics initiated by or involving a member of the department of anesthesia, an attending or resident anesthesiologist or nurse anesthetist shall be present in the room throughout the conduct of all general anesthetics, regional anesthetics, and monitored intravenous anesthetics. An exception is made when there is a direct known hazard, e.g., radiation, to the anesthesiologist or nurse anesthetist, in which case some provision for monitoring the patient must be made.

Blood Pressure and Heart Rate
Every patient receiving general anesthesia, regional anesthesia, or managed intravenous anesthesia shall have arterial blood pressure and heart rate measured at least every 5 minutes, where not clinically impractical.*

Electrocardiogram
Every patient shall have the electrocardiogram continuously displayed from the induction or institution of anesthesia until preparing to leave the anesthetizing location, where not clinically impractical.*

Continuous Monitoring
During every administration of general anesthesia, the anesthetist shall employ methods of continuously monitoring the patient's ventilation and circulation. The methods shall include, for ventilation and circulation each, at least one of the following or the equivalent:†
—*For Ventilation.* Palpation or observation of the reservoir breathing bag, auscultation of breath sounds, monitoring of respiratory gases such as end-tidal carbon dioxide, or monitoring of expiratory gas flow. Monitoring end-tidal carbon dioxide is an emerging standard and is strongly preferred.

(continued)

Table I-1. THE HARVARD MEDICAL SCHOOL STANDARDS FOR
ANESTHESIA MONITORING PRACTICE (*continued*)

—*For Circulation.* Palpation of a pulse, auscultation of heart sounds, monitoring of a tracing of intra-arterial pressure, pulse plethysmography/oximetry, or ultrasound peripheral pulse monitoring.

It is recognized that brief interruptions of the continuous monitoring may be unavoidable.

Breathing System Disconnection Monitoring
When ventilation is controlled by an automatic mechanical ventilator, there shall be in continuous use a device that is capable of detecting disconnection of any component of the breathing system. The device must give an audible signal when its alarm threshold is exceeded. (It is recognized that there are certain rare or unusual circumstances in which such a device may fail to detect a disconnection.)

Oxygen Analyzer
During every administration of general anesthesia using an anesthesia machine, the concentration of oxygen in the patient breathing system will be measured by a functioning oxygen analyzer with a low concentration limit alarm in use. This device must conform to the American National Standards Institute No. Z.79.10 standard.*

Ability to Measure Temperature
During every administration of general anesthesia, there shall be readily available a means to measure the patient's temperature.
—*Rationale.* A means of temperature measurement must be available as a potential aid in the diagnosis and treatment of suspected or actual intraoperative hypothermia and malignant hyperthermia. The measurement/monitoring of temperature during *every* general anesthetic is not specifically mandated because of the potential risks of such monitoring and because of the likelihood of other physical signs giving earlier indication of the development of malignant hyperthermia.

From Eichhorn JH, Cooper JB, Cullen DJ, et al: Standards for patient monitoring during anesthesia at Harvard Medical School. JAMA 1986; 256:1017–1020. Copyright 1986, American Medical Association.
* Under extenuating circumstances, the attending anesthesiologist may waive this requirement after so stating (including the reasons) in a note in the patient's chart.
† Equivalence is to be defined by the chief of the individual hospital department after submission to and review by the department heads. Department of Anesthesia, Harvard Medical School, Boston.

Table I-2. THE STANDARDS FOR INTRAOPERATIVE MONITORING
ACCEPTED BY THE AMERICAN SOCIETY OF ANESTHESIOLOGISTS

These standards apply to all anesthesia care although, in emergency circumstances, appropriate life support measures take precedence. These standards may be exceeded at any time based on the judgment of the responsible anesthesiologist. They are intended to encourage high-quality patient care, but observing them cannot guarantee any specific patient outcome. They are subject to revision from time to time, as warranted by the evolution of technology and practice. This set of standards addresses only the issue of basic intraoperative monitoring, which is one component of anesthesia care. In certain rare or unusual circumstances, (1) some of these methods of monitoring may be clinically impractical, and (2) appropriate use of the described monitoring methods may fail to detect untoward clinical developments. Brief interruptions of continual† monitoring may be unavoidable. *Under extenuating circumstances, the responsible anesthesiologist may waive the requirements marked with an asterisk (*); it is recommended that when this is done, it should be so stated (including the reasons) in a note in the patient's medical record.* These standards are not intended for application to the care of the obstetric patient in labor or in the conduct of pain management.

Standard I
Qualified anesthesia personnel shall be present in the room throughout the conduct of all general anesthetics, regional anesthetics, and monitored anesthesia care.

(*continued*)

Table I–2. THE STANDARDS FOR INTRAOPERATIVE MONITORING
ACCEPTED BY THE AMERICAN SOCIETY OF ANESTHESIOLOGISTS
(*continued*)

—*Objective*
Because of the rapid changes in patient status during anesthesia, qualified anesthesia personnel shall be continuously present to monitor the patient and provide anesthesia care. In the event there is a direct known hazard, e.g., radiation, to the anesthesia personnel which might require intermittent remote observation of the patient, some provision for monitoring the patient must be made. In the event that an emergency requires the temporary absence of the person primarily responsible for the anesthetic, the best judgment of the anesthesiologist will be exercised in comparing the emergency with the anesthetized patient's condition and in the selection of the person left responsible for the anesthetic during the temporary absence.

Standard II
During all anesthetics, the patient's oxygenation, ventilation, circulation, and temperature shall be continually evaluated.

Oxygenation
—*Objective*
To ensure adequate oxygen concentration in the inspired gas and the blood during all anesthetics.
—*Methods*
1. Inspired gas: During every administration of general anesthesia using an anesthesia machine, the concentration of oxygen in the patient's breathing system shall be measured by an oxygen analyzer with a low oxygen concentration limit alarm in use.*
2. Blood oxygenation: During all anesthetics, adequate illumination and exposure of the patient is necessary to assess color. Although this and other qualitative clinical signs may be adequate, there are quantitative methods, such as pulse oximetry, that are encouraged.

Ventilation
—*Objective*
To ensure adequate ventilation of the patient during all anesthetics.
—*Methods*
1. Every patient receiving general anesthesia shall have the adequacy of ventilation continually evaluated. Although qualitative clinical signs such as chest excursion, observation of the reservoir breathing bag, and auscultation of breath sounds may be adequate, quantitative monitoring of the CO_2 content and/or volume of expired gas is encouraged.
2. When an endotracheal tube is inserted, its correct positioning in the trachea must be verified. Clinical assessment is essential, and end-tidal CO_2 analysis, in use from the time of endotracheal tube placement, is encouraged.
3. When ventilation is controlled by a mechanical ventilator, there shall be in continuous use a device that is capable of detecting disconnection of components of the breathing system. The device must give an audible signal when its alarm threshold is exceeded.
4. During regional anesthesia and monitored anesthesia care, the adequacy of ventilation shall be evaluated, at least, by continual observation of qualitative clinical signs.

Circulation
—*Objective*
To ensure the adequacy of the patient's circulatory function during all anesthetics.
—*Methods*
1. Every patient receiving anesthesia shall have the electrocardiogram continuously displayed from the beginning of anesthesia until preparing to leave the anesthetizing location.*
2. Every patient receiving anesthesia shall have arterial blood pressure and heart rate determined and evaluated at least every 5 minutes.*
3. Every patient receiving general anesthesia shall have, in addition to the above, circulatory function continually evaluated by at least one of the following: palpation of a pulse, auscultation of heart sounds, monitoring of a tracing of intra-arterial pressure, ultrasound peripheral pulse monitoring, or pulse plethysmography or oximetry.

(*continued*)

Table I–2. THE STANDARDS FOR INTRAOPERATIVE MONITORING ACCEPTED BY THE AMERICAN SOCIETY OF ANESTHESIOLOGISTS (*continued*)

Body Temperature
—*Objective*
  To aid in the maintenance of appropriate body temperature during all anesthetics.
—*Methods*
  There shall be readily available a means to continuously measure the patient's temperature. When changes in body temperature are intended, anticipated, or suspected, the temperature shall be measured.

From the American Society of Anesthesiologists. With permission.
  † Note that "continual" is defined as "repeated regularly and frequently in steady succession" whereas "continuous" means "prolonged without any interruption at any time."

Standards of practice for minimal monitoring as accepted by the Harvard Medical School's Department of Anesthesia are presented in Table I–1. The House of Delegates of the American Society of Anesthesiologists accepted on October 21, 1986, a set of standards for basic intraoperative monitoring that is similar in content to the Harvard standards (Table I–2). Both of these sets of standards affirm the need to monitor oxygenation, respiration, circulation, and temperature in either a continual ("repeated regularly and frequently in steady succession") or a continuous ("prolonged without any interruption at any time") manner. However, the inability to utilize such monitoring at all times and in all patients is recognized. In fact, the "essential nature" of any given monitor may be confirmed by the unwillingness of the anesthetic caregiver to proceed in its absence. Finally, no matter how valuable, the acceptance of any particular monitor as a standard of care in the legal sense is always controversial.

ESSENTIAL NONINVASIVE MONITORING FUNCTIONS

Monitoring devices can also be classified as invasive, minimally invasive, or noninvasive, with some overlap of functions such as the use of an invasive pulmonary artery catheter to measure thermodilution cardiac output.

Inspection

Very little monitoring in perioperative patient care is by inspection only. However, the color of the skin, blood, mucous membranes, and conjunctiva can be easily noted and can provide important information about perfusion, oxygenation, and hematocrit. Pupillary reflexes, pupil size, eye movement, and presence or absence of tearing provide information about depth of anesthesia. Inspection of the nose is necessary if nasal tubes of any type are present. The chest is routinely and frequently inspected to assure adequate symmetric motion without retraction. Abdominal contraction should be absent if respiration is unobstructed and depth of anesthesia is adequate.

However, monitoring of the anesthetic equipment requires considerable inspection. The gas supply, flowmeters, pressure gauges, inspiratory and expiratory valves, cables to pressure transducers, electrocardiograph, electroencephalograph, oximeter, and automated blood pressure cuff must be inspected to ensure continuity and function.

Positioning of the patient during surgery also requires careful inspection to avoid pressure on superficial nerves, venous congestion, or arterial occlusion.[24] Airways and endotracheal tubes should be taped to avoid compression of the lip or tongue between teeth, endotracheal tube, or oropharyngeal airway. The ears should be flat against the head, without kinking or compression.[24] Neither excessive extension nor flexion of the neck should be permitted. Excessive neck flexion may cause the endotracheal tube to compress the recurrent laryngeal nerve, resulting in vocal cord paralysis. Neck extension or rotation can limit cerebral arterial blood flow, particularly in elderly patients with extracranial occlusive disease. Postoperative neck pain occurs after excessive extension in patients with cervical arthritis. The extremities should be inspected to prevent dependent edema, neural compression, arterial insufficiency, or malfunction of intravascular catheters (infiltration, extravasation, or arterial occlusion).

Palpation

Palpation of the arterial pulse for heart rate, volume, cardiac rhythm, and determination of blood pressure is a simple, readily learned monitoring task. The position of the endotracheal tube cuff can frequently be verified by laryngeal palpation. Laryngeal motion, also detected by palpation, occurs in the anesthetized patient with incomplete neuromuscular blockade.[24] Symmetry of respiratory excursion can be documented by palpation. Palpation easily reveals gastric or bladder distention, allowing drainage to be performed before gastric aspiration or the hemodynamic sequelae of a distended bladder occur. Palpation of the peripheral pulse provides an index of both blood pressure and cardiac output.

Auscultation

The heart sounds can be repeatedly assessed through a stethoscope applied over the sternal notch or precordium. Likewise, depth, rate, equality, and quality (presence of wheezing, rhonchi, rales) of breathing are similarly noted. Blood pressure can be determined using the traditional Riva Rocci method of auscultation for the onset and loss of Korotkoff sounds. More sophisticated methods of auscultation include the automated devices using Doppler or oscillotonometric methods (see Chapter 4).

Noninvasive or Minimally Invasive Methods

Most essential monitoring is either noninvasive or minimally invasive. In addition to inspection, palpation of pulses, and blood pressure determinations, essential monitoring includes such devices as cutaneous probes for monitoring tissue gases, pulse, temperature, ECG, and neuromuscular transmission. Among the minimally invasive devices are temperature probes inserted in the esophagus, nasopharynx, rectum, or tympanic membrane, esophageal stethoscopy, and needle electrodes to be inserted for electroencephalographic, electrocardiographic, and neuromuscular function monitoring. Insertion of a bladder catheter is usually minimally invasive, although it always carries the risk of urinary tract infection. External monitoring of fetal heart rate or uterine tone is minimally invasive. Highly invasive devices such as intravascular, intracranial, and intracardiac catheters or probes, which pose the greatest risks, are not usually considered as minimally essential monitors. However, the conduct of the operation may require invasive monitors as essential elements. Even when invasive monitors are present, noninvasive or minimally invasive methods to monitor the same functions should be present in the event of failure of the invasive device (e.g., placement of a manual sphygmomanometer with an automatic sphygmomanometer or arterial catheter). Such duplication also permits easy calibration of the monitor.

ELECTRICAL SAFETY

Since most of the monitoring devices used in perioperative care are electrically operated, a knowledge of the principles of electrical safety and the effect of electrocautery on monitor function is mandatory.

Intraoperative Electrical Considerations

Certain terminology is basic to the understanding of electricity. Electricity flows through "hot" wires (black) in one direction (direct current) or oscillates around zero by flowing intermittently in first one and then the opposite direction (alternating current). However, to complete a circuit electricity must flow back to the source via a neutral (white) wire, where it is grounded. A third (green) wire provides an additional ground to which leakage currents can escape.

The ampere, the quantity of electricity flowing through a conductor in 1 second, is used to measure current (the flow of electrons through a conductor). The resistance encountered by the current traveling through a conductor is measured in ohms. The electrons lost as current flows against a resistance are measured in volts. Ohm's law relates current (I), voltage (E), and resistance (R) as $E = IR$. The concentration of current traveling through a conductor is current density. Power (watts) is the product of amperes and volts and defines the rate at which work is done. Energy (joules or watt-seconds) is the product of power and time.

Shock Hazard

For a piece of monitoring equipment to function, it must have a certain amount of current that it draws through one source and returns through a second source. There is coupling to the ground between these two power sources that provides a current path or capacitive resistance between the power sources and the ground.

Electrical injury requires a closed loop or circuit in which an energy source is present to sustain a pressure differential or voltage within the circuit. The magnitude of current in a circuit depends upon the total impedance or resistance of the circuit and the pressure differential provided by the energy source. Electrocution occurs only when the victim becomes the component that closes the circuit or loop and allows lethal current to flow.[25] However, the actual injury depends upon the impedance of the victim. With intact, dry skin, the impedance is high, limiting the injury to a shock of a few milliamperes rather than a lethal injury.

Electrical current in the operating room causes either electrical shock or burns (from increased temperature from current of increased density). The shock hazard can be divided into macroshock (surface shock) or microshock (internal shock). Although both the patient and the attendants can be subjected to macroshock, only the patient is at risk for microshock.[26] The threshold for perception of a macroshock (presence of tingling) varies among individuals but usually is about 1 mA. At 5 mA, the sensation is painful and sensory nerves are stimulated, causing the individual to avoid the stimulus. Currents of 10–20 mA cause stimulation of motor nerves and muscle contraction, but the victim can release contact with the conductors (the so-called let-go current). Beyond that level, repetitive stimulation of motor nerves and their muscles prevents the victim from releasing the stimulus because the flexor muscles are stronger than the extensors.

Currents greater than 100 mA (up to 2–3 A) spread throughout the body causing ventricular fibrillation, although the respiratory center remains functional. Entrance and exit of current through the same extremity causes little effect on heart and respiratory muscles. The same current passing through the heart has greater consequences. Low-density current passing directly through the heart (from an intracardiac catheter) causes extrasystoles, whereas prolonged current exposure causes ventricular fibrillation. At currents over 6 A, cardiac rhythm may return after sustained myocardial contraction if the current stimulus is brief, but temporary respiratory paralysis, shock, and burns are likely.

The effects of electrical current on the heart depend upon the current frequency, pathway, density, and duration. Short current pulses up to 10 msec produce effects that depend upon the portion of the cardiac cycle during which they are applied. The human body is less sensitive to current frequencies beyond 1000 Hz. The response to current passing through the heart (e.g., entrance in one arm and exit in leg) depends upon current magnitude or density. For this reason, the maximum safe current allowed to pass through the heart is 10 μamp. Fibrillation has been reported with passage of 20–580 μamp of current through the heart.[27] The threshold for fibrillation decreases with closer proximity of the current to the heart (e.g., intracardiac catheters are a greater risk than are skin electrodes). The current threshold causing ventricular fibrillation is controversial since current density (current per unit area) may be the important parameter rather than threshold. Fibrillation thresholds are linked to the catheter area, with greater total current required with smaller catheters.[28]

Leakage Currents

Leakage is the escape of electricity from one conductor to another through either high- or low-resistance pathways. These currents usually involve capacitance but can result from resistive paths such as faulty insulation, electromagnetic induction, or damp terminal boards in equipment.[25] Capacitance that exists between enclosed conductors of alternating current and metal conduit permits current to flow between the conductor and the ground. A capacitor is two conductors separated by an insulator. It passes alternating current but blocks passage of direct current.

However, leakage current can also arise through high resistances. Leakage currents come from spurious impedance from the energy source rather than from the impedance of the load (the device that closes the circuit). The actual current leaking is usually quite small.

If a leakage current is present in an electrically powered monitor attached to a patient's ECG, it has two pathways to follow—either through the ground wire to earth or through the monitor case to the ECG lead and through the patient to the ground. Because current follows the path of least resistance, the path to the ground has less resistance than the patient and the leakage current is harmlessly dissipated. If the ground wire on the monitor is broken, the current has only one path, through the patient, causing a hazardous situation.

Fault currents, on the other hand, are currents passing through a spurious load impedance. A voltage generator can produce both leakage and fault currents. Leakage currents between patient leads connected together should not exceed 100 μA. Leakages between leads should not exceed 10 μA in isolated power supplies and 50 μA in nonisolated equipment. The leakage current between equipment chassis and ground should not be greater than 100 μA in cord-connected devices.[24]

A ground fault interrupter is a differential transformer and electronic amplifier, which measures the difference between the "hot" and the neutral wires in a circuit. When the difference between the two exceeds 5 A, indicating leakage from the "hot" wire to the ground wire, a circuit breaker is activated to interrupt the flow of current.

Grounding

The concept of a ground or grounding depends upon the reference point in a particular context. Technically speaking, a ground is a conducting connection to earth (a readily available conductor) or some conducting body that serves in place of earth (a water pipe in the hospital). Grounding applies to equipment, circuits, and power systems. Equipment grounding is independent of circuit or system grounding. However, grounded equipment can be used with either a grounded or an ungrounded circuit or electrical system.[25] Bruner suggests certain rules for grounding. If an item is part of the patient (e.g., pacing catheter, monitor electrode), then it should not be grounded.[25] However, the monitor or other item that is part of the electrical equipment should always be grounded.

Grounded Circuits or Systems. An electrical outlet has two insulated conductors from the power source. Across these conductors is the 120-V pressure differential. One limb of the conductors is grounded, and the voltage differential between the other conductor and the ground is 120 V.

Equipment Grounding. The third wire in the power cord, in addition to the two conductors to be connected to the power source, connects non–current-carrying metal parts of electrical appliances to ground. The grounding wire in the electrical receptacle runs with the power conductors to a bus bar in the fuse or circuit breaker box to allow interconnection of all grounding terminals or receptacles in a particular area. Such a grounding wire diverts leakage currents and provides a low-impedance path between the local ground and the metal of a piece of equipment that should not be connected to either side of a power line. However, in the absence of a competent ground, the equipment operates but produces a voltage relative to ground that can injure a person who unknowingly completes the circuit. The presence of 60-cycle "noise" on an ECG may be due to leakage current on the patient secondary to inadequate electrocardiograph electrode contact or faulty grounding.

Electrical Isolation of the Patient

Transformers. Transformers are used to isolate electrical circuits in operating rooms. A transformer transfers alternating current from one circuit to another. It consists of two separate coils of wire wound closely together around a magnetic core. An alternating current (transformers do not operate on direct current because a changing magnetic field is required) is applied to one coil, termed the primary winding, that creates a magnetic flux. As the magnetic field changes, an electric current is induced in the other coil, the secondary winding. Thus, electricity is transferred from one circuit to another by a magnetic linkage. The input and output voltages are related by the ratio of the number of turns in the secondary and primary coils. Theoretically, then, if a grounded patient comes into contact with the secondary winding terminals, no current flows through the conductor to ground. However, there is always a small amount of current leakage between the primary and secondary windings so that some of the secondary output is not isolated from ground.

Line-Isolation Monitors. One way to minimize hazards from ground faults or accidental contact with ground is by use of nongrounded or ungrounded systems monitored by line-isolation transformers (ground fault detector). However, persons in operating rooms are usually well grounded. In

INTRODUCTION

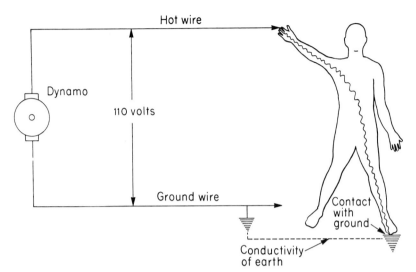

Figure I–3. A well-grounded person who contacts a single "hot" wire when the ground on a piece of equipment fails completes the circuit and receives a serious shock. (From Leonard PF, Gould AB Jr: Dynamics of electrical hazards of particular concern to operating room personnel. Surg Clin North Am 1965; 45:820.)

the isolation transformer, only the input circuit is grounded and the output circuit is "floating." A complete circuit exists only by the magnetic linkage between the two conductors. Only small amounts of leakage occur; theoretically no leakage exists between the primary and the secondary coils of an isolation transformer. Thus the "hot" and neutral wires of the hospital power supply are isolated from the electrical supply of patient monitoring equipment. If the isolation transformer is absent, a victim touching the "hot" or ungrounded wire completes the circuit and sustains a severe electrical shock (Fig. I–3). However, the isolation transformer prevents completion of the circuit even though the victim is grounded (Fig. I–4).

Nongrounded systems are often isolated from grounded systems by isolation transformers and must be continually monitored (line-isolation monitor [LIM]) to assure their effective isolation from ground by a high wire-to-ground resistance. A fault to ground in an ungrounded system converts it to a grounded one and is signaled by the LIM. The LIM is a quantitative indication of the extent of isolation of each side (conductor) of the nongrounded system. Two values are indicated: (1) the hazard current (milliamperes) and (2) the line fault impedance to ground (kilohms). The hazard current value is the milliamperes of current that would flow in the event of a direct short to ground, the maximum total hazard current (index).

A meter reading of 2 mA causes the LIM to alarm. As Leeming notes, the current causing the LIM to alarm is a hazard when the following conditions occur: (1) The patient is grounded. (2) The ground on a device is broken. (3) One power line directly contacts the ungrounded chassis of that device. (4) The patient contacts the chassis of an ungrounded device.[29] Incomplete degrees of these conditions are also hazardous because the electrically susceptible patient has to be in contact only through a sufficiently

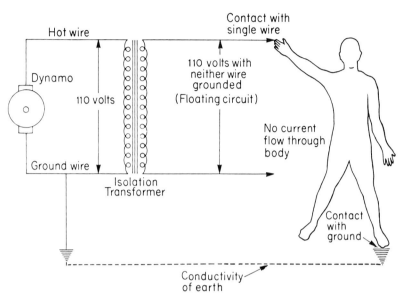

Figure I–4. When an isolation transformer is present, a grounded person contacting a "hot" wire does not complete the circuit and does not receive a shock. (From Leonard PF, Gould AB Jr: Dynamics of electrical hazards of particular concern to operating room personnel. Surg Clin North Am 1965; 45:821.)

low impedance (and grounded only through low impedance, not directly) rather than direct contact. The power line does not have to be in direct contact but also grounded through a sufficiently low impedance. The ground does not need to be completely lost but just through excessive impedance.[29]

LIMs protect only against severe macroshock not against microshock. They provide relative, not absolute, electrical isolation. The leakage current is not displayed. The hazard current exists only when there is an external conducting pathway between the power line and the ground.[29] A LIM evaluates the entire equipment-grounding complex, not any specific device, although a single device may be responsible for its activation.

Isolated Power Supply. Another way to minimize the hazard of electrical shocks is the use of isolated patient inputs on monitoring equipment. Physiologic signals from the patient (e.g., ECG) are sent through an isolation transformer to the display rather than directly to the display through conducting wires. The power supply of the circuit monitoring the patient's physiologic variable is separated from the equipment's power supply, which is highly insulated from ground. Such isolated, ungrounded systems offer nearly complete patient protection from shocks.

Electrocautery

Although the electrocautery is not a monitor, its interaction with many monitors is a source of interference and hazard. Electrocautery units produce high-frequency currents in excess of 1 A that pass from a small active electrode to the patient to produce a high current density capable of either cutting or coagulation. The high-frequency current (0.5 to 2 million Hz) returns to the machine by a dispersive electrode (patient ground plate).

Burns occur with electrocauteries when the patient ground plate is poorly applied, causing a small area of plate contact with the patient. Although the resistance at the point of contact may be low, the current density is high; this causes excessive heating of tissue (burn) at the site of plate contact. If the resistance between the patient and the dispersive electrode of the electrocautery is high, current divides and exits through the path of least resistance, such as through the ECG electrodes, a process termed the alternate path hazard. Again, if the current density is sufficiently high, burns occur at the ECG electrode or other sites.[30] Should the patient ground return plate be completely disconneted, the current generated by the electrocautery returns through paths such as indwelling catheters, temperature probes,[31] and other devices. If the current density is high, burns result from local heating as the current attempts to exit to ground. Becker and colleagues note that a current density of 1.32 mA/mm^2 causes burns, 1.05 mA/mm^2 causes severe pain in conscious humans, 0.79 mA/mm^2 causes blistering of skin, and 0.53 mA/mm^2 causes skin reddening.[30]

Such hazards are reduced by placing the dispersive electrode of the cautery as close to the surgical site as possible, insulating the patient from metal devices, applying patient dispersive electrodes over large, fleshy areas, using large ECG electrodes (never needle electrodes), and keeping ECG electrodes far from the site of cautery use.[30] Contact with tissue should always be made prior to activation of the cautery, and its use should be limited to prevent excessive heating at undesirable sites.

The presence of excessive interference from the electrocautery on monitored variables not usually so affected may indicate an improperly functioning patient return ground plate. In this situation, factors such as incorrectly applied electrodes, excessive interference from other equipment, or ground faults must also be ruled out to prevent passage of hazardous current through the patient.

Battery-Powered Monitors

Cordless, battery-powered monitors eliminate the clutter and hazard of electric cords. They are often smaller than line-operated devices and function in the event of power failure. Their low voltage generates little current, making them safer than line-operated devices. However, batteries are less reliable than line current and must be recharged to assure reliable performance. The operating expense of battery-powered monitors with recharging circuits is greater than that of line-operated devices.[1] Use of battery-operated equipment with the charger connected to the power system obviates the safety inherent in a battery-operated system.

SUMMARY

The choice of monitoring equipment must be made by the responsible anesthesiologist or critical care physician after careful consideration of the patient's disease process and anticipated perioperative changes. Since most equipment includes alarms that can be set for specific limits, the chosen equipment must be carefully programmed to warn of impending adverse conditions. Unfortunately, much of the routinely used equipment (electro-cardiograph, pulse oximeter, and blood pressure monitors) gives a high frequency of spurious alarms (75% in one study).[32] Of these incidents, the majority resulted from heart rate or blood pressure values above the preset limits and only 3% represented patient risk.[32]

Because patient monitoring is a rapidly changing field, the purchase of new devices is inevitable. In addition to the devices described in this book, equipment designed to monitor tissue metabolism—such as magnetic resonance imaging, positron emission tomography, and other spectroscopic techniques—may eventually appear for perioperative use. Specifications for purchase of new monitoring systems should be prepared jointly by physicians, nurses, and biomedical engineers. These people should determine what devices are needed, what are available, and their reliability, space requirements, service requirements, personnel, and costs. Evaluation of the equipment by these same groups is essential to avoid acquisition of unsuitable devices. Schematic wiring diagrams should be available for all electrical equipment to permit analysis of potential electrical hazards by qualified personnel.

Commonality of monitoring equipment throughout the operating suites, intensive care units, emergency rooms, and other critical care areas of a hospital should be encouraged. Interchangeability of monitors permits rapid, easy transfer of patients between hospital locations without loss of monitored data, ready replacement during calibration or repair, and rapid training of new personnel. Whenever possible, the same monitoring capability should exist during patient transport as at any other time.

Another essential feature of any monitoring operation is the presence of adequate numbers of support personnel who are expert in the care, application, trouble-shooting, and maintenance of the sophisticated monitors.[33] The duties of such personnel vary from institution to institution, as does their training. In some hospitals, these techniques may also be responsible for autotransfusion systems and intra-aortic balloon counterpulsation. They may also care for the anesthesia machine, its ventilator, anesthetic gas tanks, and anesthesia hoses and connectors. Educational requirements are a bachelor's degree at least. Some personnel maintain logs of scheduled preventive maintenance and calibration and emergency service calls. They are also responsible for the important, but often overlooked, task of keeping equipment in a clean and undamaged condition. Abuse resulting from soilage by fluid, thermal damage when heat from equipment is undissipated, and direct physical injury from collisions are common in the hospital environment.[34] Although there have been no controlled studies on the impact of technical support personnel on the efficiency of anesthesia services, the unique contributions of these people are unquestioned.[33]

References

1. Nobel JJ, Kostinsky H: Selection of monitoring equipment. *In* Saidman LJ, Smith NT (eds): Monitoring in Anesthesia. New York: John Wiley & Sons, 1978; 261.

2. Durbin CG: Personal communication. March 1, 1988.
3. Harrison GG: Anesthetic accidents. Clin Anesth 1983; 1:415–429.
4. Cooper JB, Newbower RS, Long CD, McPeek B: Preventable anesthesia mishaps: A study of human factors. Anesthesiology 1978; 49:399–406.
5. Philip JH, Raemer DB: Selecting the optimal anesthesia monitoring array. Med Instrum 1985; 19:122–126.
6. Pask EA: Hunt and signal. Proc Roy Soc Med 1965; 58:757–766.
7. Hamburger WW: Development of knowledge concerning the measurement and rhythm of the pulse. J Mt Sinai Hosp 1941; 8:585–591.
8. White PD: The evolution of our knowledge about the heart and its diseases since 1628. Circulation 1957; 15:915–923.
9. McGrew RE: Encyclopedia of Medical History. New York: McGraw-Hill, 1985; 64–66, 71–77, 126–127, 317–318.
10. Cushing H: Some principles of cerebral surgery. JAMA 1909; 52:184.
11. Lyons AS, Petrucelli RJ: Medicine. An Illustrated History. New York: Abradale, 1987; 432–436, 592.
12. Cushing H: On the avoidance of shock in major amputations by cocainization of large nerve trunks preliminary to their division. With observations on blood pressure in surgical cases. Ann Surg 1902; 36:321–345.
13. McKeson EI: The interpretation of pulse, respiration, and blood pressure with special reference to surgical shock. *In* Gwathmey JT: Anesthesia. New York: D. Appleton, 1914; 410–413.
14. Rovenstine EA: A method of combining anesthetic and surgical records for statistical purposes. Anesth Analg 1934; 13:122–128.
15. Beecher HK: The first anesthesia records (Codman, Cushing). Surg Gynecol Obstet 1940; 71:689–693.
16. Wiggers CJ: The pressure pulse in the cardiovascular system. New York: Longmans, Green, 1928; 15.
17. Einthoven W: Die galvanometrische registrirung des menschlichen capillar-elektrometers in der physiologie. Arch ges Physiol 1903; 99:472–480.
18. Hellerstein HK, Pritchard WH, Lewis RL: Recording of intracavitary potentials through single lumen, saline filled cardiac catheters. Proc Soc Exp Biol Med 1949; 71:58–60.
19. Fick A: Uber den Messung der blut quantum inden Herzentrikeln. Ver Phys Med Ges Wurzburg 1870; 16:1872.
20. Whitcher C, Ream AK, Parsons D, et al: Anesthetic mishaps and the cost of monitoring. A proposed standard for monitoring equipment. J Clin Monit 1988; 4:5–15.
21. Gravenstein JS: Essential monitoring examined through different lenses. J Clin Monit 1986; 2:22–28.
22. Eichhorn JH, Cooper JB, Cullen DJ, et al: Standards for patient monitoring during anesthesia at Harvard Medical School. JAMA 1986; 256:1017–1020.
23. Block FE: A proposed standard for monitoring equipment: What equipment should be included? J Clin Monit 1988; 4:1–4.
24. Gravenstein JS, Paulus DA: Clinical Monitoring Practice. Philadelphia: JB Lippincott, 1987; 415–425.
25. Bruner JMR: Fundamental concepts of electrical safety. Refresher Courses in Anesthesiology 1974; 2:11–25.
26. Hahn CEW: Electrical hazards and safety in cardiovascular measurements. *In* Prys Roberts C (ed): The Circulation and Anaesthesia. London: Blackwell Scientific, 1980; 605–633.
27. Bruner JMR: Hazards of electrical apparatus. Anesthesiology 1967; 28:396–425.
28. Roy OZ, Scott JR: 60-Hertz ventricular fibrillation and pump failure thresholds versus electrode area. IEEE Trans Biomed Eng 1976; 23:45.

29. Leeming MN: Protection of the electrically susceptible patient: A discussion of systems and methods. Anesthesiology 1973; 38:370–383.
30. Becker CM, Malhotra IV, Hedley-Whyte J: The distribution of radiofrequency current and burns. Anesthesiology 1973; 38:106–122.
31. Schneider AJL, Apple HP, Braun RT: Electrosurgical burns at skin temperature probes. Anesthesiology 1977; 47:72–74.
32. Kestin IG, Miller BR, Lockhart CH: Auditory alarms during anesthesia monitoring. Anesthesiology 1988; 69:106–109.
33. Frazier WT, Kelly PM, Lewis JE: The anesthesia instrumentation and monitoring specialist. Med Instrum 1985; 19:113–118.
34. Bruner JMR: Common abuses and failures of electrical equipment. Anesth Analg 1972; 51:810–820.

Monitors of Cardiovascular Function

chapter one

Electrocardiography: Monitoring for Ischemia

FIONA M. CLEMENTS, M.D.
■ NORBERT P. DE BRUIJN, M.D.

Since the discovery that ischemic myocardium produced alterations in the electrocardiogram (ECG), various ways of displaying these changes have been introduced. Advances in electronics have made ECG diagnosis more accurate and allowed for its automated analysis. This technology has resulted in the emergence of a vast amount of new information about both symptomatic and silent ischemia over the past few years. Automated on-line ECG analysis facilitates the recognition of abnormalities and trends that previously went unnoticed even in critically ill patients monitored in the operating room or intensive care unit. The significance of ST segment changes occurring in the absence of pain or hemodynamic changes is the subject of many ongoing investigations. It is the intent of this chapter to bring the reader up to date with current theory and technology pertaining to ECG monitoring for ischemia.

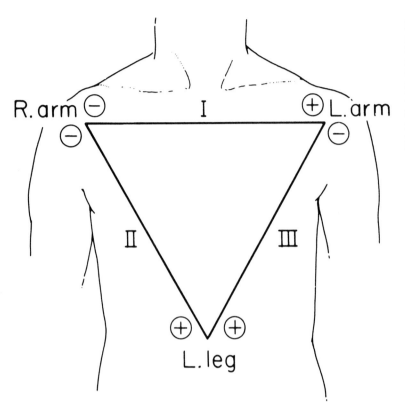

Figure 1–1. Einthoven's triangle: an equilateral triangle in the frontal plane with its corners representing the two arms and the left leg. (From Thys DM: The normal ECG. *In* Thys DM, Kaplan JA [eds]: The ECG in Anesthesia and Critical Care. New York: Churchill Livingstone, 1987; 3. By permission.)

ECG LEAD SYSTEMS USED TO MONITOR FOR ISCHEMIA

The ECG is a graphic recording of the electrical potentials produced by the beating heart. Impulse formation and conduction produce small electrical currents that may be detected over the entire body surface by applying electrodes at various places. From the infinite number of possible locations, 12 standardized leads have been defined for the standard ECG. These fall into three groups: bipolar leads I, II, and III, described by Einthoven and associates;[1] augmented unipolar leads aVR, aVL, and aVF, described by Goldberger;[2] and the unipolar precordial leads defined by Wilson.[3]

Electrodes for the standard leads are placed on the right and left arms and on the left leg. The classic approach has been to postulate geometric uniformity around the recording lead system and to construct a reference frame accordingly. Einthoven used a triangle to represent the "axis" of the bipolar limb leads I, and II, and III.[1] Einthoven's triangle is an equilateral triangle, positioned in the frontal plane, with its corners representing the two arms and the left leg (Fig. 1–1). This is obviously an oversimplification, since several factors are not taken into consideration: the inhomogeneous conducting characteristics of the body, the size and shape of the body, and the eccentric position of the heart within the chest. Nevertheless, the three

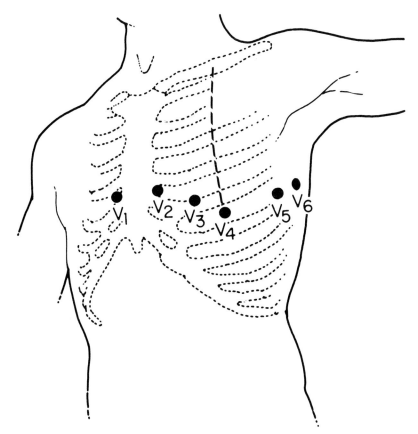

Figure 1–2. Electrode positions for the precordial unipolar leads. The dashed line indicates the midclavicular line. (From Thys DM: The normal ECG. *In* Thys DM, Kaplan JA [eds]: The ECG in Anesthesia and Critical Care. New York: Churchill Livingstone, 1987; 6. By permission.)

standard leads are extremely useful for the detection of rate and rhythm disturbances and of myocardial ischemia.

In 1932, Wilson introduced a new method to measure body surface potentials by referencing them to a "central terminal."[3] Technically this is accomplished by connecting the three "standard" electrodes by 5-KΩ resistors in series to an indifferent central terminal. The potential difference between this common electrode and one of the other active electrodes, designated the "exploring" electrode, then becomes the actual measured potential. This lead system is known as a unipolar lead system. A slightly different technique allows for approximately a 50% augmentation in amplitude of the potentials derived from the unipolar leads; this modification is now routinely employed, accounting for the leads aVR, aVL, and aVF.

The precordial leads (Fig. 1–2) also constitute a unipolar lead system, in which the standard leads form a neutral electrode. The exploring electrode is positioned in one of six locations on the chest wall:

V_1—fourth intercostal space at the right sternal border
V_2—fourth intercostal space at the left sternal border

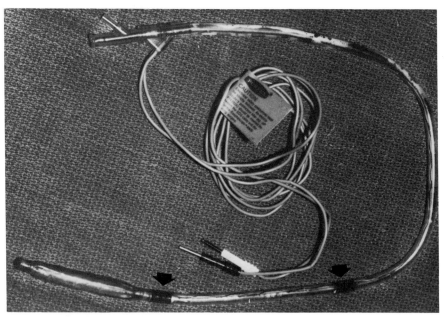

Figure 1–3. The Portex Cardioesophagoscope; a disposable esophageal stethoscope with two electrodes (arrows).

V_3—equidistant between V_2 and V_4
V_4—fifth intercostal space in the left midclavicular line
V_5—same horizontal plane as V_4, at anterior axillary line
V_6—same horizontal plane as V_4, at midaxillary line

Lead Selection

Precordial leads are more sensitive than the standard leads in the detection of ischemia and are also valuable in the diagnosis of left ventricular hypertrophy and bundle-branch block. Blackburn and Katigbak showed that 89% of all postexercise ST segment depression was detected in lead V_5, making this the most sensitive single lead for ischemia.[4] In addition to the surface leads, ischemia of the posterior surface of the heart has been shown to be more effectively detected by using an esophageally placed electrode.[5, 6] Esophageal electrodes are, however, in use primarily for the diagnosis of arrhythmias, and they are easily obtained using a commercially available esophageal stethoscope fitted with two electrodes positioned at 7 and 20 cm from the tip (Portex Cardioesophagoscope) (Fig. 1–3).

In certain specialized facilities such as the intensive care unit and the operating room, simultaneous monitoring of 12 leads is impractical. Therefore, for continuous monitoring, a number of modified bipolar chest leads have been suggested for use. Some of these are more suited to the detection of arrhythmias than ischemia. For example, MCL_1 is commonly employed in the intensive care unit because it provides a good P wave; however, CS_5, CM_5, CB_5, and CC_5 have been found more useful for the detection of

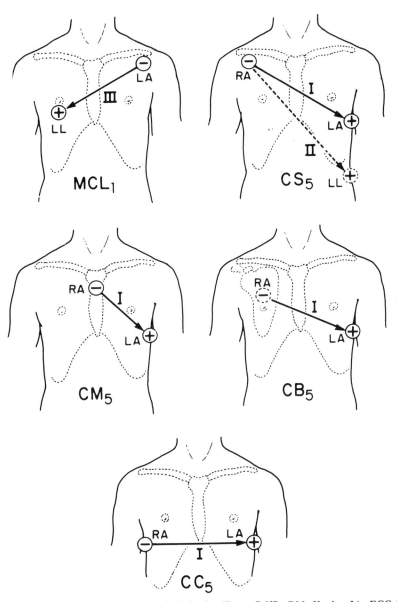

Figure 1–4. Modified bipolar standard limb leads. (From Griffin RM, Kaplan JA: ECG lead systems. *In* Thys DM, Kaplan JA [eds]: The ECG in Anesthesia and Critical Care. New York: Churchill Livingstone, 1987; 19. By permission.)

ischemia.[7, 8] It can be seen from Figure 1–4 and from the subscript "5" on each of these named leads that the positive, exploring electrode is placed in the V_5 position on the chest wall. The negative, "central" electrode is what varies, as shown. Of these leads, the CS_5 is most often used intraoperatively. Either the CS_5 or the CM_5 lead is a good alternative to a true V_5 lead. However, when feasible and available, the use of five electrodes, one on each limb and the other at a V_5 position, remains the most desirable arrangement for ischemia detection, providing the option of 7 of the 12 standard leads. This system was reported by Kaplan and King in 1976 and permits observation for both inferior and anterior ischemia of the left ventricle.[9] Simultaneous display of leads II and V_5 is currently recommended for this purpose, but continuous automated ST segment analysis of these leads may prove to be even more useful.

The localization of ischemia with the ECG has been clearly demonstrated.[10] Leads II, III, and aVF reveal disease in the right coronary artery, which supplies the basal part of the left ventricular posterior wall, the posterior third of the interventricular septum, and a large part of the right ventricle. The V leads correspond to anterior, anteroseptal, lateral, and apical ischemia, within the distribution of the left anterior descending (LAD) and circumflex coronary arteries. The LAD supplies the anterior wall of the left ventricle, the anterior two thirds of the interventricular septum, and part of the right ventricle. In a 12-lead system, V_1, V_2, and V_3 reflect anteroseptal ischemia, V_3, V_4, and V_5 suggest anteroapical ischemia, and V_4, V_5, and V_6 indicate anterolateral ischemia. True posterior wall ischemia produces changes in aVL, V_1, and esophageal leads.

ECG MANIFESTATIONS OF ISCHEMIA AND INFARCTION

The ECG manifestations of ischemia are the result of alterations in repolarization of the ischemic myocardium. Depolarization is not primarily affected. Repolarization is delayed in an area of ischemic myocardium. Decreased oxygen supply results in a delayed and abnormal electrical charging of the myocardial cells manifested as changes in the ST segment and the T wave. The sequence of repolarization, proceeding from epicardium to endocardium, is exactly opposite to that of depolarization, giving rise to an upright T wave following an upright QRS complex (Fig. 1–5A).

Symmetric T wave changes are manifestations of ischemia, abnormal ST segment changes represent an injury pattern, and abnormal Q waves show myocardial necrosis. Ischemia tends to begin in the subendocardium, which is the last region to receive blood flow from the epicardially situated coronary arteries. When ischemia is confined to the subendocardium, the forces of repolarization are increased, resulting in tall, peaked T waves (Figs. 1–5B and 1–6). However, when ischemia is transmural, implying subepicardial involvement, the direction of repolarization is reversed and travels from endocardium to epicardium. The T wave then becomes inverted (Fig. 1–5C). Note that in leads aVR, V_1, and V_2, where the QRS complex and T wave are normally negative, the polarity of the T wave is reversed and becomes upright.

Ischemic changes may be seen only in those leads that "face" the affected myocardium. Thus, anterior wall ischemia may be evident only in a V lead and not in any limb leads. However, reciprocal changes may appear in leads on the opposite side of the heart such that posterior wall ischemia,

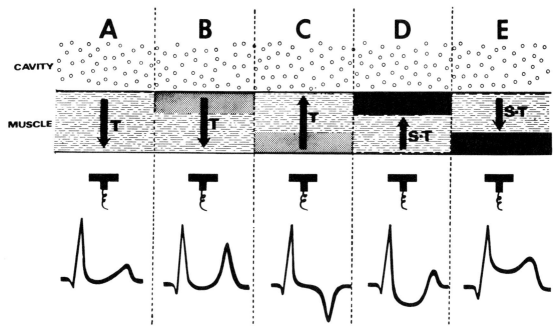

Figure 1–5. *A*, The normal endocardial to epicardial T wave vector. *B*, The T wave vector of subendocardial ischemia. *C*, The T wave vector of subepicardial ischemia. *D*, The ST segment vector of subendocardial injury. *E*, The T wave vector of subepicardial injury. (From Schamroth L: The Electrocardiology of Coronary Artery Disease. Oxford: Blackwell, 1984; 7. With permission.)

for example, may produce an upright T wave in V_1. Other factors that affect ST segment and T waves, such as digoxin, quinidine, electrolyte imbalances, or left ventricular hypertrophy, tend to affect all leads, unlike ischemia, which is almost always a localized process.

With persistent or more severe ischemia, the ECG may develop an injury pattern that is characteristic of a reversible myocardial injury, and this may precede the development of a true infarction. Two currents of injury are recognized: diastolic and systolic. The diastolic current occurs in resting cells because of the electrical gradient that exists between tissue with a normal resting potential and ischemic tissue, which has an altered, more positive, resting potential.[11] The systolic current of injury occurs during myocardial activation when the wavefront is distorted by the altered properties of the ischemic tissue. As the stimulus passes through the ischemic region, the partially depolarized cells either do not depolarize further or generate a modified action potential with an early repolarization.

Current flows from regions of relative positivity to regions of relative negativity. In the resting state, the diastolic injury current flows from ischemic to normal tissue. An ECG recording from an electrode overlying the ischemic area exhibits depression of the TP segment (Fig. 1–7) with a subepicardial injury. As electrical activation proceeds from normal into ischemic tissue, the action potentials become distorted and shortened with early repolarization. Injured tissue becomes relatively more negative than the normal tissue, and the current of injury is reversed. Thus, true ST segment

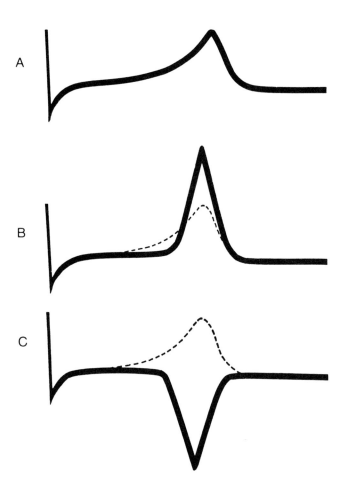

A

B

C

Figure 1–6. *A*, Normal ST segment and T wave. *B,C*, The T wave of myocardial ischemia. (From Schamroth L: The Electrocardiology of Coronary Artery Disease. Oxford: Blackwell, 1984; 5. With permission.)

elevation occurs (systolic current of injury). The ST segment elevation apparent on the surface ECG with subepicardial ischemia (see Fig. 1–5*E*) can therefore be simulated by TP or "baseline" depression, or it may involve true elevation of the ST segment. This differs from the appearance of subendocardial ischemia (see Fig. 1–5*D*), in which the recording electrode re-

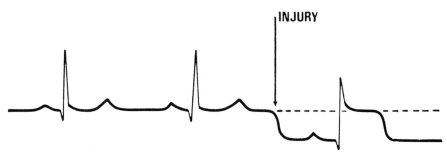

Figure 1–7. Depression of the TP segment at the onset of myocardial injury. (From Schamroth L: The Electrocardiology of Coronary Artery Disease. Oxford: Blackwell, 1984; 22. With permission.)

	Perioperative ST Segment Depression		
	None	0.10–0.19 mV	≥0.2 mV
Number of patients	646	291	86
Incidence of PMI (%)*	2.5	6.2	9.3

* *P* < 0.005 by multiple chi-square.

Figure 1–8. The relationship between the degree of ST segment depression and the incidence of perioperative myocardial infarction (PMI). (From Slogoff S, Keats AS: Does perioperative myocardial ischemia lead to postoperative myocardial infarction? Anesthesiology 1985; 62:107–114. With permission.)

cords a positive resting diastolic current (TP elevation) and a negative systolic current (ST depression). Once again, the resultant ST deviation (now depression) appears because of both of these factors. Thus, the ST segment is depressed with subendocardial ischemia and elevated with subepicardial or transmural ischemia.

Ellestad and colleagues have defined myocardial ischemia as greater than 1-mm horizontal or downsloping ST segment depression at a point 0.06 msec from the J point.[12] Much debate has centered around the importance of defining ischemic ST segment depression at a point 0.06–0.08 msec after the J point, since it is recognized that J point depression and upsloping ST segments are common occurrences, unassociated with ischemia. However, Stuart and Ellestad noted that subjects with an upsloping ST segment, but 2-mm ST segment depression measured at 0.08 msec after the J point, had the same incidence of two- and three-vessel coronary disease as did those subjects with horizontal ST depression.[13] Downsloping ST segments have been correlated with an increased mortality and with an increased number of diseased coronary vessels, when compared with horizontal ST segments.[14, 15] In addition, the degree of ST segment depression has been correlated with the amount of myocardium involved and the severity of the ischemia.[12] Similarly, the degree of ST segment depression occurring perioperatively has been related to the development of myocardial infarction in patients undergoing coronary artery bypass surgery (Fig. 1–8).[16]

In summary, depressed ST segments occur with subendocardial ischemia. As the ischemia becomes more profound, the ST segments progress from upsloping to horizontal to downsloping, at which time the ischemia may be transmural. ST elevation is also indicative of transmural ischemia, and it may occur in association with evolution of a myocardial infarction.

Progression of ischemia is associated with binding of calcium to the membranes along the intercalated disks, and it limits the potassium flux. Thus, injury current is ultimately prevented from flowing between cells, ST segment changes disappear, and they may be replaced by evidence of a completed infarction. After the disappearance of the acute ST and T wave

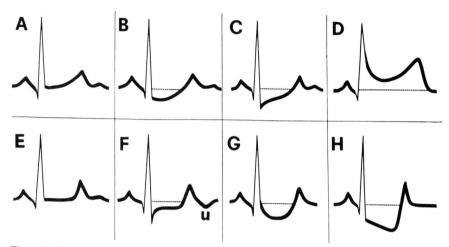

Figure 1–9. *A,* Normal P-QRS-T complex. *B,* Junctional ST segment depression. *C,* Upward sloping ST segment depression. *D,* ST segment elevation and T wave amplitude increase caused by variant angina pectoris. *E,* Horizontality of the ST segment with a sharply angled ST-T junction. *F,* Plane ST segment depression with u wave inversion. *G,* Sagging ST segment depression. *H,* Downward sloping ST segment depression. (From Schamroth L: The Electrocardiology of Coronary Artery Disease. Oxford: Blackwell, 1984; 140. With permission.)

changes, myocardial infarction is represented on the ECG only by the Q wave. A Q wave of greater than 0.03-msec duration correlates well with the presence of a myocardial infarction, except in the presence of bundle-branch block. Fortunately, when there is normal conduction, Q waves of myocardial infarction are localized to a few leads, indicating the site of the infarction. In this circumstance, the presence of Q waves are false-positive findings for infarction only 4% of the time.[17]

ST Segment Depression as a Marker for Ischemia: Confounding Factors

Many factors besides ischemia depress the ST segments, including exercise, left ventricular hypertrophy, bundle-branch blocks, digoxin therapy, hypokalemia, and even postural changes.

Exercise

Much interest has been shown in the ST segment changes induced by exercise, which causes J point depression and an upsloping ST segment (Fig. 1–9C). Unfortunately, this pattern is indistinguishable from that seen with the onset of ischemia; only continuation of exercise can separate the two. Normal subjects maintain the upsloping ST segment, whereas ischemic subjects show progressive flattening and then downsloping of the ST segment (Fig. 1–9F,H). The slope of the ST segment, therefore, has received a good deal of attention. A slope of more than 40% at a paper speed of 25 mm/

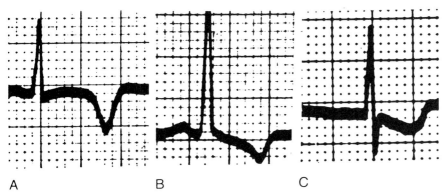

A   B   C

Figure 1–10. Electrocardiograms showing ST segment and T wave in: *A*, Coronary artery disease with a sharply pointed, symmetric, deep T wave and an ST segment that hugs the isoelectric line for a relatively long period. *B*, Left ventricular hypertrophy and strain with a depressed minimally upward concave ST segment that is not isoelectric for any period; the T wave is blunt, shallow, and asymmetric. *C*, Digitalis effect with which the ST segment is not isoelectric for any period and shows a downward slope with a sharp terminal rise ending in a blunt T wave. (From Schamroth L: The Electrocardiology of Coronary Artery Disease. Oxford: Blackwell, 1984; 313. With permission.)

second is "probably normal."[11] However, evidence has accumulated to show that the slope is less important than the presence of continued ST segment depression at a point 0.06–0.08 msec after the J point. In patients undergoing exercise stress testing, where significance was 2-mm ST segment depression 0.08 msec after the J point, Stuart and Ellestad found the same incidence of coronary disease in patients with upsloping ST segment depression as in those with horizontal ST segment depression.[13] The prognosis for patients with downsloping ST segments was worse than that for patients with either horizontal or upsloping ST segments.[13]

Left Ventricular Hypertrophy

Left ventricular hypertrophy changes many ECG features. The increased mass of the left ventricle increases the voltage of the QRS complex and alters the time course and direction of ventricular activation. A widening of the QRS-T angle can result in a shift of the ST segment opposite in direction to the QRS. In Estes' criteria for the diagnosis of left ventricular hypertrophy this carries as much weight as voltage criteria, and even more if the ST segment shift is part of a "strain" pattern.[18] Strain develops in long-standing hypertrophy, especially with the onset of left ventricular dilatation and failure. However, its mechanism and significance are not well understood. Classic "strain" is characterized by ST segments that slope downward, with an upward convexity, into an inverted T wave (Fig. 1–10*B*). It is seen in the lateral precordial leads V_5 and V_6, and in limb leads having a qS pattern.[18]

Conduction Defects

Abnormal ventricular activation sequences, such as occur with the bundle-branch blocks, alter repolarization, making the interpretation of ST segments more difficult. In addition, sudden changes in the conduction pattern in patients with Wolff-Parkinson-White syndrome simulate the onset of ischemia. On the other hand, ischemia may precipitate a right bundle-branch block. Indeed, the most common cause of bundle-branch block is coronary artery disease. Because Q waves may disappear in left bundle-branch block, the diagnosis of myocardial infarction is obscured. Bundle-branch blocks are characterized by widened QRS complexes and wide S waves. However, it appears that acute changes in the ST segments, monitored carefully, still reflect ischemia. Notably, these may not always be frank ST depression; ischemia developing in the presence of right bundle-branch block may appear as a flattening of the ST segment, restoring it closer to the baseline, whereas the T waves appear more symmetric and taller.

Digoxin

The response of the ECG to digoxin is variable. The resulting ECG may or may not reveal ST segment depression and may differ from the ECG taken during exercise. The amount of ST segment depression has not been closely correlated with the serum digoxin concentration, although in general there appears to be more ST segment depression at higher serum levels, indicating some dose-dependence.[19]

Because of the effects of digoxin on the ST segment, it is often discontinued 1–2 weeks before exercise testing. During exercise, more ST segment depression may be seen, but it does not inexorably progress with time as is typical for the ST segment depression of ischemia (Fig. 1–10C). However, the results of exercise studies done in the presence of digoxin are conflicting.

Hypokalemia

Hypokalemia produces significant flattening and depression of the ST segment. In addition, however, the T wave is usually diminished in amplitude, the Q-T interval becomes prolonged, and a U wave may appear (Fig. 1–11).

Posture

Postural changes affect the ECG. Shifting of the heart within the chest alters the axis of the ECG. Older literature suggests that a number of leads may show ST-T wave changes during movement from supine to sitting or standing positions.[20] With improvements in electrodes, electronic amplification, and filtering techniques, the relative importance of this problem has diminished.

Artifacts Due to Electronic Filtering Mechanisms

Electronic-related artifacts are more likely to be encountered with the use of bedside monitoring than during performance of the 12-lead standard ECG, during which the patient does not move or speak. A bedside monitor

ST   T   U

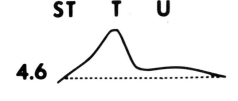

4.6

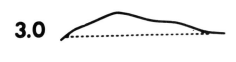

3.0

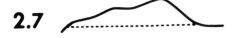

2.7

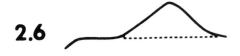

2.6

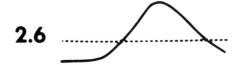

2.6

Figure 1–11. The ECG effects of hypokalemia. There is progressive development of the U component of the ST-T-U wave as the serum potassium levels decrease. The T wave itself becomes progressively flatter. (From Braunwald E: Heart Disease: A Textbook of Cardiovascular Medicine. Philadelphia: WB Saunders, 1980; 247.)

PROGRESSIVE HYPOKALEMIA

filters out extraneous signals derived from movement of the patient and preserves the general pattern of the ECG. The potential difference generated by the heart between two surface electrodes is approximately 1 mV, whereas there may be 20 mV across the skin. The latter, however, is a much lower frequency signal that can be excluded by a filter with a low-frequency cut-off of 0.5 Hz. This frequency cut-off unfortunately may interfere with reproduction of the ST segment, which is a relatively low-frequency portion of the ECG complex and may be as low as 0.14 Hz.[21] Thus, for closer examination of the ST segment it is desirable to have a frequency cut-off below this level. Many ECG monitors allow for the manual selection of one of two levels: a monitor mode with a frequency cut-off of 0.5 Hz and a diagnostic mode with a cut-off of 0.05 Hz. The diagnostic mode allows for a more faithful display of the ST segment but may also introduce more baseline wandering owing to other low-frequency signals.

In addition to filtering artifacts, other interference may appear on the ECG. Intraoperatively, electrocautery is the most frequent problem, but one that is generally intermittent and short-lived. More sustained artifacts are created by other machinery in the operating room such as the roller pumps of an extracorporeal oxygenator and suction devices.

Sensitivity of ST Segment Change for the Detection of Ischemia

Much experimental work has been done to compare the onset of ST segment changes with other indexes of ischemia such as lactate production and regional wall motion abnormalities.[22] Much work has been done with graded occlusions of a coronary artery in animal studies, but with the advent of percutaneous transluminal coronary angioplasty, a human model of ischemia has also become available for study.

On the basis of many studies, it appears that ST segment changes occur within 30–60 seconds of an acute, total coronary occlusion. With epicardially placed electrodes, the center of the infarct zone generates more marked ST elevation than does the periphery, reaching a maximum 5–7 minutes after occlusion. In clinical practice, using surface leads, the onset of ischemia is more frequent and of more interest than a completed myocardial infarction.

Regional lactate production and wall motion abnormalities develop when coronary flow has been reduced to about 48% of its normal value (using graded reductions in coronary flow in dogs), and they precede the onset of ST segment abnormalities. With approximately 75% reduction in coronary flow, ECG changes begin to develop (Fig. 1–12).[23–25] This evidence that ST segment changes are less sensitive than regional wall motion abnormalities for the detection of ischemia has been supported by a clinical study of patients with coronary disease undergoing major vascular surgery.[26] Of 50 patients studied, 24 developed new wall motion abnormalities intraoperatively, but only 6 showed ST segment changes. The six patients with ST segment changes also had regional wall motion abnormalities. There were three perioperative myocardial infarctions; only one of these patients had intraoperative ST segment changes, but all of them exhibited new regional wall motion abnormalities.

The pulmonary capillary wedge pressure waveform has also been studied as an early indicator of ischemia. In 40 patients undergoing coronary artery bypass grafting, ischemia was defined as 1-mm ST depression or the development of an abnormal wedge tracing with an A and C wave greater than 15 mmHg, or a V wave greater than 20 mmHg. Ten patients met wedge tracing criteria only, three met ECG criteria only, and five met both. The authors concluded that a wedge pressure tracing could be more sensitive than the ECG for the detection of ischemia.[27]

Properly applied, the ECG remains both a cheap and convenient way to monitor patients for ischemia and a standard of care unlikely to be replaced. It is clear, however, that it is not the most sensitive tool available and that certain patients benefit from additional monitoring.

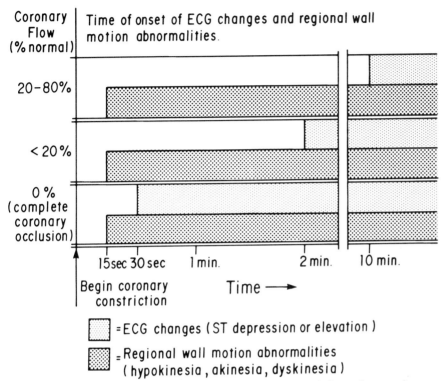

Figure 1–12. Temporal relationship between acute coronary constriction and onset of electrocardiogram (ECG) and regional wall motion abnormalities. This figure summarizes data from several animal and human studies (Lachman, Semler, Gustafson, Circulation 1965; Berson, Pipberger, Am Heart J 1966; Clements, de Bruijn, Anesth Analg 1987).

ST SEGMENT ANALYSIS

Routine observation of a bedside ECG monitor fails to detect many episodes of ischemia.[28, 29] Transient small changes in ST depression are difficult to detect unless hard-copy waveforms are painstakingly compared over time. Until recently, continuous ECG display has been more useful for the rapid detection of arrhythmias rather than specifically for ischemia monitoring. As newer ECG monitors have gained credibility for their accuracy in recording the ST segment, interest has developed in automated on-line ST analysis and trend recordings. In the critical care setting, this provides not only enhanced detection of ischemia but also continuous feedback following therapeutic interventions.

Equipment

Automated ST analysis systems require a computer algorithm to recognize the QRS complex and to identify a point along the baseline trace that

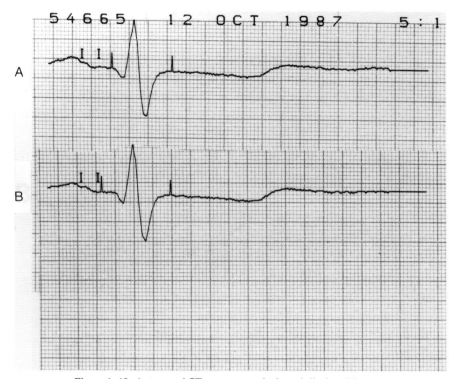

Figure 1–13. Automated ST segment analysis and display (Marquette system): *A,* The default isoelectric and ST segment points are shown. *B,* The isoelectric point has been manually shifted to select an earlier point prior to the QRS complex.

can be compared with a point along the defined ST segment. Various methods of accomplishing this have been developed.

Marquette System

Marquette Electronics has computer software with their standard bedside monitor that has already undergone various refinements. Many other manufacturers are now beginning to introduce their own ST analysis systems. The Marquette system continuously measures and trends the depression or elevation of the ST segment in three selected leads, currently leads I, II, and V_5. An isoelectric point is selected 16 msec prior to the onset of the QRS complex and compared with a point on the ST segment 40 msec after the onset of the QRS. These points are also manually adjustable, which is useful when the QRS complex is widened (Fig. 1–13*A,B*). The deviation of the ST segment from baseline, whether as elevation (positive) or depression (negative), is converted to a positive number for all leads, and these are added together. The summation of ST deviation is then plotted on a trend line. This "ST deviation plot" provides up to 28 minutes of trend display, an upward deflection indicating more ST deviation, and a downward trend indicating a return to baseline (Fig. 1–14). With a strip-chart recorder, a hard copy of the ST deviation plot can be obtained for permanent record.

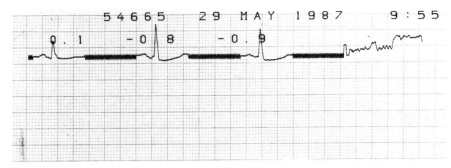

Figure 1–14. ST deviation plot display (Marquette system). ST deviation for the previous 28 minutes is shown. The rising line on the right indicates recent development of ischemia, with ST depression in leads II and V. (See text.)

In addition to the trend line, the QRS complex of each of the three leads is also displayed with a numeric value of the ST segment depression or elevation in millimeters, and this is updated every 32 beats.

Results. Kotrly, Kotter, and coworkers[30, 31] reported on the use of the Marquette ST analysis system in 312 patients over a 2.5-year period, during which time the incidence of ischemic events and their relationship to hemodynamic events was noted for the prebypass phase of open heart surgery. The ST segment analysis system became familiar to the anesthesiologists involved during this time and was used in their clinical care of the patients. Among their findings, the authors reported that the incidence of ischemia decreased significantly from 17% to 6% after the first 6 months of the study, making the overall incidence of ischemia 8.1% for the completed study. They noted that the acceptance of the ST analysis system with a reliable and sensitive trend line increased awareness of small ST segment changes and prompted interventions to correct them. Thus, the system may have contributed to the reduction in ischemia noted over the course of the study. In addition, they noted that the overall incidence of ischemia was considerably lower than the 26–69% reported in other studies of comparable patient populations.[16] Among the possible factors responsible for this discrepancy are the accuracy of the ECG monitor and the definition of ischemic changes.

Ambulatory ECG Monitoring Systems

Soon after the introduction of ambulatory ECG monitors, it was noted that patients with documented coronary artery disease manifested frequent episodes of ST segment deviation, only 25% of which were accompanied by angina.[32, 33] On the basis that 80% of these episodes could be reduced by administration of nitroglycerin, it was felt that these ST deviations truly represented ischemia.[34] However, the ability of amplitude-modulated (AM) recording systems to record frequencies below 10 Hz was found to be limited. Indeed, narrow bandwidths used to eliminate baseline wandering and other artifacts tended to specifically distort the frequency spectrum that includes the ST segment.[35] Thus, ambulatory monitors were somewhat discredited for the purpose of ST segment monitoring. Further doubt of their usefulness was engendered by studies that did not distinguish between J point depression and horizontal or downsloping ST segment depression persisting for 60 or 80 msec.

Recently, however, ambulatory monitoring has regained favor, by virtue of improvements in technology and validation studies of various systems. For example, studies comparing the detection of ST segment depression by simultaneous two-channel Holter monitoring and 12-lead ECG during exercise testing have shown a concordance of 96%.[36] The sensitivity of the two methods was similar—81% and 84%, respectively—and the specificity for both was 85%.

Portable ST Segment Monitors. Because of the vast amount of ECG data that is generated by long-term monitoring, automated ST segment analysis has become essential. Although tape-recorded ECG traces can be computer-scanned after a period of monitoring, real-time analysis offers the opportunity for providing instant notification of an ischemic episode and thus correlation with activity and therapeutic intervention. This capability makes such monitors useful in the care of hospitalized patients as well as ambulatory outpatients. A number of commercially available portable monitors have now been developed; some use frequency-modulated (FM) or AM tape recordings, and others use solid-state memory. Some offer real-time analysis with an interactive capability in addition to a printed report that is generated at the end of the monitoring period. Some monitors allow simultaneous recording of two leads rather than one.

The QMed System. The monitor marketed by QMed, Inc., rather than storing continuous ECG traces for the entire period of monitoring, saves only significant events. Thus, events of tachycardia, bradycardia, premature ventricular contractions, wide complex tachycardia, and ST segment depressions are saved and displayed on the final report as 5-second ECG tracings. Histograms showing the trends of heart rate and ST segment and other significant data are also retrievable.

The computer used to derive the information first defines the QRS complex, interrogating the incoming ECG signal at a frequency of 256 Hz. A QRS complex is defined when the three inflection points representing the Q, R, and S points are found within a time of 120 msec. The Q is noted when the slope of the line increases beyond a threshold value; similarly, the J point is defined when the slope falls to zero following the QRS complex. A point 60 msec after the J point is then taken for comparison with the isoelectric segment of the PR interval (Fig. 1–15). Tracings rejected by the algorithm as QRS complexes and those for which an ST segment cannot be analyzed are shown in Fig. 1–16. When ST segment depression persists for 40–60 seconds, an ischemic event is recorded.[37]

The QMed monitor has been used during the perioperative period in patients undergoing vascular surgery. In one patient who sustained an acute anterior wall myocardial infarction, the monitor revealed four episodes of silent ischemia (1-mm ST segment depression) during the 4 hours preceding the infarction (Fig. 1–17).[38] In addition, trends of heart rate and premature ventricular beats indicated a persistent tachycardia and more frequent ectopia preceding the infarct (Fig. 1–18). Although the patient was in an intensive care unit during the same period of time, these events were unap-

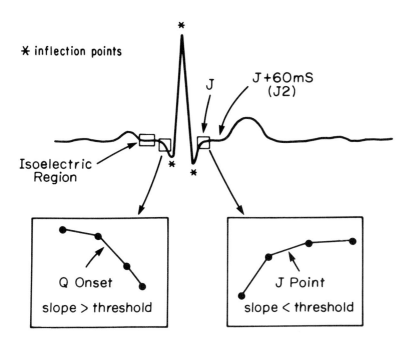

Figure 1–15. QRS analysis by computer algorithm in the Qmed system marks the inflection points (*) of the complex. The Q and J points are identified by the changing slope of the analogue signal (see text). (From Levin RI, Cohen D, Frisbie W, et al: Potential for real-time processing of the continuously monitored electrocardiogram in the detection, quantitation, and intervention of silent myocardial ischemia. Cardiol Clin 1986; 4:735–745.)

preciated by routine observation of the bedside ECG display, which did not feature ST segment analysis. The audible alarm, which can be programmed to sound for episodes of ST segment depression, alerts the intensive care unit staff to the presence of ST segment depression in patients with severe coronary disease.

In a group of 24 patients undergoing peripheral vascular reconstructions monitored pre-, intra-, and postoperatively, for a mean time of 74.5 hours, there was a 37% incidence of ischemia.[39] All ischemic events were unaccompanied by angina except for some episodes in one patient. The occurrence of ischemia was significantly correlated with unfavorable outcomes ($p < 0.02$). In many instances, ST segment depression occurred in conjunction with increased heart rate, but not invariably. In patients with heart rate–related ischemia, the effects of beta blockade were easily demonstrated (Fig. 1–19).

CHARACTERISTICS AND SIGNIFICANCE OF SILENT ISCHEMIA

With the arrival of reliable monitors for ST segment analysis, the concept of silent ischemia has emerged as a prominent feature of coronary artery disease. Several studies have shown that the majority of episodes of ST segment depression are painless in patients with coronary disease. However, silent ischemia appears to carry the same prognosis as painful ischemia.[40, 41] Thus, symptoms of coronary artery disease are recognized to be only "the tip of the iceberg"; the new concept of the "total ischemic burden" has

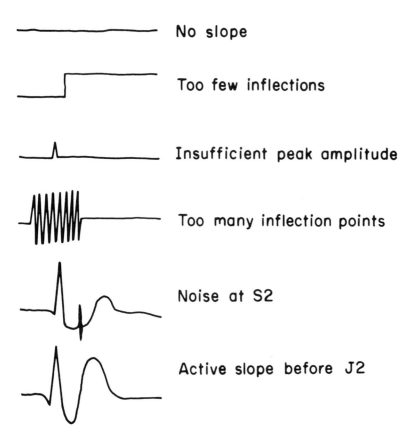

No slope

Too few inflections

Insufficient peak amplitude

Too many inflection points

Noise at S2

Active slope before J2

Figure 1–16. Examples of "beats" rejected for QRS-1 analysis by the computer algorithm (Qmed system). The first four traces would be rejected as QRS complexes; the last two would be recognized as QRS complexes but rejected for ST analysis. (From Levin RI, Cohen D, Frisbie W, et al: Potential for real-time processing of the continuously monitored electrocardiogram in the detection, quantitation, and intervention of silent myocardial ischemia. Cardiol Clin 1986; 4:735–745.)

evolved as a more accurate indicator of myocardial oxygen balance in the long term. The goal of medical therapy may therefore be a significant reduction in the total ischemic burden, or the total duration of ischemic time, rather than merely the amelioration of symptoms. As more attention is directed toward silent ischemia in the perioperative period, it is useful to examine the data pertaining to silent ST segment depression in subjects with and without coronary disease and in those with and without anginal symptoms.

About 70–85% of ischemic episodes are silent, or painless.[40, 41] Sixty to 80% of patients with chronic stable angina have daily episodes of ischemia or 5–10 episodes of ischemia per week, with a median duration of 17 minutes (range 1–90).[42] Painful episodes of ischemia tend to last longer than painless episodes, e.g., 21 ± 7 minutes versus 16 ± 5 minutes, but there has been no correlation between the degree of ST depression and the occurrence of pain.[43] Also, 70% of ischemic episodes occur with only minimal physical activity and may be more related to levels of mental activity. Interestingly, the heart rate at onset of ischemia during ambulatory monitoring is significantly lower than the heart rate at onset of ischemia during exercise testing. Thus, factors other than increased myocardial oxygen demand alone must play a significant role. Patients with early positive stress tests experience more silent ischemia during ambulatory monitoring. Episodes occur most

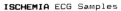

ISCHEMIA ECG Samples

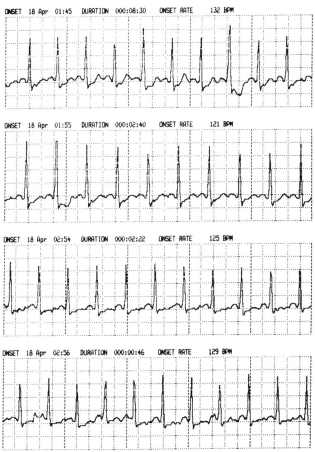

Figure 1–17. Five-second ECG traces recorded by a Qmed ambulatory monitor during ischemic episodes (1-mm ST segment depression) occurring shortly before an extensive anterior wall myocardial infarction. (From Clements FM, McCann RL, Levin RI: Continuous ST-segment analysis for the detection of perioperative myocardial ischemia. Crit Care Med 16(7):710–711, © by Williams & Wilkins, 1988.)

frequently between the hours of 6:00 A.M. and 10:00 A.M., which mirrors the peak time of occurrence of myocardial infarction and sudden death.[44]

In patients with coronary disease but without prior myocardial infarction or angina, the prevalence of silent ischemia is 2.5–10%.[45, 46] Patients with unstable angina and transient ECG evidence of ischemia, receiving maximum medical therapy in a coronary care unit, have demonstrated a 50% incidence of silent ischemia.[47] Moreover, silent ischemia was a better predictor of poor outcome than was the presence of continued chest pain.[47] In the group of patients exhibiting ischemia, duration of ischemia was significant in that those patients with more than 60 minutes of ischemia per 24 hours were more likely to have unfavorable outcomes than were those with less. In normal patients without cardiovascular disease, typical ST segment changes of ischemia are extremely rare.[48, 49] However, many factors, such as digoxin or quinidine therapy, left ventricular hypertrophy, and even postural changes, can affect the ST segment. Provided the computer analysis program truly measures planar ST segment depression, ambulatory monitors appear to be reliable for the detection of ischemia. The computer interpre-

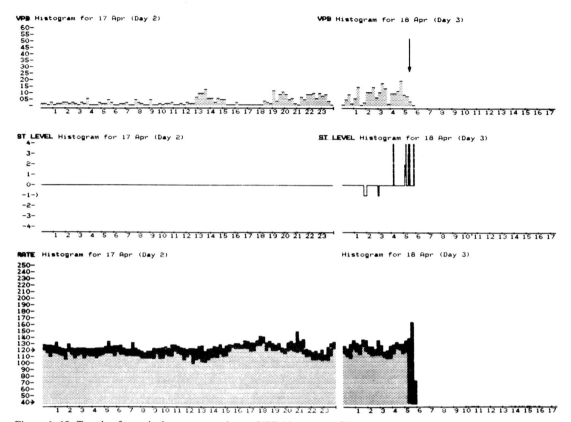

Figure 1–18. Trends of ventricular premature beats (VPB histogram), ST segments (ST level histogram), and heart rate (HR histogram) over the 30 hours preceding an anterior wall myocardial infarction (Qmed report). (Hard-copy traces of the ischemic episodes recorded prior to the myocardial infarction are presented in Fig. 1–17.) The apparent ST elevation noted in this report could not be confirmed in hard-copy form with the monitor used and may have been artifactual. The patient arrested at 05:30 and required electrical defibrillation several times before sinus rhythm was restored. (From Clements FM, McCann RL, Levin RI: Continuous ST-segment analysis for the detection of perioperative myocardial ischemia. Crit Care Med 16(7):710–711, © by Williams & Wilkins, 1988.)

tation of ST segments in the presence of digoxin or quinidine therapy and with left ventricular hypertrophy still remains controversial, however.

SIGNIFICANCE OF INTRAOPERATIVE ISCHEMIA

For patients with proven coronary artery disease, the incidence of intraoperative myocardial ischemia detected by the ECG has been reported to range from 26% to 67%. In a recent study by Slogoff and Keats examining 1023 patients, ischemia occurred in 36.9% of all patients undergoing coronary artery bypass grafting (CABG), and perioperative myocardial infarction was three times as frequent in patients with ischemia, 6.9% versus 2.5%.[16] More recently, Kotter and coworkers reported ischemic ECG changes before car-

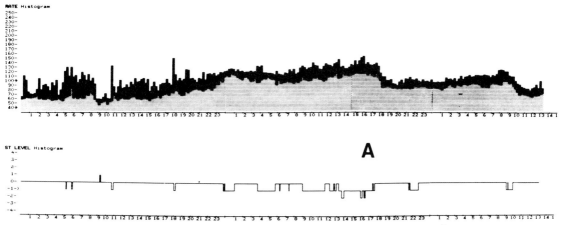

Figure 1–19. Histograms for heart rate (above) and ST level (below), for 2.5 days of monitoring. The effect of atenolol 50 mg, given twice at *A*, can be seen in this patient with multiple episodes of painless ischemia postoperatively.

diopulmonary bypass in 11.9% of patients. In their study, the incidence was lower in patients undergoing initial CABG (8.1%) than in patients having repeat CABG (23.5%). The highest incidence was observed in patients with combined CABG-valve operations (35.3%).[31] In Kotter and coworkers' study, nitrates, calcium blockers, or beta blockers did not affect the occurrence of ischemia.[31] An interesting difference between these two studies is the incidence of myocardial ischemia present at the time of arrival in the operating room—18% of the patients in the study of Slogoff and Keats versus only 0.3% in Kotter and coworkers' study.[16, 31] In a group of patients with coronary artery disease undergoing noncardiac surgery, Coriat and associates found an incidence of myocardial ischemia of 42%, using ST segment criteria.[50]

The use of prophylactic nitroglycerin to prevent myocardial ischemia is controversial. Coriat and colleagues reported that 1 μg/kg/minute of nitroglycerin was effective in preventing intraoperative ischemic events.[51] However, other investigators noted that nitroglycerin was ineffective in preventing intraoperative ischemia.[52, 53]

The incidence of perioperative myocardial ischemia in patients with coronary artery disease is substantial, and the consequences of such ischemic episodes are serious, with a significant percentage of these patients developing myocardial infarction. The role of pharmacologic interventions to prevent myocardial ischemia remains unclear, but interventions to control myocardial oxygen supply and demand via manipulation of hemodynamic parameters are probably effective.

In spite of its limitations, electrocardiography remains one of the most important tools to detect intraoperative ischemia episodes. Recent technologic improvements and the development of reliable automated ST segment analysis have significantly enhanced its value and facilitated early diagnosis of perioperative myocardial ischemic events.

References

1. Einthoven W, Fahr G, de Waart A: On the direction and manifest size of the variations of potential in the human heart and on the influence of the position of the heart on the form of the electrocardiogram. Am Heart J 1950; 40:163–178.
2. Goldberger E: Unipolar lead electrocardiography and vector cardiography. Philadelphia: Lea & Febiger, 1953.
3. Johnson FD, Lepeschkin E (eds): Selected papers of Dr. Frank N. Wilson. Ann Arbor: JW Edwards, 1955.
4. Blackburn H, Katigbak R: What electrocardiographic leads to take after exercise? Am Heart J 1964; 67:184–185.
5. Kates RA, Zaidan JR, Kaplan JA: Esophageal lead for intraoperative electrocardiographic monitoring. Anesth Analg 1982; 61:781–785.
6. Copeland DG, Tullis IF, Brody DA: Clinical evaluation of a new esophageal electrode, with particular reference to the bipolar esophageal electrogram. Part I. Normal sinus mechanism. Am Heart J 1959; 57:862–873.
7. Griffin RM, Kaplan JA: Comparison of ECG leads V_5, CS_5, CB_5 and II by computerized ST segment analysis. Anesth Analg 1986; 65:S65.
8. Bazaral MG, Norfleet EA: Comparison of CB_5 and V_5 leads for intraoperative electrocardiographic monitoring. Anesth Analg 1981; 60:849–853.
9. Kaplan JA, King SB III: The precordial electrocardiographic lead (V_5) in patients who have coronary-artery disease. Anesthesiology 1976; 45:570–574.
10. Robertson D, Kostok WJ, Ahuja SP: The localization of coronary artery stenosis by 12-lead ECG response to graded exercise test. Am Heart J 1976; 91:437–444.
11. Braunwald E: Heart Disease: A Textbook of Cardiovascular Medicine. Philadelphia: WB Saunders, 1980.
12. Ellestad MH, Cooke DM Jr, Greenberg PS: Stress Testing: Principles and Practice. Philadelphia: FA Davis, 1980; 85.
13. Stuart RJ, Ellestad MH: Upsloping ST segments in exercise stress testing. Am J Cardiol 1976; 37:19–22.
14. Robb GP, Marks H: Post-exercise electrocardiogram in arteriosclerotic heart disease. JAMA 1967; 200:918–926.
15. Goldschlager N, Selzer A, Cohn K: Treadmill stress tests as indicators of presence and severity of coronary artery disease. Ann Intern Med 1976; 85:277–286.
16. Slogoff S, Keats AS: Does perioperative myocardial ischemia lead to postoperative myocardial infarction? Anesthesiology 1985; 62:107–114.
17. Horan LG, Flowers NC, Johnson JC: Significance of the diagnostic Q wave of myocardial infarction. Circulation 1971; 43:428–436.
18. Marriott HJ: Practical Electrocardiography. Baltimore: Williams & Wilkins, 1983.
19. Sundqvist K, Atterhog JH, Jogestrand T: Effect of digoxin on the electrocardiogram at rest and during exercise in healthy subjects. Am J Cardiol 1986; 57:661–665.
20. Lachman AB, Semler HJ, Gustafson RH: Postural ST-T wave changes in the radioelectrocardiogram simulating myocardial ischemia. Circulation 1965; 31:557–563.
21. Berson AS, Pipberger HV: The low-frequency response of electrocardiographs, a frequent source of recording errors. Am Heart J 1966; 71:779–789.
22. Clements FM, de Bruijn NP: Perioperative evaluation of regional wall motion by transesophageal two-dimensional echocardiography. Anesth Analg 1987; 656:249–261.
23. Waters DD, da Luz P, Wyatt HL, et al: Early changes in regional and global

left ventricular function induced by graded reductions in regional coronary perfusion. Am J Cardiol 1977; 39:537–543.

24. Tomoiki H, Franklin D, Ross J Jr: Detection of myocardial ischemia by regional dysfunction during and after rapid pacing in conscious dogs. Circulation 1978; 58:48–56.

25. Tomoiki H, Franklin D, McKown D, et al: Regional myocardial dysfunction and hemodynamic abnormalities during strenuous exercise in dogs with limited coronary flow. Circ Res 1978; 42:478–496.

26. Smith JS, Cahalan MK, Benefiel DJ, et al: Intraoperative detection of myocardial ischemia in high risk patients; electrocardiography vs two-dimensional transesophageal echocardiography. Circulation 1985; 75:1015–1021.

27. Kaplan JA, Wells PH: Early diagnosis of myocardial ischemia using the pulmonary artery catheter. Anesth Analg 1981; 60:789–793.

28. Roy WL, Edelist G, Gilbert B: Myocardial ischemia during non-cardiac surgical procedures in patients with coronary artery disease. Anesthesiology 1979; 51:393–397.

29. Coriat P, Daloz M, Bousseau D, et al: Prevention of intraoperative myocardial ischemia during non-cardiac surgery with intravenous nitroglycerin. Anesthesiology 1984; 61:193–196.

30. Kotrly KJ, Kotter GS, Mortara D, et al: Intraoperative detection of myocardial ischemia with an ST segment trend monitoring system. Anesth Analg 1984; 63:343–345.

31. Kotter GS, Kotrly KJ, Kalbfleisch JH, et al: Myocardial ischemia during cardiovascular surgery as detected by an ST segment trend monitoring system. J Cardiothorac Anesth 1987; 1:190–199.

32. Bellet S, Roman L, Kostis J, et al: Continuous electrocardiographic monitoring during automobile driving. Am J Cardiol 1968; 22:856–862.

33. Cohn PF: Severe asymptomatic coronary artery disease: A diagnostic, prognostic and therapeutic puzzle. Am J Med 1977; 62:565–568.

34. Schang SJ, Pepine CJ: Transient asymptomatic ST segment depression during daily activity. Am J Cardiol 1977; 39:396–402.

35. Balasubramanian V, Lahiri A, Green HL, et al: Ambulatory ST-segment monitoring. Problems, pitfalls, solutions, and clinical application. Br Heart J 1980; 44:419–425.

36. Tzivoni D, Benhorin J, Gavish A, Stern S: Holter recording during treadmill testing in assessing myocardial ischemic changes. Am J Cardiol 1985; 55:1200–1203.

37. Levin RI, Cohen D, Frisbie W, et al: Potential for real-time processing of the continuously monitored electrocardiogram in the detection, quantitation, and intervention of silent myocardial ischemia. Cardiol Clin 1986; 4:735–745.

38. Clements FM, McCann RL, Levin RI: Continuous ST-segment analysis for the detection of perioperative myocardial ischemia. Crit Care Med 1988; 16:710–711.

39. Clements FM, McCann RL: Perioperative silent ischemia: Prevalence and significance in patients undergoing peripheral vascular surgery. (Abstract.) Society of Cardiovascular Anesthesiologists 10th Annual Meeting 1988; 101.

40. Deanfield JE, Kensett M, Wilson RA, et al: Silent myocardial ischaemia due to mental stress. Lancet 1984; 2:1001–1005.

41. Shea MJ, Deanfield JE, Wilson R, et al: Transient ischemia in angina pectoris: Frequent silent events with everyday activities. Am J Cardiol 1985; 56:34E–38E.

42. Deanfield JE, Selwyn AP, Chierchia S, et al: Myocardial ischaemia during daily life in patients with stable angina: Its relation to symptoms and heart rate changes. Lancet 1983; 2:753–758.

43. Schang SJ Jr, Pepine CJ: Transient asymptomatic ST depression during daily activity. Am J Cardiol 1977; 39:396–402.
44. Mullen JE, Stone PH, Turi ZG, et al: Circadian variations in the frequency of onset of acute myocardial infarction. N Engl J Med 1985; 313:1315–1322.
45. Langou RA, Huang EK, Kelley MJ, et al: Predictive accuracy of coronary artery calcification and abnormal exercise test for coronary artery disease in asymptomatic men. Circulation 1980; 62:1196–1203.
46. Eriksson J, Thoulaw E: Follow-up of patients with asymptomatic myocardial ischemia. *In* Rutishauser W, Roskamm H (eds): Silent Myocardial Ischemia. Berlin: Springer-Verlag, 1980; 154–164.
47. Gottlieb SO, Weisfeldt LM, Ouyant P, et al: Silent ischemia as a marker for early unfavorable outcomes in patients with unstable angina. N Engl J Med 1986; 314:1214–1219.
48. Stern S, Tzivoni D: Dynamic changes in the ST-T segment during sleep in ischemic heart disease. Am J Cardiol 1973; 32:17–20.
49. Deanfield JE, Ribeiro P, Oakley K, et al: Analysis of ST segment changes in normal subjects: Implications for ambulatory monitoring in angina pectoris. Am J Cardiol 1984; 54:1321–1325.
50. Coriat P, Harari A, Daloz M, Viars P: Clinical predictors of intraoperative myocardial ischemia in patients with coronary artery disease undergoing non-cardiac surgery. Acta Anaesthesiol Scand 1982; 26:287–290.
51. Coriat P, Daloz M, Rousseau D, et al: Prevention of intraoperative myocardial ischemia during noncardiac surgery with intravenous nitroglycerin. Anesthesiology 1984; 61:193–196.
52. Gallagher JD, Moore RA, Jose AB: Prophylactic nitroglycerin infusions during coronary artery bypass surgery. Anesthesiology 1986; 64:785–789.
53. Thompson IR, Mutch WAC, Culligan JD: Failure of intravenous nitroglycerin to prevent intraoperative myocardial ischemia during fentanyl-pancuronium anesthesia. Anesthesiology 1984; 61:385–393.

chapter two

Electrocardiography: Monitoring for Arrhythmias

MARK J. RICE, M.D.
■ JOHN L. ATLEE III, M.D.

Intraoperative arrhythmias may be quite common, with incidences up to 84%[1] reported during general anesthesia. Since many of these dysrhythmias are hemodynamically significant or are harbingers of serious physiologic disturbances, their prompt recognition is of the utmost importance.

The chapter covers the incidence and significance of dysrhythmias, the mechanism underlying their formation, and methods for monitoring the electrocardiogram (ECG)—including discussion of means to reduce the risk of microshock and minimize electrocautery interference, recognition of specific dysrhythmias and electrocardiographic changes resulting from physiologic derangements, and finally, consideration of electronic pacemaker electrocardiography (normal as well as abnormal function).

INCIDENCE OF DYSRHYTHMIAS

The exact incidence of intraoperative dysrhythmias is unknown. The reported incidence depends on the methods used for detection, the anesthetic and surgical procedure, and associated diseases and physiologic derangements.

Intuitively, young, healthy patients have a lower incidence of dysrhythmias than older persons undergoing similar procedures. Intrathoracic surgery, which often results in manipulation of the myocardium, has a higher incidence of dysrhythmias than does extremity surgery. The most important factor in comparing the studies concerning incidence is, however, the method or procedure of monitoring for dysrhythmias.

Studies that do not continuously record or monitor the ECG ("incomplete" studies) may miss transient rhythm disturbances and provide a lower incidence for dysrhythmias related to a particular procedure. To qualify as a "complete" incidence study, the ECG should be *continuously monitored and recorded*.

In the first of two reported complete studies, Kuner and coworkers[2] studied 154 patients undergoing either general or regional anesthesia and found evidence of arrhythmias in 62% overall. The recording of sinus tachycardia, which would probably have increased the incidence, was not included in this percentage. The use of general anesthesia was associated with a higher incidence of dysrhythmias than was regional anesthesia, 66% versus 52%. In thoracic surgery (93%) there was a higher incidence than in extremity operations (56%). There was little difference between patients with (62%) and without (59%) pre-existing heart disease. Intubated patients (72%) had more arrhythmias than did nonintubated (44%) patients.

In the second complete study, Bertrand and colleagues[1] found an overall dysrhythmia incidence of 84% in 100 surgical patients. They found the highest incidence of dysrhythmias during intubation and extubation. Sixty-five of the 90 patients intubated displayed dysrhythmias during either intubation or extubation but not during other parts of the surgical or anesthetic procedure.

To enhance the likelihood of dysrhythmia detection, the anesthesiologist must do everything possible to increase her or his ability to detect rhythm disturbances during the patient's intraoperative course. The electrocardiograph should be among the first monitors applied when the patient enters the operating room. After placement of other necessary monitoring devices, the ECG should be recorded from *all available leads* for future intra- and postoperative comparisons. The audible R wave detector should be turned to an easily identified level. Throughout the course of the anesthetic, the ECG should be consulted frequently, even when the audible tone of the heartbeat is regular. If any change in rhythm is detected, an immediate permanent ECG should be recorded for comparison with ECGs obtained at the beginning of the case.

Any patient exhibiting significant intraoperative dysrhythmias or who is at increased risk for postanesthesia complications should have continuous ECG monitoring during transport from the operating room to the postanesthesia recovery room or the intensive care unit. Transport ECG monitors should be readily available for this purpose. Also, ECG monitors should be placed at each recovery station for immediate postoperative dysrhythmia surveillance. Nursing personnel should be trained to detect and diagnose common rhythm disturbances and immediately consult the anesthesiologist concerning management.

SIGNIFICANCE OF ARRHYTHMIAS

The majority of intraoperative dysrhythmias are not severe and usually require no treatment. Such relatively "benign" dysrhythmias rarely require specific drug or electrical management, but obvious correctable causes should be removed. Often dysrhythmias are the result of some physiologic derangement or adverse drug action.

Some dysrhythmias, however, can be deleterious and require immediate recognition, correct diagnosis, removal or correction of causes, and possible specific drug or electrical management. Aberrations of rhythm may be dangerous because (1) adverse hemodynamic consequences result, (2) tachycardia is associated with myocardial ischemia, or (3) they are likely to deteriorate into dangerous ventricular arrhythmias.

A variety of rhythm disturbances reduce cardiac output because of decreased diastolic ventricular filling volumes. This results from either a dyssynchrony between atria and the ventricles or inadequate atrial contractions. Dysrhythmias associated with atrioventricular (AV) dissociation include *type II second-degree AV block, third-degree AV block, AV junctional rhythm,* and *any ectopic ventricular rhythm.* Sufficiently rapid supraventricular tachyarrhythmias provide little time for atrial filling and consequently lower ventricular diastolic filling volumes.

There is a delicate balance between myocardial oxygen supply and utilization. An unfavorable balance can cause ischemia, which if left untreated could lead to myocardial injury, infarction, or lethal dysrhythmias. Major determinants of myocardial oxygen demand are heart rate, wall tension, and contractility. The supply of oxygen for myocardial tissue is often relatively fixed in each patient. Consequently, there is the potential for ischemia with large increases in demand produced by tachycardia. Factors that increase the likelihood of significant myocardial ischemia secondary to tachycardia include occlusive coronary artery disease, anemia, hypovolemia, myocardiopathies, ventricular hypertrophy, and chamber enlargement.

Finally, certain dysrhythmias are likely to deteriorate into *lethal ventricular arrhythmias.* Frequent, multiform, or "R on T" ventricular ectopic beats may trigger sustained ventricular tachycardia or ventricular fibrillation. Any supraventricular tachyarrhythmia in patients with the capability of antegrade fast pathway conduction (e.g., ventricular pre-excitation syndromes) can lead to ventricular tachycardia and fibrillation if sustained and if the ventricular rate is in excess of 150 beats/minute (adults). Ventricular dysrhythmias occur under these conditions even in the absence of demonstrable myocardial or coronary artery disease.

MECHANISMS OF ARRHYTHMOGENESIS

A basic understanding of the mechanisms thought to cause dysrhythmias is required for correct management and is also helpful for recognition. Dysrhythmias result from abnormalities of impulse formation (automaticity) or propagation (re-entry of excitation) or both, discussed later.

Normal Electrical Activity of the Heart

The sinoatrial (SA) node (dominant pacemaker), subsidiary atrial pacemaker cells found along the sulcus terminalis, AV junctional pacemakers, and His-Purkinje cells are capable of spontaneous impulse formation—*automaticity*. The propagated action potential proceeds from the sinus node via functional, but probably not anatomic, preferential atrial conducting pathways to the AV node. Here, conduction is greatly slowed, allowing for optimal ventricular filling. From the AV node, the action potential proceeds to the His (common) bundle, the Purkinje system, and then to the ventricular myocardial cells.

The action potentials of cells found in the SA and AV nodes are characterized by a slow upstroke velocity, maximum diastolic transmembrane potential of -60 to -80 mV, and low amplitude.[3] Cells with these action potential characteristics are termed slow-response cells. In contrast, fast action potentials are characterized by a fast upstroke velocity, resting membrane or maximum diastolic potentials of -80 to -95 mV, and larger amplitudes owing to positive overshoots (reversal $+$ 15–30 mV). Fast action potentials are characteristic of atrial and ventricular muscle and Purkinje (fast-response) cells. Both fast and slow action potentials are depicted schematically in Figure 2–1.

The slow-inward current carried mainly by calcium is responsible for the upstroke of slow action potentials, whereas the fast-inward (predominantly sodium) current is responsible for the upstroke of fast-response cells. The slow-inward current (activated during depolarization at -50 to -40 mV in fast-response cells) is responsible for the action potential plateau (phase 2). Phase 3 (repolarization) is mediated by potassium-outward (K^+) currents, whereas an adenosine triphosphatase (ATPase)–dependent sodium-potassium exchange pump (Na^+–K^+) restores the sodium and potassium gained or lost, respectively, by the interior of the cell during the action potential. The Na^+–K^+ exchange pump functions mainly during the latter part of repolarization and electrical diastole (phase 4). Action potential phases are shown in Figure 2–1.

Spontaneous diastolic depolarization from a physiologic (normal level) diastolic membrane potential is a normal property ("normal automaticity") of cells found in the SA and AV nodes and the His-Purkinje system. Atrial and ventricular muscle can manifest automaticity under nonphysiologic circumstances ("abnormal automaticity," discussed later). The ionic basis for

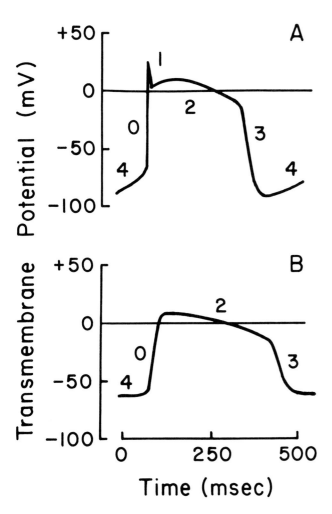

Figure 2–1. Fast and slow action potentials. *A,* Fast potential: phase 0—rapid depolarization; phase 1—early rapid repolarization; phase 2—plateau; phase 3—final repolarization; phase 4—resting membrane potential. *B,* Slow potential: initiated from less negative potential and lacks phase 1. (From Atlee JL III: Perioperative Cardiac Dysrhythmias: Mechanisms, Recognition and Management. Chicago: Year Book Medical, 1985; 27. With permission.)

normal automaticity has not been firmly established. Membrane properties leading to such activity can be identified in a general way.[4] The K^+ permeability of the membrane makes its potential more negative, closer to the K^+–equilibrium potential (E_K), whereas a small Na^+ permeability holds it away from E_K in a delicately balanced fashion. A third process is activated that tips the delicate balance toward depolarization, either by a time-dependent fall in K^+ conductance or by a time-dependent rise in Na^+ or Ca^{2+} conduction. Consequently, the net positive-inward current slightly exceeds the net positive-outward current, resulting in slow diastolic depolarization. This net positive-inward current is termed the pacemaker current. Although the mechanism for the pacemaker current in SA node and His-Purkinje cells is probably similar, it is likely that the relative contribution of changes in Na^+, K^+, or Ca^{2+} conductance differs between these types of cells since spontaneous diastolic depolarization begins from different levels of maximum diastolic potential.

Abnormal Electrical Activity of the Heart

Enhanced Automaticity

As stated previously, the normal heartbeat originates from the SA node. Under usual conditions, the sinus node overdrive suppresses latent pacemaker activity in other areas of the heart, even though other conduction tissues can display automaticity. Ectopic beats or abnormal rhythms may originate from latent pacemakers if automaticity in the SA node is suppressed, as by disease or drugs, or if automaticity in the latent pacemakers is enhanced, as by catecholamines. Alternatively, abnormal forms of automaticity may arise from His-Purkinje or atrial and ventricular muscle fibers when their normally high resting membrane potentials are reduced below -60 mV by disease processes.[5] As with normal automaticity (described previously), abnormal automaticity also depends on the balance between depolarizing and repolarizing currents, although the relative contribution of different ionic species (particularly an increased role of Ca^{2+}) probably differs.

Some sustained rhythmic membrane activity is triggered by a propagated or stimulated action potential. Such triggered activity must be distinguished from true spontaneous automatic activity, previously discussed. The latter arises in the absence of a direct cause, although it may be influenced by drugs or altered physiologic states. Triggered sustained rhythmic activity arises from *early* (before transmembrane potential has returned to its maximum diastolic level) or *late afterdepolarizations* (after membrane potential has returned to greater than its maximum diastolic level—hyperpolarization). Afterdepolarizations, with or without sustained rhythmic activity, may occur at virtually any level of membrane potential and are caused by numerous physiologic, pathologic, and pharmacologic states or interventions in almost all fiber types.[4] Arrhythmias due to triggering may be difficult to distinguish from those due to re-entry of excitation, since both can be initiated or terminated by single or paired extrasystoles.[4]

Re-entry

Re-entry depends on interrelationships among anatomic substrate, initiating source (active membrane generation properties, e.g., ionic currents dependent on metabolic processes), characteristics of the sink (passive membrane properties, e.g., resistance, capacitance, electronic interactions), conduction velocity, and refractoriness.[4] Re-entry of excitation is depicted in Figure 2–2 for a branching Purkinje fiber, the classic Schmitt-Erlanger model. In this model, some alteration in active or passive membrane properties creates a functionally isolated segment of tissue that blocks conduction in one direction but permits slowed conduction in the other direction. Conduction is slowed sufficiently to permit previously activated tissue to regain excitability and be reactivated. Calculations using the Schmitt-Erlanger model with an area of unidirectional block, but normal conduction velocity for Purkinje fibers (about 3 m/second), indicate a minimal circuit length for re-entry of 1 m.[4] If conduction is slowed to 0.1 m/second, as in depressed

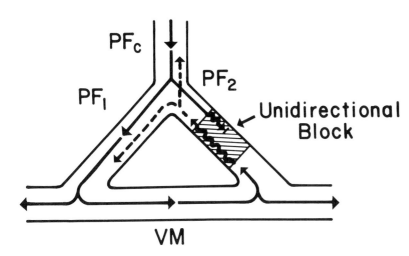

Figure 2–2. Re-entry using model of unidirectional block. (PF = Purkinje fiber, VM = ventricular muscle [myocardium].) See text for explanation. (From Fozzard HA, Arnsdorf MR: Cardiac physiology. *In* Fozzard HA, Haber E, Jennings RB, et al [eds]: The Heart and Cardiovascular System. New York: Raven Press, 1986; 24. With permission.)

Purkinje or other fast-response fibers (discussed later), then the minimal circuit length becomes several millimeters and re-entry is anatomically feasible.

A re-entrant circuit may be anatomic or functional (depressed fast-response fiber as a result of myocardial ischemia, injury, or spontaneous depolarization in adjacent fibers); may involve supraventricular, AV junctional, or ventricular tissue; and may be large, as in bundle-branch re-entry, or small, such as reflection with a single strand of a Purkinje fiber. Since action potentials of the sinus and AV nodes depend on the slow-inward (mainly Ca^{2+}) current and have slow conduction velocities, it is not surprising that re-entrant beats or sustained re-entrant rhythms utilize the AV or SA nodes as the site of unidirectional block. Finally, conduction velocity can be slowed in fast-response fibers (atrial and ventricular muscle, Purkinje fibers) by a decrease in maximal sodium conductance. The latter occurs as the result of loss of membrane potential in "depressed" fast-response fibers.

Mechanistic Approach to Diagnosis and Treatment

When a dysrhythmia is noted, it is important that correct electrocardiographic diagnosis be made as quickly as possible. Only from correct interpretation of the ECG can the underlying mechanism causing the dysrhythmia be determined. Management of rhythm disturbances is more often successful when the correct mechanism (re-entry, normal versus abnormal automaticity, triggered sustained rhythmic activity) initiating the dysrhythmia is identified.

Monitoring Technique

Electrical Hazards. There is always the danger of ventricular fibrillation when electrical current passes through the myocardium. If a potential difference is applied across two areas of skin, a current flows between them, and the amount transferred depends on the resistance to this flow of electrical energy (*voltage = current × resistance; Ohm's law*). As an example, if 100 V is applied across each arm and the resistance (dry skin) is 200,000 Ω, then the current flowing through the body would be 5×10^{-4} A (0.5 mA). This amount of current would barely be perceived and falls into the category of *macroshock*. Approximately 100 mA is required during macroshock to cause ventricular fibrillation.[6] The line-isolation monitor (LIM) that constantly tests operating room circuits for leakage current alarms at 2 mA and guards against macroshock.

If an electrode catheter or a central access catheter filled with a conducting solution (e.g., normal saline) is placed against the myocardium, a much smaller amount of current is required to cause ventricular fibrillation. This amount of current is termed *microshock*. The microshock threshold for ventricular fibrillation is approximately 0.1 mA (100 μA). The microshock threshold for esophageal electrodes has not been established, but the prudent physician should assume it to be close to 100 μA. The anesthesiologist must take great care to ensure that *no electrical bridge be made between any piece of monitoring equipment and a catheter or lead that is in proximity to the myocardium*. Remember, the LIM only alarms at a leakage current greater than 2 mA, which surely would cause ventricular fibrillation upon direct application to the heart. A rubber glove around exposed electrodes (e.g., pacemaker leads) is useful in protecting against microshock.

P Wave Monitoring. During general anesthesia, complex dysrhythmias are often observed. The most common mistake made during the diagnosis of the complex rhythms is misinterpretation of atrial activity. Normal QRS complexes mean only that the impulse originated above the bifurcation of the His bundle, but they do not imply SA node origin. The relationship of the P wave to the QRS (AV sequence) or the P wave to the R wave (ventriculoatrial [VA] sequence) should be established. Therefore, during electrocardiographic monitoring of patients intraoperatively, identification of atrial activity (P waves) should be maximized.

Conventional P wave monitoring from the 12-lead electrocardiograph is best done through leads II, aVF, and V_1, since the normal axis of atrial activity parallels these leads. During most anesthetic techniques, lead aVF is not monitored, which leaves leads II and V_1 as the primary intraoperative P wave monitors. Lead V_1 lies directly over the right atrium, and lead II parallels the axis of the atrial impulse, under normal circumstances.

Surface electrodes (II and V_1) are sometimes limited and ineffective as adequate P wave monitors. Patients who suffer from obesity, chronic obstructive lung disease, and "thick chests" have attenuated waveforms that make their ECG, particularly atrial activity, difficult to interpret. In these patients it becomes especially necessary to find another lead to monitor for dysrhythmias.

Intra-atrial Leads. The closer the electrodes are placed to the atrium, the better the atrial activity appears on the electrocardiographic tracing. The *intra-atrial* electrogram is probably the "gold standard" for monitoring P wave activity. However, this method[7] is mostly confined to the electrophysiologic laboratory or used after cardiac surgery.

Esophageal Leads. A close approximation to the intra-atrial system is

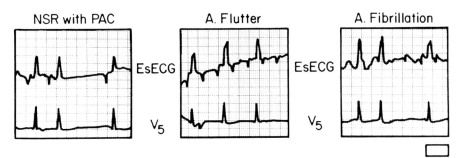

Figure 2–3. Comparison of dysrhythmia progression between esophageal lead (EsECG) and lead V_5. The rhythm progresses from sinus rhythm with premature atrial contractions (PACs) to atrial flutter and then to atrial fibrillation. The diagnosis is only evident from the esophageal lead. (From Kates RA, Zaiden JR, Kaplan JA: Esophageal lead for intraoperative electrocardiographic monitoring. Anesth Analg 1982; 61:781–785. With permission.)

the *esophageal ECG*.[8, 9] The lead, which has been used for many years, has only recently been introduced into the operating room.[10] P waves that are undetectable in a conventional 12-lead system are often easily seen with the esophageal lead. As compared with lead II, the esophageal lead is superior in the elucidation of complex arrhythmias.[11]

Kates and colleagues[10] compared leads II and V_5 with the esophageal ECG, using an intra-atrial lead as the standard. They were able to correctly diagnose dysrhythmias with leads II and V_5, 54% and 42%, respectively. The esophageal lead provided information that led to the correct diagnosis 100% of the time. Three examples of their comparisons are shown in Figure 2–3. Not only is this lead valuable in detecting dysrhythmias, but the esophageal electrode has also been noted to be valuable in detecting ischemia (especially posterior wall ischemia).[12]

An esophageal electrode can be made from an 8-F red Robinson catheter and a J guidewire. The J wire is threaded through the red Robinson catheter so that just the J portion of the distal wire is exteriorized at the tip of the catheter. This unit is taped to an esophageal stethoscope and placed in the esophagus. The proximal end of the J wire is attached (alligator clip lead) to the V lead input of the electrocardiograph. An electrocautery protection filter must be positioned between the esophageal lead and the electrocardiographic machine if electrocautery is to be used in close proximity to the tip of the esophageal lead. The electrocautery grounding pad should be far removed from the chest. Esophageal stethoscopes with electrocardiographic leads are also available commercially.

Diagnostic versus Monitoring Mode. Many electrocardiographic oscilloscopes have a toggle switch to choose between *monitoring* and *diagnostic* modes while observing and recording the electrocardiographic trace. The difference between the two modes is the frequency level at which the signal is attenuated.[5]

In the monitoring mode, all signals below 0.5 Hz are eliminated, which leaves a "clean" electrocardiographic trace. However, the amplitude of the P wave (as well as T wave) may be decreased, which sometimes makes P wave detection difficult. This mode provides a steady baseline and a good waveform for dysrhythmia monitoring.

The diagnostic mode filters frequencies below 0.14 Hz and provides the detail necessary for accurate interpretation of the ST segment and T wave changes often seen with ischemia, injury, or infarction. This mode transfers more artifact to the tracing (making P wave identification quite difficult) and often allows for a wandering baseline with respiration. This fact makes the diagnostic mode less favorable for routine dysrhythmia monitoring.

COMMON PERIOPERATIVE DYSRHYTHMIAS

Marriott[13] makes the following suggestions for using the electrocardiograph for dysrhythmia monitoring:

1. Use the lead with maximal information. If you are interested in P waves, monitor the best leads to identify them (II, V_1, or esophageal leads).
2. Try to ensure maximal mechanical convenience. Although it is true that if the lead system is quite complicated, it falls into disuse, a standard three-lead system *plus* an esophageal lead (pre-existing dysrhythmias or likely to have dysrhythmias) is quite practical for everyday operating room utilization.
3. One lead is insufficient. Always check one lead against the others and record ECGs with dysrhythmias so that they may be closely compared with other leads and against recordings taken at the beginning of the anesthetic.
4. Know when to use other leads. This stems directly from principle number 3.

Supraventricular Dysrhythmias

Bradydysrhythmias

Sinus bradycardia is present when normal P waves occur at a rate of less than 60 beats/minute in an adult, with a P-R interval more than 0.12 second. It is commonly seen in young adults and well-trained athletes. Distance runners quite often have rates at rest between 30 and 40 beats/minute. It is also noted with increased vagal tone (e.g., edrophonium administration) or decreased sympathetic discharge (high spinal block). For children, intrinsic rates are higher, and 100 beats/minute may be bradycardia in a neonate. Intravenous atropine can be used to increase sinus rate by vagolysis.

Sinus dysrhythmia (Fig. 2–4) is common in young adults. Sinus dysrhythmia occurs in phasic or nonphasic forms. In the *phasic variation* the P-P interval cycles with respiration, and the difference in the maximum and minimum cycle lengths exceeds 120 msec. The *nonphasic* form of sinus dysrhythmia does not cycle with respiration. *Sinus arrest* is simply a pause

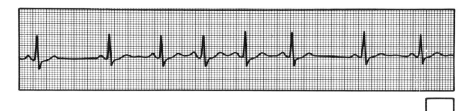

Figure 2–4. Sinus dysrhythmia with cycle lengths from 560 msec to 960 msec. (From Atlee JL III: Perioperative Cardiac Dysrhythmias: Mechanisms, Recognition and Management. Chicago: Year Book Medical, 1985; 226. With permission.)

in the normal sequence of P waves caused usually by increased vagal tone or by digoxin toxicity.

SA exit block is like sinus arrest with a pause in the P wave series. However, the new P-P interval is often some *exact multiple* of the patient's normal P-P interval. Presumably, it is caused by the failure of propagation of the SA impulse in the perinodal tissue, and it may be associated with normal SA node automatic function. The etiology of SA exit block is similar to that of sinus arrest.

The *sick sinus syndrome* is a term referring to patients who exhibit any or all of the following dysrhythmias: (1) paroxysmal sinus bradycardia, (2) sinus arrest or exit block, (3) AV conduction disturbances, or (4) atrial tachydysrhythmias. The cause is usually a diseased sinus node, most often secondary to coronary artery disease and subsequent ischemia. Patients with symptomatic sick sinus syndrome require insertion of a pacemaker.

Tachydysrhythmias

The most common intraoperative dysrhythmia is *sinus tachycardia*. The diagnosis is made from morphologically normal P waves at a nearly constant rate of over 100 beats/minute in adults. There are numerous causes, including catecholamine excess, surgical stress (sometimes with inadequate anesthesia), hypovolemia, hypercapnia, hypoxia, sepsis, and reduced vagal tone.

Another very common dysrhythmia during anesthesia is *wandering atrial pacemaker*. As shown in Figure 2–5, it is characterized by variation in the P wave morphology along with a changing P-R interval (Fig. 2–5 also

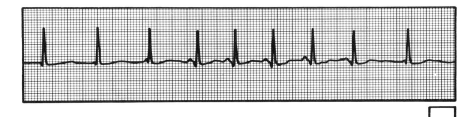

Figure 2–5. Wandering atrial pacemaker with variation of P-R interval and changing morphology of P waves (beats four to eight). The first three and the last two beats are atrioventricular (AV) junctional rhythm and illustrate the phenomenon of "isorhythmic dissociation" (see text).

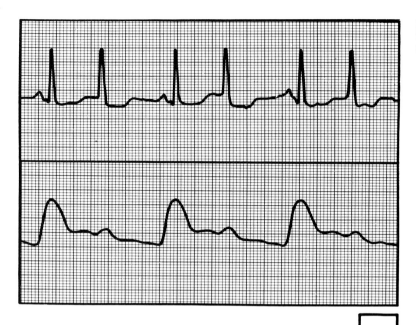

Figure 2–6. Premature atrial beats reduce ventricular filling, decreasing the arterial pressure.

illustrates AV junctional rhythm). Similar to sinus dysrhythmia, the R-R interval also changes in cyclic fashion. This dysrhythmia is often seen in healthy patients anesthetized with a potent volatile anesthetic (halothane, enflurane, or isoflurane).

Premature atrial beats (PABs) are also quite common during general anesthesia and are noted by occasional premature P waves, with the P-R interval being greater than or equal to 0.12 second. Figure 2–6 is an example of this rhythm. The morphology of the P wave is usually different from the patient's normal P wave. PABs are precipitated by increased catecholamine levels, myocardial ischemia, chronic pulmonary disease, and intra-atrial catheters. Often they are of little clinical significance and require no treatment.

Atrial flutter (F) is characterized by "sawtooth" atrial flutter waves with no isoelectric interval between them. The usual rate of flutter is 250–350 beats/minute (300 beats/minute is most common), and the diagnosis should be suspect if the atrial rate is less than 250 beats/minute. The ratio of ventricular conduction of these beats usually varies from 2:1 to 4:1 (atrial flutter to ventricular beat) with 3:1 conduction very uncommon. Therefore, the usual ventricular rate is about 75 or 150 beats/minute. Recognizing flutter is quite dependent on monitoring leads II, III, V_1, or aVF, where the P waves are easily noted. As shown in Figure 2–7, flutter is sometimes missed in lead V_5 but usually not in lead II. Carotid sinus pressure increases vagal tone and slows the rate.

Atrial fibrillation (AF) is another commonly observed rhythm disturbance recognized by the irregular R-R interval and irregular, chaotic baseline (F waves). The F waves are sometimes noted only in intra-atrial or esophageal leads. Patients with long-standing hypertension, hyperthyroidism, mi-

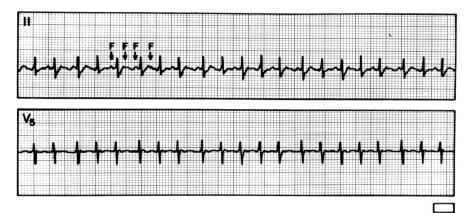

Figure 2–7. Atrial flutter with 2:1 AV block. The flutter (F) waves are noted in lead II but not lead V₅. (From Atlee JL III: Perioperative Cardiac Dysrhythmias: Mechanisms, Recognition and Management. Chicago: Year Book Medical, 1985; 231. With permission.)

tral valve disease, or ischemic heart disease often have AF. Digitalis slows ventricular response in both F and AF by prolonging the functional refractory period of the AV node.

AV junctional rhythms encompass a variety of rhythm disturbances originating in the AV junctional area. *AV junction escape beats* occur when the discharge from the SA node slows and the junctional pacemaker is no longer overridden. On the ECG, this is recognized by a long R-R interval followed by a normal QRS complex that is not preceded by a P wave. Junctional escape beats are quite common during anesthesia in young, healthy, "vagotonic" patients.

When the junctional pacemaker tissue completely takes over the genesis of the heartbeat owing either to the failure of the SA node to generate impulses or to nonpropagated impulses, a junctional rhythm is present (Fig. 2–8). The rate is usually 50–70 beats/minute. If the sinus rate is nearly the same as that of the junctional pacemaker, and the sinus impulses are blocked at the AV junction because of physiologic refractoriness induced by adjacent

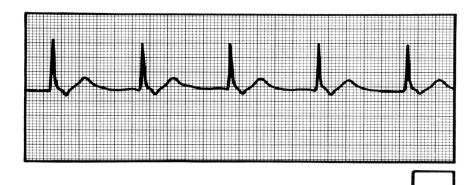

Figure 2–8. AV junctional rhythm. Note the probable retrograde P waves in the ST segment.

pacemaker discharge, the P waves, while remaining upright, appear to march in and out of the QRS complex. This phenomenon is termed isorhythmic AV dissociation (see Fig. 2–5). The latter phenomenon is quite common during general anesthesia with halothane, isoflurane, or enflurane.

AV junctional tachycardia is distinguished by normal (supraventricular) QRS complexes without antecedent P waves and a rate of 70–110 beats/minute. It is seen in patients with significant underlying heart disease or digoxin overdose, and it is common after open heart surgery.

Ventricular Arrhythmias

The ventricular arrhythmias include *premature ventricular beats* (PVBs) and *ventricular tachycardia* caused by electrical activation originating below the bifurcation of the bundle of His. PVBs are characterized by an early, *bizarre-appearing QRS complex* wider than 0.12 second and with the T wave opposite the QRS deflection. The impulse originating in the ventricle may provoke a retrograde P wave (inverted in lead II, III, or aVF). Retrograde (VA) conduction of the PVB may reset automaticity in the SA node so that the PVB is often followed by a compensatory pause.

It may be quite difficult (sometimes impossible) to distinguish a PVB from a PAB with aberrant ventricular conduction. Such beats may be as bizarre-looking as a PVB but often are not followed by a compensatory pause. PABs with aberrant conduction can be distinguished from PVBs by examination of the QRS in several leads and by the relationship of P waves to the QRS complex (AV association = PAB; VA association = PVB).

When two PVBs occur consecutively, the term couplet is used; three beats in a row is called triplet. Uniform PVBs in association with beats from another focus in a recurring fashion is termed bigeminy (Fig. 2–9); three such beats, trigeminy. Figure 2–10 is an example of quadrigeminy. If the PVBs appearing on a rhythm strip have different morphologies, the term multiform is used.

Causes of PVBs include coronary artery disease, hypertension, hypothyroidism, or valvular heart disease. Some patients without demonstrable heart disease have this rhythm disturbance secondary to drugs or some acute physiologic derangement. Hypokalemia, hypoxia, or hypercapnia often triggers new onset PVBs during anesthesia. During thoracic and cardiac surgery, PVBs are very common with direct myocardial manipulation and usually cease when such stimulation is stopped. Lidocaine, 1 mg/kg intravenously, is used to terminate PVBs when inciting causes have been controlled. PVBs refractory to lidocaine are treated with propranolol, procainamide hydrochloride, phenytoin, or newer antidysrhythmic drugs.

Ventricular tachycardia (VT) is characterized by three or more PVBs in a row. The usual rate is between 110 and 250 beats/minute. Distinguishing this dysrhythmia from supraventricular tachycardia (SVT) with aberrant conduction is sometimes quite difficult. The diagnosis of SVT with aberrant conduction is suggested when the tachycardia slows with vagal maneuvers

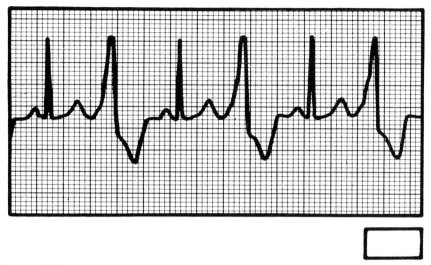

Figure 2–9. Bigeminy: Premature ventricular beats (PVBs) alternating with sinus beats.

or is initiated by premature P waves or there are short R-P intervals (VA association).

VT is likely if occasional *capture* or *fusion beats* are present. Capture beats may or may not have a manifest, associated P wave and normal QRS complexes with an interval between beats less than that of the wide QRS complexes. This indicates supraventricular capture of the ventricle. Fusion beats may also have a manifest P wave and a QRS complex that is wider than normal beats but not of the same duration or morphology as QRS complexes with ventricular origin beats. Fusion beats result from simultaneous activation of the ventricles by beats originating below and above the common bundle. Also, compensatory pauses and AV dissociation favor VT. If VT is unresponsive to lidocaine intravenously or hemodynamic compromise is present, direct current cardioversion should be performed.

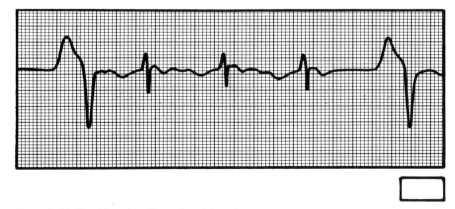

Figure 2–10. Quadrigeminy: Every fourth beat is a PVB.

AV Conduction Block

Heart block is defined as a conduction delay anywhere along the path of normal impulse propagation. The most common sites of block are the AV node, His bundle, or bundle branches.

First-Degree AV Block

A prolongation of the AV conduction time (P-R interval) beyond 0.21 second is called *first-degree AV block.* This can occur in healthy young patients or may be observed during anesthesia with any of the potent volatile anesthetic agents known to prolong or delay AV conduction, especially in patients receiving beta-adrenergic or calcium channel blockers.[14] With this dysrhythmia, as well as with other types of heart block, it is important to maximize the P wave morphology using an esophageal lead if necessary.

Second-Degree AV Block

When some, but not all, P waves are transmitted to the ventricle, second-degree heart block is present. There are two distinct types of second-degree AV block, Mobitz types I and II.[13]

Second-Degree AV Block, Type I. Second-degree block, type I, also termed Wenckebach block, usually occurs in the AV node and consists of progressively lengthening P-R intervals prior to a nonconducted P wave. The P-R interval prior to dropped beats may be as long as 0.60 second. Second-degree AV block, type I, is common in healthy patients with high vagal tone and is also occasionally observed during inhalation of volatile anesthetics. It is relatively benign unless associated with bradycardia and hypotension.

Second-Degree AV Block, Type II. Second-degree AV block, type II, is more serious than type I and usually results from block below the AV node. In this dysrhythmia some of the P waves are not followed by a QRS complex. However, the P-R interval for conducted beats is relatively constant and of normal duration. Second-degree AV block, type II, is almost always indicative of severe underlying heart disease. It is frequently observed during the warming phase of cardiopulmonary bypass. Treatment for type II block is required if hemodynamic compromise results. Pacemaker therapy, using transthoracic, esophageal, or intravenous routes, effectively controls second-degree AV block, type II.

Third-Degree Heart Block

There is no transmission of impulses from the atrium to the ventricles in third-degree heart block. The P waves and the QRS complexes, both of normal morphology, have separate and independent rates. An example of third-degree heart block is shown in Figure 2–11. The ventricular rate is usually about 40 beats/minute or less. The sudden appearance of third-degree heart block during anesthesia may cause profound hypotension and circu-

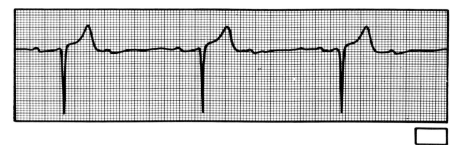

Figure 2–11. Third-degree heart block with the P waves and QRS complexes each having separate and independent rates. (Courtesy of Steven Croy, MD.)

latory collapse. Consequently, it demands immediate attention. Electrocardiographic leads that accentuate P wave morphology make the diagnosis easier. Intravenous atropine for vagolysis and isoproterenol to stimulate idioventricular pacemakers are used until a pacemaker can be inserted.

Ventricular Pre-excitation

Pre-excitation occurs when the ventricle is activated by cardiac impulses that travel from the atrium via anomalous conduction pathways. Figure 2–12 shows a diagram of these types of anomalous pathways. Kent fibers are thought to contribute to *Wolff-Parkinson-White (WPW) syndrome.* The James fibers are responsible for *Lown-Ganong-Levine (LGL) syndrome.*

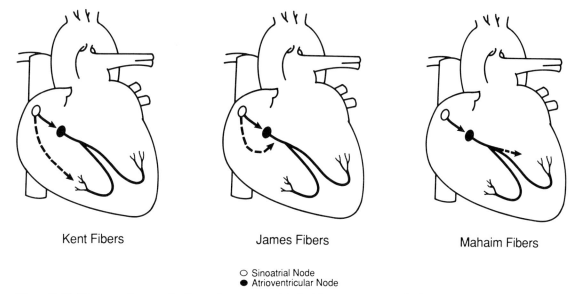

Kent Fibers   James Fibers   Mahaim Fibers

○ Sinoatrial Node
● Atrioventricular Node

Figure 2–12. The anomalous conduction pathways associated with common pre-excitation syndromes: Kent fibers (Wolff-Parkinson-White [WPW] syndrome), James fibers (Lown-Ganong-Levine syndrome), and Mahaim fibers. (From Goodloe SL: Abnormalities of cardiac conduction and cardiac rhythm. *In* Stoelting RK, Dierdorf SF [eds]: Anesthesia and Co-existing Disease. New York: Churchill Livingstone, 1983; 87. By permission.)

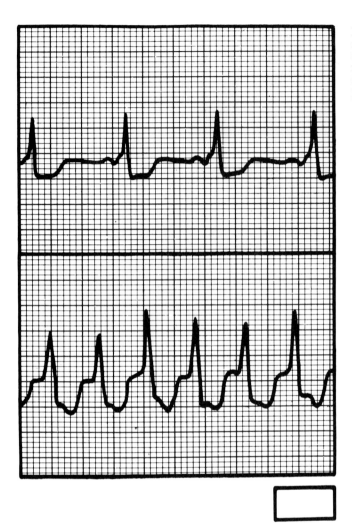

Figure 2–13. The upper portion is the baseline rhythm of WPW in an intensive care unit (ICU) patient (note delta wave). The lower figure is supraventricular tachycardia (SVT) initiated during intubation in this nonsedated patient. The dysrhythmia reverted to normal before treatment could be instituted.

WPW Syndrome

WPW syndrome is the most common of the pre-excitation syndromes, seen in about 0.3% of the general population.[15] The syndrome is characterized on the ECG by a short P-R interval (< 0.12 second), a delta wave (the early upsloping R portion of the QRS complex), and a wide QRS complex (caused by the summation of stimulation from the Kent fibers and the AV node). The most common dysrhythmia associated with WPW syndrome is a *reciprocating SVT.*

Figure 2–13 shows reciprocating tachycardia during intubation in the intensive care unit in an unanesthetized patient with underlying WPW syndrome. Reciprocating tachycardia in patients with WPW syndrome is characterized by a normal QRS complex and rates between 130 and 150 beats/minute. It requires both the atria and the ventricles to sustain re-entry and usually begins and terminates rather abruptly.

Pharmacologic intervention for supraventricular dysrhythmias secondary to WPW syndrome depends upon the electrophysiologic properties of the drug to be used. Verapamil or propranolol, which prolongs AV nodal conduction and refractoriness (depresses the normal AV pathway), is the treatment for SVT with normal QRS complexes. When anomalous conduction is present, lidocaine terminates SVT in patients with WPW syndrome. Digitalis should probably be avoided because, although it prolongs conduction in the AV node, it shortens the refractory period in the accessory pathway. Surgical ablation of the accessory tract is used in patients with drug-resistant tachyarrhythmias.

LGL Syndrome

The ECG in patients with LGL syndrome has normal P waves, normal QRS complexes, and short P-R intervals. The James fibers bypass the AV node, allowing the sinus or other supraventricular impulses to reach the ventricles earlier than normal. Ventricular activation via the bundle of His and its branches is normal, giving a normal QRS complex. Patients with LGL syndrome tend to develop paroxysmal tachycardias.

ECG MANIFESTATIONS OF ALTERED PHYSIOLOGIC STATES

The first step in arrhythmia management is recognition and then the removal or correction of causes. Altered physiologic states are frequently the cause for dysrhythmias, and they often are associated with specific ECG patterns. Drugs (including anesthetics), acid-base abnormalities, and central nervous system (CNS) disorders are implicated as the etiology of some arrhythmias.

Electrolyte Disturbances

Potassium

Hypokalemia. Hypokalemia is a common problem in surgical patients because of diuretic therapy for hypertension or hyperventilation. With the possible exception of the potassium-sparing diuretics, diuretics cause an obligate renal potassium loss frequently uncorrected by diet or potassium replacement.

Hypokalemia increases resting membrane potential and, more importantly, increases the duration of the action potential and also the length of the refractory period. The length of the refractory period is extended to a much greater degree than is the action potential duration. This effect of hypokalemia provides the setting for *re-entry-type arrhythmias*.[16] Hypokalemia also increases the threshold of the action potential, which increases abnormal automaticity.

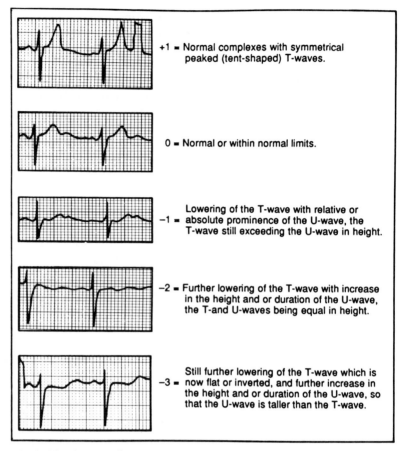

+1 = Normal complexes with symmetrical peaked (tent-shaped) T-waves.

0 = Normal or within normal limits.

−1 = Lowering of the T-wave with relative or absolute prominence of the U-wave, the T-wave still exceeding the U-wave in height.

−2 = Further lowering of the T-wave with increase in the height and or duration of the U-wave, the T-and U-waves being equal in height.

−3 = Still further lowering of the T-wave which is now flat or inverted, and further increase in the height and or duration of the U-wave, so that the U-wave is taller than the T-wave.

Figure 2–14. The electrocardiogram (ECG) during various degrees of hypokalemia. (From Helfant RH: Hypokalemia and arrhythmias. Am J Med 1986; 80:16. With permission.)

Electrocardiographic evidence of hypokalemia is often exhibited prior to the occurrence of dysrhythmia. Weaver and Burchel[17] have given the following criteria for diagnosis of hypokalemia via the ECG: (1) a T wave to U wave ratio of less than or equal to 1, (2) a U wave greater than 0.5 mm in lead II or greater than 1.0 mm in lead V_3, and (3) ST segment depression equal to or greater than 0.5 mm. Figure 2–14 depicts the electrocardiographic effects of mild to severe hypokalemia.

The most common dysrhythmia noted in hypokalemic patients is *PVBs*. Also reported are PABs and AV junctional disturbances. In a recent study by Cohen and coworkers,[18] a strong relationship was shown between diuretic use (and accompanying hypokalemia) and PVBs. In this study, two groups of hypertensive patients were randomized into either "special intervention" (they received counseling on diet, smoking, and techniques for lowering cholesterol) or "usual care" groups. Decreases in potassium were analyzed using regression coefficients. A decrease of 1.0 mEq/L of potassium was associated with a 28% increase in PVBs in the usual care group and an 18% increase in the special intervention group. Moderate hypokalemia is associated with PVBs, AV dissociation, and atrial tachycardia with block. Ventricular tachycardia and fibrillation have been reported with severe hypokalemia.[5]

Hyperventilation is another common cause of hypokalemia in the operative setting. With the ever-increasing use of neuromuscular blocking drugs as part of the anesthetic technique, mechanical ventilation is frequently used to free the anesthesiologist's hands during a long anesthetic procedure. With the advent of continuous end-tidal CO_2 monitoring, the problem of hyperventilation is now quite evident. Edwards and coworkers[19] characterized the relationship between hyperventilation (with lowered P_{CO_2}) and serum potassium concentrations as seen in Figure 2–15.

Hyperkalemia. Dysrhythmias are not often seen with hyperkalemia until the serum potassium increases above 7.5 mEq/L. With mild hyperkalemia, tall, peaked T waves appear. However, as the level of serum potassium increases, widening of the QRS complex, ST elevation, and slowing of the sinus rhythm become evident. In extreme cases, the rhythm looks like a sine wave but not until serum potassium is very high. The dysrhythmia most noted with hyperkalemia is an AV conduction disturbance (heart block, aberrant conduction). With severe hyperkalemia, heart block can deteriorate into *ventricular fibrillation*, but this is very uncommon.

Calcium

Variations in serum ionized calcium are well tolerated by the cardiac conduction system, and dysrhythmias are rarely seen with aberrations of calcium homeostasis. *Hypocalcemia* prolongs the Q-T interval and ST segment. With very low calcium concentrations, there may be T wave inversion. Hypocalcemia has been reported to be antidysrhythmic, and no dysrhythmias have been described.

The Q-T interval is shortened by *hypercalcemia*, and there is associated prolongation of the P-R interval. Severe hypercalcemia may lead to ventricular fibrillation, but this is said to be rare. After cardiac bypass, when transient serum ionized calcium concentrations can be elevated (iatrogenic hypercalcemia), arrhythmias have rarely been noticed.

Magnesium

Hypermagnesemia. Hypermagnesemia slows AV node and intraventricular conduction.[20] Aberrations in cardiac conduction occur when serum magnesium increases, as during treatment of pre-eclampsia. Normal serum magnesium is 2 mEq/L. The cardiac complications occur at higher magnesium concentrations than does respiratory depression, which is noted at about 10 mEq/L. Cardiac conduction disturbances begin at about 20 mEq/L.

Hypomagnesemia. Ventricular dysrhythmias may be associated with hypomagnesemia. Havestadt and colleagues[20] compared the serum magnesium level in 35 elderly patients suffering from ventricular arrhythmias with the magnesium levels in 41 control patients (age and sex matched) without dysrhythmias. The mean plasma magnesium level in the dysrhythmia group was

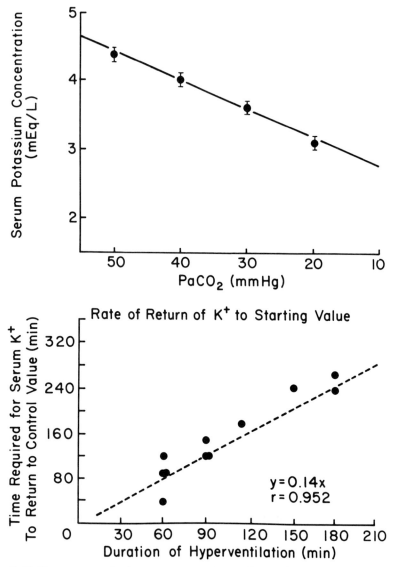

Figure 2–15. The upper panel relates serum potassium to the arterial CO_2 tension (Pa_{CO_2} in mmHg). Hyperventilation produced Pa_{CO_2} values <40 mmHg. The lower graph displays the time required for the potassium concentration to return to baseline following hyperventilation. (From Edwards R, Winnie AP, Ramamurthy S: Acute hypocapneic hypokalemia: An iatrogenic anesthetic complication. Anesth Analg 1977; 56:788. With permission.)

0.79 ± 0.1 mmol/L compared with 0.85 ± 0.07 mmol/L in the control group. Half of the hypomagnesemic group was then treated with magnesium for 5 days. The reduction in arrhythmias correlated with increased serum magnesium. In this study, erythrocyte electrolytes were measured, and it was found that the concentrations of calcium and sodium, which were markedly elevated in the high dysrhythmia group, decreased after magnesium therapy. The authors concluded that the dysrhythmias were caused by sodium and calcium imbalance rather than directly related to magnesium concentration. The time course of dysrhythmia reduction supports this theory, since the rhythm disturbances did not disappear within the time frame of the magnesium increase; rather, they followed the decreases in intracellular (erythrocyte) calcium and sodium.

The Effect of Pharmacologic Agents

Digitalis

Digitalis (most widely used preparation—digoxin) decreases the effectiveness of the sodium-potassium ATPase pump, decreasing intracellular potassium and increasing intracellular sodium concentrations. The increase in sodium displaces intracellular calcium from common binding sites and thus increases the available calcium, which enhances contractility and contributes to a loss of resting membrane potential.

Almost any dysrhythmia can be produced by digitalis toxicity. The classic example of a dysrhythmia caused by digoxin toxicity is *atrial tachycardia with AV block*. PABs and PVBs are common with digitalis toxicity. Serum levels are not always helpful in the diagnosis and management of digitalis toxicity since effective digoxin levels differ among patients. Other factors, in addition to the absolute serum drug level, increase the incidence of dysrhythmias in digitalized patients. Hypokalemia is perhaps the most common, but increased catecholamines, hypercalcemia, hypoxia, hypercapnia, and acid-base imbalance were also important. Therefore, it is imperative that dysrhythmia treatment in patients receiving digitalis include a thorough search for other aggravating causes.

Therapy for digitalis intoxication includes normalization of serum potassium, since potassium delays additional myocardial binding of digitalis. Antidysrhythmia therapy includes lidocaine, procainamide hydrochloride, phenytoin, or propranolol. Direct current countershock may be hazardous secondary to ventricular arrhythmias but is indicated when circulatory collapse is present.

Theophylline

Theophylline, used to treat bronchospastic disease, inhibits phosphodiesterase and thus increases intracellular cyclic adenosine monophosphate (cAMP) by reducing its metabolism. Cyclic AMP as a "second messenger" acts on bronchial smooth muscle to cause bronchodilation and increases automaticity in the heart. Rhythm disturbances noted with theophylline toxicity include *AF, multifocal atrial tachycardia, F, SVT,* and, of course, *sinus tachycardia*. Serum theophylline levels over 20 μg/L are associated with dysrhythmias. However, as the serum theophylline level increases above 20 μg/L, the incidence of arrhythmias does not increase further.[21]

It is well known that theophylline potentiates halothane's effect of lowering the threshold for epinephrine-induced arrhythmias.[22] To our knowledge, this interaction has not been investigated with enflurane or isoflurane.

Since these agents are commonly used to produce bronchodilation in patients suffering from bronchospastic disease, the interaction of these agents with theophylline is likely to be encountered. Consequently, in these circumstances, one must be especially careful to monitor for dysrhythmias and also strive to reduce endogenous as well as exogenous catecholamine levels.

Lithium

The most common agent used to treat bipolar affective disorders is lithium. It is thought to replace sodium in generating the action potential but cannot be extruded by the sodium-potassium ATPase pump from the cell during repolarization.[23] Lithium accumulates in the cell, lowering resting membrane potential and leading to AV conduction disturbances, the most common dysrhythmias seen with lithium toxicity. Usually this manifests as first-degree AV block, which is considered benign and warrants no treatment.[24] With the resurgence of electroconvulsive therapy for depression, anesthesiologists care for increasing numbers of patients on lithium therapy.

Tricyclic Antidepressants

Tricyclic antidepressants are widely used to treat clinical depression. This class of drug, which has strong anticholinergic properties, has the potential for severe cardiac toxicity.

At therapeutic levels, the tricyclics are "quinidine-like" and display antiarrhythmic properties. At higher levels, conduction through the Purkinje fibers is delayed, and a widened QRS complex is observed. At toxic levels, a *wide QRS complex* (>100 msec), *AV conduction abnormalities* (even third-degree heart block), *ventricular ectopy*, and *ventricular fibrillation* may occur.[25] Toxic levels of these drugs following overdose are not uncommon, since patients being treated for severe depression are likely to be suicidal.

Volatile Anesthetic Agents

A discussion of the dysrhythmic potential of halothane, enflurane, and isoflurane is beyond the scope of this chapter. Briefly, it is well known that these agents equally reduce the SA node discharge rate.[26] Halothane and enflurane decrease AV node as well as His-Purkinje fiber conduction times. Isoflurane has little effect on AV nodal but prolongs His-Purkinje conduction time.[27] The dysrhythmias seen most often with these agents are *bradycardia* and *AV junctional rhythms*.

Importantly, any of these agents can potentiate the dysrhythmic effect of epinephrine (sensitization), although enflurane and isoflurane are less likely to do so.[28] Furthermore, thiopental sodium may increase the likelihood of sensitization.[29] In a frequently quoted study, Johnston and colleagues[30] injected epinephrine into patients undergoing transsphenoidal hypophysectomies with halothane, enflurane, or isoflurane anesthesia. Halothane was most dysrhythmic (mean dose of epinephrine for ventricular dysrhythmias 2.1 μg/kg), with enflurane (6.7 μg/kg) and isoflurane (10.9 μg/kg) far less so.

However, none of these doses should be considered "safe" under clinical circumstances, since there was considerable variance in the dose of epinephrine for dysrhythmia, particularly with enflurane and to some extent with isoflurane.[30] It is prudent to keep the dose of epinephrine used for surgical hemostasis below 1.0 μg/kg, monitor closely for dysrhythmias, and avoid halothane if possible. Of the available potent anesthetics, isoflurane would appear to be the most compatible with epinephrine.

Pathophysiologic Alterations

Acid-Base Abnormalities

Clinically observed derangements in acid-base physiology have never been conclusively shown to directly cause dysrhythmias. Associated autonomic and electrolyte imbalance and cellular hypoxia are the more likely causes.

CNS Disease

The most common ECG abnormalities associated with CNS lesions, particularly acute subarachnoid hemorrhage, are Q-T interval prolongation, ST segment elevation or depression, inverted or tall T waves, and, uncommonly, Q waves that mimic myocardial infarction.[31] Common dysrhythmias include PVBs, *ventricular tachycardia*, and *sinus tachycardia*. Cushing's reflex, associated with elevated intracranial pressure (ICP), includes *bradycardia* and *hypertension*. This is noted only with ICP greater than 50 mmHg. Taylor and Fozzard suggest that the mechanism behind many dysrhythmias related to CNS dysfunction is autonomic imbalance, since beta blockers are often effective treatment.[31]

ARTIFACTS OF THE ECG

As one considers the cause(s) for an apparent dysrhythmia, *artifacts* should be considered as causes of abnormal ECGs. Good contact must be made between the electrode and the patient when applying the electrodes. Disposable electrodes work well, but the gel dries if the patch is exposed to air for an extended period of time. Leads are damaged with frequent use and can result in faulty tracings (switching leads or looking at different leads clinches the diagnosis of lead-wire defects). Patient movement as well as skeletal muscle contractions (voluntary or involuntary) produces interference leading to incorrect diagnoses. A frequent source of interference is the electrocautery. Most currently used oscilloscopes have filters to reduce electrocautery noise. Placing the grounding pad so that the path of current from the surgical area to the ground is far from the chest greatly reduces electrocautery interference. Figure 2–16 has examples of common artifacts seen

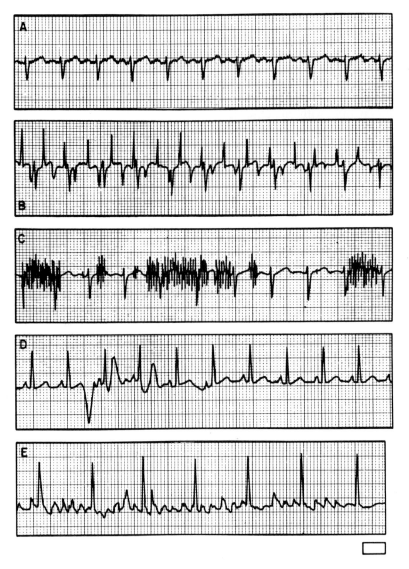

Figure 2–16. Common ECG artifacts: *A*, 60-Hz interference secondary to poor electrode contacts. *B*, Lead motion artifact. *C*, Electrocautery interference. *D*, Electrode movement artifact simulating PVBs. (Note: These do not affect the sinus cycle.) *E*, Succinylcholine chloride–induced fasciculations simulating atrial fibrillation. (From Atlee JL III: Perioperative Cardiac Dysrhythmias: Mechanisms, Recognition and Management. Chicago: Year Book Medical, 1985; 268. With permission.)

in the operating room setting. Hiccups may be the source of artifact, as depicted in Figure 2–17.

PACEMAKER ELECTROCARDIOGRAPHY

Approximately 100,000 new pacemakers are placed into patients in the United States each year.[32] Most anesthesiologists care for patients with pacemakers during anesthesia and surgery. Cardiac pacemakers are devices that impart an electrical impulse to the heart. They are placed in patients suffering from AV block, sinus node dysfunction, other bradydysrhythmias,

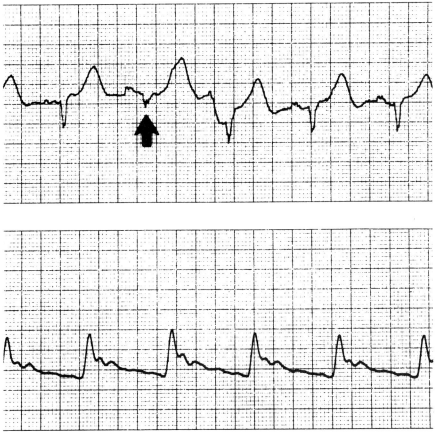

Figure 2–17. ECG interference from a patient with hiccups. (Courtesy of Karen J. Schwenzer, MD.)

and some tachydysrhythmias. Pacemaker components include a power source (battery), leads that then conduct current from the power source to the heart, and electronic circuitry that senses the native rhythm (most current pacemakers) and regulates the paced rhythm.

Pacemaker Terminology

An impulse of electrical energy is imparted in a circuit through the heart by the electrodes of the pacemaker. The circuit includes that portion of the myocardium that is stimulated. If one lead is placed against the heart and one lead is remote from the heart (usually the pacemaker case), it is in a *unipolar* configuration. If both leads are in contact with the heart, the system is in a *bipolar* configuration. Leads can be *epicardial* (surface of the heart) or *endocardial* (transvenous). The latter is most common today.

Pacemakers designed to deliver an electrical impulse at a certain rate regardless of native cardiac electrical activity are termed *asynchronous* (fixed rate) pacemakers. Asynchronous pacemakers are most commonly

Table 2–1. INTER-SOCIETY COMMISSION FOR HEART DISEASE RESOURCES FIVE-POSITION PACEMAKER CODE

I	II	III	IV	Sp
Chamber Paced	Chamber Sensed	Mode of Response	Programmable Functions	Antitachy Fun
V = Ventricle	V = Ventricle	T = Triggered	P = Simple Programmable	B = Bursts
A = Atrium	A = Atrium	I = Inhibited	M = Multiprogrammable	N = Normal
				S = Scannin
D = Double	D = Double	D = Double	C = Communicating	E = Externa
	0 = None	0 = None	0 = None	
		R = Reverse		

R = Pacemaker activated at fast rates only (i.e., upon sensing a tachyarrhythmia as opposed to br
P = Rate or output only.
C = Telemetry, interrogation (P or M implicit).
N = Paces at normal rate upon sensing tachyarrhythmia (underdrive pacing).
S = Scanning response (such as timed extrasystoles).
E = External control (activated by a magnet, radiofrequency, or other means).

used following cardiopulmonary bypass and for the emergency treatment of asystole. Asynchronous pacing impulses may induce dysrhythmias by competing with the intrinsic rhythm. *Demand* pacemakers, which sense the heart's native rhythm, only respond with an electrical impulse if no native beats are sensed during a specified time period.

There are a multitude of pacing modalities, depending on the chamber(s) paced, chamber(s) sensed (in demand units), responses of the pacemaker to sensed events, programmability, and special functions. The delineations of these parameters are given by the five-position pacemaker code.

Pacemaker Identification Code

The *five-position pacemaker code* was introduced by the Inter-Society Commission for Heart Disease Resources in 1983 to identify available pacing modes. The code is shown in Table 2–1.[33] The first position names the heart chamber that is paced, either the atrium or the ventricle, or both (double). The second position identifies the chamber that is sensed. This only applies to demand pacemakers, as the asynchronous type does not sense cardiac electrical activity (specified as none). The mode of response is given in position three. Triggered signifies that the pacer output is in response to sensed events. Inhibited means that the pacemaker does not fire upon sensing spontaneous activity. Double indicates that one chamber is inhibited and one is triggered. Reverse signifies that the pacer is activated at fast heart rates and deactivated at slow rates (reverse of usual activity). Position four gives the extent of programmability. Special antitachyarrhythmia functions of the pacemaker are shown in position five.

Diagnosis of Pacemaker Function

Normal Pacemaker Function

Prior to anesthetizing a patient who has a pacemaker, the anesthesiologist must be assured that the unit is properly functioning. The first step is to obtain the record of the pacemaker insertion; from this information the type of pacemaker can be determined. If the old records are not available, many patients carry pacemaker identification cards that contain the essential information. A third possible source of information is the physician who placed the unit.

The electrocardiograph can be very useful for ascertaining proper pacemaker function. When the pacemaker is functioning properly, unless inhibited, a pacemaker spike should be seen immediately preceding the P wave or QRS, or both, depending on the chamber(s) paced. The rate of nonadjustable pacemakers should be within 2 beats/minute of the manufacturer's specific recommendations. If the rate differs, there may be impending power source depletion. If the patient is in normal sinus rhythm and no pacemaker spikes are noted, then the patient's heart rate is most likely higher than the rate set in the pacemaker. Preoperatively, under electrocardiographic guidance, the patient's rate should be slowed to determine if the pacemaker is functioning. This can be done with either edrophonium or vagal maneuvers (carotid massage). If the pacemaker's function is questionable, an electrophysiologist should be consulted.

Abnormal Pacemaker Function

Pacemakers are usually quite dependable, but they may fail to function normally owing to interference from electrocautery, threshold alterations from drugs and physiologic states, or failure of the pulse generator or leads.

Electromagnetic Interference. Most current pacemakers contain sensing mechanisms so that pacing occurs only in the absence of sensed cardiac events (demand mode). There are instances, however, when the pacemaker can misinterpret extraneous electrical interference as spontaneous cardiac impulses. Such electrical interference (electromagnetic interference [EMI]) can either inhibit or trigger pacemaker output, depending on the mode of operation. *Unipolar* pacemakers are most susceptible to EMI because of the larger interelectrode distance. *Bipolar* units are much less susceptible because of the shorter interelectrode distance.

Electrocautery units are the most common cause of EMI in the operative setting, especially if the instrument is used in proximity to the pacemaker case or electrodes. Many demand pacemakers automatically switch to the *asynchronous mode* upon sensing *continuous EMI*, but this may not happen with *intermittent EMI*. As electrocautery is most often used in an intermittent manner, one should not rely on the pacemaker to automatically revert to the asynchronous mode.

If electrocautery is to be used, patients with demand units should have their units converted to an asynchronous mode by placing a magnet over the pulse generator. The risk of inducing tachydysrhythmia with competing rhythms is possible with some programmable pacemakers with magnet application.[34]

If the pacemaker is left in the demand mode, several measures reduce the risk of EMI-induced malfunction: (1) The grounding pad should be as far as possible from the chest. (2) Intermittent electrocautery may be used. If interference is present, the pacemaker still maintains a reasonable heart rate. (3) Heart sounds or pulse pressure should be monitored continuously. EMI renders the electrocardiograph useless for the detection of malfunction. (4) Reprogram the unit, if possible (random or phantom reprogramming),[34] with a magnet (it is better to reprogram the unit to the asynchronous mode prior to the procedure).

Other potential sources for interference with demand pacemaker function include *myotonic potentials* (pectoralis muscle, and with unipolar pacemakers) and *ionizing beams of radiation* (diagnostic x-rays are not a problem).

Failure of the Pacemaker. Failure of the unit to generate a stimulus can be caused by lead-wire fracture, misconnection of the leads into the pulse generator, or power source depletion. Impending or actual power source depletion is denoted by a reduction in rate (asynchronous mode) from a specified rate set (see particular rate information for the specific pacemaker unit). Cross-talk, the ventricular sending of atrial impulses, can lead to failure to pace. It can be corrected by reprogramming the atrial sensing refractory period. Lead dislodgment can provide an ineffective stimulus from the pacemaker. Also, a change in functional properties of the myocardium (myocardial infarction, hypothermia, and hyperkalemia) causes the stimulus to be ineffective.

Pacing at an Altered Rate. Pacing at an altered rate occurs with (1) *power source depletion* with subsequent reduction in rate, (2) *oversensing* that induces rate slowing (or, with triggered modes, acceleration), and (3) *rate drift*, which is seen with aging pacemakers (differs from impending power source depletion).

Improper Sensing. *Failure to sense* is often caused by lead dislodgment or lead-wire fracture. The *misdiagnosis of sensing failure* may be made when pacemaker impulses fall on intrinsic cardiac beats, causing fusion beats.

Oversensing occurs when the pacemaker senses signals other than those it is supposed to sense. For example, large T waves (as with hyperkalemia or hypocalcemia) may be sensed as another QRS complex. Ventricular electrodes may inappropriately sense atrial activity (cross-talk), which triggers additional beats or inhibits output.

Anesthesia for Pacemaker Insertion

The anesthesiologist is frequently asked to care for patients during permanent pacemaker placement.[35] Almost all permanent pacemakers can be placed with the patient under local anesthesia, with light sedation as required. The routine use of general anesthesia is to be discouraged, since anesthetics could have unpredictable and dangerous effects on marginal native rhythms (e.g., produce asystole). If general anesthesia is required, then temporary transvenous leads should be placed prior to anesthesia and proper pacing function obtained. Regardless of the anesthetic technique, atropine and isoproterenol should be readily available in case of bradycardia or heart block associated with pacemaker failure.

References

1. Bertrand CA, Steiner NV, Jameson AG, Lopez M: Disturbances of cardiac rhythm during anesthesia and surgery. JAMA 1971; 216:1615–1617.
2. Kuner J, Enescu V, Utsu F, et al: Cardiac arrhythmias during anesthesia. Dis Chest 1967; 52:580–587.
3. Hoffman BF, Cranefield PF: Electrophysiology of the Heart. New York: McGraw-Hill, 1960.
4. Fozzard HA, Arnsdorf MF: Cardiac physiology. *In* Fozzard HA, Haber E, Jennings RB, et al (eds): The Heart and Cardiovascular System. New York: Raven, 1986; 1–30.
5. Atlee JL III: Perioperative Cardiac Dysrhythmias: Mechanisms, Recognition and Management. Chicago: Year Book Medical, 1985.
6. Litt L, Rampil IJ: Physics and anesthesia. *In* Miller RD (ed): Anesthesia. New York: Churchill Livingstone, 1986; 111.
7. Goldreyer BNL: Intracardiac electrocardiography in the analysis and understanding of cardiac arrhythmias. Ann Intern Med 1972; 77:117–136.
8. Kistin AD, Bruce JC: Simultaneous esophageal and standard electrocardiographic leads for the study of cardiac arrhythmias. Am Heart J 1957; 53:65–73.
9. Brown WH: A study of the esophageal lead in clinical electrocardiography, part II. Am Heart J 1936; 12:306–338.
10. Kates RA, Zaidan JR, Kaplan JA: Esophageal lead for intraoperative electrocardiographic monitoring. Anesth Analg 1982; 61:781–785.
11. Copeland GD, Tullis IF, Brody DA: Clinical evaluation of a new esophageal electrode, with particular reference to the bipolar esophageal electrocardiogram. Am Heart J 1959; 53:862–873.
12. Scherlis L, Sandberg AA, Wener J, et al: RS-T segment displacement in induced coronary insufficiency as studied with esophageal leads. Circulation 1950; 2:598–603.
13. Marriott HJ: Practical Electrocardiography. Baltimore: Williams & Wilkins, 1983; 109–128.
14. Atlee JL III, Brownless SW, Burstrom RE: Conscious-state comparisons of the effects of inhalation anesthetics on specialized atrioventricular conduction times in dogs. Anesthesiology 1986; 64:703–710.
15. Chung EK: Wolff-Parkinson-White syndrome: Current views. Am J Med 1977; 62:252–266.
16. Helfant RH: Hypokalemia and arrhythmias. Am J Med 1986; 80:13–22.
17. Weaver WF, Burchel H: Serum potassium and the electrocardiogram and hypokalemia. Circulation 1973; 47:408–418.
18. Cohen JD, Neaton JD, Prineas RJ, Daniels KA: Diuretics, serum potassium and ventricular arrhythmias in the multiple risk factor intervention trial. Am J Cardiol 1987; 60:548–554.
19. Edwards R, Winnie AP, Ramamurthy S: Acute hypocapneic hypokalemia: An iatrogenic anesthetic complication. Anesth Analg 1977; 56:786–792.
20. Havestadt C, Ising H, Günther T, et al: Electrolytes and ventricular arrhythmias. Magnesium 1985; 4:29–33.

21. Bertino JS, Walker JW: Reassessment of theophylline toxicity. Arch Intern Med 1987; 147:757–760.
22. Stirt JA, Berger JM, Ricker SM: Arrhythmogenic effects of aminophylline during halothane anesthesia in experimental animals. Anesth Analg 1980; 59:410–416.
23. Carmelict EE: Influence of lithium ions on trans-membrane potential and cation content of cardiac cells. J Gen Physiol 1964; 47:501–530.
24. Martin CA, Piascik MT: First degree A-V block in patients on lithium carbonate. Can J Psychiatry 1985; 30:114–116.
25. Salzman C: Clinical use of antidepressant blood levels and the electrocardiogram. N Engl J Med 1985; 313:512–513.
26. Bosnjak ZJ, Kampine JP: Effects of halothane, enflurane, and isoflurane on the SA node. Anesthesiology 1983; 58:314–321.
27. Blitt CD, Raessler KL, Wightman MA, et al: Atrioventricular conduction in dogs during anesthesia with isoflurane. Anesthesiology 1979; 50:210–212.
28. Atlee JL III, Roberts FL: Thiopental and epinephrine-induced dysrhythmias in dogs anesthetized with enflurane or isoflurane. Anesth Analg 1986; 65:437–443.
29. Atlee JL III, Malkinson CE: Potentiation by thiopental of halothane-epinephrine-induced arrhythmias in dogs. Anesthesiology 1982; 57:285–288.
30. Johnston RR, Eger EI II, Wilson C: A comparative interaction of epinephrine with enflurane, isoflurane and halothane in man. Anesth Analg 1976; 55:709–712.
31. Taylor AL, Fozzard HA: Ventricular arrhythmias associated with CNS disease. Arch Intern Med 1982; 142:232–233.
32. Parsonnet V, Bernstein AD: Cardiac pacing in the 1980s: Treatment and techniques in transition. J Am Coll Cardiol 1983; 1:339–354.
33. Parsonnet V, Furman S, Smyth NPD: Optimal resources for implantable cardiac pacemakers. Circulation 1983; 68:224–244A.
34. Domino KB, Smith TC: Electrocautery-induced re-programming of a pacemaker using a precordial magnet. Anesth Analg 1983; 62:609–612.
35. Atlee JL III: Pacemakers and cardioversion. *In* Kaplan JA [ed]: Cardiac Anesthesia. Orlando: Grune & Stratton, 1987:855–879.

chapter three

Intravascular Pressure Monitoring Systems

■ ROBERT G. LOEB, M.D.

Arterial blood pressure monitoring, along with pulse rate, is historically and currently one of the most frequently monitored physiologic parameters during anesthesia. Invasive monitoring of arterial blood pressure in anesthesia and critical care is common. Invasive monitoring is more advantageous than noninvasive monitoring because continuous observation of the waveform is possible, arterial blood samples can be readily obtained, and it is the gold standard. Invasive blood pressure monitoring is deceptively simple, as exemplified by the misnomer "direct pressure monitoring." As explained in this chapter, clinical monitoring of intravascular pressure is not direct but indirect through transducers, filters, amplifiers, and displays. Attention to detail and an understanding of the frailties of such systems are necessary to avoid inaccuracy and misinterpretation.

COMPONENTS OF A PRESSURE MEASUREMENT SYSTEM

Common clinical pressure measurement systems consist of four main subsystems (Fig. 3–1): the mechanical coupling system, the transducer, the

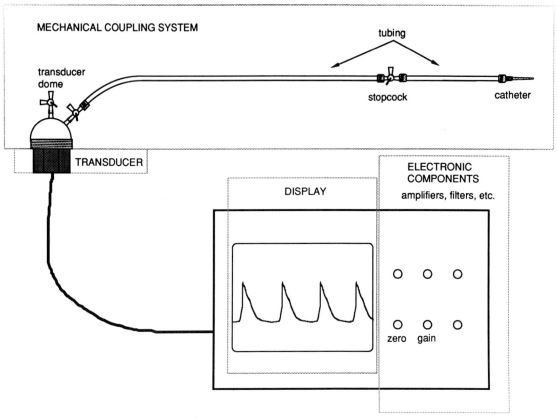

Figure 3–1. The four subsystems of a clinical pressure measurement system: mechanical coupling system, transducer, display, and electronic components.

electronic components, and the display. The mechanical coupling system transmits the pressure from the source to the transducer. The transducer converts the pressure into an electrical analog (usually voltage). The electronic components change the electrical analog into a form suitable for display and extract features of the waveform. The display converts the electrical signal and features into a visible form. The mechanical coupling system consists of an intravascular catheter, tubing, stopcocks, and sometimes a transducer dome. The electronic components include amplifiers, filters, and analog or digital circuits for peak detection and averaging.

CALIBRATION AND PERFORMANCE

Static Calibration

The most important factor for ensuring the accuracy of a blood pressure measurement is the calibration of the system. Static calibration refers to the calibration of the system against a known static pressure. Clinical pressure monitoring systems are assumed to be linear; that is, the pressure input versus the system output is described by a straight line. Therefore, a two-point calibration is sufficient.

Two-Point Calibration

Static calibration is performed by first exposing the mechanical coupling system to atmospheric pressure (this is usually performed by opening a stopcock to air). The electrical "zero" control is then adjusted to bring the displayed pressure to zero. On digital systems, a "zero" button is pressed. Either way, this results in balancing of the preamplification circuitry to produce a zero voltage. Second, a known pressure is presented to the mechanical coupling system at the same site and level that the zero reading was taken. The known pressure is usually generated with a mercury manometer, but a water manometer (1.35 cm H_2O = 1 mmHg) or any calibrated manometer is acceptable. With the system exposed to a known pressure, the electrical "gain" control is adjusted to bring the displayed pressure to the calibrated value. This adjusts the gain of the preamplifier circuits to match the sensitivity of the transducer.

Two-point calibration should be performed prior to attaching a patient to the system. Since pressure transducers have a standard sensitivity of 5.0 μV/V/mmHg, it can be argued that one-point calibration is sufficient. However, reusable transducers are subject to abuse, and, when used with transducer domes containing a diaphragm, the method of applying the dome affects the sensitivity.[1] The only way to verify accuracy is by two-point calibration of the entire system. Disposable transducers are calibrated at the factory but may be damaged during shipping. Although the quality control of these devices seems to be good, two-point calibration prior to use identifies the rare defective unit.[2] Two-point calibration should be repeated during use if it is suspected that the transducer has malfunctioned.[3]

Drift. The system should be rezeroed, without changing the gain, periodically during use. Transducer drift occurs over time. Usually, the zero drifts with little change in sensitivity.[2] Drift may lead to inaccuracy, especially when low pressures (e.g., venous or intracranial) are being measured. Two main causes of drift are thermal effects on the transducer[2] and the effect of transducer domes containing diaphragms. Temperature changes of 10°C usually change the measured pressure by less than 1 mmHg.[2]

Transducer domes with diaphragms create larger inaccuracies. Gradual drifts of the baseline of 15 mmHg over 3 hours have been reported.[4] Inadvertent loosening of the transducer dome during use has caused 80 mmHg negative offsets.[5] It is recommended, therefore, that the system be rezeroed and transducer domes be tightened at frequent intervals during use. Transducer offset may also occur during electrocautery.[6] Therefore, pressure values obtained while electrosurgical units are active may not be accurate.

Reference Points. The pressure reference point varies with the pressure being measured and the position of the patient. Central venous pressure is measured at the level of the middle of the right atrium. Intracranial pressure is measured at the tragus of the ear. The pressure reference point for arterial blood pressure may be the middle of the right atrium when the patient is in the supine position or the level of the brain in neurosurgical procedures performed with the patient in a sitting position.

The column of fluid between the transducer and the pressure reference point represents a static pressure.[7] This static pressure can be zeroed mechanically or electrically. Mechanical zeroing is achieved by ensuring that the transducer is at the level of the pressure reference point. Electrical zeroing is achieved by rezeroing the system with a stopcock open at the pressure reference point, disregarding the level of the transducer. Either procedure needs to be repeated whenever the level of the transducer changes with respect to the pressure reference point.

Dynamic Calibration

Measuring static pressure is relatively straightforward. Accurately measuring dynamic pressures is more difficult by an order of magnitude. Fundamental to understanding the potential distortion is a conceptual knowledge of the behavior of oscillating systems. (For a mathematical description of the behavior of oscillating systems, see this chapter's appendix.)

There are many examples of oscillating systems: vibrating strings, pendulums, and waves on a pool of water. The vascular tree, the mechanical coupling subsystem, the pressure transducer, and electrical amplifier circuitry are also oscillating systems.

All oscillating systems have two energy storage compartments between which energy is transferred. In mechanical systems, the energy storage compartments are mass (which stores kinetic energy as inertia when in motion) and elasticity (which stores potential energy when distorted). Oscillations decrease with time, owing to friction, when no energy is added to the system (there are no perpetual motion machines). Damping or viscosity is a measure of the friction that counteracts the kinetic energy of the mass. To summarize, an oscillating system can be described by the coefficients of mass, stiffness (the inverse of elasticity), and damping.

Natural Frequency

All oscillating systems have a natural frequency. The natural frequency is the oscillating frequency of the undamped system. Oscillations at the natural frequency generate the largest displacement for a given input energy. The qualitative effects of changes in mass and stiffness on natural frequency are demonstrated by observations of piano strings. The low notes (slow oscillations) are generated by long, heavy, thick strings that are loosely stretched to be less stiff; high notes are generated by short, thin, light strings that are tightly stretched to be more stiff. Natural frequency decreases with increased mass and decreased stiffness.

Damping

Damping can be understood qualitatively by imagining a vibrating string immersed in honey. Two things would be noticed when comparing oscil-

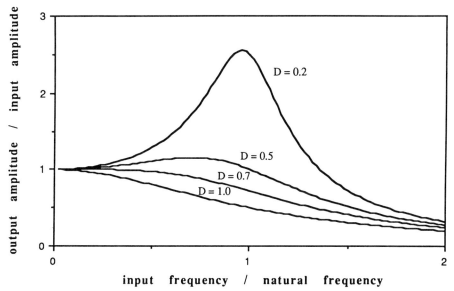

Figure 3–2. The effect of damping on the frequency response. Increasing the damping coefficient (D) results in less overshoot from oscillations near the natural frequency of the system. It also decreases the oscillating frequency. A damping coefficient around 0.7 is optimal because it yields an output-to-input amplitude ratio close to unity over the widest frequency range.

lations in honey with those in air; the oscillations in honey extinguish more quickly and the string oscillates at a lower frequency. That the oscillating frequency increases as damping decreases can also be demonstrated by the increasing pitch of the voice after inhaling a low-density gas such as helium. The resonant frequency is the oscillating frequency of a damped system. It is a function of the natural frequency and the damping coefficient (Fig. 3–2).

Figure 3–3 illustrates the effect of increasing the coefficient of damping on the response of an oscillating system to a sudden input of energy. Increasing the coefficient of damping decreases the overshoot but increases the response time of the system (response time is the time required to reach some fraction of the final value).

MECHANICAL COUPLING SUBSYSTEM

The mechanical coupling subsystem (i.e., catheter, stopcock, tubing, dome) contains the elements of an oscillating system. The mass is represented by the mass of fluid within the system. The distensibility of the plastics from which the components are made gives the system its elasticity. Damping is a function of the frictional resistance to movement of the fluid and distortion of the plastics.

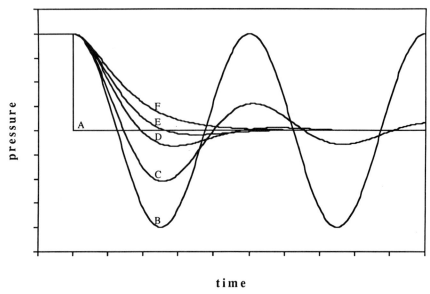

Figure 3–3. The effect of damping on the system response to a step change in pressure: *A*, The input signal. *B*, Response of a system with zero damping. *C*, Response of a system with a damping coefficient of 0.2. *D*, Response of a system with a damping coefficient of 0.5. *E*, Response of a system with an optimal damping coefficient of 0.7. *F*, Response of a system with a critical damping coefficient of 1.0. Note that a damping coefficient around 0.7 yields the best compromise between fast response time and small overshoot.

Natural Frequency

Numerous studies have described the natural frequency and damping coefficient of commercial pressure monitoring systems. Bare transducers have resonant frequencies of 100–500 Hz.[1, 8] Transducer-tubing systems have much lower natural frequencies of 5–50 Hz.[9–12] The length of the tubing has a profound influence on the natural frequency.[11] Five feet of low-compliance tubing results in a natural frequency of 6.5 Hz compared with 33 Hz for 6 inches of tubing. This may be especially important when using disposable systems with an option of patient- versus pole-mounted transducers. In one study, the natural frequencies of seven brands of pole-mounted disposable units ranged from 19 to 28 Hz; mounting the same transducers on the patient resulted in increased natural frequencies in a range from 41 to 73 Hz.[13]

The presence of a diaphragm in a disposable transducer dome also causes a decrease in natural frequency. A study of five transducer models showed natural frequencies of 270–545 Hz when domes without diaphragms were used; the same transducers had natural frequencies of 54–423 Hz when used with domes containing diaphragms.[1] More important, the method of application of the transducer dome significantly affected the natural frequency. Consistently, the lowest natural frequencies resulted when the dome was applied without water between the diaphragm and the dome.[1]

The final factor influencing the natural frequency of the mechanical coupling system, and a factor that is too frequently ignored by clinicians, is the presence of air bubbles. Air bubbles are compressible and increase the elasticity of the system. Most clinicians only know that air bubbles increase the damping coefficient of the mechanical coupling system. However, air bubbles also cause a significant decrease in the natural frequency. The addition of 0.03 ml of air to pole-mounted disposable pressure transducer systems decreases the natural frequency from a range of 18–28 Hz to a range of 8–13 Hz.[13]

Damping Coefficient

The length of tubing, the presence of diaphragms in transducer domes, and the presence of air bubbles also affect the damping coefficient. Five feet of low-compliance tubing results in a damping coefficient of 0.1 compared with 0.3 for 6 inches of tubing.[11] The damping coefficients for five transducers without diaphragms ranged from 0.023 to 0.1; the same transducers had damping coefficients from 0.035 to 0.125 when used with domes containing diaphragms.[1] The addition of 0.3 ml of air to pole-mounted disposable pressure transducer systems increases the damping coefficient from a range of 0.14–0.22 to a range of 0.16–0.28.[13]

Frequency Content

To predict the effect of any combination of resonant frequency and damping coefficient on the accuracy of reproduction of a pressure waveform, one first needs to know the frequency content of the pressure waveform. Fourier analysis is a mathematical method of extracting the simple sine and cosine waves that sum to form a complex wave. Fourier analysis of blood pressure waveforms is demonstrated in Figure 3–4. Multiple studies have concluded that the original blood pressure waveform can be accurately reproduced by summing the first five to ten harmonics.[8, 14] Because heart rate normally is in the range of 60–180 beats/minute (1–3 Hz), the fifth to tenth harmonics encompass a range of 5–30 Hz. Re-examination of Figure 3–2 reveals that amplitude distortion occurs around the natural frequency of the system. Small damping factors allow amplitude overshoot, whereas large damping coefficients result in low relative amplitudes below the natural frequency.

Two methods to preserve an accurate amplitude response are to increase the natural frequency of the system and to optimize the damping coefficient. Gardner published a study that experimentally derived the adequate dynamic response range of invasive blood pressure measurement systems used for monitoring in intensive care units and operating rooms.[9] His results indicate the combinations of natural frequency and damping coefficient that accurately reproduce arterial blood pressure waveforms (Fig. 3–5). Two ranges are depicted. Systems with adequate response accurately reproduce pressures at slow heart rates. Systems with optimum response may be necessary to accurately reproduce blood pressure waveforms at fast heart rates or when fast upstrokes are present in the pressure waveform.[13]

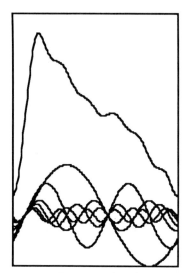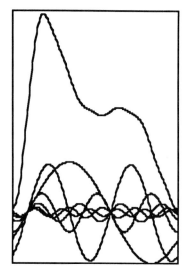

Figure 3–4. Two examples of Fourier analysis of a blood pressure waveform. The upper trace in each example is the original waveform. The lower traces in each example are the sine wave harmonics, which sum to yield the original waveform. The period of each sine wave is an integral multiple of the period of the original waveform. The only difference between the examples is the relative amplitude of each sine wave harmonic.

The largest error introduced by inadequate dynamic response is an inaccurate systolic pressure. Because the systolic upstroke of the pressure waveform contains the highest frequency components, these components are the most difficult to reproduce accurately. Figure 3–5 demonstrates the effect of dynamic response on the measured systolic pressure. Systolic pressure is underestimated by an overdamped system and overestimated by an underdamped system. Diastolic pressure is less sensitive to suboptimal dynamic response, but it is underestimated by underdamped systems and overestimated by overdamped systems. Mean pressure is least affected by the dynamic response of the measuring system.

Clinical Determination of Dynamic Response

There are two methods of determining the natural frequency and damping coefficient of a blood pressure measurement system. In the clinical laboratory, a pressure generator can be used to produce a constant amplitude sine wave pressure at progressively increasing frequency (sine wave method). Natural frequency and damping coefficient can be determined by comparing the pressure tracing recorded by the system under investigation with the pressure tracing recorded by a reference transducer (Fig. 3–6). In the operating room or intensive care unit, the natural frequency and damping coefficient of a pressure measurement system can be determined by the response of the system to a square wave pressure input. A square wave pressure can be generated by opening then quickly closing the fast-flush valve of a continuous flush mechanism (square wave method). Figure 3–7

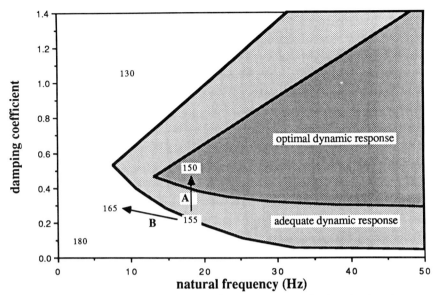

Figure 3–5. The adequate and optimal dynamic response ranges for invasive blood pressure measurement systems. The numbers are examples of output systolic pressures for a systolic input pressure of 150 mmHg. Increasing the damping coefficient decreases the systolic pressure. Systems with a high natural frequency have a wider range of acceptable damping coefficients. Systems with a natural frequency below 7.5 Hz are never adequate. *Arrow A* shows the effect of changing the damping coefficient of the mechanical coupling system with a commercial device for that purpose. *Arrow B* shows the effect of introducing an air bubble into the mechanical coupling system. (Modified from Gardner RM: Direct blood pressure measurement: dynamic response requirements. Anesthesiology 1981; 54:227–236.)

demonstrates this method of determining the dynamic response of the system from the measured pressure waveform. Figure 3–8 provides a graph and table for determining the damping coefficient from the amplitude ratio.[9] The sine wave and square wave methods of determining dynamic response yield identical results.[13]

Methods to Improve Dynamic Response

Most commercial blood pressure measurement systems are underdamped, with a borderline natural frequency for arterial blood pressure measurement.[12] What can the clinician do if the measured dynamic response of his or her system is outside the acceptable range? To optimize the dynamic response, the natural frequency should be as high as possible; a natural frequency below 7.5 Hz is never acceptable.[9] This is accomplished by using the shortest practical tubing (definitely less than 4 feet) and the fewest number of stopcocks (not more than one) between the transducer and the patient.[11] Tubing should be noncompliant; compliant devices such as T-connectors with injection ports should not be used.

Air bubbles should be meticulously removed from the mechanical coupling system.[15] Bubbles often hide in stopcocks and transducer domes. Air embolization through arterial and venous catheters is associated with sig-

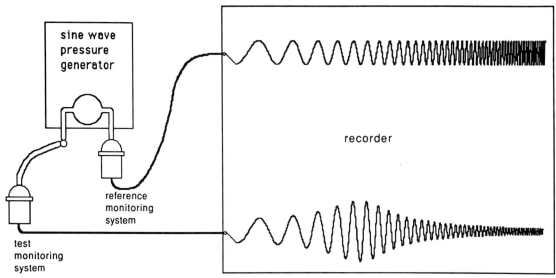

Figure 3–6. The sine wave method of determining dynamic response. A sine wave pressure of increasing frequency is simultaneously measured by a reference and a test system. The reference system should have a flat response; the test system should have an output defined by the natural frequency and damping coefficient. Two measurements are made: the frequency at which there is peak amplitude from the test system (oscillating frequency), and the ratio of test system amplitude to reference system amplitude at the oscillating frequency. The damping coefficient and natural frequency can be calculated from these numbers (see this chapter's appendix for formulas).

nificant patient morbidity, especially in children;[16, 17] air should be aspirated into a syringe when it is detected.[16] To reduce the incidence of invisible bubbles, air should be removed from the intravenous bag before it is pressurized, the intravenous solution may be warmed or exposed to ultrasonic waves prior to use, and a filter may be used to trap air distal to the fast-flush mechanism.[16, 18]

After all measures have been taken to increase the natural frequency of the system, the dynamic response may still be inadequate owing to suboptimal damping. A number of devices are commercially available to increase the damping coefficient of the system without decreasing the natural frequency. This effect is illustrated in Figure 3–5. These devices, which are available with fixed or adjustable output, can be easily used to bring the dynamic response into the optimal range.[9, 10]

TRANSDUCERS

A transducer is a device that converts one form of energy into another. All pressure transducers first convert pressure into movement. An elastic device, such as a Bourdon tube or a diaphragm, is exposed to the pressure, and its deflection is measured.

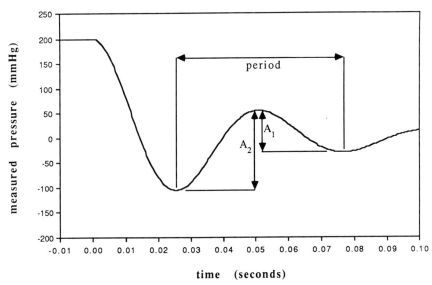

Figure 3–7. The square wave method of determining dynamic response. A square wave is generated by opening then quickly closing the fast flush valve of a continuous flush mechanism. Two measurements are then made from the recorded output: the oscillating frequency, which is the inverse of the period; and the amplitude ratio of two successive peaks, A_1/A_2. In this example the oscillating frequency is 19 Hz (1/0.052 second), and the amplitude ratio is 0.51. The damping coefficient and natural frequency can be derived from these numbers (see this chapter's appendix and Fig. 3–8).

Historical Development

Geddes has written a fascinating summary of the historical development of blood pressure transducers.[8] Early transducers measured the deflection of a Bourdon tube using mechanical linkages, a method still used today in blood pressure manometers. However, purely mechanical manometers have a very low frequency response owing to the need for a large sensing element with a large displacement volume. This is an inherent requirement, because the energy to move the mechanical parts must come from the event being measured. A significant advance was made in the fidelity of blood pressure measurement with the development of mechano-optical transducers. These devices, developed between 1903 and 1945, further transduced the movement of the sensing element to the deflection of a beam of light. Ultimately, high fidelity was achieved using miniature low-elasticity glass membrane sensing elements to deflect the light beam. These devices, although useful in the physiology laboratory, were never clinically used because pressure recordings required a darkened room and photographic techniques.

Given the advanced state of electrical technology, it is not surprising that modern blood pressure transducers convert movement of the sensing element into current or voltage. This conversion is usually accomplished by inducing a change in capacitance, inductance, or resistance. High-frequency response is achieved using small sensing elements with low fluid displacement.

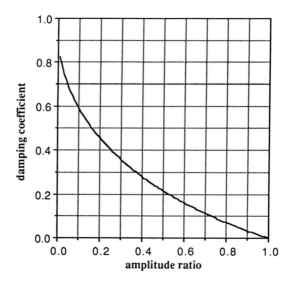

	0.00	**0.01**	**0.02**	**0.03**	**0.04**	**0.05**	**0.06**	**0.07**	**0.08**	**0.09**
.0	1.000	0.826	0.780	0.745	0.716	0.690	0.667	0.646	0.627	0.608
.1	0.591	0.575	0.559	0.545	0.531	0.517	0.504	0.491	0.479	0.467
.2	0.456	0.445	0.434	0.424	0.414	0.404	0.394	0.385	0.376	0.367
.3	0.358	0.349	0.341	0.333	0.325	0.317	0.309	0.302	0.294	0.287
.4	0.280	0.273	0.266	0.259	0.253	0.246	0.240	0.234	0.228	0.221
.5	0.215	0.210	0.204	0.198	0.192	0.187	0.181	0.176	0.171	0.166
.6	0.160	0.155	0.150	0.146	0.141	0.136	0.131	0.126	0.122	0.117
.7	0.113	0.108	0.104	0.100	0.095	0.091	0.087	0.083	0.079	0.075
.8	0.071	0.067	0.063	0.059	0.055	0.052	0.048	0.044	0.041	0.037
.9	0.034	0.030	0.027	0.023	0.020	0.016	0.013	0.010	0.006	0.003
1.0	0.000									

Figure 3–8. Two methods of determining the damping coefficient from the square wave method amplitude ratio. The conversion can be read from the graph or, if greater accuracy is desired, from the table. For example, an amplitude ratio of 0.51 yields a damping coefficient of 0.210.

Types

Capacitance Transducers

In a capacitance transducer, the sensing element is one plate of the capacitor (Fig. 3–9). As pressure is applied, the two plates of the capacitor move closer together and capacitance increases. An oscillating voltage is applied across the plates of the capacitor, and an alternating current that varies with the pressure on the sensing element results. This alternating current is then demodulated (converted to direct current) for further processing. Capacitance transducers have a number of practical problems.[8, 19, 20] They have poor temperature stability and require separate temperature-compensating circuitry. Electrical cables are themselves capacitors; therefore, the oscillator and demodulator must be built into the transducer housing to avoid interference. This increases the size of the unit.

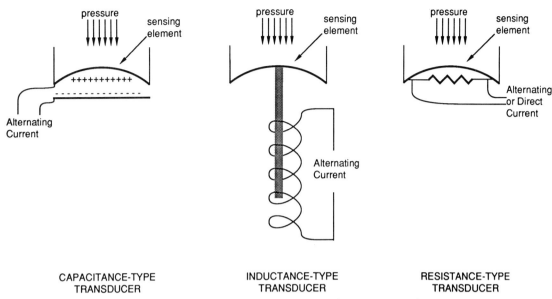

Figure 3–9. The three common types of electronic pressure transducers.

Further, in order to be used with biologic amplifiers, the current produced must first be converted to voltage.

Inductance Transducers

Inductance is an electrical property of coils produced by the forces of an induced magnetic field that causes the coil to resist changes in current flow. The inductance of a coil is affected by the position of an iron core within the coil. Inductance transducers have a core attached to the sensing element (Fig. 3–9). As pressure is applied, the core is displaced into the coil and inductance increases. Like capacitance, inductance is measured with an oscillating current. Therefore, the transducer housing usually contains oscillators and demodulators. Inductance transducers have a number of advantages. They are stable over a useful temperature range and can be designed to have a large electrical output for a small mechanical displacement. The most sensitive transducers based on the property of inductance use a miniature linear variable differential transformer. These units use a core and four coils to produce a multivolt output for 0.001-inch deflection of the sensing element.

Resistance Transducers

Change in resistance is the most common way of measuring displacement of the sensing element. The principle of measurement is based on the fact that the resistance of a wire increases as it is stretched (Fig. 3–9). Nondisposable pressure transducers are usually bonded strain gauges. In these, a resistor or a group of resistors is bonded to the back of the diaphragm. As pressure is applied to the diaphragm, the resistors are distorted and their resistance changes. Resistive-type transducers have a major advantage over capacitance- and inductance-type transducers. Change in resistance is easily converted to change in voltage by use of a Wheatstone bridge. Therefore, bulky circuits for modulation-demodulation are not necessary. Strain gauges are temperature-sensitive, but the Wheatstone bridge can be designed with two or four active arms to be temperature-compensated. Recently, disposable pressure transducers have become popular. These are resistive-type transducers. The diaphragm is a piece of silicon with the resistive elements etched onto it.

Intravascular Transducers

Most clinical pressure transducers are for external use, but intravascular transducers can be of the inductive, capacitance, or resistive type. The advantage of intravascular transducers is that there is no mechanical coupling system to distort the pressure waveform. The frequency response of an intravascular transducer system can be flat to over 100 Hz.

Unfortunately, intravascular transducers have a number of drawbacks. They are expensive and fragile, a bad combination for clinical devices. Although they are miniature compared with external transducers, they are too large to be passed through a catheter smaller than 18 gauge. Finally, they cannot be recalibrated during use. The result is that intravascular transducers are not widely used for clinical measurement of intravascular pressures.

Standardization

Manufacturers have adopted a standard blood pressure transducer output of 5 microvolts per volt excitation per mmHg input pressure (5 μV/V/mmHg). This standardization means that transducers from different manufacturers are functionally interchangeable. The interface plug between the transducer and the preamplifier has not been standardized, so a conversion unit may still be required to connect any particular combination of transducer and monitor.

AMPLIFIERS AND FILTERS

Electrical amplification and filtering occurs between the generation of the electrical analog at the transducer and the display of the pressure waveform. Many modern monitors also perform analog-to-digital conversion of the signal at this point. The actual mechanism of this "electronic massage" for any given monitor is unimportant and proprietary, but the specifications of the amplifiers, filters, and analog-to-digital convertors are important since they influence the waveform and derived values. Amplifiers are used to increase the voltage and power of the signal. They contain oscillating electronic circuits but have a frequency response 100 times better than that of the mechanical coupling sysem.

Low-pass filters are included for three reasons: to remove high-frequency noise due to electrocautery; to smooth the waveform, which is often reconstructed from discretely sampled points; and to give the waveform a more pleasant appearance. Removal of electrocautery noise is clinically necessary. However, filtering to yield a more rounded appearance of the waveform is unwarranted. It is a serious problem because it is not standardized and the filters affect the frequencies of interest. For example, Hewlett-Packard monitor models 78353/4 and 78833/4 (Hewlett-Packard Co., Waltham, MA) have a bandwidth of 0–12 Hz, whereas the Tektronix model 414 monitor (Tektronix, Inc., Beaverton, OR) has a bandwidth of 0–20 Hz. (Bandwidth is the frequency range over which the output has between 70% and 140% the power of the input.) Nonstandardization may cause discrepancies, especially in systolic values and derived cardiovascular parameters, whenever a patient is moved from one monitor to another.

There are two reasons that a waveform may be sampled as discrete points and then reconstructed. Some monitors electronically disconnect the transducer hundreds of times per second (chop the signal) and subtract any baseline voltage during that time to maintain baseline stability of the internal electronic components. More important, most modern monitors convert the analog voltage to a digital value. This process, known as analog-to-digital conversion, occurs 60 to a few hundred times per second. The advantages of having the information in a digital form are that it can be stored and manipulated. Stored values allow display of frozen waveforms and trends. Digital computer manipulation of the values allows feature detection, automatic calculation of derived variables, and other sophisticated algorithms discussed later.

ELECTRONIC SIGNAL ANALYSIS

The shape of the pressure waveform is important to detect artifact, to judge the effect of arrhythmias on blood pressure (see Chapter 2), and perhaps to estimate the inotropic and volume status of the cardiovascular system. In addition to displaying the waveform, clinical monitors extract and digitally display four features: rate, systolic pressure, diastolic pressure, and mean pressure. These values are used, either directly or in derived parameters, to guide diagnostic and therapeutic decisions. These values are affected by dynamic and static calibration and electronic filtering as well as by the method of signal analysis.

What information is important from a physiologic viewpoint? Heart rate is one description of cardiovascular status. Cardiac output is affected by heart rate, especially in children. Heart rate also affects the oxygen supply-to-demand ratio of the heart. Heart rate variability with respiration indicates active autonomic control, and variability with surgical stimulus is helpful to evaluate depth of anesthesia. Therefore, the absolute value of heart rate and some measure of heart rate variability are clinically useful parameters.

The systolic blood pressure, that is, the average aortic pressure during systole, estimates left ventricular afterload. The mean blood pressure indicates tissue perfusion pressure. Perfusion pressure of the coronary arteries is influenced by the diastolic pressure, that is, the average aortic pressure during diastole. Normally these systemic pressures are relatively uniform, beat to beat, over the respiratory cycle. However, hypovolemia is associated with increased variability with respiration. For systemic pressures, the clinically useful values are the average systolic pressure, the average diastolic pressure, the average mean pressure, and some measure of blood pressure variability.

Central vascular pressures (central venous pressure, pulmonary artery pressure, and pulmonary capillary wedge pressure) are used as correlates of atrial filling pressure and end-diastolic volume. These pressures are dramatically affected by respiration, especially in critically ill patients. The physiologically important values occur at end-expiration when the intrathoracic pressure is closest to atmospheric pressure. Therefore, for central vascular pressure the average end-expiratory mean pressure is the most desirable measurement.

In the past two decades, there has been a shift in technology in clinical monitors from analog to digital techniques of signal analysis. However, there are still many monitors in use that employ analog technology. Analog averaging is usually accomplished by using a resistor-capacitor circuit. These circuits output a voltage that is the exponentially weighted average of the input voltage. The effect is that all previous values are averaged, the more recent values being weighted exponentially more than the older values. A step change in input results in an exponential approach to the change in output. The response time of the circuit can be adjusted by changing the relative values of the resistor and capacitor. The output of these circuits is not very different from a moving average for an oscillating signal, but their response to a step change is quite different. There are also analog circuits that detect and hold a peak or nadir voltage. These circuits are used to detect systolic and diastolic values, actually maximum systolic and minimum diastolic pressures. In the older equipment, the averaging and peak detection circuits were reset every few seconds; the output was then a mean, peak, or nadir presure detected over a constant period of time. This tended to emphasize the highest systolic and lowest diastolic pressures during the respiratory cycle and was especially inaccurate at slow heart rates.

More recent analog devices reset the averaging and peak detection circuits in synchrony with the heart rate. This allows calculation of beat-to-beat values of mean, peak, and nadir pressures that are averaged prior to display. Heart rate can be determined from the blood pressure waveform by taking the first derivative of the waveform and counting the rate of strongly positive values or by counting the number of times the pressure changes from a value below the mean pressure to a value above the mean pressure. Either event triggers an electronic pulse that is fed into an averaging circuit whose output voltage then correlates with the average heart rate. In summary, monitors using analog signal processing to extract waveform parameters display the exponentially weighted average of heart rate, maximum systolic pressure, minimum diastolic pressure, and exponentially weighted mean pressure. Maloy and Gardner have experimentally demonstrated that these values may not equal those determined by a clinician reading from a calibrated strip-chart recording.[21] The systolic pressure is the most inaccurate value displayed, especially in patients with hypertension, pulsus paradoxus, or arrhythmias.

Digital Processing Algorithms

Digital signal processing is also used in most of the new blood pressure monitors. It is performed by one or more internal microprocessors. Digital processing algorithms are proprietary, and manufacturers rarely reveal the details of their methods. In general, algorithms are used to determine the beginning and end of a cardiac cycle. The maximum and minimum pressures during that cycle are then selected as systolic and diastolic values. These values, averaged over a constant period of time, are displayed. Mean pressures are also calculated beat to beat. Digital algorithms do perform better than analog algorithms. Maloy and Gardner found that the numeric values displayed by monitors using digital technology agreed more closely with clinicians' readings than did monitors using analog technology.[21] Even using current digital algorithms, systolic values are less reliable than diastolic values, and machine-generated values are sensitive to artifacts in the waveform.

New algorithms are being devised to remove the effect of respiratory artifact on central vascular pressures. Currently, the recommendations are for the clinician to determine these pressures from a calibrated paper-strip recording at end-exhalation.[22, 23] Simultaneous measurement of airway pressure accurately identifies end-expiration.[24] Alternatively, stable digital values can be obtained during a prolonged expiratory pause in the paralyzed and anesthetized patient.[3] However, this procedure has the risk of morbidity from failure to reinitiate mechanical ventilation. With current algorithms, the displayed mean value of central vascular pressures during mechanical ventilation is completely inaccurate and should not be used as either an absolute value or a trend.[23–25]

A number of methods have been described in an attempt to automatically determine end-expiratory values of pulmonary artery pressures. The in goal of each of these algorithms is to detect end-expiration. This is done most accurately by measuring the pressure, temperature, flow, or carbon dioxide concentration in the respiratory gas.[24, 26] Unfortunately, these techniques require additional measuring equipment.

An alternative method is described by Ellis.[27] He noted that the beat-to-beat mean pressure fluctuates least during end-expiration whenever expiratory time exceeds or equals inspiratory time. He used this observation to develop an algorithm that identifies end-expiration from information present in the pressure waveform itself.[27]

After end-expiration is identified, end-expiratory pressures can be estimated in a number of ways. One way is to average all values but to give greater weight to the values with less beat-to-beat variability.[27] This method is currently used in some monitors. Another way is to average only the end-expiratory values.[26] These methods are slightly more accurate than simple averaging techniques but become inaccurate at high respiratory rates. They also have the disadvantage that they do not display the pressure waveform with the respiratory artifact removed.

Mitchell and coworkers have recently reported a microprocessor-based method of removing the respiratory artifact from the pressure waveform.[28] To separate the cardiac and respiratory components, they use an adaptive filter that changes its characteristics based on the measured heart rate. They then determine the mean intravascular pressure using Ellis's algorithm and add this offset to the cardiac component. The result is a continuous pulmonary artery pressure waveform with the respiratory artifact removed. The method is equally applicable to central venous pressure and pulmonary capillary wedge pressures.

Commercially available monitors use simple analog or digital methods, or both, to determine average systolic, mean, and diastolic pressures. Algorithms are being developed to remove or identify artifact in invasive pressure waveforms. It is hoped that future commercial monitors will use more sophisticated electronic signal analysis.

DISPLAYS

Most clinicians are familiar with the variety of displays available on commercial monitors. Early blood pressure monitors used a simple oscilloscope to display the waveform. Systolic, diastolic, and mean values were displayed on separate analog or digital meters. Today, monitor displays have increased in complexity and sophistication. Waveforms and numbers are displayed simultaneously on a cathode ray tube. Display format can be partially defined by the user and can automatically change as different combinations of transducers are connected to the monitor. Remote displays are available; these are classified as "smart" or "dumb." Dumb terminals simply echo the monitor's integrated display. They are usually large screens used in operating rooms so that all members of the surgical team can observe cardiovascular parameters. Smart terminals allow various levels of display control from a remote location. These are most frequently used in intensive care units to display information from multiple monitors in a central location.

Two major improvements in displays have become available: color and trend displays. Color displays help the user to find and focus her or his attention on a particular waveform or value. This is important since displays often contain multiple waveforms and values from a number of sources. Many commercial monitors now have the ability to store a few hours of information and display it on a compressed time scale. The immediate advantages are twofold: (1) A clinician who has not been in constant attendance has access to an accurate record of the patient's physiologic status during the clinician's absence. (2) The clinician can view physiologic parameters on a compressed time scale to detect trends that may not be apparent in real time. Trend displays are underutilized by clinicians. Most clinicians are used to the standard monitor display of real-time waveforms; this is the most frequently selected display for continual observation in the operating room and intensive care unit.

No studies have been done to determine whether physiologic stability can be better maintained by a clinician using real-time waveforms or trend displays as feedback, but trend displays may be the better choice under many circumstances. Humans are very effective in detecting patterns, but their memory limits their ability to detect patterns occurring over a span of time. By allowing the clinician to focus on the changes in relevant physiologic variables over a relevant period of time, trend displays aid in the detection and treatment of undesirable conditions.

EFFECTS OF CATHETERS

Superficial arteries are commonly cannulated for arterial pressure measurement. Barr first reported the use of an over-the-needle catheter that is inserted percutaneously for indwelling use.[29] Central arteries and veins are commonly cannulated using the method first described by Seldinger (see Chapters 4 and 5).[30]

Catheter Size and Type

The size of the catheter influences the rate of complications and the dynamic response of the system. Bedford studied the incidence of temporary radial artery occlusion as a function of catheter size. He found a 34% incidence of occlusion 24 hours after insertion with 18-gauge catheters compared with 8% with 20-gauge catheters.[31] The incidence of arterial occlusion is directly related to the percentage of the vessel lumen that is occupied by the catheter. Wrist circumference is a noninvasive measurement that is well correlated with the risk of radial arterial occlusion; a wrist circumference less than 18 cm is associated with a greater than 25% incidence of occlusion using an 18-gauge catheter.[32] Although radial artery occlusion is usually temporary, persistent occlusion can result.[33] The lower incidence of thrombosis with smaller catheters is an advantage to the clinician. Distal occlusion of the radial artery causes overshoot of the measured systolic pressure owing to increased wave reflection, whereas proximal occlusion causes a reduction in measured pulse pressure owing to overdamping.[34] Small catheters have an additional effect of increasing the dynamic accuracy of the system. Although small catheters have a slightly lower resonant frequency than do large catheters, they have a significantly larger damping coefficient.[35, 36] Because most blood pressure monitoring systems are underdamped, this results in increased accuracy of the system. The major clinical disadvantage of smaller catheters is that they kink more easily.

Catheter Composition

The material from which the catheter is made also influences the rate of complications. Intravascular catheters are commonly manufactured from polyethylene, polypropylene, polyvinylchloride, or polytef (Teflon). Numerous studies have documented the increased thrombogenicity of polypropylene and polyethylene over Teflon.[34, 37–40] Polyvinylchloride is comparable to Teflon in its incidence of thrombus formation.[39, 41] Thrombogenicity is also affected by the smoothness of the catheter surface; roughened Teflon catheters are more thrombogenic than polyethylene catheters.[38] This may be clinically important, since pulmonary artery catheters have a higher incidence of thrombus formation when they are passed through introducers or protective sleeves.[42] Heparin impregnation of catheters decreases the incidence of thrombus formation initially, but the effect is lost after 48 hours, probably because the heparin leeches out of the catheter.[39] In addition to initial thrombus formation, polyethylene catheters cause injuries to the vessel, which could serve as a nidus for atherosclerotic plaques.[43]

A notable exception to the findings presented here are the data from Slogoff and coworkers. In their study of 1699 patients after radial artery cannulation, they were unable to find any correlation between the risk of thrombus and catheter size (18 or 20 gauge) or catheter composition (Teflon or polypropylene).[44] They did report a statistically higher incidence of thrombosis in women (who tend to have a smaller wrist circumference).[44]

Maintenance of Catheter Patency

Catheters for pressure monitoring are kept patent by one of three methods: intermittent bolus of heparin-containing solution, continuous flush of heparin-containing solution, or continuous flush of non–heparin-containing solution.

Intermittent Bolus Technique

Historically, intermittent boluses of heparin-containing solution was the only method available. There are two major problems with the intermittent bolus technique. The first is that it is not particularly effective in preventing catheter thrombosis, leading to waveform damping.[39] Wesseling and Smith report that the duration of waveform loss owing to damping with the intermittent bolus technique is 2–10 times that with the continuous flush technique.[45] More important, significant patient morbidity can result from a manual bolus when thrombotic or air emboli are forced retrograde into the central or cerebral circulation.[17] The volume of the bolus necessary to reach the central circulation correlates with the height of the patient. Therefore, extreme care is necessary during bolus injection in pediatric patients.

Continuous Flush Technique

In 1970, Gardner and colleagues published a report of the first commercial continuous flush device for clinical use.[46] Such devices, which infuse fluid through the catheter at a nominal rate of 3–6 ml/hour, are now widely used. Advantages of continuous flush include effectiveness, ease of use, and the ability to maintain a closed sterile system. An additional advantage is that constantly wedged pulmonary artery catheters may be identified by a steady rise in the measured pulmonary artery pressure with loss of the waveform.[47]

There are, of course, some disadvantages with continuous flush. A static error is introduced in the pressure measurement. The magnitude of the error is dependent on the infusion rate and the resistance to flow through the catheter. Static errors between 0.1 and 2.5 mmHg have been reported.[18, 46] For arterial pressure monitoring this error is clinically insignificant. A more important disadvantage is the potential for inadvertent excess fluid administration. This can occur if the flush mechanism is defective.[48] However, in neonates and children, even a flow of 3–6 ml/hour through multiple pressure monitoring lines may exceed the fluid requirements for that patient. In such cases the standard system can be modified so that the fluid for the flush device is dispensed from a syringe pump or volumetric infusion pump.[49] A final potential problem of continuous flush is the introduction of air into the pressure monitoring system. If the fluid source for the flush device is a pressurized bag of fluid that contains air, an air embolism may occur when the bag empties. This may be avoided if all the air is removed from the bag prior to applying pressure. Smaller amounts of air can also be introduced during a fast flush. This occurs owing to the vortex created when a stream of fluid enters the drip chamber. The best solution is to inspect the system for air after a fast flush or to use an appropriate filter.

The final issue in maintaining catheter patency is whether to use heparin in a continuous flush solution. Most practitioners use 1 or 2 U of heparin/ml of flush solution. There are no studies reported to justify this practice, and there are practitioners who do not add heparin. Because of the possibility of heparin overdose, this is an issue that merits further investigation.

PRESSURE ALTERATION IN VASCULATURE

The preceding discussions imply that systems with an optimal dynamic response accurately measure blood pressure. However, although the pressure at the site of measurement is accurately reproduced, the pressure may already be distorted at the site where it is measured. The vascular tree is a complex oscillating system that acts to change the blood pressure at different areas of the body. Usually the pressures in peripheral arteries contain more high-frequency components than do central arteries; the systolic pressure is usually higher in peripheral arteries.[50, 51] However, there are exceptions. Multiple studies have demonstrated that the systolic pressure is often lower in peripheral arteries than it is in central arteries immediately after cardiopulmonary bypass.[50, 52, 53] Iatrogenic compression of an upstream artery can also cause a falsely low peripheral blood pressure, for example, during sternal retraction.[54, 55] In neonates the peripheral pressure correlates well with the central umbilical artery pressure.[56]

Three major factors cause the vascular tree to change peripheral blood pressure: oscillations, wave reflections, and phase shift. The effects of oscillation on pressure measurements have been discussed previously. The vascular tree acts like many oscillating segments connected in series.[57] The damping coefficient and resonant frequency of each segment are functions of the vascular tone and blood volume. Computer modeling demonstrates how changes in vascular compliance and resistance alter the radial artery pressure independent of central aortic pressure. Not only are the systolic, diastolic, and mean pressures affected, the entire shape of the pressure waveform is changed.[57] The dicrotic notch of the radial artery pressure waveform is an artifact;[51, 57] there is no correlation between it and the dicrotic notch of the central aortic pressure waveform.

The influence of wave reflection and phase shift on the resultant peripheral pressure is probably less than that of oscillations. Wave reflections occur when the pressure wave reaches the resistance arterioles.[58] At the arterioles, some of the energy of the pressure wave forces blood past the resistance, some of the energy is absorbed by the vessel, and the remainder is reflected. The tone of the arterioles influences the amount of energy reflected. Normal femoral vascular beds reflect 80% of the incident wave; reflections are decreased to almost zero after intra-arterial vasodilator injections.[58] The location of the pressure measurement site with respect to the wave reflection site and the elasticity of the arterial tree influence the effect of reflected waves on the measured pressure. Reflected waves coincident with the systolic part of the incident waveform cause an increased systolic pressure; those transmitted slower or detected a farther distance away contribute to a diastolic peak.[58]

Wave reflection is easily demonstrated. When pressure is applied with the finger over the intravascular portion of an arterial catheter, an increase in the systolic pressure is observed.[34] This is because a situation is created in which there is 100% energy reflection coincident with the systolic pressure. A similar situation occurs when there is thrombosis obstructing the artery distal to the site of measurement.[34]

Phase shift occurs because higher frequencies are transmitted at different rates than lower frequencies.[59] This distorts the peripheral pressure, causing the leading edge of the systolic pressure to be exaggerated.[14]

Because the pressure waveform in peripheral vessels is so different from that in the central aorta, care should be used in interpreting peripheral invasive blood pressures. The pressures in peripheral arteries differ from the aortic pressures to which the heart is exposed. Derived values that are meaningful when calculated from aortic pressures are meaningless when calculated from peripheral pressures. For example, the ratio of the area under the diastolic portion of the aortic pressure to the area under the systolic aortic pressure (DPTI/SPTI) has been used to predict the myocardial oxygen supply-to-demand ratio. This ratio is magnified by 25% when peripheral instead of aortic pressures are used.[60] Similarly, derivations of myocardial contractility and stroke volume from the peripheral blood pressure are inaccurate.[57]

Invasive blood pressure measurements are used clinically to judge the cardiovascular status of the patient. Extrapolations are made from arterial blood pressure to flow conditions in the brain, heart, kidney, and other organs, to the work of the heart, and even to cardiovascular volume status. The vascular tree and measurement devices modulate the pressure waveform in complex and dynamic ways. It is appropriate to use blood pressure trends to direct therapy; however, one should avoid placing too much confidence in the absolute value displayed on the blood pressure monitor.

APPENDIX

The oscillating behavior of the mechanical coupling system can be described by this differential equation

$$M \frac{d^2x}{dt^2} + R \frac{dx}{dt} + Ex = P(t) \qquad \text{Equation 3-1}$$

which describes the displacement of the fluid (x) for a given pressure waveform, P(t). M is the kinetic fluid mass of the system, R is the viscous damping, and E is the effective modulus of volume elasticity.

With zero damping, the system oscillates at the natural frequency (f_n) in response to a sudden input pressure

$$f_n = \frac{1}{2\pi} \sqrt{\frac{E}{M}} . \qquad \text{Equation 3-2}$$

E can be calculated from the physical characteristics of the transducer

$$E = A^2 \frac{\Delta P}{\Delta V} \qquad \text{Equation 3-3}$$

where A is the exposed area of the transducer sensing element and $\Delta P/\Delta V$ is the change in pressure required to cause a volume of fluid to enter the transducer.

M can also be related to the physical characteristics of the system

$$M = \frac{4}{3} \left(\frac{A}{a}\right)^2 la\rho + LA\rho \qquad \text{Equation 3-4}$$

where a is the cross-sectional area of the tubing, ρ is the density of the fluid, and L and l are the lengths of the columns of fluid in the transducer and tubing, respectively. Of course, the cross-sectional area is related to the diameter of the tubing, d, by,

$$a = \frac{\pi d^2}{4} . \qquad \text{Equation 3-5}$$

Thus the natural frequency is increased by decreasing the elasticity and surface area of the transducer sensing element, by using short wide-bore tubing, and by using a fluid of low density.

The damping coefficient (D) is the viscous damping of the system expressed as a fraction of the critical damping. The damping coefficient can be calculated from the physical characteristics of the system

$$D = \frac{16\eta}{d^3} \sqrt{\frac{3L}{\pi\rho E}} \qquad \text{Equation 3-6}$$

109

where η is the fluid viscosity. Note that damping is inversely related to the cube of the diameter of the tubing.

The natural frequency and damping coefficient can be calculated by measuring the output of the system for a step pressure input or an increasing frequency sine wave input. In either case, the damped resonant frequency (f_d) of the system is measured. The damped resonant frequency is related to the natural frequency by

$$f_d = f_n(1 - 2D^2). \qquad \text{Equation 3–7}$$

Using the step pressure method, the damping coefficient is calculated by measuring the amplitude ratio of two successive peaks (A_s) (see Fig. 3–7)

$$D = -\ln\left[\frac{A_s}{\sqrt{\pi^2 + (\ln A_s)^2}}\right]. \qquad \text{Equation 3–8}$$

Using the sine wave method, the damping coefficient is calculated by measuring the amplitude ratio of the test system to the reference system at the frequency of test system peak amplitude (Ar_{fd})

$$D = \sqrt{\frac{1 - \sqrt{1 - \frac{1}{(Ar_{fd})^2}}}{2}}. \qquad \text{Equation 3–9}$$

Once the damping coefficient and natural frequency have been determined, the response of the system to a step pressure input and an increasing frequency sine input can be predicted. The output of the system over time to a step pressure input is

$$P(t) = P_0 - \frac{P_0}{\sqrt{1 - D^2}} e^{-D2\pi f_n t} \sin\left(2\pi f_n t\sqrt{1 - D^2} + \sin^{-1}\sqrt{1 - D^2}\right). \qquad \text{Equation 3–10}$$

for $0 < D \leq 1$. The output-to-input amplitude ratio (A_r) for any sine wave input frequency (f) (Fig. 3–2) is

$$A_r = \frac{1}{\sqrt{\left(\frac{f}{f_n}\right)^4 + 2\left(\frac{f}{f_n}\right)^2 (2D^2 - 1) + 1}}. \qquad \text{Equation 3–11}$$

References

1. Fox F, Morrow DH, Kacher EJ, Gilleland TH: Laboratory evaluation of pressure transducer domes containing a diaphragm. Anesth Analg 1978; 57:67–76.
2. Disposable Pressure Transducers—Evaluation. Health Devices 1984; 13:268–290.
3. Barbieri LT, Kaplan JA: Artifactual hypotension secondary to intraoperative transducer failure. Anesth Analg 1983; 62:112–113.
4. Gordon VL, Welch JP, Carley D, et al: Zero stability of disposable and reusable pressure transducers. Med Instrum 1987; 21:87–91.
5. Sisko F, Hagerdal M, Neufeld GR: Artifactual hypotension without damping, a hazard of disposable diaphragm domes. Anesthesiology 1979; 51:263–264.
6. Milne B, Cervenko FW, Henderson MB, Westra PJ: Transducer offset by electrocautery resulting in erroneous blood pressure measurement. Can J Anaesth 1986; 33:234–236.
7. Fernandez-Cano F: A simple accurate technique for establishing zero reference levels for pressure measurements. (Letter.) Anesthesiology 1984; 61:478.
8. Geddes LA: The Direct and Indirect Measurement of Blood Pressure. Chicago: Year Book Medical, 1970; 1–69.
9. Gardner RM: Direct blood pressure measurement—dynamic response requirements. Anesthesiology 1981; 54:227–236.
10. Abrams JH, Olson ML, Marino JA, Cerra FB: Use of a needle valve variable resistor to improve invasive blood pressure monitoring. Crit Care Med 1984; 12:978–982.
11. Boutros A, Albert S: Effect of the dynamic response of transducer-tubing system on accuracy of direct blood pressure measurement in patients. Crit Care Med 1983; 11:124–127.
12. Shinozaki T, Deane RS, Mazuzan JE: The dynamic responses of liquid-filled catheter systems for direct measurements of blood pressure. Anesthesiology 1980; 53:498–504.
13. Hunziker P: Accuracy and dynamic response of disposable pressure transducer-tubing systems. Can J Anaesth 1987; 34:409–414.
14. Geddes LA, Baker LE: Principles of applied biomedical instrumentation. New York: John Wiley & Sons, 1968; 446–467.
15. Wade LD, Krejcie TC: The effect of air bubbles on the dynamic response of invasive pressure monitoring systems. (Abstract.) Anesth Analg 1983; 62:289.
16. Soule DT, Powner DJ: Air entrapment in pressure monitoring lines. Crit Care Med 1984; 12:520–522.
17. Lowenstein E, Little JW, Lo HH: Prevention of cerebral embolization from flushing radial-artery cannulas. N Engl J Med 1971; 285:1414–1415.
18. Gardner RM, Bond EL, Clark JS: Safety and efficacy of continuous flush systems for arterial and pulmonary artery catheters. Ann Thorac Surg 1977; 23:534–538.
19. Rushmer RF: Cardiovascular Dynamics. Philadelphia: WB Saunders, 1976; 36–75.
20. Lee APB: Biotechnological principles of monitoring. Int Anesthesiol Clin 1981; 19:197–207.
21. Maloy L, Gardner RM: Monitoring systemic arterial blood pressure: Strip chart recording versus digital display. Heart Lung 1986; 15:627–635.
22. Schmitt EA, Brantigan CO: Common artifacts of pulmonary artery and pulmonary artery wedge pressures: Recognition and interpretation. J Clin Monit 1986; 2:44–52.

23. Maran AG: Variables in pulmonary capillary wedge pressure: Variation with intrathoracic pressure, graphic and digital recorders. Crit Care Med 1980; 8:102–105.

24. Berryhill RE, Benumof JL, Rauscher LA: Pulmonary vascular pressure reading at the end of exhalation. Anesthesiology 1978; 49:365–368.

25. Riedinger MS, Shellock FG, Swan HJC: Reading pulmonary artery and pulmonary capillary wedge pressure waveforms with respiratory variations. Heart Lung 1981; 10:675–678.

26. Oden R, Mitchell MM, Benumof J: Detection of end-exhalation period by airway thermistor: An approach to automated pulmonary artery pressure measurement. Anesthesiology 1983; 467–471.

27. Ellis DM: Interpretation of beat-to-beat blood pressure values in the presence of ventilatory changes. J Clin Monit 1985; 1:65–70.

28. Mitchell MM, Meathe EA, Jones BR, et al: Accurate, automated, continuously displayed pulmonary artery pressure measurement. Anesthesiology 1987; 67:294–300.

29. Barr PO: Percutaneous puncture of the radial artery with a multi-purpose Teflon catheter for indwelling use. Acta Physiol Scand 1961; 51:343–347.

30. Seldinger SI: Catheter replacement of the needle in percutaneous arteriography. Acta Radiol 1953; 39:368–376.

31. Bedford RF: Radial arterial function following percutaneous cannulation with 18- and 20-gauge catheters. Anesthesiology 1977; 47:37–39.

32. Bedford RF: Wrist circumference predicts the risk of arterial occlusion after cannulation. Anesthesiology 1978; 48:377–378.

33. Weiss BM, Gattiker RI: Complications during and following radial artery cannulation: A prospective study. Intensive Care Med 1986; 12:424–428.

34. Kim JM, Arakawa K, Bliss J: Arterial cannulation: Factors in the development of occlusion. Anesth Analg 1975; 54:836–841.

35. Browning DH, Graves SA, van der Aa J: Catheters for arterial pressure monitoring in pediatrics. Anesthesiology 1981; 55:A131.

36. Goodwing SR, Graves SA, van der Aa J: Umbilical catheters and arterial blood pressure monitoring. J Clin Monit 1985; 1:227–231.

37. Davis FM, Stewart JM: Radial artery cannulation. Br J Anaesth 1980; 52:41–47.

38. Mortensen JD, Schaap RN: Further experience with an acute intra-arterial implantation screening test for thrombogenicity of intravascular catheters. Trans Am Soc Artif Intern Organs 1980; 26:284–288.

39. Downs JB, Chapman RL Jr, Hawkins IF Jr: Prolonged radial-artery catheterization. Arch Surg 1974; 108:671–673.

40. Bedford RF: Percutaneous radial-artery cannulation—increased safety using Teflon catheters. Anesthesiology 1975; 42:219–222.

41. Brown AE, Sweeney DB, Lumley J: Percutaneous radial artery cannulation. Anaesthesia 1969; 24:532–536.

42. Youngberg JA, Texidor M, Cantrell C, et al: Introducers and protective sleeves increase thrombogenicity of pulmonary artery catheters. Anesthesiology 1985; 63:A181.

43. Madsen JK, Garbarasch C, Nielsen PE: Endothelial injury of arteries following catheterization with polyethylene tubes: Experimental studies on rabbit aorta using the Seldinger technique. Cardiovasc Res 1979; 13:541–546.

44. Slogoff S, Keats AS, Arlund C: On the safety of radial artery cannulation. Anesthesiology 1983; 59:42–47.

45. Wesseling KH, Smith NT: Availability of intraarterial pressure waveforms from catheter-manometer systems during surgery. J Clin Monit 1985; 1:11–16.

46. Gardner RM, Warner HR, Toronto AF, Gaisford WD: Catheter-flush system for continuous monitoring of central arterial pulse waveform. J Appl Physiol 1970; 29:911–913.

47. Shin B, Ayella RJ, McAslan C: Pitfalls of Swan-Ganz catheterization. Crit Care Med 1977; 5:125–127.

48. Morray J, Todd S: A hazard of continuous flush systems for vascular pressure monitoring in infants. Anesthesiology 1983; 58:187–189.

49. Johnson DL: Invasive pressure monitoring: A modified system for pediatrics. Dimensions of Critical Care Nursing 1986; 5:93–96.

50. Gallagher JD, Moore RA, McNicholas KW, Jose AB: Comparison of radial and femoral arterial blood pressures in children after cardiopulmonary bypass. J Clin Monit 1985; 1:169–171.

51. Bruner JMR: Handbook of blood pressure monitoring. Littleton, MA: PSG, 1978.

52. Mohr R, Lavee J, Goor DA: Inaccuracy of radial artery pressure measurement after cardiac operations. J Thorac Cardiovasc Surg 1987; 94:286–290.

53. Stern DH, Gerson JI, Allen FB, Parker FB: Can we trust the direct radial artery pressure immediately following cardiopulmonary bypass? Anesthesiology 1985; 62:557–561.

54. Saka D, Lin TY, Oka Y: An unusual cause of false radial-artery blood-pressure readings during cardiopulmonary bypass. Anesthesiology 1975; 43:487–489.

55. Diamant M, Arkin DB: False radial-artery blood-pressure readings. Anesthesiology 1976; 44:273.

56. Butt WW, Whyte H: Blood pressure monitoring in neonates: Comparison of umbilical and peripheral artery catheter measurements. J Pediatr 1984; 105:630–632.

57. Schwid HA, Taylor LA, Smith NT: Computer model analysis of the radial artery pressure waveform. J Clin Monit 1987; 3:220–228.

58. O'Rourke MF, Yaginuma T: Wave reflection and the arterial pulse. Arch Intern Med 1984; 144:366–371.

59. Remington JW: Contour changes of the aortic pulse during propagation. Am J Physiol 1960; 199:331–334.

60. Reitan JA, Martucci RW, Levine NA: A computer evaluation of the ratio of the diastolic pressure-time index to the time-tension index from three arterial sites in dogs. J Clin Monit 1986; 2:95–99.

chapter four

Monitoring of Arterial Pressure

■ CAROL L. LAKE, M.D.

PHYSIOLOGY

Arterial Pulse

The arterial pulse results from the wave of vascular distention initiated by the impact of the stroke volume of each heartbeat ejected into a closed system. This wave begins at the base of the aorta and radiates throughout the arterial system. There is both a fast-moving (10 m/second) pressure wave and a slower (0.5 m/second) flow element in the pressure pulse.[1] The pulse waveform results from both the forward-propagating pressure wave and its reflectance back toward the heart from various portions of the circulation. The major source of wave reflection is the arteriole, which provides the majority of peripheral vascular resistance.[2] Peak aortic blood flow acceleration produces the initial rate of rise of the pressure pulse, whereas the ejection of ventricular volume fills out and sustains the pulse waveform.[1] The initial peak of the arterial waveform is the direct continuation of its initial upstroke. It is followed by a more or less well defined notch and subsequently by a second peak. The second peak falls away to the descending limb of the waveform, which often contains a dicrotic notch (Fig. 4–1).[1]

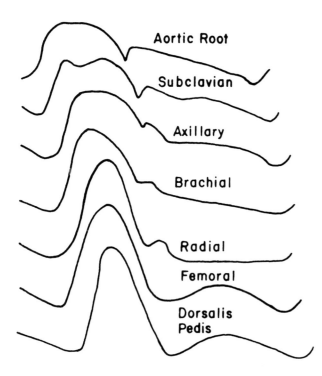

Figure 4-1. The pulse waveform changes as it moves from the central circulation to the periphery because of forward wave propagation and wave reflection. In the periphery, systolic pressure is higher, diastolic and mean pressures are lower, and the waveform displays greater amplitude. (From Bedford RF: Invasive blood pressure monitoring. *In* Blitt CD [ed]: Monitoring in Anesthesia and Critical Care Medicine. New York: Churchill Livingstone, 1985; 50. By permission.)

The height of the dicrotic notch is unrelated to systemic vascular resistance.[3] The lowest point of the waveform is diastolic pressure.

As it moves peripherally, the arterial waveform changes dramatically (Fig. 4-1). The pulse waveform becomes more peaked and increases in amplitude because the initial slope of the upstroke continues for a longer time. Systolic pressure is higher and diastolic pressure lower. The waveform has a greater amplitude, lower mean pressure, more pronounced diastolic wave, and a delayed foot.[2] Mean pressure must decrease peripherally in order for flow to continue, although it changes less than either systolic or diastolic pressure.

Pulse contour also varies with physiologic conditions. In the aged as compared with children, wave reflection occurs earlier in the cardiac cycle, increasing systolic and decreasing diastolic pressure. Although pulse pressure increases as the pressure wave travels from the central aorta to the periphery in young subjects, there may be little change in elderly persons because the loss of elasticity with age reduces the degree of waveform amplification. Pulse waveforms vary during atrial fibrillation, with beats having accentuated systolic peaks if they have a long systolic duration.

Pulse wave velocity depends upon vessel elasticity, with the more rapid transit in the least distensible arteries such as the aortic arch (3–5 m/second). The pulse wave travels about 7–10 m/second in large distensible arteries such as the subclavian artery. In small nondistensible peripheral arteries, wave velocity increases to 15–30 m/second. Thus, the aortic waveform precedes the brachial by 0.05 second. Shock decreases pulse wave velocity because of hypotension, peripheral vasoconstriction, and increased heart rate (decreases duration of systole).

Table 4–1. CAUSES OF INACCURACY IN NONINVASIVE MEASUREMENT OF ARTERIAL PRESSURE

Improper cuff size (too small or large)
Observer error (hearing of sounds, visualization of meter needle oscillation)
Improper cuff application to limb (too tight or loose)
Too rapid cuff deflation (difficulty assessing sound disappearance)
Too slow cuff deflation (venous congestion)
Uncalibrated gauges
Circulatory alterations (shock, vasoconstriction)

Blood Pressure

Blood pressure is the lateral pressure exerted on the walls of the vessels by blood contained within the vascular system. Mean arterial pressure is the product of systemic vascular resistance (in resistance units) and cardiac output. If the arterial waveform is normal, mean pressure is approximately one third of the difference between systolic and diastolic pressures. Mean arterial pressure probably best estimates total perfusion. Systolic pressures are particularly useful in the assessment of myocardial oxygen demand, whereas diastolic pressures relate to supply. Pulse pressure, the difference between systolic and diastolic pressures, narrows with hypovolemia or hemorrhage. Increased pulse pressure opens collapsed capillary beds.[4]

INDICATIONS FOR ARTERIAL PRESSURE MONITORING

Although arterial pressure was measured in an animal in 1731, indirect recordings in humans were not made until 1855, and in 1904, a committee at the Massachusetts General Hospital recommended *against* the adoption of routine blood pressure monitoring during surgery. Today it is essential to use either noninvasive or invasive methods to measure systolic, diastolic, mean, and pulse pressures during all surgical procedures.

Invasive methods are usually reserved for the critically ill, for situations in which hemodynamic compromise is likely as a result of the surgical procedure, or when multiple blood specimens are required. Because of measurement errors, the higher energy required to generate a Korotkoff sound than a direct signal, changes in arterial compliance, and differences in equipment, pressures measured by the various methods often fail to correlate (Table 4–1).[1, 4]

INDIRECT MEASUREMENT OF ARTERIAL PRESSURE

Methods used to measure arterial pressure indirectly include (1) palpation, (2) detection of Korotkoff sounds with an occlusive cuff (Riva Rocci method), (3) Doppler, (4) oscillotonometry using either a standard oscillo-tonometer or an automated method, and (5) plethysmography. The American Heart Association recommends standard procedures and methods to minimize errors in noninvasive determination of blood pressure (Table 4–1).[5]

Palpatory Method

The simplest method of blood pressure determination is by palpating the pulse while an occluding cuff is inflated to a pressure above expected arterial pressure and then gradually deflated until the first pulse is palpable. In infants, the "flush" method is a variation of the palpation method in which the pressure at which limb color returns is noted. The flush method is highly dependent upon speed of cuff deflation, peripheral perfusion, and operator skill.[6] Oscillations of aneroid manometers during cuff deflation provide very subjective endpoints of flicker oscillation start and flicker oscillation maximum that roughly estimate blood pressure.[1]

More sophisticated modifications of the palpatory method are observation of return of the pulse by Doppler, direct arterial cannula, or oximeter when cuff deflation is performed.[7] Measurements of arterial pressure by return of oximeter saturation correlate satisfactorily with Doppler-measured pressures only in infants under 1 year of age.[7] Likewise, augmentation of systolic pressure measured directly occurs with inflation and deflation of a cuff proximal to an arterial cannula.[1]

Korotkoff Method

Technique

The best-known method of noninvasive determination of arterial blood pressure is the auscultatory method using Korotkoff sounds.[8] Stethoscopes and sphygmomanometers are relatively inexpensive, readily available, and reasonably reliable and accurate. Korotkoff sounds are produced with resumption of blood flow through a previously collapsed artery. Inflation of the cuff to a pressure above the expected systolic pressure and gradual deflation permit identification of the maximum audible (systolic) and minimum audible (diastolic) pressures. The inflation device is a simple rubber bulb with a one-way valve that is reliable and easily replaced. Attached to the inflation device is the deflation valve, allowing deflation at 2–4 mmHg/heartbeat. Very rapid deflation decreases the resolution of the pressure determination.[9] Too rapid deflation underestimates systolic pressure and either overestimates or underestimates diastolic pressure, depending upon individual assessment of sound disappearance.[9] Too slow deflation allows venous congestion to occur, which attenuates the Korotkoff sounds near the diastolic pressure.[9]

Use of a transducer with a wide frequency response reveals the presence of three components to the pulse recorded during cuff deflation.[10] These components are K_1, K_2, and K_3, with K_2 a triphasic signal appearing at

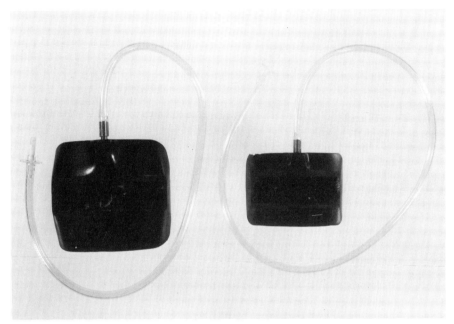

Figure 4–2. The Diasyst sensor for recording Korotkoff's sounds in the auscultatory method is a modified stethoscope bell in which the skin functions as the diaphragm. The smaller size is for use with infants and children.

systolic pressure and disappearing at diastolic pressure, roughly corresponding to the audible Korotkoff sounds. The K_2 signal is more accurate than standard auscultatory methods and is similar to intra-arterial measurements.[10]

Equipment

The pressure sensor in the sphygmomanometer is either a mercury manometer or an aneroid gauge. For accuracy, the mercury manometer must be vertical and have a clean, unbroken column of mercury resting at the zero point. The aneroid gauge is a simple device containing a diaphragm of hollow, corrugated metal disks, which expands or contracts as pressure changes. Diaphragmatic motion is transmitted to a rod connected to a gear operating a pointer. Aneroid gauges must be calibrated against mercury to ensure accuracy, since the diaphragm and transmitting parts malfunction over time or after mechanical or thermal shocks.

A stethoscope placed over the artery is the signal detector. Other sensors used to auscultate the pulse include the Diasyst (Fig. 4–2) piezoelectric microphones, and foil electret sensors. The Diasyst is a modified stethoscope bell in which the skin serves as the diaphragm.

Appropriate cuff size is essential to sphygmomanometric pressure measurements. The artery is collapsed by an occlusive cuff, which must be 20% larger than the diameter of the limb. If the cuff is too small, the systolic and diastolic pressures are artificially increased, and vice versa.[11] All air should

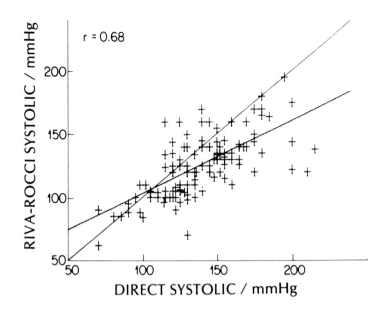

Figure 4–3. The comparison of direct intra-arterial systolic pressures with those measured by the Riva-Rocci auscultatory method shows considerable scatter (r = 0.68). (Modified from Bruner JMR, Krenis LJ, Kunsman JM, Sherman AP: Comparison of direct and indirect methods of measuring arterial blood pressure, part III. Med Instrum 1981; 15[2]:182–188, © by Association for the Advancement of Medical Instrumentation.)

be expelled from the cuff when it is applied. Snug application to the limb is essential, since loosely fitting cuffs falsely elevate pressure measurements.[9] Tight application of the cuff causes venous distention and patient discomfort.

Compared with intra-arterial pressures, auscultatory pressures differ by 1–7 torr systolic and 8–18 torr diastolic (Fig. 4–3).[12–16] Inaccuracies also result from the continuous nature of the task of blood pressure measurement in an operating room or intensive care unit. When the caregiver's attention is diverted to other tasks, recordings are not made, incorrect numbers are recorded, and the human ear is unattuned to the Korotkoff sounds.[17] Finally, changes in the circulation affect pressure measurement. Detection of the Korotkoff sounds is difficult when peripheral vasoconstriction or hypotension is present. When the patient is in shock, Korotkoff sounds are gradually attenuated until they are inaudible.[9] Auscultation is also impossible in the absence of pulsatile flow, as it is during cardiopulmonary bypass. In a hyperdynamic circulatory state, auscultatory sounds are present before the systolic pressure is reached, overestimating systolic and underestimating diastolic pressure.[9]

Doppler Methods

Technique

The Doppler effect is the principle by which frequency is changed when waveform energy is reflected from a moving surface. The pitch of the sound is proportional to the velocity of the reflective surface. The volume of the sound is proportional to the area of the moving reflective surface.[18] Blood pressure is measured with a 10-Hz ultrasound device, which is a radiofrequency oscillator driving a crystal in a transducer and receiver assembly

---

Table 4–2. DIFFERENCES BETWEEN KOROTKOFF AND DOPPLER
SOUNDS

---

1. Korotkoff sounds heard only during opening of artery; Doppler sounds heard during opening
   and closure.
2. Korotkoff sounds require vibratory motion in audible range; any arterial motion generates
   a Doppler signal.
3. Korotkoff sounds depend upon the properties of the resonant biologic system in which it
   operates; Doppler signals are altered by changes in operating frequency.

Data from Stegall HF, Kardon MB, Kemmerer WT: Indirect measurement of arterial blood
pressure by Doppler ultrasonic sphygmomanometry. J Appl Physiol 1968; 25:793.

that detects the difference in frequency between the transmitted and the
reflected ultrasound in response to occlusion and deflation of a proximally
located cuff.[18, 19]

A Doppler-shift signal is detected when blood flow causes movement
of the arterial wall at systolic pressure. No Doppler-shift signal is detected
while the artery is closed. Diastole is a soft sloshing sound, which is described by Stegall and coworkers but is difficult to detect clinically.[20] Differences between Korotkoff sounds and Doppler-shift sounds are listed in
Table 4–2.[20]

Doppler measurements of blood pressure are higher than those obtained
with palpation or flush techniques but lower than those obtained with direct
arterial pressures.[21] Figure 4–4 demonstrates the close correlation of Doppler pressures with intra-arterial measurements. One of the major advantages

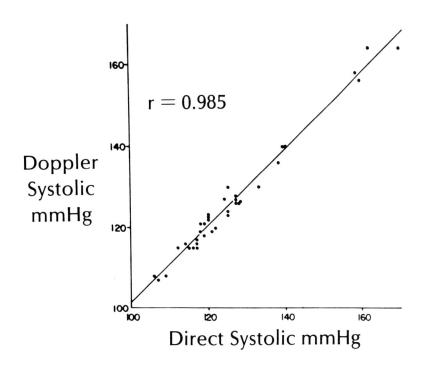

Figure 4–4. The relationship of systolic arterial pressures measured using a Doppler-shift signal is compared with direct intra-arterial measurements. Good correlation with an r = 0.985 is seen. (Modified from Stegall HF, Kardon MB, Kemmerer WT: Indirect measurement of arterial blood pressure by Doppler ultrasonic sphygmomanometry. J Appl Physiol 1968; 25:796.)

of the Doppler technique is the ability to measure pressure during low flow states, such as the mean arterial pressure during cardiopulmonary bypass and cardiopulmonary resuscitation.[22]

Semiautomated Doppler Method

A semiautomated device using the Doppler principle is the Arteriosonde (Kontron, Everett, MA). Initial cuff inflation pressure is set manually in this equipment. A deflation valve is attached to the inflation bulb, permitting controlled, continuous decreases in pressure. A 2-Hz ultrasound beam (the signal sensor, chosen because arterial walls reflect that frequency) is directed at the brachial artery while the cuff is deflated at adjustable intervals between 2 and 5 mmHg/second. At arterial opening the compressed arterial wall produces a Doppler frequency shift of about 135 Hz. The pressure sensor is an aneroid gauge. The Arteriosonde accurately measures pressures in most clinical situations, including during hypotensive techniques.[23] At low pressures, ultrasound and palpatory techniques are more accurate than auscultatory methods.[23-25] As with the auscultatory method, appropriate cuff size is essential for accurate pressure measurement. Speed of cuff deflation affects the accuracy of pressure determination as discussed previously (Korotkoff method). Disadvantages of the Arteriosonde include the susceptibility to motion and electrocautery, the requirement for accurate placement over the artery, and the need to use a coupling gel.[18]

Oscillometric Method

Standard Technique

Von Recklinghausen first described the oscillotonometer in 1931, although similar devices had been used earlier in infants.[26] The oscillotonometer consists of a double-cuff system, with the proximal cuff occluding the artery while the distal cuff senses the onset of arterial pulsation. Systolic and diastolic pressures are obtained by noting the oscillation of a mercury column or an aneroid manometer. Slow deflation of the cuff is essential for accurate measurement of systolic pressure,[27] since there is considerable observer variation in the detection of needle oscillation.[27] Fast rates of deflation produce a greater decrease in cuff pressure between heartbeats, making the change in oscillation of the needle more apparent.

Oscillometry is the only noninvasive method that directly estimates mean blood pressure. The minimum occlusive pressure at which maximum oscillation occurs is the mean arterial pressure. Diastolic measurements, regardless of deflation rate, are quite inaccurate.[27] The pressure waves do not change dramatically but only decrease in amplitude, making recognition of a diastolic endpoint impossible. Several cardiac cycles are required for oscillotonometric determination of arterial blood pressure because the measurement depends upon the heart rate, blood pressure, initial cuff inflation pressure, and rate of cuff deflation.[18]

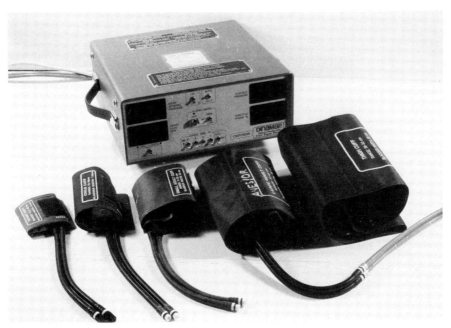

Figure 4–5. The Dinamap is an automated noninvasive device for measurement of arterial blood pressure by the oscillometric technique. Cuffs suitable for use in infants, children, and adults (arm or thigh) are shown. A switch alters the algorithm controlling cuff inflation pressures to ranges suitable for infants and adults.

Automated Technique

Automated techniques have the advantages of independence from Korotkoff sounds, greater accuracy, and limited operator intervention.

In the automated oscillometric technique using the Dinamap (*d*evice for *i*ndirect *n*oninvasive *a*utomatic *m*ean *a*rterial *p*ressure; Critikon, Tampa, FL), the cuff is both actuator and transducer (Fig. 4–5). An electric pump generates pressure to inflate the single-bladder cuff, initially to a pressure above systolic pressure. A solenoid valve incrementally deflates the cuff. The pressure-sensing function is performed by a pressure transducer enclosed within the instrument case. The cuff has two tubes, one to inflate the cuff from a pump and the other to transmit the sensed pressure to the pressure transducer within the instrument. A microprocessor controls the cuff inflation-deflation sequence. The cuff itself is the signal sensor that responds to pressure oscillations in the limb. Specific placement of the cuff over an artery is unnecessary. However, an appropriately sized cuff for the extremity must be used, as described previously.

Two cardiac cycles are compared at each increment if "noise" conditions are low. With increased "noise" (patient or cuff movement), inflation is held until successive comparative beats occur. Under these conditions, measurement becomes time-dependent, although normally the entire sequence from measurement to display is 20 – 45 seconds.[17] The averaged pairs of oscillations and the corresponding cuff pressures are stored and analyzed electronically to determine the systolic, diastolic, and mean pressures. Sys-

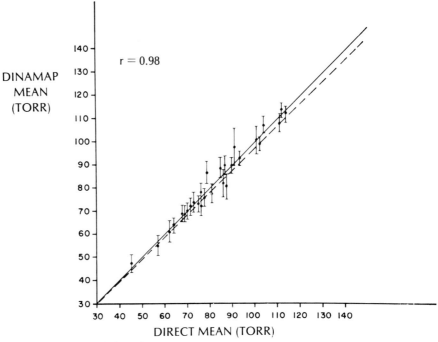

Figure 4–6. The correlation of direct intra-arterial measurement of mean arterial pressures with those measured by Dinamap shows a correlation coefficient of 0.98. (Modified from Ramsey M III: Noninvasive automatic determination of mean arterial pressure. Med Biol Eng Comput 1979; 17:11–18.)

tolic pressures correspond to the rapid increase in the amplitude of oscillation, and diastolic to the rapid decrease in oscillation after maximum oscillation. The lowest cuff pressure at which maximum oscillation occurs is the mean arterial pressure.[28] The heart rate is the median of those obtained by analysis of all pressure pulses in a given determination.

Problems with Measurement. The accuracy of the automated oscillometric technique to measure pressures similar to those pressures measured directly in the aorta or a peripheral artery has been documented (Fig. 4–6).[28–31] Under ideal conditions, automated noninvasive methods are accurate to ± 10 mmHg. Other investigators[32] noted good correlations only for systolic pressures. Diastolic pressures are 8–13 mmHg higher when measured by Dinamap as compared with those obtained by direct arterial measurements.[31] Oscillometric measurements are also accurate in premature or term infants.[33, 34] However, noninvasive devices cannot replace direct arterial measurements when substantial beat-to-beat variability in the pressure is present.[29] Pressure measurement with a Dinamap is difficult during patient movement because the instrument considers the movement a large oscillation. Failure to evacuate air from the cuff prior to application to a vasoconstricted patient results in attenuation of oscillations by the residual air volume. Although mean arterial pressure is measured under these conditions, systolic and diastolic pressures are usually not.[9]

Plethysmography

Technique

Peñaz used the principle of unloading of the arterial wall to measure a calibrated pressure waveform in the finger.[35] Further modification of the cuff and other components by Wesseling and associates led to the currently available device known as the Finapres (*fin*ger *a*rterial *pres*sure; Ohmeda, Englewood, CO).[36, 37] The Finapres consists of a small finger cuff containing an infrared photoplethysmograph volume transducer and an inflatable bladder. The photoplethysmograph diode and the light detector are positioned on the medial and lateral aspects of the finger near the digital arteries to record finger volume. A servo control system regulates the pressure applied by the cuff to the arterial wall. As the arterial wall expands with an increase in blood pressure, the volume differential is measured by the transducer. In response to the increasing volume, cuff pressure increases until original arterial blood volume and pressure are restored (the so-called closed-loop or servo mode of operation). The external pressure of the cuff closely matches the arterial pressure of the finger so that the external pressure is a function of arterial blood pressure. Both the arterial waveform and pressures are displayed.

Problems with Measurement

The accuracy of this device compared with conventional Riva Rocci technique,[37] direct brachial,[38] or radial arterial pressure[39] has been documented. Recent evidence shows that pressures measured in the thumb correlate with intra-arterial pressure better than do those from other digits.[40] Changes in hemoglobin saturation affect the transmission of light to the device but not the pressure readings.[40]

Safety with long-term use has been confirmed, although the pressure in the cuff is at or near mean arterial pressure for prolonged periods of time.[41] Pressures are above venous levels, resulting in slight swelling of the finger.[42] Capillary oxygen tension decreases significantly within 2.5 minutes of cuff inflation, and oxygen saturation determined by oximetry demonstrates desaturation.[42] Numbness of the finger after 60 minutes of monitoring has been noted but resolved within 1 minute of discontinuation.[42] The possibility of digital nerve injury must be considered. Whether the interposition of periods without monitoring alters neural ischemia is unclear, since capillary Po_2 is actually reduced by rest periods.[42]

Arterial spasm may preclude measurements in some patients, particularly those with cardiopulmonary bypass or other circulatory stresses (administration of phenylephrine hydrochloride, peripheral vasoconstriction).[40, 41] During peripheral vasoconstriction, systolic pressures measured with Finapres were 7 mmHg above and diastolic and mean pressures 9 mmHg below those of the upper arm.[43]

Risks of Noninvasive Measurements

Despite their noninvasive nature, cuff techniques for blood pressure measurement are not without risk. With electrically operated devices, the possibility of shock hazards always exists. Failure of cuff deflation permits increasing venous congestion as well as lack of arterial perfusion, causing tissue ischemia and nerve damage. Ulnar nerve damage has been reported when the cuff is applied too distally on the arm, causing direct compression of the ulnar artery in the ulnar groove by the edge of the cuff.[44] Intravenous injection of an irritating substance during cuff inflation might cause tissue damage owing to a locally increased concentration. Accidental injection of succinylcholine chloride into a vein distal to the inflated cuff of an automated device during a rapid-sequence anesthetic induction may preclude timely intubation in a patient with a full stomach.

INVASIVE MEASUREMENT OF BLOOD PRESSURE

Although indirect measurements of blood pressure by palpation, oscillometry, and auscultation demonstrate close agreement, the values are always lower than directly measured pressures (underestimating systolic and overestimating diastolic pressure).[1, 45] Direct techniques measure arterial pressure, whereas indirect methods often depend upon detection of blood flow beneath an occlusive cuff.[1]

With the exception of the plethysmographic technique, noninvasive methods of pressure determination usually do not display an arterial pressure waveform. Arterial pressure waveforms provide a qualitative approximation of alterations in the circulation. The area beneath the curve is affected by myocardial performance, peripheral vascular resistance, and stroke volume.

Indwelling arterial cannulas are utilized in all procedures requiring cardiopulmonary bypass, most major vascular surgery, intrathoracic procedures, and other critically ill patients (adult respiratory distress syndrome, treatment with vasodilator drugs, or positive end-expiratory pressure). Single uncomplicated radial arterial punctures produce no changes in blood flow.[46] However, if more than 3–4 arterial blood specimens are required daily, a indwelling arterial catheter should be inserted.[47]

Technique of Cannulation

A technique for percutaneous cannulation of an artery was first reported by Peterson and colleagues in 1949.[48] Cannulation techniques are similar in all sites (Fig. 4–7). The technique described here is specific to the radial artery, and pertinent details for other sites are discussed elsewhere in this chapter.

Adequate preparation is essential for successful arterial cannulation. The patient's arm should be comfortably supported on an armrest. Good lighting over the site is helpful, and the operator should be seated. The patient's wrist should be dorsiflexed over a folded towel or other support. The course of the artery is traced on the skin. Povidone-iodine skin preparation is performed without removal of the mark. Local anesthesia is infil-

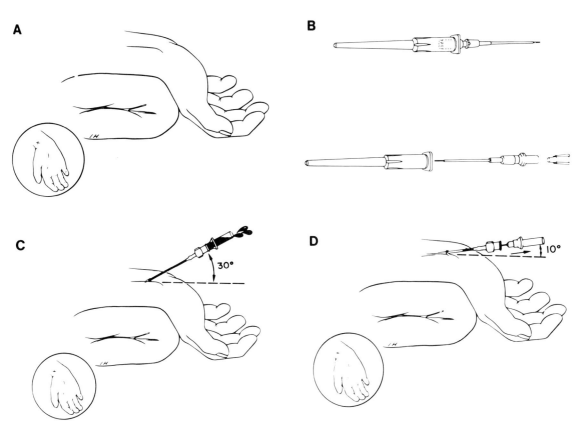

Figure 4–7. The technique of cannulation of a peripheral artery is similar for almost all arteries. The direct technique for the radial artery is demonstrated. *A*, Proper hand position is demonstrated with the hand dorsiflexed over a small roll. *B*, The technique of placing the catheter cover over the end of the catheter is shown. This technique allows visualization of free flow of blood without environmental contamination. (Personal communication, KR Grosslight, MD.) *C*, The catheter is inserted at a 30–40-degree angle to the plane of the wrist until spurting blood flow is obtained. *D*, The angle of the catheter is reduced to 10° while the plastic catheter is advanced into the artery. (From Lake CL: Cardiovascular Anesthesia. © 1985 Springer-Verlag New York; 54. With permission.)

trated into the area over the artery, taking care not to puncture the artery or to obliterate its pulsation. A small nick with a 20-gauge needle is made in the skin over the anticipated puncture site to prevent catheter damage. Through the skin nick, a 20-gauge catheter is introduced at an angle of 30° to the skin.[49] Twenty-two-gauge catheters are commonly used in children under the age of 5 years. Some workers prefer tapered catheters in small infants because they are less flexible and pass easily into the artery, the snugly fitted catheter and stylet make puncture easier, and the transparency of the catheter makes arterial entry apparent during the puncture (Fig. 4–8).[50]

Three techniques for arterial cannulation are commonly used: direct cannulation, Seldinger technique, and transfixion technique. In the direct technique, the cannula is advanced until arterial pulsation is transmitted to the cannula. The artery is then pierced, the angle of the cannula to the skin is reduced to 10°, and the cannula is advanced from the needle into the artery (see Fig. 4–7). A pressure transducer is then connected to verify the arterial

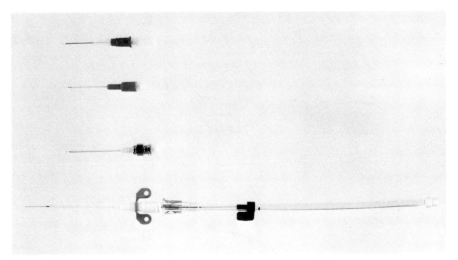

Figure 4–8. Various types of arterial catheters are commonly used. Twenty-two-gauge catheters (*top*), either tapered or straight, are used in infants and children under the age of 5 years. In adults, 20-gauge catheters are placed either directly or using a wire guide (*bottom*).

waveform. Aspiration of blood to ensure free flow should be performed. The Seldinger technique requires passage of a guidewire through the cannula after arterial puncture, followed by advancement of the cannula over the guidewire (Fig. 4–8 [bottom]; and see Chapter 5). In the transfixion method, the posterior wall of the artery is punctured before the needle is withdrawn from the cannula. The cannula is slowly withdrawn until free-flowing blood is obtained. At that point, the cannula is advanced into the vessel lumen and connected to a pressure transducer (see Chapter 3). Success rates for cannulation at the initial radial artery site have been reported at 92%.[51]

Fixation of the catheter to the skin with the Venigard system or tape to prevent accidental removal is essential. Iodophor ointment is applied to the puncture site after successful cannulation. The support used to dorsiflex the wrist is removed to prevent median nerve damage.

Difficult Arterial Cannulation

If passage of the catheter-needle unit to a distance of 2 cm beneath the skin fails to obtain freely spurting blood flow, the stylet should be removed and the catheter slowly withdrawn. Inadvertent penetration of the posterior wall of the artery is common and often recognized only during withdrawal. Once free flow is obtained, an attempt to advance the catheter should be made.

If no blood flow is obtained on withdrawal, the catheter-needle unit should be reassembled, the needle flushed with heparinized saline solution, and another attempt made after confirming the palpable course of the artery. The number of attempts should be limited in order to reduce trauma to the artery. Catheters that give a grating sensation on passage through tissue or artery should be removed since the catheter tip may be damaged, causing intimal arterial injury.[52] Doppler transducers have been used to guide cannulation of weakly palpable arteries or those in infants.[53-55] Placement of a pulse oximeter distal to the proposed cannulation site and repeated palpation over the area determine the arterial course by observation of cessation of the distal pulse.[56] This technique is particularly useful in obese patients.

Flushing of an intra-arterial catheter causes one of two responses: a localized area of a few square centimeters of intense blanching or a generalized transient area of slight pallor (the preferable response).[57] Careful adjustment of the position of the catheter tip usually converts response 1 to response 2, which suggests less interference with local cutaneous circulation by the flushing solution.

Arterial Cannulation Sites

Cannulation of the arterial circulation is performed most commonly in the radial artery. Other sites that have been safely used include the femoral, dorsalis pedis, posterior tibial, brachial, axillary, ulnar, dorsal radial, superficial temporal, internal mammary, and umbilical arteries (Fig. 4–9).[58-67]

Radial

Evaluation of Collateral Flow. Both radial arteries should be assessed to determine equality of pulsation prior to cannulation. In patients with generalized arteriosclerosis, determination of blood pressure in both arms prevents inadvertent cannulation of a radial artery distal to an innominate or subclavian stenosis. Likewise, cannulation distal to a brachial or axillary cannulation site (as after angiography) should be avoided because pulse volume is often diminished.

In almost 90% of humans, the ulnar artery provides most of the arterial perfusion to the hand.[68] However, the arterial anatomy of the hand is quite variable.[69] The adequacy of ulnar collateral flow is assessed using Allen's test. Allen's test determines the dominant vessel supplying the hand. Whenever possible, the nondominant vessel should be cannulated. To perform Allen's test, the examiner compresses both radial and ulnar arteries while the patient flexes and extends his or her fingers four or five times to blanch the hand. If the palmar arterial arch is intact, release of either artery permits rapid restoration of color to the hand (within 5–7 seconds).[69]

However, if the arterial circulation is compromised, release of the occluded artery prevents the normal reactive hyperemia. In addition to observation of reflow, Husum and Berthelsen suggest measurement of the blood pressure in the thumb, since the arterial pressure in the thumb can be inadequate in the presence of an Allen test demonstrating adequate collateral flow.[70] Chronic occlusion of both radial and ulnar arteries with the only blood supply through numerous palmar collaterals has been reported.[71] Some investigators suggest that arterial occlusion be performed where the tip of the arterial cannula will lie.[72] Such a technique avoids subsequent occlusion of aberrant arteries supplying the palmar arterial arch.[72] In one series, almost 22% of hands had an incomplete palmar arch.[73]

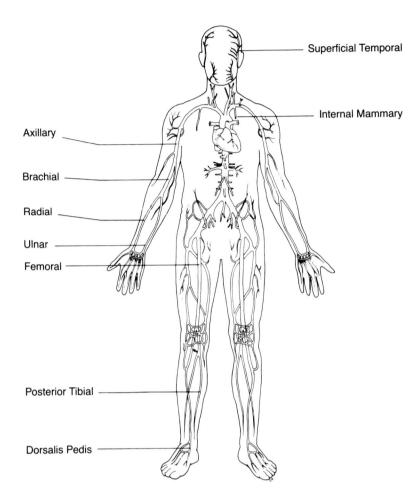

Figure 4–9. Sites for cannulation of the systemic arterial circulation. Although the most common location for catheterization is the radial artery, axillary, brachial, femoral, dorsalis pedis, superficial temporal, and other sites are used when radial collateral circulation is inadequate or radial pressures may be erroneous. Not demonstrated is the umbilical artery cannulation site.

In anesthetized patients, Allen's test is modified by having an assistant passively clench the fist while the radial and ulnar arteries are compressed. Alternatively, the pulse in a finger is checked using a Doppler or pulse oximeter during radial and ulnar compression to document patency of the transpalmar arch.[74,75] The time for return of a pulse oximeter reading with release of ulnar compression should be less than 15 seconds.[76]

Wide separation or marked hyperextension of the fingers permits the palmar fascia to occlude the transpalmar arch so that flow appears inadequate.[77, 78] Another cause of apparently inadequate collateral flow is arterial spasm in the ulnar artery caused by compression of the radial artery.[71]

The necessity for performance of Allen's test has been questioned by Slogoff and colleagues.[79] They cannulated the radial artery in 16 patients who required longer than 15 seconds for refill without ischemic damage. Another large series in which Allen's test was routinely used to determine the cannulation site demonstrated a similar incidence of ischemic complications and flow abnormalities after decannulation as seen in the series of Slogoff and colleagues.[80] Conversely, hand ischemia requiring amputation has been reported in the presence of adequate collateral circulation demonstrated by Allen's test.[81] However, there has not been a large prospective study performing radial arterial cannulation in patients without ulnar pulses or flow except through the cannulated radial artery.

Ulnar

The technique and complications of ulnar cannulation are similar to those of the radial artery, described previously. However, it should be noted that the ulnar artery is usually the primary source of blood flow in the hand.

Brachial

Cannulation of the brachial artery is performed with either an 18- or 20-gauge catheter at the elbow where it lies medial to the biceps tendon. Although one of the major risks is median nerve damage because the nerve lies just medial to the artery at the elbow,[82] the safety of brachial cannulation in cardiac surgical patients has been documented.[58, 66, 83] Another risk is thrombosis, necessitating surgical exploration. Brachial arterial pressures are usually similar to femoral pressures.[84]

Axillary

Axillary arterial catheters are inserted at the junction of the pectoralis major with the deltoid muscle. The patient's arm is placed as for the axillary approach to the brachial plexus.[58, 66] The Seldinger technique (see Chapter 5) is recommended to place an 18- or 20-gauge 12–15-cm catheter.[67] The left axillary artery is preferentially used to minimize the possibility of cerebral air embolism during flushing of the catheter. Axillary arterial cannulation is a useful option in patients with severe peripheral vascular disease.[85] Concomitant sympathetic blockade of the upper extremity using continuous brachial plexus blockade further protects the arm by increasing its blood flow.[85]

Femoral

The femoral artery is cannulated directly in adults with an 18-gauge catheter, 5–15 cm in length. Alternatively, the Seldinger technique of passing a wire through a 20-gauge 2–3 cm catheter is used to cannulate the vessel with a larger, longer catheter.

Minor complications such as local hemorrhage or ecchymoses are occasionally seen.[58] Disadvantages of the femoral approach are its position within the surgical field during cardiovascular surgery and its temporary discontinuation if an intra-aortic balloon must be placed in the same artery. Massive retroperitoneal hematoma has been reported after unsuccessful femoral cannulation.[86]

In children, 18- or 20-gauge 5–10-cm catheters are often more easily placed in the femoral than in the radial arteries. However, cannulation of the femoral artery is often avoided in children because of its proximity to the peritoneum, the risk of hip capsule puncture, and the potential for decreased limb growth with thrombosis. In the series reported by Glenski and coworkers, femoral catheterization was performed in 151 children undergoing cardiac surgery, with only a 3.6% failure rate.[87] Decreased limb perfusion occurred in 25% of neonates, but the overall rate was only 6 in 165 catheterizations. No permanent complications were noted. Rosenthal and colleagues noted no reduction in leg growth after femoral cannulation.[88]

Dorsalis Pedis

Evaluation of Collateral Flow. The major arterial supply to the foot consists of the anterior tibial, posterior tibial, and peroneal arteries. Anterior and posterior tibial arteries are terminal branches of the popliteal artery. The posterior tibial artery divides near the medial malleolus to form the lateral and medial plantar arteries. In the foot, the anterior tibial artery continues as the dorsalis pedis artery, which divides to form the deep plantar and first dorsal metatarsal arteries. A plantar arterial arch is formed by the connections between the deep and the lateral plantar arteries. However, the pedal circulatory pattern is quite variable.[89, 90]

Collateral circulation via the posterior tibial artery is evaluated by occlusion of the dorsalis pedis and compression of the great toenail. Adequate flow via the lateral plantar artery is present if flushing of the toe occurs. An alternative method suggested by Youngberg and Miller is compression of both dorsalis pedis and posterior tibial arteries together with compression of great and second toes.[91] Adequate collateral flow is verified by both flushing of the toes and a Doppler probe on the dorsalis pedis when posterior tibial compression is released. Flow can also be evaluated by pulse plethysmography.[90]

Cannulation should not be performed unless circulation is restored within 10 seconds of posterior tibial release.[92] Palm and Husum also recommend measurement of great toe pressure with compression of the dorsalis pedis. In 99 of 200 feet studied, blood pressure in the great toe decreased to 44% of control with dorsalis pedis compression.[92]

Technique of Cannulation. A 20-gauge catheter is used to cannulate the artery as it lies subcutaneously on the dorsum of the foot, parallel and lateral to the extensor hallucis longus tendon.[93] An alternative site is the anterior peroneal artery, which is cannulated just medial and above the anterior aspect of the lateral malleolus.[62]

Problems and Complications. Systolic and pulse pressures in the dorsalis pedis artery are higher than either the brachial or the radial pressures (systolic and pulse). However, mean arterial and diastolic pressures are higher in the radial than in the dorsalis pedis artery. Severe peripheral vascular disease often causes the dorsalis pedis to be nonpalpable or have inadequate collateral flow. The incidence of thrombosis ranges from 6.7% to 25%.[65, 91] Arterial recannulation occurs but often fails to restore the vessel to its previous condition.[65]

Superficial Temporal

The temporal artery is a branch of the external carotid artery, which passes anterior to the tragus of the ear. Cannulation of the superficial temporal artery is performed by first delineating the often variable arterial course with a Doppler probe.[63] Arterial puncture is performed at the superior edge of the helix of the ear,[64] either percutaneously or through a 0.3–2-cm incision (depending upon the patient's size) with the catheter-needle device in a bevel-down position.[63] The bevel-down position prevents posterior arterial perforation. Proper positioning of the catheter tip is critical. An optimal location is in the external carotid at the junction with the external maxillary artery.[63, 64] The superficial temporal artery is often quite tortuous and difficult to cannulate. Other risks include thrombosis, with scalp ischemia and catheter malposition permitting emboli to reach the cerebral circulation via the internal carotid artery. Because of the site, it is often difficult to secure the catheter so it does not become dislodged.[64]

Internal Mammary

Occasionally the internal mammary artery is cannulated in children during intrathoracic procedures such as Blalock-Taussig shunts or banding of the pulmonary artery. An occluding suture is placed around the artery to prevent bleeding when the catheter is removed. Direct cannulation of the artery is performed using PE50 polyethylene tubing.[61]

Umbilical

Technique. The umbilical arteries branch from the internal iliac arteries, crossing over the ureters and passing inferiorly on either side of the dome of the bladder to course in the anterior abdominal wall to the umbilicus. Either a percutaneous or a cutdown technique is used to cannulate the umbilical artery of infants soon after birth. With the percutaneous method, a 16-gauge short catheter is initially inserted; through this a longer 3.5- or 5-F catheter is guided into the aorta. The cutdown method requires placement of a suture at the base of the umbilicus prior to cutting the umbilical cord several millimeters above the skin. An umbilical artery is identified and a probe inserted to dilate the vessel prior to passage of the catheter (a 3.5- or 5-F feeding tube or catheter). Spasm at the junction of hypogastric and iliac arteries is the most common cause for failure to catheterize the umbilical artery.[94] After the catheter is successfully inserted, the suture at the umbilical base is tied around the catheter.

Optimal locations for the catheter tip are just above bifurcation,[95] below the inferior mesenteric artery, or the middorsal aorta above the diaphragm. Undesirable locations include the celiac plexus or renal or superior mesenteric arteries (Fig. 4–10).[60]

Complications of umbilical arterial cannulation include abdominal organ ischemia, if the catheter becomes dislodged into specific intra-abdominal vessels; aortic thrombosis; embolism; lower extremity ischemia secondary to arterial vasospasm; and vascular perforation causing hemorrhage.[60, 96, 97] Factors contributing to complications include protracted catheter use and repeated manipulation. Methods to avoid complications include radiographic confirmation of catheter tip location, avoidance of catheter manipulation,

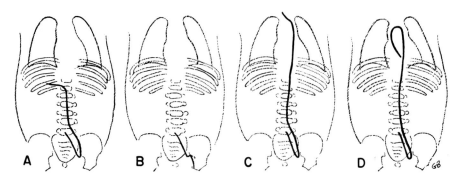

Figure 4–10. Abnormal locations of umbilical arterial catheters are demonstrated. *A*, The tip of the catheter has been displaced into one of the abdominal vessels, hepatic, superior mesenteric, or renal. *B*, The catheter coursed downward to lie in the external iliac artery. *C*, Excessive passage of the catheter so that its tip is in carotid or innominate arteries. *D*, The excessive length of catheter inserted results in passage around the aortic arch, across the aortic valve, and into the left ventricle. (From Paster SB, Middleton P: Roentgenographic evaluation of umbilical artery and vein catheters. JAMA 1975; 231:742–746. Copyright 1975, American Medical Association. With permission.)

use of nonthrombogenic catheters, and timely removal of catheters when no longer indicated.[98]

Indications for Removal of Intra-arterial Catheters

Arterial cannulas can remain for 3 or more days in the absence of infection, arterial insufficiency, or hematoma. However, after prolonged cannulation they become nonfunctional because of thrombus accumulation. Feeley described a technique for thrombectomy if continued arterial pressure monitoring is required.[98]

Technique for Removal of Intra-arterial Catheters

Bedford suggested that radial arterial cannulas be removed with continuous aspiration during proximal and distal arterial occlusion.[99] Thrombotic material, potentially contributing to arterial occlusion, might be removed from other cannulation sites as well. After decannulation, compression is applied for 10 minutes or longer to prevent formation of hematoma (Fig. 4–11).

Complications

Although most of the studies of complications concern radial artery cannulation, complications such as hematomas, decreased peripheral circulation distal to the cannula site, infection, vasospasm, thrombosis, embolism, aneurysm formation, and infection are applicable to all sites. Em-

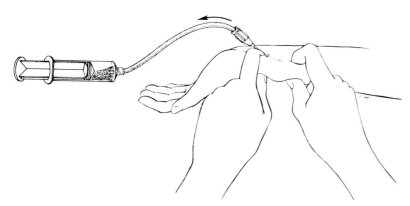

Figure 4–11. The technique recommended by Bedford for removal of arterial cannulas includes compression of the artery proximal and distal to the catheter site while the catheter is removed during continuous aspiration. This method allows aspiration of thrombotic material surrounding the catheter.[99]

bolism due to clots or air flushed into the cerebral circulation is most likely in radial, brachial, axillary, and temporal cannulation sites. From the radial artery, 3–12 ml of flushing solution in adults and 0.3–5 ml in children produce retrograde flow.[100–102] Chang and associates document passage of air from a radial arterial cannula into the vertebral artery of an animal.[101] The volume of flush solution necessary to reach the central circulation correlates well with the patient's height.[100] Another source of emboli are bubbles in the constant infusion system, particularly with rapid flushing or the use of a microdrip chamber.[103, 104]

Hemorrhage resulting from inadvertent disconnection of an arterial catheter from the transducer tubing is potentially lethal since about 500 ml of blood/minute is lost if cardiac output is normal.[47] Ischemic complications may be more likely in patients with severe atherosclerosis, diabetes, low cardiac output, and peripheral vasoconstriction, particularly from vasoactive drugs.

Reported complications specific to the radial artery include pseudo-aneurysm,[105] expanding aneurysm,[106] forearm amputation in patients with type V hyperlipoproteinemia,[107] vasospasm,[108] ecchymoses and induration of the skin,[109, 110] arteriovenous fistula, and median and radial nerve injuries (from compression by hematomas). Neural compression is more common after arterial punctures than with indwelling catheters.[111]

Thrombosis

Thrombosis of the radial artery is a common complication occurring in 34% of patients when 18-gauge catheters are used and decreasing to 8% with use of 20-gauge catheters (Figs. 4–12 and 4–13).[110, 112] During ulnar compression a decrease in the arterial pressure to 10 mmHg or less in the thumb is diagnostic of occlusion.[113] Other factors contributing to an increased incidence of thrombosis include use of polypropylene rather than polytef (Tef-

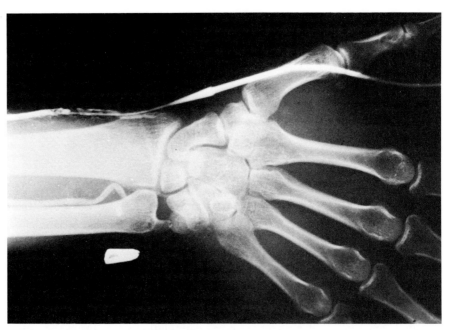

Figure 4–12. Radial artery occlusion after cannulation with a tapered polypropylene catheter is demonstrated in this arteriogram performed through the catheter. There is no antegrade flow around or beyond the catheter, only retrograde flow toward the brachial artery. (From Bedford RF: Percutaneous radial-artery cannulation. Increased safety using Teflon catheters. Anesthesiology 1975; 42:221. With permission.)

lon) catheters,[114] use of tapered rather than straight catheters,[115] increased duration of cannulation,[109] increased proportion of vessel lumen occupied by catheter,[112] and smaller wrist circumference (47% incidence of occlusion with wrist circumferences less than 18 cm versus 21% with larger wrists (Figs. 4–14 and 4–15).[116] In contrast to Bedford's study in adults,[49] Marshall and colleagues noted no increased incidence of thrombosis with use of tapered polypropylene 20- or 22-gauge catheters in children.[50] However, thrombosis is unaffected by the method of cannulation (perforation of the posterior arterial wall versus nonperforation).[117] Pretreatment with aspirin prior to cannulation decreases the incidence of thrombosis from 39% to 13%.[118] This effect is particularly prominent in women (smaller arteries) in whom the incidence of thrombosis was decreased from 63% to 22%.[118] Thrombosis can be delayed for several days after decannulation (Table 4–3).[109] Recanalization eventually occurs after occlusion but requires an average of 13 days (Fig. 4–16).[57, 119]

The etiology of ischemia of the hand in the presence of a radial artery catheter can be difficult to determine.[120] Proximal pulses should be examined, and, if they are absent, an arteriogram should be performed to eliminate embolism. Vessel occlusion distal to an arterial cannula has been demonstrated by Kim and coworkers.[119] The presence or absence of a change in the arterial waveform during occlusion of the cannulated artery distal to the puncture site is noted. When arterial flow is obstructed to a patent artery, the arterial pressure increases and the configuration of the waveform changes

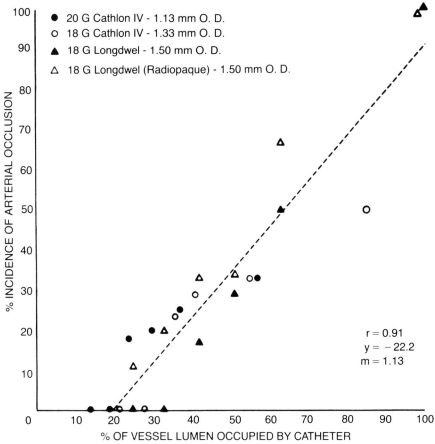

Figure 4–13. The incidence of occlusion of the radial artery after cannulation is increased by the use of 18-gauge compared with 20-gauge catheters. This results from the increased proportion of the vessel lumen that is occupied by the catheter. (From Bedford RF: Radial arterial function following percutaneous cannulation with 18- and 20-gauge catheters. Anesthesiology 1977; 47:39. With permission.)

as the blocked flow is converted to increased pressure. However, if the artery is occluded, additional occlusion distal to the occluded segment fails to alter either pressure or arterial waveform.

Infection

Bacteremia and positive blood cultures have been reported after catheters remained *in situ* for more than 4 days.[121, 122] Other factors contributing to catheter-related infections are use of nondisposable transducer domes, use of dextrose instead of saline for the flushing solution, and location of the continuous flush device near the insertion site instead of just distal to the transducer.[121, 123, 124] However, a recent study in 68 children demonstrated no positive catheter or fluid cultures after 59 hours of cannulation.[125]

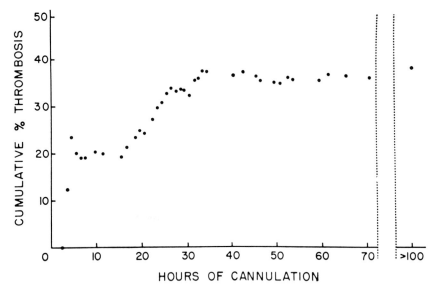

Figure 4–14. The incidence of radial artery thrombosis increases with the duration of cannulation from no thrombosis with cannulations of less than 2 hours to a 38% incidence with more than 40 hours of cannulation. (From Bedford RF, Wollman H: Complications of percutaneous radial-artery cannulation: An objective prospective study in man. Anesthesiology 1973; 38:231. With permission.)

Special Problems with Radial Arterial Catheters

Problems with measurement of direct arterial pressure are sufficiently frequent to warrant the presence of a second measuring device such as a noninvasive automated blood pressure monitor. Despite widespread use of radial catheters for 2 decades, occasional difficulties with accurate pressure measurement occur. Placement of self-retaining chest wall retractors for dissection of internal mammary arteries to use as coronary artery bypass grafts distorts normal arterial anatomy, resulting in damping of the arterial pressure waveform.[126, 127] However, the mean arterial pressure remains accurate.[128] Factors contributing to this problem include lateral tilt of the operating table, compression of the arm, and position of the retractor. Although measurement of arterial pressure in the opposite extremity obviates the immediate problem, concern about the adequacy of blood flow to the arm warrants retractor repositioning. Similar problems have been noted with opening of sternal retractors, particularly in obese patients of short stature.[129] Retractor opening in these patients causes a condition similar to the thoracic outlet syndrome.[129]

The inaccuracy of the pressure measured in the radial artery immediately after discontinuation of cardiopulmonary bypass has been reported in both children and adults.[130–132] Both central aortic and femoral arterial pressures are commonly higher than radial pressures for 45–60 minutes after termination of extracorporeal circulation in some patients. When vigorous cardiac contractility is directly observed but peripherally measured pressures are disproportionately low, arterial pressure should be measured in the aorta or femoral artery or by using a cuff on the brachial artery until the

Figure 4–15. The incidence of thrombosis increases with duration of arterial cannulation. After 1–3 days the incidence is 11%, whereas after 4–10 days it is 29%. Cannula dysfunction also increases after more than 3 days of cannulation. (From Bedford RF: Longterm radial artery cannulation. Effects on subsequent vessel function. Crit Care Med 1978; 6[1]:64–67, © by Williams & Wilkins, 1978. With permission.)

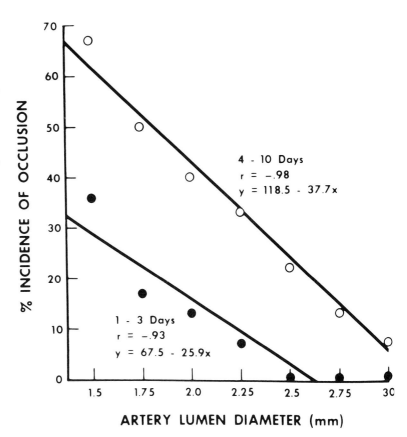

peripheral circulation returns to normal.[130] Gradients usually resolve within 10–60 minutes after bypass is terminated.

The etiology of these gradients may be peripheral vasoconstriction,[132] decreased forearm vascular resistance during rewarming from bypass,[83, 132] hypothermia, hypovolemia, or proximal shunting.[83, 130–132] Additional volume replacement eliminated the gradient associated with decreased cardiac index and mixed venous oxygen saturation (previously abnormally increased) and increased systemic vascular resistance in Mohr and associates' series of patients.[131] Patients without gradients between femoral and radial

---

Table 4–3. FACTORS CONTRIBUTING TO ARTERIAL THROMBOSIS*

Catheter size[116]
? Tapered catheters[49,50,115]
Increased duration of cannulation[109]
Increased proportion of vessel lumen occupied by catheter[112]
Smaller size of wrist[116]
Polypropylene catheters[50,114,115]

---

* Thrombosis is unaffected by method of cannulation but is decreased by aspirin pretreatment.[117,118]

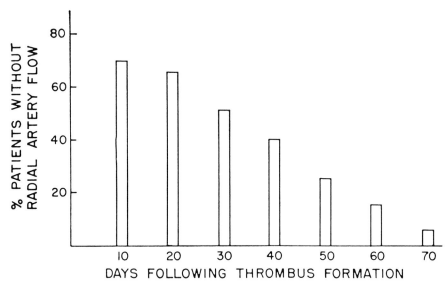

Figure 4–16. The time to recanalization of the radial artery after thrombosis ranges from 3 to 75 days, with the majority recanalized by 40 days after cannula removal. (From Bedford RF, Wollman H: Complications of percutaneous radial-artery cannulation: An objective prospective study in man. Anesthesiology 1973; 38:232. With permission.)

artery pressures did not demonstrate alteration in systemic resistance after discontinuation of bypass. Another possibility is previously unrecognized Raynaud's syndrome. Carter and colleagues report a marked decrease or loss of finger systolic pressure associated with the sympathetic vasoconstriction induced by cooling.[133]

References

1. Bruner JMR, Krenis LJ, Kunsman JM, Sherman AP: Comparison of direct and indirect methods of measuring arterial blood pressure. Med Instrum 1981; 15:11–21 (part I); 15:97–101 (part II); 15:182–188 (part III).
2. O'Rourke MF, Yaginuma T: Wave reflections and the arterial pulse. Arch Intern Med 1984; 144:366–371.
3. Gerber MJ, Hines RL, Barash PG: Arterial waveforms and systemic vascular resistance: Is there a correlation? Anesthesiology 1987; 66:823–825.
4. Ream AK: Systolic, diastolic, mean or pulse: Which is the best measurement of arterial pressure? *In* Gravenstein JS, et al (eds): Essential Noninvasive Monitoring in Anesthesia. New York: Grune & Stratton, 1980; 53–74.
5. Kirkendall WN, Feinleib M, Freis ED, Mark AL: Recommendations for human blood pressure determination by sphygomomanometers. Circulation 1980; 62:1145A–1155A.
6. Darnall RA: Noninvasive blood pressure measurement in the neonate. Clin Perinatol 1985; 12:31–49.
7. Wallace CT, Baker JD, Alpert CC, et al: Comparison of blood pressure measurement by Doppler and by pulse oximetry techniques. Anesth Analg 1987; 66:1018–1019.

8. Korotkoff NS: On the subject of methods of determining blood pressure. Bull Imperial Med Acad 1905; 11:365.

9. Ramsey M III: Noninvasive blood pressure monitoring methods and validation. *In* Gravenstein JS, et al (eds): Essential Noninvasive Monitoring in Anesthesia. New York: Grune & Stratton, 1980; 37–51.

10. Blank SG, West JE, Muller FB, et al: Wideband external pulse recording during cuff deflation: A new technique for evaluation of the arterial pressure pulse and measurement of blood pressure. Circulation 1988; 77:1297–1305.

11. Manning DM, Kuchirka C, Kamienski J: Miscuffing: Inappropriate blood pressure cuff application. Circulation 1983; 68:763–766.

12. Ragan C, Bordley J: The accuracy of clinical measurements of arterial blood pressure. Bull Johns Hopkins Hosp 1941; 69:504–528.

13. Holland WW, Humerfelt S: Measurement of blood pressure, comparison of intra-arterial and cuff values. Br Med J 1964; 2:1241–1243.

14. Simpson JA, Jamieson G, Dickhaus DW: Effect of size of cuff bladder on accuracy of measurements of indirect blood pressure. Am Heart J 1965; 70:208–215.

15. Nielsen PE, Janniche H: The accuracy of auscultatory measurement of arm blood pressure in very obese subjects. Acta Med Scand 1974; 195:403–409.

16. Breit SN, O'Rourke MF: Comparison of direct and indirect arterial pressure measurements in hospitalized patients. Aust NZ J Med 1974; 4:485–491.

17. Apple HP: Automatic noninvasive blood pressure monitors: What is available? *In* Gravenstein JS et al (eds): Essential Noninvasive Monitoring in Anesthesia. New York: Grune & Stratton, 1980:7–24.

18. Morgan JL, Kemmerer WT, Halber MD: Doppler shifted ultrasound. Minn Med 1969; 52:503–506.

19. Kirby RR, Kemmerer WT, Morgan JL: Transcutaneous Doppler measurement of blood pressure. Anesthesiology 1969; 31:86–89.

20. Stegall HF, Kardon MB, Kemmerer WT: Indirect measurement of arterial blood pressure by Doppler ultrasonic sphygmomanometry. J Appl Physiol 1968; 25:793–798.

21. Hernandez A, Goldring D, Hartman AF: Measurement of blood pressure in infants and children by the Doppler ultrasound technique. Pediatrics 1971; 48:788.

22. Waltemath CL, Preuss DD: Determination of blood pressure in low-flow states by the Doppler technique. Anesthesiology 1971; 34:77–79.

23. Poppers PJ, Epstein RM, Donham RT: Automatic ultrasound monitoring of blood pressure during induced hypotension. Anesthesiology 1972; 35:431–435.

24. Pederson RT, Vogt FB: Korotkoff vibrations in hypotension. Med Instrum 1973; 7:251–256.

25. Perlman LV, Chiang BN, Keller J, Blackburn H: Accuracy of sphygmomanometers in hospital practice. Arch Intern Med 1970; 125:1000–1003.

26. Von Recklinghausen H: Neue Wege zur blutdruckmessung. Berlin: Springer-Verlag, 1931.

27. Hutton P, Prys-Roberts C: The oscillotonometer in theory and practice. Br J Anaesth 1982; 54:581–591.

28. Ramsey M III: Noninvasive automatic determination of mean arterial pressure. Med Biol Eng Comput 1979; 17:11–18.

29. Borrow KM, Newburger JW: Noninvasive estimation of central aortic pressure using the oscillometric method for analyzing systemic artery pulsatile blood flow: Comparative study of indirect systolic, diastolic, and mean brachial artery pressure with simultaneous direct ascending aortic pressure measurements. Am Heart J 1982; 103:879–896.

30. Yelderman M, Ream AK: Indirect measurement of mean blood pressure in anesthetized patient. Anesthesiology 1979; 50:253–256.
31. Hutton P, Dye J, Prys-Roberts C: An assessment of the Dinamap 845. Anaesthesia 1984; 39:261–267.
32. Nystrom E, Reid KH, Bennett R, et al: A comparison of two automated indirect arterial blood pressure meters: With recordings from a radial arterial catheter in anesthetized surgical patients. Anesthesiology 1985; 62:526–530.
33. Friesen RH, Lichtor JL: Indirect measurement of blood pressure in neonates and infants utilizing an automatic noninvasive oscillometric monitor. Anesth Analg 1981; 60:742–745.
34. Kimble KJ, Darnall RA, Yelderman M, et al: An automated oscillometric technique for estimating mean arterial pressure in critically ill newborns. Anesthesiology 1981; 54:423–425.
35. Peñaz J: Photoelectric measurement of blood pressure volume and flow in the finger. Digest, 10th International Conference of Medical Biological Engineers 1973; 104.
36. Wesseling KH, de Wit B, Snoeck B, et al: An implementation of the Peñaz method for measuring arterial blood pressure in the finger and first results of an evaluation. Inst Med Physics TNO Prog Rep 1978; 6:168–173.
37. Wesseling KH, van Bemmel R, van Dieren A, et al: Two methods for the assessment of hemodynamic parameters of epidemiology. Acta Cardiol 1978; 33:84–87.
38. Smith NT, Beneken JEW: An overview of arterial pressure monitoring. *In* Gravenstein JS et al (eds): Essential Noninvasive Monitoring in Anesthesia. New York: Grune & Stratton, 1980; 75–88.
39. Molhoek GP, Wesseling KH, Settels JJ, et al: Evaluation of the Peñaz servo-plethysmo-manometer for the continuous, noninvasive measurement of finger blood pressure. Basic Res Cardiol 1984; 79:598–609.
40. Kurki T, Smith NT, Head N, et al: Noninvasive continuous blood pressure measurement from the finger: Optimal measurement conditions and factors affecting reliability. J Clin Monit 1987; 3:6–13.
41. Smith NT, Wesseling KH, DeWit B: Evaluation of two prototype devices producing noninvasive, pulsatile, calibrated blood pressure measurement from a finger. J Clin Monit 1985; 1:17–29.
42. Gravenstein JS, Paulus DA, Feldman J, McLaughlin G: Tissue hypoxia distal to a Peñaz finger blood pressure cuff. J Clin Monit 1985; 1:120–125.
43. Dorlas JC, Nijboer JA, Butijn T, et al: Effects of peripheral vasoconstriction on the blood pressure in the finger, measured continuously by a new noninvasive method (the Finapres[R]). Anesthesiology 1985; 62:342–345.
44. Sy WP: Ulnar nerve palsy possibly related to use of automatically cycled blood pressure cuff. Anesth Analg 1981; 60:687–688.
45. Van Bergen FH, Weatherhead DS, Treloar AE, et al: Comparison of indirect and direct methods of measuring arterial blood pressure. Circulation 1954; 10:481–490.
46. Noreng MF: Blood flow in the radial artery before and after arterial puncture. Acta Anaesthesiol Scand 1986; 30:281–282.
47. Pierson DJ, Hudson LD: Monitoring hemodynamics in the critically ill. Med Clin North Am 1983; 67:1343–1360.
48. Peterson LH, Dripps RD, Risman GC: A method for recording the arterial pressure pulse and blood pressure in man. Am Heart J 1949; 37:771–782.
49. Bedford RF: Percutaneous radial-artery cannulation. Increased safety using Teflon catheters. Anesthesiology 1975; 42:219–222.
50. Marshall AG, Erwin DC, Wyse RKH, Hatch DJ: Percutaneous arterial cannulation in children. Anaesthesia 1984; 39:27–31.

51. Gardner RM, Schwartz R, Wong JC, Burke JP: Percutaneous indwelling radial-artery catheters for monitoring cardiovascular function. N Engl J Med 1974; 290:1227–1231.

52. Talmage EA: Shearing hazard of intra-arterial Teflon catheters. Anesth Analg 1976; 55:597–598.

53. Brodsky JB, Wong AL, Meyer JA: Percutaneous cannulation of weakly palpable arteries. Anesth Analg 1977; 56:448.

54. Buakham C, Kim JM: Cannulation of a nonpalpable artery with the aid of a Doppler monitor. Anesth Analg 1977; 56:125–126.

55. Chinyanga HM, Smith JM: A modified Doppler flow detector probe: An aid to percutaneous radial arterial cannulation in infants and small children. Anesthesiology 1979; 50:256–258.

56. Introna RPS, Silverstein PI: A new use for the pulse oximeter. (Letter.) Anesthesiology 1986; 65:342.

57. Johnson RW: Complication of radial artery cannulation. Anesthesiology 1974; 40:353–355.

58. Gordon LH, Brown M, Brown OW, Brown EM: Alternative sites for continuous arterial monitoring. South Med J 1984; 77:1498–1500.

59. Pyles ST, Scher KS, Vega ET, et al: Cannulation of the dorsal radial artery: A new technique. Anesth Analg 1982; 61:876–878.

60. Paster SB, Middleton P: Roentgenographic evaluation of umbilical artery and vein catheters. JAMA 1975; 231:742–746.

61. Laks H, Rongey K, Schweiss J, William VL: Internal mammary artery cannulation. Ann Thorac Surg 1977; 24:488–490.

62. Moorthy SS: Cannulation of the anterior peroneal artery in adults. Anesth Analg 1981; 60:360–361.

63. Prian GW: New proximal approach works well in temporal artery catheterization. JAMA 1976; 235:2693–2694.

64. Hegemann CO, Rappaport I, Berger WJ: Superficial temporal artery cannulation. Arch Surg 1969; 99:619–624.

65. Husum B, Palm T, Eriksen J: Percutaneous cannulation of the dorsalis pedis artery. Br J Anaesth 1979; 51:1055–1058.

66. Barnes RW, Foster EJ, Janssen GA, Boutros AR: Safety of brachial arterial catheters as monitors in the intensive care unit: Prospective evaluation with Doppler ultrasonic velocity detector. Anesthesiology 1976; 44:260–264.

67. Adler DC, Bryan-Brown CW: Use of the axillary artery for intravascular monitoring. Crit Care Med 1973; 1:148–150.

68. Mozersky DJ, Buckley CJ, Hagood C, et al: Ultrasonic evaluation of the palmar circulation. Am J Surg 1973; 126:810–812.

69. Allen EV: Thromboangiitis obliterans: Methods of diagnosis of chronic occlusive arterial lesions distal to the wrist with illustrative cases. Am J Med Sci 1929; 178:237–244.

70. Husum B, Berthelsen P: Allen's test and systolic arterial pressure in the thumb. Br J Anaesth 1981; 53:635–637.

71. Hirai M, Kawai S: False positive and negative results in Allen test. J Cardiovasc Surg 1980; 21:353–360.

72. Gandhi SK, Reynolds AC: A modification of Allen's test to detect aberrant ulnar collateral circulation. Anesthesiology 1983; 59:147–148.

73. Coleman SS, Anson BJ: Arterial patterns in the hand based upon a study of 650 specimens. Surg Gynecol Obstet 1961; 113:409–424.

74. Brodsky JB: A simple method to determine patency of the ulnar artery intraoperatively prior to radial artery cannulation. Anesthesiology 1975; 42:626–627.

75. Ramanathan S, Chalon J, Turndorf H: Determining patency of palmar arches by retrograde radial pulsation. Anesthesiology 1975; 42:756–758.

76. Nowak GS, Moorthy SS, McNiece WL: Use of pulse oximetry for assessment of collateral arterial flow. (Letter.) Anesthesiology 1986; 64:527.

77. Greenhow DE: Incorrect performance of Allen's test: Ulnar artery flow erroneously presumed inadequate. Anesthesiology 1972; 37:356–357.

78. Kamienski RW, Barnes RW: Critique of the Allen test for continuity of palmar arch assessed by Doppler ultrasound. Surg Gynecol Obstet 1976; 142:861–864.

79. Slogoff S, Keats AS, Arlund C: On the safety of radial artery cannulation. Anesthesiology 1983; 59:42–47.

80. Mandel MA, Dauchot PJ: Radial artery cannulation in 1000 patients: Precautions and complications. J Hand Surg 1977; 2:482–485.

81. Mangano DT, Hickey RF: Ischemic injury following uncomplicated radial artery catheterization. Anesth Analg 1979; 58:55–57.

82. Macon WL IV, Futrell JW: Median-nerve neuropathy after percutaneous puncture of the brachial artery in patients receiving anticoagulants. N Engl J Med 1973; 288:1396.

83. Pauca AL, Meredith JW: Possibility of A-V shunting upon cardiopulmonary bypass discontinuation. Anesthesiology 1987; 67:91–94.

84. Pascarelli EF, Bertrand CA: Comparison of blood pressures in the arms and legs. N Engl J Med 1964; 270:693–698.

85. Yacoub OF, Bacaling JH, Kelly M: Monitoring of axillary arterial pressure in a patient with Buerger's disease requiring clipping of an intracranial aneurysm. Br J Anaesth 1987; 59:1056–1058.

86. Christian CM, Naraghi M: A complication of femoral arterial cannulation in a patient undergoing cardiopulmonary bypass. Anesthesiology 1978; 49:436–437.

87. Glenski JA, Beynen FM, Brady J: A prospective evaluation of femoral artery monitoring in pediatric patients. Anesthesiology 1987; 66:227–229.

88. Rosenthal A, Anderson M, Thomson SJ, et al: Superficial femoral artery catheterization in infants and small children. Circulation 1977; 56:102–105.

89. Spoerel WE, Deimling P, Aitken R: Direct arterial pressure monitoring from the dorsalis pedis artery. Can Anaesth Soc J 1975; 22:91–99.

90. Huber JF: The arterial network supplying the dorsum of the foot. Anat Rec 1941; 80:373–391.

91. Youngberg JA, Miller ED: Evaluation of percutaneous cannulation of the dorsalis pedis artery. Anesthesiology 1976; 44:80–83.

92. Palm T, Husum B: Blood pressure in the great toe with simulated occlusion of the dorsalis pedis artery. Anesth Analg 1978; 57:453–456.

93. Johnstone RE, Greenhow DE: Catheterization of the dorsalis pedis artery. Anesthesiology 1973; 39:654–655.

94. Vidyasagar D, Downes JJ, Boggs TR: Respiratory distress syndrome of newborn infants: II. Technic of catheterization of umbilical artery and clinical results of treatment of 124 patients. Clin Pediatr 1970; 9:332–336.

95. Cole AFD, Rolbin SH: A technique for rapid catheterization of the umbilical artery. Anesthesiology 1980; 53:254–255.

96. McFadden PM, Ochsner JL: Neonatal aortic thrombosis: Complication of umbilical artery cannulation. J Cardiovasc Surg 1983; 24:1–4.

97. Marsh JL, Fonkalsrud EW: Serious complications after umbilical artery catheterization for neonatal monitoring. Arch Surg 1975; 110:1203–1208.

98. Feeley TW: Re-establishment of radial-artery patency for arterial monitoring. Anesthesiology 1977; 46:73–75.

99. Bedford RF: Removal of radial-artery thrombi following percutaneous cannulation for monitoring. Anesthesiology 1977; 46:430–432.

100. Lowenstein E, Little JW, Lo HH: Prevention of cerebral embolization from flushing radial-artery cannulas. N Engl J Med 1971; 285:1414–1415.
101. Chang C, Dughi J, Shitabata P, et al: Air embolism and the radial arterial line. Crit Care Med 1988; 16:141–143.
102. Edmonds JF, Barker GA, Conn AW: Current concepts in cardiovascular monitoring in children. Crit Care Med 1980; 8:548–553.
103. Gardner RM, Bond EL, Clark JS: Safety and efficacy of continuous flush systems for arterial and pulmonary artery catheters. Ann Thorac Surg 1977; 23:534–538.
104. Harbort RA, Dalgetty RG: Bubble formation in flush systems. Ann Thorac Surg 1978; 25:179–180.
105. Wolf S, Mangano DT: Pseudoaneurysm, a late complication of radial-artery catheterization. Anesthesiology 1980; 52:80–81.
106. Mathieu A, Dalton B, Fischer JE, Kumar A: Expanding aneurysm of the radial artery after frequent puncture. Anesthesiology 1973; 38:401–403.
107. Cannon BW, Meshier WT: Extremity amputation following radial artery cannulation in a patient with hyperlipoproteinemia type V. Anesthesiology 1982; 56:222–223.
108. Dalton B, Laver MB: Vasospasm with an indwelling radial artery cannula. Anesthesiology 1973; 34:194–197.
109. Bedford RF, Wollman H: Complications of percutaneous radial-artery cannulation: An objective prospective study in man. Anesthesiology 1973; 38:228–236.
110. Miyasaka K, Edmons JF, Conn AW: Complications of radial artery lines in the pediatric patient. Can Anaesth Soc J 1976; 23:9–14.
111. Gauer PK, Downs JB: Complications of arterial catheterization. Respir Care 1982; 27:435–444.
112. Bedford RF: Radial arterial function following percutaneous cannulation with 18- and 20-gauge catheters. Anesthesiology 1977; 47:37–39.
113. Palm T: Evaluation of peripheral arterial pressure on the thumb following radial artery cannulation. Br J Anaesth 1977; 49:819–824.
114. Davis FM, Steward JM: Radial artery cannulation. Br J Anaesth 1980; 52:674–684.
115. Downs JB, Rackstein AD, Klein EF, Hawkins IF: Hazards of radial-artery catheterization. Anesthesiology 1973; 38:283–286.
116. Bedford RF: Wrist circumference predicts the risk of radial-arterial occlusion after cannulation. Anesthesiology 1978; 48:377–378.
117. Jones RM, Hill AB, Nahrwold ML, Bolles RE: The effect of method of radial artery cannulation on postcannulation blood flow and thrombus formation. Anesthesiology 1981; 55:76–78.
118. Bedford RF, Ashford TP: Aspirin pretreatment prevents post-cannulation radial-artery thrombosis. Anesthesiology 1979; 51:176–178.
119. Kim JM, Arakawa K, Bliss J: Arterial cannulation: Factors in the development of occlusion. Anesth Analg 1975; 54:836–841.
120. Vender JS, Watts RD: Differential diagnosis of hand ischemia in the presence of an arterial cannula. Anesth Analg 1982; 61:465–468.
121. Band JD, Maki DG: Infection caused by arterial catheters used for hemodynamic monitoring. Am J Med 1979; 67:735–741.
122. Freeman R, King B: Analysis of results of catheter tip culture in open-heart surgery patients. Thorax 1975; 30:26–30.
123. Shinozaki T, Deane R, Mazuzan JE, et al: Bacterial contamination of arterial lines: A prospective study. JAMA 1983; 249:223–225.
124. Weinstein RA, Stamm WE, Kramer L: Pressure monitoring devices: Overlooked sources of nosocomial infection. JAMA 1976; 236:936–938.

125. Ducharme FM, Gauthier MK Lacroix J, Lafleur L: Incidence of infection related to arterial catheterization in children. A prospective study. Crit Care Med 1988; 16:272–276.
126. Kinzer JB, Lichtenthal PR, Wade LD: Loss of radial artery pressure trace during internal mammary artery dissection for coronary artery bypass graft surgery. Anesth Analg 1985; 64:1134–1136.
127. Daimant M, Arkin DB: False radial-artery blood-pressure readings. (Letter.) Anesthesiology 1976; 44:273.
128. Nicolson SC, Jobes DR: Arterial pressure monitoring during internal mammary artery harvesting. (Letter.) Anesth Analg 1986; 65:821.
129. Saka D, Lin YT, Oka Y: An unusual cause of false radial-artery blood-pressure readings during cardiopulmonary bypass. Anesthesiology 1975; 43:487–489.
130. Stern DH, Gerson JI, Allen FB, Parker FB: Can we trust the direct radial artery pressure immediately following cardiopulmonary bypass? Anesthesiology 1985; 62:557–561.
131. Mohr R, Lavee J, Goor DA: Inaccuracy of radial artery pressure measurement after cardiac operations. J Thorac Cardiovasc Surg 1987; 94:286–290.
132. Gallagher JD, Moore RA, McNicholas KW, Jose AB: Comparison of radial and femoral arterial blood pressures in children after cardiopulmonary bypass. J Clin Monit 1985; 1:168–171.
133. Carter SA, Dean E, Kroeger EA: Apparent finger systolic pressures during cooling in patients with Raynaud's syndrome. Circulation 1988; 77:988–996.

chapter five

Venous and Pulmonary Pressures

■ KAREN J. SCHWENZER, M.D.

Access to the central venous circulation is widely used in the perioperative management of critically ill patients in order to administer fluids and vasoactive drugs, obtain blood samples, and monitor central vascular pressures. Central venous pressure (CVP) reflects left ventricular preload in healthy hearts. However, in many clinical situations, this relationship between CVP and left ventricular preload is not valid. With the development of a flow-directed, balloon-tipped pulmonary artery catheter, left ventricular preload and function are better assessed by monitoring pulmonary artery pressure (PAP) and pulmonary capillary wedge pressure (PCWP). This chapter reviews the literature and discusses the indications, risk, and benefits of the important methods used to monitor CVP and PAP in the evaluation of hemodynamic function in critically ill patients in the operating room and the intensive care unit.

MONITORING OF CVP

Left Ventricular Function

The goal of hemodynamic management is to assure that tissue perfusion is adequate to meet aerobic metabolic needs. A balance among intravascular

147

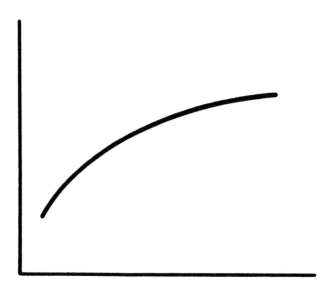

Figure 5–1. The Frank-Starling law states that ventricular performance (i.e., force of contraction) depends upon preload (i.e., fiber length, ventricular end-diastolic volume [VEDV]). (From Benumof JL: Anesthesia for Thoracic Surgery. Philadelphia: WB Saunders, 1987; 181.)

blood volume, cardiac output, and vascular resistance must be achieved. The vital component is the maintenance of an adequate cardiac output.

The Frank-Starling law of myocardial function states that as the initial myocardial fiber length increases, the force of contraction of that fiber increases. In the intact heart, myocardial fiber length is represented by left or right ventricular end-diastolic volume or preload (Fig. 5–1). Measurement of preload permits accurate assessment of intravascular volume in relation to myocardial performance. However, measurement of cardiac performance is also required. This is accomplished by evaluation of stroke volume or cardiac output, urine output, capillary refill, and the patient's level of consciousness. In addition, the construction of a Frank-Starling myocardial function curve relating stroke volume to left ventricular preload is clinically useful in assessing therapeutic protocols in critically ill patients.

Preload

It is technically difficult to repeatedly measure accurate, quantitative ventricular volumes. Therefore, left ventricular end-diastolic pressure (LVEDP) is used as an approximation of left ventricular preload. The relationship between ventricular volume and pressure is myocardial compliance.

In the normal heart, the thick, muscular left ventricle is relatively noncompliant as compared with the thin-walled right ventricle. The difference in compliance of the two ventricles, as a consequence of their anatomic structure, is responsible for the changes in the slopes of their corresponding

P_{CV} versus P_{pad} and P_{paw}

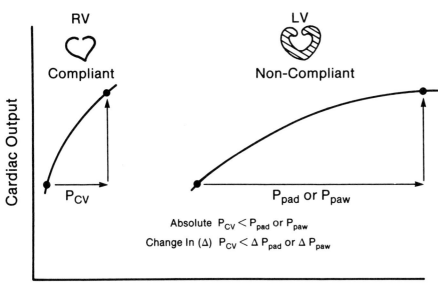

Figure 5–2. The relationship between central venous pressure (P_{CV}) and pulmonary artery wedge pressure (P_{paw}) and pulmonary artery diastolic pressure (P_{pad}) is normally based on the differences in compliance between the right ventricle (RV) and the left ventricle (LV). The right ventricle is relatively compliant because of its thin musculature, whereas the left ventricle is relatively noncompliant because of its thick musculature. Thus, when preload changes in a normal heart, the P_{CV} (as a reflection of RVEDV) increases only a small amount for a given increase in cardiac output, whereas the P_{paw} and P_{pad} (as reflections of LVEDV) increase a large amount for the same increase in cardiac output. Thus, owing to the differences in compliance between the two ventricles, the absolute P_{CV} is always less than the P_{paw} and P_{pad}, and the change in the P_{CV} is always less than the change in P_{paw} and P_{pad}. (From Benumof JL, Anesthesia for Thoracic Surgery. Philadelphia: WB Saunders, 1987; 190.)

Frank-Starling curves (Fig. 5–2) and PCWP versus CVP as an index of preload. When compliance is normal, LVEDP is a good index of left ventricular preload. However, in a very stiff, noncompliant ventricle, LVEDP does not accurately reflect left ventricular end-diastolic volume.[1] In such situations, LVEDP may be increased, whereas end-diastolic volume is normal.

The relationship of LVEDP and other CVPs is diagrammed in Figure 5–3. The use of CVP to assess left-sided heart filling pressures has its limitations because CVP reflects right atrial pressure, which primarily reflects changes in right ventricular end-diastolic pressure (RVEDP) and only secondarily reflects changes in pulmonary venous and left-sided heart pressures. However, if one recognizes that comparative changes in preload and stroke volume in response to therapy or disease are more important than absolute values of CVP or PCWP, the CVP can serve as a reliable indicator of intravascular blood volume. In addition, in patients with good ejection

VENOUS AND PULMONARY PRESSURES

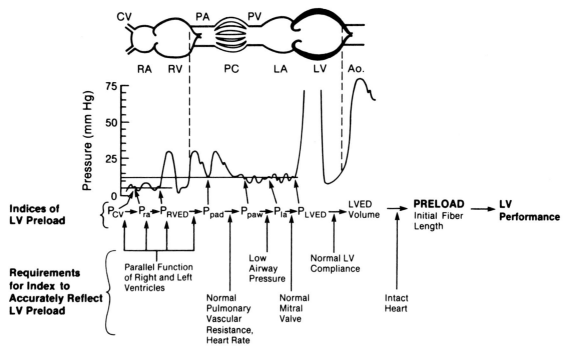

Figure 5–3. The relationship of LVEDP and other central venous pressures (CVP). In the top portion of the diagram the various central vascular and cardiac chambers are portrayed in the sequence that blood flows through them. The cardiac valves portray the end-diastolic moment, the pulmonary and aortic valves are closed, and the mitral and tricuspid valves are open. The graph depicts the characteristic vascular pressure waveforms. Below this graph the various indexes of left ventricular preload are indicated and the requirements for each of the indexes to accurately reflect left ventricular preload described. (From Benumof JL: Anesthesia for Thoracic Surgery. Philadelphia: WB Saunders, 1987; 182.)

fractions, the CVP approximates LVEDP in absolute number as well as change.[2-4]

In an abnormal heart, the left and right ventricular function curves are markedly different from one another, and the CVP is a poor reflection of left-sided preload. In the presence of left ventricular failure, a higher LVEDP is needed to generate an adequate stroke volume (Fig. 5–4). In such situations, a "normal" CVP results in a suboptimal intravascular volume and a low cardiac output. The CVP may not only be an inadequate index of intravascular volume but can also be quite misleading. For instance, the presence of tricuspid valvular stenosis interferes with the correlation between CVP (or mean right atrial pressure) and RVEDP. A better reflection of LVEDP would be obtained by monitoring PCWP.

At end-diastole the left ventricle, left atrium, pulmonary veins, pulmonary capillaries, and pulmonary artery function as a single, fluid-filled chamber. In the absence of mitral valve disease, left atrial pressure equals LVEDP. Bedside measurement of PCWP is obtained with a flow-directed, balloon-tipped pulmonary artery catheter. When the balloon is properly placed in a pulmonary artery, its inflation completely obstructs blood flow through the artery and forms a static column of blood distal to the catheter tip. This column of blood allows the catheter tip to measure pulmonary

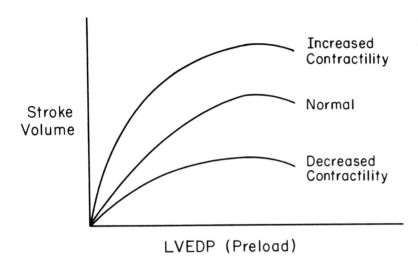

Figure 5–4. A family of Frank-Starling curves is demonstrated. The horizontal axis shows preload, and the vertical axis shows myocardial work.

venous circulation. Because there are normally no pressure gradients between the pulmonary veins and the left atrium, the pulmonary artery obstruction pressure or, more familiarly, PCWP, reflects left atrial pressure and left ventricular preload. In the presence of mitral valve disease, however, the correlation between mean left atrial pressure (or PCWP) and LVEDP is lost.

Another index of left-sided heart preload is the pulmonary artery diastolic pressure (PADP), which is obtained with a flow-directed pulmonary artery catheter or a transthoracic pulmonary artery catheter. In the absence of elevated pulmonary vascular resistance, PADP is an excellent estimate of LVEDP.

Clinical Uses

Assessment of Venous Return and Hypovolemia

The CVP monitors the adequacy of central venous return, intravascular blood volume, and right ventricular function. The CVP actually reflects the pressure in the great veins as blood returns to the heart. If blood return decreases, venous pressure also decreases. In general, a decreased venous pressure reflects decreased blood volume and indicates the need for additional fluid or blood to expand the intravascular space. The administration of fluid in such situations increases CVP, indicating restoration of intravascular volume. No predetermined number for CVP should be used; instead, the goal of volume repletion is the restoration of tissue perfusion. For this reason, serial measurements, rather than single, absolute ones, are highly valued in the assessment of cardiovascular performance.

Surgical Indications for Monitoring CVP

During anesthesia and surgery, assessment of cardiovascular performance and intravascular volume is paramount to a patient's well-being. Failure to recognize inadequately replaced preoperative losses, hemorrhage, intraoperative fluid shifts, and faulty fluid management leads to hypovolemia. Depending upon the clinical scenario, frequent assessment of pulse pressure, systolic pressure, heart rate, capillary refill, and urine output alerts the anesthesiologist to the presence of hypovolemia.

The decision to use invasive CVP monitoring during surgery is based on a patient's preoperative condition and intraoperative requirements. A patient with pre-existing cardiorespiratory disease or one who is undergoing surgical procedures causing further derangement in cardiorespiratory function during the perioperative period benefits from invasive measurement of CVP. Operative procedures with anticipated massive blood and fluid transfusion (trauma), those associated with significant intravascular fluid shifts (hemicolectomy), those associated with decreased venous return (performed in the lateral decubitus position), and those near the great vessels, heart, or other mediastinal structures (portacaval shunt) warrant the use of invasive monitoring to assess intravascular volume. Measurement of CVP is especially prudent if the surgical procedure is complicated by the presence of sepsis, heart disease, or respiratory failure.

Other Indications for Central Venous Catheterization

Central venous catheterization is often accomplished for the sole purpose of obtaining venous access when peripheral veins are unavailable. A central venous catheter allows access to the central circulation for fluid and drug infusions during the perioperative period. At other times, intravenous administration of vasoactive drugs and other drugs likely to injure peripheral veins and tissues requires central venous access. Hypertonic parenteral hyperalimentation must be administered directly into the central venous circulation. Central venous catheters are used in the diagnosis and aspiration of venous air emboli as well as in the transvenous insertion of temporary pacing leads. In all these cases, the precautions and risks discussed here are applicable. Blood samples may be obtained from a central venous catheter as long as the intravenous fluids are aspirated from the catheter prior to sampling. Failure to do this can lead to abnormal values, which should be suspected when eccentric laboratory reports are received (see Chapters 17 and 18).

INSERTION OF CENTRAL VENOUS CATHETERS

Proper skills for insertion of central venous catheters are best learned from a tutor skilled in the procedure. Percutaneous insertion is the preferred technique, although venous cutdowns are occasionally necessary in infants and some adults. Vascular cutdowns are used for insertion of long-term central venous catheters such as the Hickman, Broviac, or Groschong catheters.

Table 5–1. EQUIPMENT NEEDED FOR PLACEMENT OF CENTRAL
VENOUS CATHETERS

Povidone-iodine preparatory solution
Sterile drape or towels
25-gauge needle for local anesthetic infiltration
Local anesthetic without vasoconstrictor
Filter needle to draw up local anesthetic
22-gauge seeker needle
18-gauge 6.35-cm thin-walled needle with radiopaque catheter over it
18-gauge 6.35-cm thin-walled needle
Two 5-ml syringes
Stainless steel guidewire with flexible tip on one end and J-tip on the other
Scalpel
Venous dilator
Radiopaque polyurethane central venous catheter
Luer-Lok injection caps
Suture material with needle
Sterile gauze

Patient Preparation

Proper equipment is essential for central venous catheterization. Table
5–1 outlines the necessary supplies, although there are numerous prepackaged central venous catheterization kits containing the necessities available.
The assistance of a technician or nurse familiar with the procedure is also
recommended. Patient sedation with any number of drugs such as the benzodiazepines or narcotics is helpful. Insertion into the internal jugular, external jugular, and subclavian veins is facilitated by placing the bed in the
Trendelenburg position to distend the veins for ease of puncture and to
prevent the entrainment of air during insertion. With these approaches, the
patient's head is turned to the side opposite the insertion site to increase
exposure.

Sterile technique must be maintained throughout the procedure. This
is facilitated by the use of sterile gloves, a sterile gown, face mask, and an
appropriate hair covering. Central venous catheter–related infections are
minimized by proper preparation of the skin surface prior to catheter insertion. The skin site is shaved, if needed, and an iodine preparation, such
as povidone-iodine (Betadine), is applied and allowed to dry. A solution of
70% alcohol is then applied and allowed to dry. The area is draped with
sterile towels. The insertion site is infiltrated with a local anesthetic, such
as 0.5–1.0% lidocaine without vasoconstrictor.

Choice of Technique

There are three basic methods of gaining access to the central circulation: catheter-over-the-needle, catheter-through-the-needle, and catheter-
over-a-guidewire (Seldinger) techniques.

Catheter-over-the-Needle Technique

With a catheter-over-the-needle technique, once the needle tip is located within the lumen of the vein, the central venous catheter is advanced directly over it. The entire needle-catheter assembly must be of adequate length to reach the central circulation. There are a number of prepackaged catheter-over-the-needle products available to perform this direct approach to the central circulation. The most common length is 5.5–6 inches, which allows the catheter to reach the superior vena cava from the jugular or subclavian vein. The entire insertion is relatively simple and done in one step. In addition, the catheter completely occupies the puncture made in the vessel wall by the needle, minimizing bleeding. However, many clinicians find the length of the device cumbersome, especially when a syringe is attached to the hub during insertion. Another disadvantage is that the needle tip may be within the vein while the leading edge of the catheter is still extraluminal. Consequently, the catheter cannot be successfully advanced.

Catheter-through-the-Needle Technique

Catheter-through-the-needle also employ prepackaged devices. With this technique, once the needle is within the lumen of the vein, the catheter is passed through it and advanced to its proper position. Since the needle cannot be removed past the hub of the catheter, a protective sheath must fix the needle to the catheter to ensure that the catheter is not cut by the sharp edge of the needle. Any attempts to withdraw the catheter into the needle can result in shearing of the catheter with subsequent embolism, and this must be avoided. In addition, the catheter diameter is smaller than the needle puncture, so leakage of blood around the catheter is common.

Seldinger Technique

The preferred technique is the one described by Seldinger,[5] using a catheter-over-a-guidewire technique. Once the needle tip (18 or 20 gauge) is located in the lumen of the vein and venous blood is seen in the syringe, the syringe can be removed and a guidewire inserted through the needle. Guidewires are available in many sizes, shapes, and lengths. One end of the guidewire is flexible, either with a straight configuration or with a J-tip to facilitate advancement of the wire into the central circulation using the external jugular vein approach. The J-tip may be used with other approaches as well. The guidewire is prepackaged with a short sheath that is used to straighten the J-tip in order to ease insertion into the needle. The outside diameter of the guidewire must be smaller than the inside of the needle or cannula through which it must pass (Table 5–2). The wire should be at least 10 cm longer than the central catheter, although one twice as long as the catheter is generally used. During catheterization of the central circulation, the guidewire should be firmly grasped to prevent embolism of the wire.

Once the wire is inserted 15–20 cm into the vein, the needle is removed over the wire, leaving the wire in the vein. The puncture site and vein are dilated to accommodate the central catheter by advancing a tapered obtur-

Table 5–2. RELATIVE SIZES OF ANGIOGRAPHIC WIRES, CANNULAS, AND NEEDLES

Outer Diameter of Wire (Inches)*	Smallest Thin-Walled Needle through Which Wire Fits (Gauge)	Smallest Cannula through Which Wire Fits (Gauge)
0.018–0.021	21	22
0.022–0.025	19	20
0.028	19	18
0.035	18	16
0.038	18	16

* A 0.025-inch or smaller wire fits through the lumina of most pulmonary artery catheters.
From Blitt CD (ed): Monitoring in Anesthesia and Critical Care Medicine. New York: Churchill Livingstone, 1985; 136. By permission.

ator over the guidewire. Then, the central venous catheter is passed over the guidewire and advanced to the central circulation, with the guidewire always grasped. The guidewire is removed, and venous blood is aspirated from the catheter lumen. One modification of the Seldinger technique uses a short over-the-needle cannula, which is advanced off the needle into the vein after the initial venous puncture. The guidewire is then threaded through the cannula. Utilization of this guidewire technique allows the initial venipuncture to be accomplished with a small needle or cannula, minimizing the risk of traumatizing adjacent structures.[6] Either technique permits a wide variety of central venous catheters or vascular sheaths to be inserted over the guidewire.

Choice of Catheter

The decision to choose one type of central venous catheter over another is based on the intended use. For instance, some catheters are designed to be flexible and nonirritating and are ideal for long-term central hyperalimentation. Others are easy to insert and are preferred for emergency fluid resuscitation.

Central venous catheters are available in a variety of materials. The most common materials are polyvinylchloride, polypropylene, polyethylene, polyurethane, polytef (Teflon), and polymeric silicone (silastic). Most are chemically inert, although the risk of thrombus formation is variable (Table 5–3). Some polyvinylchloride pulmonary artery catheters are coated with heparin to reduce the incidence of thrombus formation on the catheter.

Multilumen central venous catheters have gained wide acceptance for use in the operating room and intensive care units. These devices have two to three lumina, enabling simultaneous continuous CVP monitoring and fluid or drug administration. However, the lumen sizes are one 16 gauge and one or two 18 gauges. When using multilumen central venous catheters, the proximal lumina are flushed with heparinized saline solution (1 U/ml) prior to insertion and capped with syringes or Luer-Loks to prevent thrombus formation and air entrainment during insertion. The distal port is then

Table 5–3. COMPARISON OF CENTRAL VENOUS CATHETER MATERIALS

Type of Material	Chemical Inertness	Thrombogenicity	Flexibility	Transparent
Polyvinylchloride (PVC)	− − −	+ + +	+ + +	Yes
Siliconized PVC	−	+ +	+ +	Yes
Polyethylene	− −	+ + +	+ +	Yes
Polypropylene	− −	+ + +	+ +	Yes
Siliconized polypropylene	0	+	+ +	Yes or no
Teflon	−	+	+	No
Silastic	0	0	+ + + +	No
Polyurethane	− −	+	+ + +	No

Key: 0 = none, + = minimal, + + = moderate, + + + and + + + + = large, − = less, − − = much less, − − − = markedly less.
From Blitt CD (ed): Monitoring in Anesthesia and Critical Care Medicine. New York: Churchill Livingstone, 1985; 136. By permission.

threaded over the guidewire. Once the catheter is properly positioned within the central venous circulation, blood should be able to be aspirated from all the ports.

Choice of Site

A number of sites are available for central venous catheterization. The choice of a particular site is determined by the experience of the physician, accessibility, convenience, success rate in directing the catheter to the central venous circulation, risk to the patient, and probably duration of use.

Anatomy and Technique

Internal Jugular Vein. The internal jugular vein is often the site of choice because the site is clean, the incidence of thrombophlebitis is low, and the patient is allowed freedom of movement. It is a favored site for anesthesiologists because of its easy accessibility during operative procedures.

The highest success rate of localizing the catheter in the superior vena cava or right atrium is achieved through the right internal jugular vein. This provides a straight path into the superior vena cava. Disruption of anatomic relationships by tumor or trauma, the inability to position the patient's head properly, and systemic anticoagulation are contraindications to this approach. Previous neck surgery is a relative contraindication, although the potential success rate (using echo guidance) after carotid endarterectomy is 79%.[7]

Despite the multiplicity of techniques that have been described for catheterization of the internal jugular vein, there are three basic approaches as determined by the venous relation to the sternocleidomastoid muscle, namely, posterior, central, and anterior routes. With all these techniques, the anatomic landmark is the sternocleidomastoid muscle and its two heads (Fig. 5–5). From its origin at the jugular foramen, the internal jugular vein

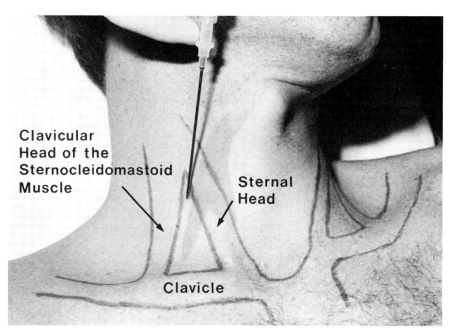

Figure 5–5. Anatomic landmarks and needle approach to the internal jugular vein.

runs directly caudad, under the clavicle, to join the subclavian vein. The internal jugular vein, carotid artery, and vagus nerve run together within the carotid sheath. Initially in its course through the neck, the vein lies posterior to the carotid artery but then becomes lateral to it near the clavicle.

The most widely accepted route is the central approach to the right internal jugular vein. The patient is prepared, as described previously, with the head turned away from the site of catheterization. The triangle formed by the sternal and clavicular heads of the sternocleidomastoid muscle and the clavicle is identified. The course of the vein follows a line connecting the mastoid process and the clavicular head of the sternocleidomastoid muscle, which is the lateral wall of the triangle. The puncture site is made at the apex of the triangle, and the needle is directed along this line at a 45° angle to the skin. Prior to puncture, the carotid artery is palpated to ensure its medial location. Attempts to "slide" the artery out of the path of the needle are not recommended since the artery and vein lie in a common sheath. Rather, the risk of cannulating the carotid artery can be reduced to a minimum by careful adherence to proven technique and utilization of a small-caliber needle (22 gauge) or catheter (18 or 20 gauge) to localize the internal jugular vein prior to insertion of a large-bore catheter or sheath introducer.

As the needle is passed, gentle negative pressure is applied to the syringe until venous blood is easily aspirated. If the vein is not entered, the needle is withdrawn slowly and completely with gentle aspiration. If, as occasionally occurs, the vein has been punctured through and through, a return of blood into the syringe is seen during withdrawal. Verification of the venous nature of the punctured vessel can be performed by connecting the needle or catheter to a pressure transducer *prior* to insertion of the definitive central venous catheter. Both the waveform and the pressure should confirm venous puncture.[8] Once venous access is obtained, catheter placement proceeds as previously described.

Multiple variations on the landmarks and insertion point have been described, all with very good success rates.[9] However, catheterization of the internal jugular vein necessitates cannulating a central vein that cannot be visualized or palpated. The most frequent complication is carotid artery puncture. This is usually not a serious problem, except when a large catheter or introducer is inadvertently passed into the artery. In such cases, surgical exploration and repair may be necessary.[8]

Subclavian Vein. Subclavian venipuncture as a venous access route was first described by Aubaniac over 35 years ago.[10, 11] It offers the same advantages of the internal jugular approach, but the potential development of a pneumothorax must be considered.

The infraclavicular approach to the subclavian vein requires that the patient's head be turned slightly away from the side of catheterization and rested flat on the bed. A small, rolled towel placed longitudinally between the scapulae allows the shoulders to fall back onto the bed and brings the subclavian vein closer to the clavicle (Fig. 5–6). The clavicular head of the sternocleidomastoid muscle as it inserts on the clavicle and the anterior scalene muscle as it passes behind the clavicle are identified (Fig. 5–7). The location of the subclavian vein in this area is constant as it passes beneath the clavicle. If it is displaced, it is only more cephalad, as in the case of the patient with emphysema. It does not lie posterior to the scalene muscle.

After proper patient preparation, skin puncture is done just inferior to the clavicle at the junction of its middle and inner thirds, with the needle aimed at a point behind the sternal manubrium. The puncture site should permit a horizontal approach to the vein, with the needle tip always anterior to the anterior scalene muscle. As the needle passes under the clavicle, gentle negative pressure is applied to the syringe until venous blood is easily aspirated. If the vein is not entered, the needle is withdrawn slowly and completely with gentle aspiration. If unsuccessful, the landmarks are re-evaluated, and re-entry is directed slightly more cephalad or medially. The temptation to direct the needle more posteriorly should absolutely be avoided, as the vein does not lie behind the anterior scalene muscle but the subclavian artery and the cupula of the lung do. Upon puncture of the subclavian vein and free return of blood into the syringe, the catheter is inserted as described previously.

In 1965, Yoffa described a supraclavicular approach to the subclavian vein.[12] He and others reported a decreased number of complications associated with inadvertent puncture of arterial and pulmonary structures.[13]

The important landmarks for the supraclavicular approach to the subclavian vein are the clavicular head of the sternocleidomastoid muscle as it inserts upon the clavicle, the anterior scalene muscle behind the clavicle, and the subclavian artery behind the anterior scalene muscle (Fig. 5–8). After proper patient preparation, skin puncture is directed just behind the clavicle at a 45° angle to the sagittal plane and pointed 15° forward of the coronal plane. While gently aspirating the syringe, the needle is advanced, moving

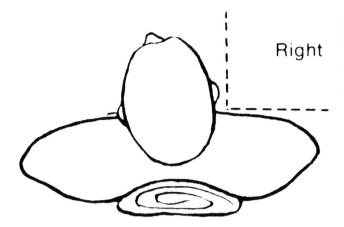

Figure 5–6. Correct placement of the patient for insertion of subclavian catheter is in the Trendelenburg position with the arms by the side. A rolled towel is placed along the thoracic spine to extend the shoulders. (From Grant JP: Handbook of Total Parenteral Nutrition. Philadelphia: WB Saunders, 1980; 50.)

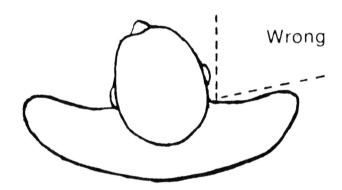

safely away from the structures of the subclavian artery and the lung. Once venous access is obtained, the syringe is lowered toward the shoulder to align the needle with the vein. Catheter placement then proceeds as previously described.

External Jugular Vein. The external jugular vein runs obliquely across the body of the sternocleidomastoid muscle toward the middle of the clavicle and into the subclavian vein. In spite of this vein's superficial location, successful placement of central venous catheters using this approach is often difficult owing to the two sets of valves within it and the acute angle with which it joins the subclavian vein. A guidewire with a flexible J-tip can be directed past the valves, bends, and branching vessels of the vein and can increase the success rate of properly positioning central venous catheters.[14, 15]

Blitt and coworkers' description of external jugular vein cannulation required a 5.5- or 6-inch over-the-needle cannula.[15] However, a variation of this method using a modified Seldinger technique with a short over-the-

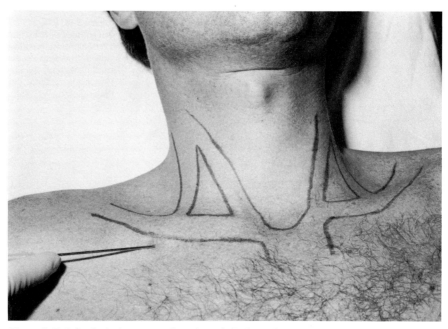

Figure 5–7. Infraclavicular approach to the subclavian vein.

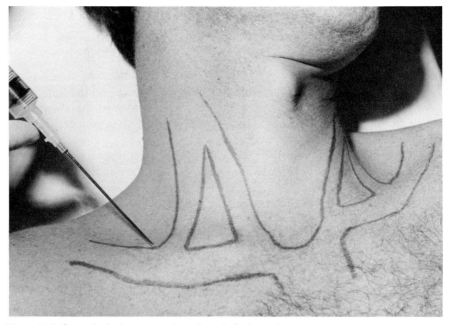

Figure 5–8. Supraclavicular approach to the subclavian vein.

needle cannula is less cumbersome and enables the clinician to insert a variety of catheters over the guidewire. After proper patient preparation, skin
puncture is made slightly distal to the midpoint of the vein. Cannulation
should only be attempted if the vein is easily visible or palpable. Applying
pressure just above the clavicle may help distend the vein. The patient's
performance of a Valsalva maneuver or use of gentle hepatic pressure also
distends the external jugular vein. The needle is advanced while applying
gentle aspiration until free flow of venous blood is obtained. The short over-
the-needle cannula is advanced off the needle into the vein, and the needle
is then removed. Blood should be easily aspirated from the cannula prior to
the insertion of the J-tipped guidewire. This may require some manipulation
until free flow is obtained. Then the guidewire is advanced through the short
cannula. If difficulties are met in advancing the wire into the central circulation, the wire can be rolled between the thumb and the index finger while
simultaneously moving the wire in and out 1–2 cm.[6] Once the guidewire is
advanced into the central circulation, the short cannula is removed and the
central catheter inserted in the usual fashion.

The external jugular vein is a popular site for access to the central
circulation, since its use is associated with a low complication rate and a
high success rate and it is easily accessible to the anesthesiologist during an
operative procedure.[15, 16] Catheterization of the external jugular vein avoids
the risks of inserting a needle deep into the neck and is a safe technique for
the patient with a bleeding diathesis or on anticoagulants. Thrombosis of
the vein occurs in 2–3% of cases.[17] Pulmonary artery catheterization can
be accomplished with this approach, although the large venous introducers
occasionally cannot be successfully passed under the clavicle. At other
times, the introducer cannot turn the acute angle as it enters the subclavian
vein; this causes it to kink, so that the pulmonary artery catheter cannot pass
through it. Therefore, even in experienced hands, the rate of successful
placement of central venous catheters and introducers is higher with the
internal jugular and subclavian vein approaches than with the external jugular vein approach.[6]

Femoral Vein. The femoral vein is used to gain access to the central
circulation, provided the catheter is sufficiently long to reach the mediastinal
level of the vena cava. It accompanies the femoral artery and becomes the
external iliac vein, which flows into the inferior vena cava. The femoral vein
is easily cannulated percutaneously in the femoral triangle just below the
inguinal ligament. The major structures in the triangle, from lateral to medial,
are the femoral nerve, femoral artery, femoral vein, and lymph tissue (Fig.
5–9). The structures are superficial, and the arterial pulse can be easily
identified just below the inguinal ligament. Skin puncture is made about 1
cm medial to the arterial pulse with a short over-the-needle cannula directed
slightly medially, parallel to the palpated pulse. Gentle aspiration is maintained with a syringe attached to the needle as it is advanced until free flow
of venous blood is obtained. The short cannula is advanced off the needle
into the vein. Free flow of blood is confirmed, and the guidewire is advanced
through the cannula into the central circulation. The chosen central catheter
is then threaded over the wire in the usual fashion. The Seldinger technique,

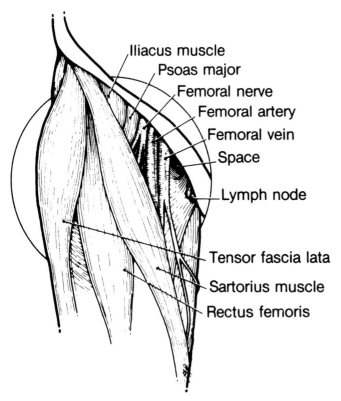

Iliacus muscle
Psoas major
Femoral nerve
Femoral artery
Femoral vein
Space
Lymph node
Tensor fascia lata
Sartorius muscle
Rectus femoris

Figure 5–9. Anatomy of the femoral region. The femoral artery is medial to the femoral nerve, and the femoral vein is medial to the artery. (From Blitt CC: Monitoring in Anesthesia and Critical Care Medicine. New York: Churchill Livingstone, 1985; 160. By permission.)

consisting of a wire passed directly through a thin-walled needle, may also be used.

Catheterization of the femoral vein is simple and has a reported high success rate.[18] However, femoral vein catheterization is associated with a high incidence of complications. Deep vein thrombosis or thrombophlebitis occurs in 5–50% of cases, and pulmonary embolism occurs in approximately 2%.[17, 19] Catheter-related septicemia has been reported in 2–20% of cases.[17, 19, 20] Therefore, it is recommended that catheterization of the femoral vein be avoided except for short-term use or in unusual circumstances.

Antecubital Veins. The veins of antecubital fossae are used frequently because of their ease of puncture and their size and because of the minimal discomfort to the patient. However, the success rate for central placement by this route is low.[21]

The medial basilic vein is preferred over the more lateral cephalic vein because of the difficulty that may occur when the catheter is advanced through the shoulder region using the lateral cephalic vein (Fig. 5–10). A catheter-through-the-needle method is the most common technique employed for basilic vein cannulation, and numerous prepackaged devices are available in appropriate lengths. Many have a removable, flexible guidewire within the catheter for ease of insertion. A modified Seldinger technique may also be used for insertion of introducers when pulmonary artery catheterization is indicated.

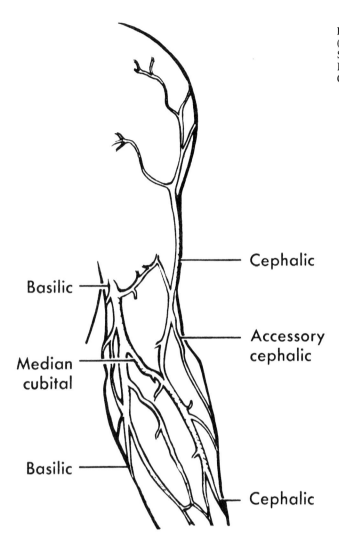

Figure 5–10. Anatomy of the antecubital fossa. (Reproduced by permission from Daily EK, Schroeder JS [eds]: Techniques in Bedside Hemodynamic Monitoring. St Louis, 1985, The CV Mosby Co; 58.)

Basilic

Median cubital

Basilic

Cephalic

Accessory cephalic

Cephalic

The puncture site is prepared as described previously, a tourniquet applied, and the needle puncture made. Free flow of venous blood into the catheter is the best evidence that the needle is free within the vein. The tourniquet is removed, and the catheter is advanced through the needle. Any early resistance or early cessation of advancement suggests that the catheter is extraluminal or even located within the venous wall. This indicates that the needle and catheter should be withdrawn and a new puncture made. The catheter should not be withdrawn through the needle to avoid shearing and embolism of the catheter. Difficulty with continued advancement may occur at the shoulder region, particularly if the cephalic vein is used. Manipulating the arm by rotating, adducting, abducting, or straightening it often permits further advancement of the catheter tip. The catheter may also meet some resistance at the venous valves, which can be overcome with gentle manipulation of the catheter. Sometimes, the catheter passes into the ipsilateral internal jugular vein. The chance of this occurring can be reduced by turning the patient's head toward the side of the needle puncture.[22-24] After insertion, care must be taken to fix the needle tip so that it cannot sever the catheter.

Catheter Care

To prevent inadvertent removal or advancement of the catheter, it is sutured in place and taped securely. Finally, a sterile dressing with antimicrobial ointment is applied. A chest roentgenogram is always obtained following central venous catheterization to ascertain the position of the catheter tip and to check for pneumothorax.

In the operating room, verification of catheter position is performed by observation of the waveform and aspiration of blood through the lumen. The proper position of a central venous catheter depends upon its purpose. For measurement of right ventricular filling pressures, a right atrial placement would be indicated. However, owing to the thinness of the atrial wall, it is recommended that a catheter not be left within the right atrium because of the danger of perforation and resultant cardiac tamponade. The ideal location of a central venous catheter is within the superior vena cava, just proximal to its entry into the right atrium.

Care of central venous catheters includes a constant infusion source to maintain catheter patency. However, the use of high-pressure bags with a continuous flush device has the potential risk of fluid overload, particularly in children. It is recommended that a syringe or Harvard pump system be used to maintain catheter patency in infants and small children and that fluid infusions be controlled at 1 ml/hour. When pulmonary hypertension is present, a constant infusion of 2 ml/hour is recommended to maintain catheter patency. Anticoagulation of flush solutions with heparin is usually a personal decision, although an hourly infusion of 1 U of heparin should not cause a coagulopathy.

Monitoring of CVP in Pediatric Patients

General Considerations

Invasive hemodynamic monitoring with central venous and pulmonary artery catheters has become routine in critically ill children for the diagnosis and management of hemodynamic problems. However, pediatric patients who require hemodynamic monitoring present a wide range of problems that are absent in the adult patient. The clinician must recognize the unique physiologic characteristics of children that make them different from adults (Table 5-4). These differences influence the choice of monitoring used, whether noninvasive or invasive. In addition, certain basic considerations should be understood. A child's small vascular lumen makes cannulation difficult. The quality of pressure tracings from small catheters inserted into these lumina are less than optimal. Blood loss occurring during the insertion procedure and during the sampling of central venous blood may represent a significant proportion of a small infant's total blood volume. Fluid overload

Table 5–4. HEMODYNAMIC VARIABLES: COMPARISON OF PEDIATRIC AND ADULT PATIENTS

Variable	Pediatric	Adult
Estimated Blood Volume	80 ml/kg	65 ml/kg
Heart Rate (Age-related)		50–80 beats/minute
Infants	120–160 beats/minute	
Toddlers	90–140	
Preschoolers	80–110	
School age children	75–100	
Adolescents	60–90	
Systemic Arterial Pressure (Age-related)		90–140/60–90 mmHg
Neonates	60–90/20–60 mmHg	
Infants	74–100/50–70	
Toddlers	80–112/50–80	
Preschoolers	82/100/50–78	
School age children	84–120/54–80	
Adolescents	94–140/62–80	
Stroke Volume		50–120 ml/beat
Neonates	5 ml/beat	
Preschoolers	15 ml/beat	
School age children	35 ml/beat	
Cardiac Index	3.5–4 L/minute/m^2	2.5–4 L/minute/m^2
Systemic Vascular Resistance	800–1600 dynes/sec/cm^5	1200–1500
Pulmonary Vascular Resistance	80–240 dynes/sec/cm^5	100–300
Right Atrial Pressure	3 mmHg	5 mmHg
Right Ventricular Pressure	30/3 mmHg	25/4 mmHg
Pulmonary Artery Pressure	30/10 mmHg	25/12 mmHg
Pulmonary Capillary Wedge or Left Atrial Pressure	8 mmHg	10 mmHg
Left Ventricular Pressure	100/6 mmHg	120/10 mmHg
Aortic Pressure	100/6 mmHg	120/80 mmHg

Reproduced by permission from Daily EK, Schroeder JS (eds): Techniques in Bedside Hemodynamic Monitoring. St Louis, 1985, The CV Mosby Co.

can occur quite insidiously in small children when standard flush devices and high-pressure bags are used. Children are also more susceptible to infection, and strict adherence to sterile technique must be maintained. The potential for paradoxical air embolus is real in children with right-to-left shunts, and strict adherence to proven technique is necessary. Finally, children are usually unable to cooperate with central venous catheterization and require physical or pharmacologic restraints in order to maintain safe and sterile technique.

Physiology

As with normal adults, there is good correlation between CVP, PADP, and LVEDP in children. However, many situations invalidate this relationship. Severe pulmonary disease, such as neonatal respiratory distress syndrome and other forms of respiratory failure, and use of positive pressure ventilation at high pressures, cardiopulmonary bypass, hypothermia, and massive blood transfusion all alter the relationship between CVP and LVEDP. In addition, sepsis, hypoxemia, and acidosis increase pulmonary vascular resistance, which poses additional difficulties in monitoring left ventricular function. Although central venous catheters can be used for infusion of large volumes of fluid and vasoactive drugs, for the measurement of right-sided filling pressures, for parenteral alimentation, and for venous access, the use of pulmonary artery catheters in small children and infants has gained wide acceptance for evaluation of LVEDP and cardiac function in such situations.

Technique

Central venous access in pediatric patients is obtained either by cutdown or by percutaneous use of the Seldinger technique after induction of general anesthesia or administration of sedation. The most commonly used insertion sites are the femoral, internal jugular, subclavian, and antecubital veins, although central venous catheters can be placed in the umbilical vein in the newborn infant (Fig. 5–11). The choice of site is often determined by the experience of the physician.

Anatomic studies at autopsy in pediatric patients less than 1 year of age and 6 kg of weight suggest that the internal and external jugular veins should be considered for access into the central venous system because they enter the superior vena cava with a straight course. The right and left subclavian veins appear to enter the central venous system at acute angles, which become less acute as the child grows.[25] Percutaneous access to the internal jugular vein can be obtained by either a high[26] or a low[27,28] approach. Success in either approach to the internal jugular vein is probably related more to the experience of the physician than to the choice of technique.

Some physicians prefer access to the central circulation of the child through an easily visualized external jugular vein. This avoids blind needle puncture in the neck and decreases the risk of pneumothorax from a subclavian vein approach. However, this must be weighed against the significant occurrence of improper positioning of the tip of the catheter within the central venous circulation. Success of proper intrathoracic position increases with the experience of the physician and the age of the child.[29, 30]

The infraclavicular approach to the subclavian vein is often preferred for long-term catheterization in children, although there is significant risk of pneumothorax, hydrothorax, and hemothorax.[31–35] The basilic vein has the advantages of being peripheral and easily visible or palpable. However, the success rate in reaching a central venous location is limited in small children. In children weighing over 20 kg, a removable guidewire within the prepackaged catheter, using a direct through-the-needle approach, can increase the rate of successful placement from the antecubital veins. The femoral vein provides a large vein that is easily identified in the femoral triangle. A wide variety of central venous catheters (including pulmonary artery catheters from the femoral approach) can be inserted using the traditional or modified Seldinger technique.

Complications

Erroneous Data

Calibrated Transducer versus Water Manometer. Measurement of CVP can be done with a simple manometer filled with an isotonic aqueous solution

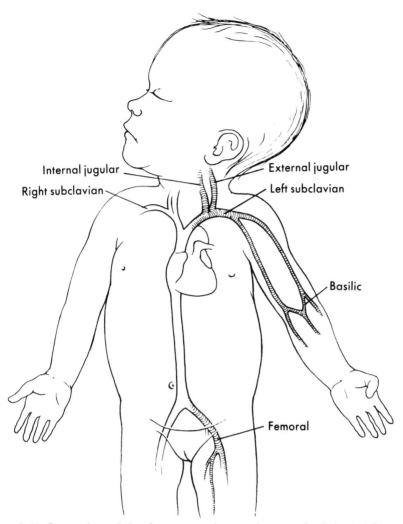

Figure 5–11. Commonly used sites for access to the central venous circulation in infants.

or with a pressure transducer system with a high-frequency response. The saline manometers are more commonly reported in centimeters of water, which is converted to millimeters of mercury by dividing by 1.36 (1 mmHg = 1.36 cmH$_2$O). The zero point of the manometer or transducer must be positioned exactly if low venous pressures are to be measured accurately. The right atrium is usually considered as the zero level, and it corresponds to the midaxillary line in the supine patient who has normal anatomy of the spine and thorax.

Although simple to use, water manometers have been replaced by more accurate, calibrated pressure transducers in the operating room and the intensive care unit. To obtain accurate CVP measurements, proper interpretation of the waveform must be made. Central venous waveforms obtained by electronic transducers show respiratory and cardiovascular fluctuations (Fig. 5–12). A digital display averages these fluctuations and gives inaccurate information if there are large intrapleural pressure changes with spontane-

EKG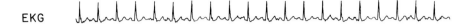

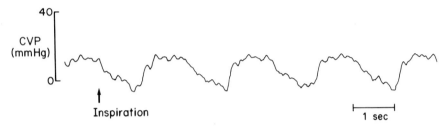

Figure 5–12. Large negative deflection in CVP waveform with inspiration.

ous or mechanical ventilation. Therefore, it is recommended that CVP waveforms be interpreted using a strip-chart recorder rather than a digital display.[36]

Alterations of the Central Venous Waveform. The normal central venous waveform is diagrammed in Figure 5–13. The best way to recognize waves is to look for descents or venous collapse. The A wave corresponds to atrial contraction and comes just before the systolic collapse or X′ descent. A large A wave in sinus rhythm implies the presence of a stronger-than-normal right atrial contraction such as occurs with an obstruction at the tricuspid valve or with a stiff, noncompliant right ventricle. If the atrium contracts when the tricuspid valve is closed, atrial pressure is transmitted backward into the vena cava to form a large A wave, called a cannon wave. Cannon waves occur with early P waves, such as with premature atrial depolarization or a junctional pacemaker or with atrioventricular dissociation. In atrial fibrillation, there is no atrial contraction and, therefore, no A wave.

The systolic collapse, or the X′ descent, is produced by the right ventricle drawing down the floor of the atrium during systole. A poor right ventricular contraction, such as with right ventricular infarction or failure, may attenuate or even eliminate the X′ descent. Atrial fibrillation decreases the X′ descent owing to loss of the atrial kick (decreased ventricular volume). In the presence of tricuspid regurgitation, the right atrium fills during systole, and the regurgitant volumes encroach on the X′ descent. This is seen as a

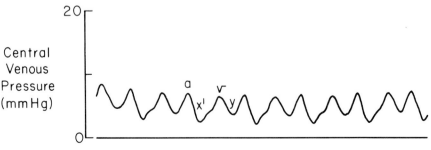

Figure 5–13. A normal CVP waveform.

higher-than-normal V wave. Normally, the V wave is built up during the end of ventricular systole while the tricuspid valve is still closed. As the strength of right ventricular contraction weakens, flow from the vena cava into the right atrium is unimpeded. This increased flow is seen as the V wave. Therefore, any increased flow into the right atrium during ventricular systole, such as with atrial septal defects and tricuspid regurgitation, increases the size of the V wave. The V wave begins earlier in atrial fibrillation, and only a prominent Y descent is seen on the CVP waveform.[37]

The Y descent occurs with opening of the atrioventricular valves following ventricular contraction. When the tricuspid valve opens in diastole, the atria and ventricles act as a single chamber. Pulmonary hypertension or pulmonary stenosis increases the resistance to right ventricular ejection, causing right ventricular hypertrophy and decreased compliance. The decreased compliance increases the diastolic pressure in this atrioventricle. If there is a higher pressure in this common chamber in diastole, the V wave builds up in the atrium from this increased base line. This results in an increased V wave.

Effects of Intrathoracic Pressure. Changes in the CVP occur with ventilation because changes in intrathoracic pressure are readily transmitted through the pericardium and relatively thin-walled atria and venae cavae. During spontaneous ventilation, inspiration lowers the CVP. All forms of positive pressure ventilation increase CVP, as does coughing or any Valsalva maneuver. In order to minimize the effects of respiration, CVP measurements are made at end-expiration using a calibrated pressure transducer and a strip-chart recorder.

Positive End-expiratory Pressure. The use of positive end-expiratory pressure (PEEP) presents additional problems in interpreting CVP in critically ill patients. The application of PEEP to a patient's airway is transmitted to the central vascular structures and increases right atrial pressure, measured CVP, and intrapleural pressure. The increase in right atrial pressure decreases venous return, resulting in a decreased cardiac output, making interpretation of a high CVP and cardiac function difficult. Ideally, transmural right atrial pressure (intravascular right atrial pressure minus intrathoracic pressure) reflects the true filling pressure. PEEP causes a decreased true filling pressure and cardiac output with an increase in measured CVP.[38]

A possible solution is to temporarily remove the patient from PEEP to make hemodynamic measurements. However, the beneficial effects on gas exchange that PEEP provides are quickly lost. When PEEP is reapplied, recovery time is prolonged. If PEEP is compromising cardiac output, temporary removal increases venous return and alters the patient's cardiovascular condition. Monitoring the patient in such a way does not reflect her or his true hemodynamic state when PEEP is present. Therefore, it is recommended that the patient's cardiovascular performance be monitored with PEEP present, recognizing that the CVP measurements obtained are slightly higher than those obtained without PEEP.

Physical Damage during Insertion of the Catheter

The potential for complications when inserting central venous catheters in critically ill patients is related to needle injury of adjacent tissues and vessels. The most common injury is inadvertent arterial puncture, with an incidence of approximately 2%.[39] The potential for vascular injury is decreased with the initial use of a small (22-gauge) needle to locate the internal jugular or subclavian vein. Few complications follow arterial puncture if the needle is immediately withdrawn and local pressure is applied. Inadvertent arterial puncture, and some venous punctures, can lead to localized hematoma formation. Observing the patient's vital signs should indicate more serious sequelae, such as pericardial tamponade from a subclavian artery puncture. The needle may also damage nerves at multiple sites, particularly the brachial plexus, stellate ganglion, and phrenic nerve. Inexperience with central venous catheterization procedures and poor attention to proper technique favor such complications.

Complications associated with the needle puncturing the pleura include pneumothoraces, hemothoraces, and chylothoraces. Mediastinal structures can be injured as well from the subclavian approach resulting in pneumomediastinum, hemomediastinum, pneumopericardium, and pericardial tamponade.

Entry of a bolus of air into the venous system is a potentially fatal event associated with insertion of central venous catheters. Air embolism occurs when the syringe is removed from the needle, when intravenous tubing is changed or accidentally disconnected, or when the subcutaneous track fails to close immediately following removal of a catheter.[40] Proper attention to detail at insertion and meticulous care of central venous catheters prevent air embolism.

Plastic catheters are easily sheared off into the central circulation by traction on the beveled tip of the inserting needle. There are numerous reports of catheter shearing and inevitable cardiac embolization.[41-47] To avoid this complication, plastic catheters should be inserted with the distal beveled tip of the needle introducer facing the patient. Unsuccessful catheterization necessitates simultaneous withdrawal of the catheter and needle to avoid shearing. No attempts should be made to manipulate the catheter in and out through the insertion needle during catheter placement. If embolization to the heart occurs, the retained catheter fragments must be removed because of the problems of myocardial thrombi, recurrent episodes of sepsis, and cardiac arrhythmias. Catheter fragments can be removed by a variety of percutaneous transvenous techniques. If transvenous techniques using fluoroscopy are unsuccessful, a simple incision may suffice. For right-sided heart fragments, cardiopulmonary bypass occasionally becomes necessary.[48,49]

Improper Position of the Catheter

It is very important that the central venous catheter tip be located properly in the superior vena cava for safe use. Catheters that enter small venous tributaries or the contralateral internal jugular or subclavian vein should be repositioned. Catheter tips located in the right atrium or right ventricle have been reported to perforate these chambers[50-53] or cause arrhythmias.[54] Extravascular catheter tips can lead to hydrothorax, hemothorax, and hemomediastinum. Checking for free flow of venous blood from the catheter lumen aids early detection of extravascular catheter tips.

Long-Term Complications

Late complications associated with central venous catheterization include infection, thrombosis, and perforation of vascular or cardiac structures.

Local and Systemic Infections. Central venous catheters are important causes of nosocomial infections and sepsis. Contamination can occur at the time of insertion owing to poor sterile technique with secondary bacterial migration from the skin after catheter placement, from hematogenous spread from distant infected foci, or from infected intravenous fluids, tubings, or transducers. Once the catheter is colonized, it may become a nidus for disseminated infection, particularly in the seriously ill and immunocompromised host. Identifying microbial colonization is a sensitive index of catheter-associated bacteremia, although standard broth culture methods lack specificity. The specificity of catheter cultures improved when Maki and colleagues[55] developed a semiquantitative solid agar culture technique that distinguishes colonized catheters from contaminated catheters. A positive semiquantitative culture (greater than 15 colonies) denotes infection, usually only locally, but a precursor of catheter-related septicemia. Other methods for the rapid diagnosis of intravascular catheter–related infection include Gram's staining of the catheter[56] and an impression smear.[57] The use of scanning electron microscopy to identify the presence of bacterial-glycocalyx biofilms on right-sided heart flow–directed catheters also reveals bacterial colonization.[58]

The risk of catheter-related bloodstream infections is approximately 4% when central venous catheters are used, as compared with the 1% risk for Teflon peripheral venous catheters.[59,60] Previous studies have suggested that most bloodstream infections related to intravascular devices originate from the patient's flora or from organisms on the hands of the personnel inserting the catheter.[61] At least two studies have demonstrated an association between the organisms present on the skin at the cannula insertion site and the organisms causing the bloodstream infection.[61,62] Although rigorous aseptic measures preclude the introduction of organisms at the time of catheter insertion, additional measures, such as careful maintenance of sterile technique during dressing changes and the prudent use of an appropriate antimicrobial ointment, are needed to prevent the invasion of organisms into the wound site after catheter insertion.

Thrombophlebitis. Complications associated with the presence of central venous catheters include venous thrombosis and thrombophlebitis. Most patients with thrombosis display edema of the involved arm, neck, and face. Infrequently, the first sign of central vein thrombosis is inability to catheterize a previously cannulated vein. No other symptoms may be present. An unknown source of sepsis may be the presenting sign of central vein thrombosis after secondary colonization with bacteria or fungi.[63]

When there is central vein thrombosis, microembolization and significant pulmonary embolization can occur.[64–67] If the clinical situation indicates pulmonary embolism, thrombosis of the central veins should be suspected and venograms considered. Treatment of central vein thrombosis requires removal of the catheter, culturing of the tip, and initiation of intravenous heparin therapy. Local symptoms should resolve in 24–48 hours, although eventual recannulation of the vein is difficult to document.

MONITORING OF PULMONARY ARTERY AND CAPILLARY WEDGE PRESSURES

When used judiciously, pulmonary artery catheters assist in the management of critically ill patients by allowing bedside determination of left ventricular filling pressure and cardiac output. However, the enthusiasm for invasive central monitoring in the 1970s and early 1980s has been tempered by the recognition of multiple associated complications, such as ventricular arrhythmias, pulmonary artery rupture, pulmonary infarction, and systemic or local infections. Therefore, a pulmonary artery catheter is only indicated when the data obtained will improve therapeutic decision making without unnecessary risk.

The pulmonary artery catheter measures CVP, PAP, and PCWP. It is balloon-tipped, allowing bedside placement without the aid of fluoroscopy.

Pulmonary artery systolic, diastolic, and mean pressures are easily determined with pulmonary artery catheters. Measurement of PADP is used to estimate LVEDP. At the end of diastole, the pulmonary arteries, pulmonary veins, left atrium, and left ventricle form a single chamber with a small pressure gradient in the direction of flow. When the pulmonary vascular bed, mitral valve, and left ventricle function normally, PADP, PCWP, mean left atrial pressure, and LVEDP are approximately equal.[68–70]

The distal thermistor can be used for the rapid determination of cardiac output using the thermodilution method. Numerous other parameters, such as cardiac index, systemic and pulmonary vascular resistance, and ventricular function curves, can be derived from these data. The catheter can be used to sample mixed venous blood, allowing determination of physiologic intrapulmonary shunting, oxygen consumption, and lactate levels. Finally, the pulmonary artery can be used for the administration of drugs or agents likely to cause phlebitis in the peripheral vasculature or which must be directed in a concentrated form into the heart or great vessels.

PCWP

Although measurement of CVP is valuable in determining right ventricular preload, in evaluating right ventricular dysfunction in right ventricular infarcts, and as a clue to the diagnosis of cardiac tamponade, CVP is of limited value in assessing left ventricular hemodynamics. Studies in a variety of clinical settings have demonstrated a poor correlation between right and left atrial filling pressures.[71, 72] In order to look at LVEDP, one of its correlates, PCWP[73] or PADP,[74] is used as an estimate of left-sided preload.

Equating PCWP with left atrial pressure assumes an open circuit from

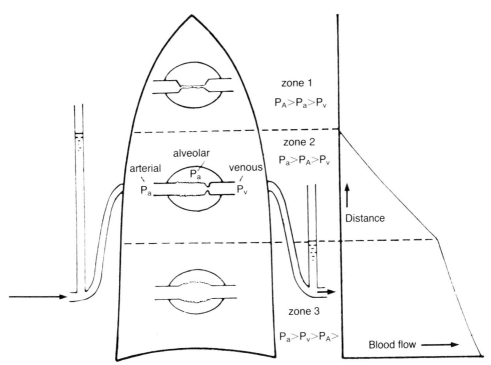

Figure 5–14. West's zones of lung and distribution of blood flow in the upright lung. (From West JB, Dollery CT, Naimark A: Distribution of blood flow in isolated lung: Relation to vascular and alveolar pressures. J Appl Physiol 1964; 19:723. With permission.)

the catheter tip to the left atrium with minimal pressure gradients. This is not the case if the vessel is filled with blood clots or if the catheter is located in West and associates' zones I and II in the pulmonary vascular tree, where alveolar pressure is greater than arterial pressure (zone I) or venous pressure (zones I and II) (Fig. 5–14).[75]

In zone III, where both pulmonary arterial and venous pressures exceed alveolar pressure, there is continuous flow, and conditions are met for accurate measurement of PCWP. Fortunately, most of the lung enters zone III when the patient is supine, and most pulmonary artery catheters float into zone III since most of the blood is flowing into this zone.[76] However, during low-flow states, such as hypovolemia,[77] or when PEEP increases alveolar pressure above pulmonary venous pressure, zone III may be converted to zone II.[78] If the tip of the catheter is at or below the left atrium, the conditions in zone III exist even if PEEP values are as high as 30 cmH_2O.[78,79] A cross-table lateral chest film aids in confirmation of the location of the catheter tip relative to the left atrium when its position is in doubt.[78-80] If the tip is above the atrium, the catheter should be repositioned to ensure zone III placement.

Effects of Ventilatory Mode

Transmural distending pressure determines ventricular inflow and stroke volume and is equal to the difference between intravascular pressure and extravascular pressure. In the majority of pulmonary blood vessels, extravascular pressure is atmospheric; therefore, when a measurement from a pulmonary artery catheter is referenced to atmospheric pressure, the recorded intravascular pressure equals the transmural pressure. If the extravascular pressure becomes positive, as with positive pressure ventilation without PEEP, transmural pressure is reduced by the amount of extravascular pressure. Negative extravascular pressure, as with spontaneous ventilation, increases transmural pressure and tends to dilate the vessel and increase flow. In both situations, transmural pressure is not reflected by the measured intravascular pressure. The solution is to measure the PADP and PCWP at end-expiration when extravascular pressure is closest to atmospheric pressure. This assures that pulmonary vascular pressures are not influenced by changes in pleural pressure. Measurements are made manually using a strip-chart recorder or from a calibrated screen so that the expiratory phase can be identified.

There are additional problems due to PEEP-induced changes in vascular and pleural pressures. As discussed previously, when positive pressure is applied to the airway at end-expiration, the increased alveolar pressure can convert a zone III to zone II or I. In addition, PEEP alters pleural pressure and pressures within the intrathoracic vessels.[38, 78] The amount of pressure transmitted to the pleural space and intrathoracic vessels depends on the level of PEEP and the compliance of the lungs and chest wall. A stiff, noncompliant lung does not transmit as much airway pressure to intrathoracic vessels as a noncompliant lung. As long as a zone III location of the pulmonary artery catheter is maintained, the measured intravascular PCWP approximates left atrial pressure. In fact, one study reports that PEEP up to 30 cmH2O does not markedly affect intravascular pressures in patients with very poor lung compliance.[81] The understanding is that the stiffer the lungs, the less the transmitted pressure. When high levels of PEEP are used in compliant lungs, more pressure is transmitted to the vessels, making interpretation of pressure measurements quite difficult. Other studies, however, suggest that in patients with noncompliant lungs, measured vascular pressures increase with increasing PEEP, as do pleural pressures and the true transmural distending pressure. The difference between the intravascular pressure and the pleural pressure may actually decline.[38]

One potential solution to this problem is to disconnect the patient from the ventilator and measure all the pressures referenced to atmospheric pressure at end-expiration. This is not always safe and is not recommended. The second solution is to place a pulmonary artery catheter in zone III of the lung and to keep the level of PEEP below 10 cmH2O. If the PEEP level is higher, the measured vascular pressures may rise 1–2 mmHg for every 5 cm of PEEP applied above 10 cmH2O.[76] Thus, although a PCWP or 18 mmHg in a patient breathing spontaneously would be associated with interstitial pulmonary edema, it may be an acceptable value in a patient receiving PEEP at 20 cmH2O.

The third alternative is to take direct measurement of intrapleural pressure as a means of assessing the transmural PCWP gradient.[82] This can be accomplished by inserting catheters into the pleural space or by using an esophageal balloon. Intrapleural pressure measurement is not feasible in all patients. Readings are always consistently made at end-expiration. Over-interpretation of pressure readings in patients receiving PEEP should be avoided.

Effects of Cardiac Pathology

Left atrial pressure is not equal to LVEDP in the presence of mitral valve disease or markedly reduced ventricular compliance.[68, 74, 76] In such a setting the PCWP is less helpful in assessing left ventricular function. LVEDP does not accurately reflect left ventricular end-diastolic volume.[1] A very stiff, noncompliant ventricle may allow a high end-diastolic pressure to accompany a normal end-diastolic volume. This poor correlation between PCWP and left ventricular end-diastolic volume is present in a broad group of critically ill patients, demonstrating the heterogeneity of myocardial compliance in the septic shock syndrome, ischemic heart disease,[83–87] and hemorrhagic shock.[88]

Pulmonary Hypertension

Jenkins and coworkers[89] and Scheinman and colleagues[90] correlated PADP to left atrial pressure in patients with heart disease but normal pulmonary vascular resistance. When pulmonary vascular resistance is abnormal, as with pulmonary hypertension, this correlation is lost. An elevated pulmonary vascular resistance is usually associated with elevated PAPs and increases right ventricular afterload. This may cause right ventricular failure and elevated CVP as well. Despite these changes, left atrial pressure remains in the normal range. Thus, in the presence of pulmonary hypertension, one must determine PCWP and not use PADP as an approximation of LVEDP.[70, 74]

The pulmonary artery catheter can aid in diagnosing pulmonary hypertension and evaluating intracardiac pressures. The administration of vasoactive drugs directly into the right-sided heart chamber or pulmonary vasculature can be guided by the hemodynamic information obtained during pharmacologic intervention.

Clinical Uses

Use in Cardiac Surgery

Pulmonary artery catheters are used in the perioperative management of patients with compromised ventricular function undergoing valve replacement, coronary artery bypass grafting, resection of ventricular aneurysms, and repair of congenital heart defects. The accurate reflection of left- and right-sided preload and the rapid determination of cardiac output by the thermodilution technique permit mechanical and pharmacologic therapy to optimize cardiac function and tissue perfusion in the perioperative period.[91] The no. 7-F, quadruple-lumen, balloon-tipped thermodilution catheter is inserted percutaneously in adults and advanced into the pulmonary artery by continuous pressure monitoring preoperatively.

Thermodilution catheters without balloon tips may be inserted directly into the right atrium during cardiac surgical procedures. This technique is applicable to the pediatric population or to patients with disease of tricuspid or pulmonic valves.

Use in General Surgery

Induction of anesthesia, endotracheal intubation, and other circumstances associated with marked alteration in left ventricular afterload or in blood volume represent periods of intense stress to the surgical patient. Extensive surgical procedures, such as large abdominal resections and transurethral prostatic resections, are associated with changes in blood volume that may be poorly tolerated in patients with prior myocardial infarction, angina pectoris, or pulmonary hypertension. Accurate assessment of volume status and cardiac performance is especially helpful in elderly patients or patients with severe cardiac or pulmonary disease. Vascular procedures, such as surgery for resection of thoracic or abdominal aortic aneurysms, are facilitated by perioperative control of preload and cardiac output to limit the cardiac and renal complications associated with these procedures.[92] Prolonged orthopedic procedures, débridement and grafting of severe burns, and surgery for multitrauma may all indicate the need for invasive hemodynamic monitoring with a pulmonary artery catheter.

Use in Intensive Care Units

Hemodynamic Monitoring. The flow-directed, balloon-tipped catheter is commonly used in intensive care units for patients with septic or anaphylactic shock, multisystem organ failure, instability during hemodialysis, intra-aortic balloon counterpulsation, and acute vasodilator therapy. Pulmonary artery catheterization has not been shown to decrease mortality in the critically ill, although it provides data useful for diagnosis and therapy. Pulmonary artery catheters distinguish cardiogenic from noncardiogenic pulmonary edema and guide treatment in patients with adult respiratory distress syndrome, pulmonary embolus, cor pulmonale, and fat embolism syndrome.

Patients with acute myocardial infarction complicated by perforated ventricular septum, mitral regurgitation, severe pulmonary congestion, or cardiogenic shock benefit from invasive hemodynamic monitoring.[93, 94] When clinical shock is present after acute myocardial infarction, the short-term mortality and morbidity rates are reduced from 85–90% to 50% or less with measurement of PAPs.[95] In contrast to these findings, a community-wide study of 3263 patients with validated acute myocardial infarction failed to demonstrate a beneficial effect in hospital stay or mortality rate associated with the use of a pulmonary artery catheter in the management of patients with congestive heart failure, hypotension, or cardiogenic shock.[96] A randomized controlled clinical trial to assess the efficacy of the pulmonary artery catheter in patients with acute myocardial infarction is indicated as more pulmonary artery catheters are used to manage this high-risk population.

A pulmonary artery catheter guides preload and afterload therapy in patients with severe congestive heart failure or unstable angina. Constrictive pericarditis or cardiac tamponade due to a variety of causes is effectively recognized by the near equality of right atrial pressure, right ventricular diastolic pressure, PADP, and PCWP. Acute bacterial endocarditis and congestive cardiomyopathy are additional indications for hemodynamic monitoring in the intensive care unit.

Sampling of Mixed Venous Blood. The capability of obtaining true mixed venous blood from the distal port of the pulmonary artery catheter for analysis of oxygen consumption, intrapulmonary shunt fraction, arterial minus mixed venous oxygen content difference, and lactate levels is an advantage of the pulmonary artery catheter over simple central venous catheters. Although the partial pressure of oxygen in the superior vena cava of normal persons is close to the true mixed venous partial pressure, it is much higher in patients in shock because blood flow is redistributed away from the renal and splanchnic beds.[97] Blood from the inferior vena cava is also a poor reflection of true mixed venous oxygen tension ($P\bar{v}O_2$) because of the large nonmetabolic blood flow from the kidneys. Use of blood from the right atrium for determination of $P\bar{v}O_2$ also may yield an inaccurate measurement since there may be inadequate mixing of the three sources of mixed venous blood (the inferior vena cava, superior vena cava, and coronary sinus) in the atrium.[98]

Since the true $P\bar{v}O_2$ reflects the difference between the oxygen delivered and the oxygen consumed, it is important to obtain an accurate sample in the critically ill patient to make important assessment of the adequacy of perfusion. The normal $P\bar{v}O_2$ is 40 mmHg. Because of regional difference in blood flow, a normal $P\bar{v}O_2$ does not necessarily indicate adequate perfusion in each organ system. This is especially evident in patients with multisystem organ failure associated with adult respiratory distress syndrome,[99] although it is safe to say that the finding of a reduction in mixed venous oxygen does suggest poor tissue oxygenation. A decreased $P\bar{v}O_2$ is found whenever the oxygen delivery system fails, whether from decreased arterial oxygen tension, decreased hemoglobin, or decreased cardiac output. For instance, in patients with congestive heart failure, the mixed venous oxygen content declines and decreases further with the onset of cardiogenic shock as the myocardial pump fails.[100] A reduction in $P\bar{v}O_2$ also occurs when there are increased tissue requirements, such as with sepsis, severe burns, and seizures.

Myocardial Ischemia. Left ventricular ischemia decreases left ventricular compliance, increasing LVEDP, left atrial pressure, PCWP and PADP. When the myocardium is ischemic and noncompliant, the PCWP waveform reveals a large A wave during atrial contraction. In addition, ischemia may cause dysfunction of the mitral papillary muscles, allowing intermittent mitral regurgitation (Fig. 5–15). These signs of myocardial ischemia and the effects of therapeutic interventions such as intravenous nitroglycerin on the size of an A or V wave are assessed with a pulmonary artery catheter.

Measurement of Thermodilution Cardiac Output. The modification of

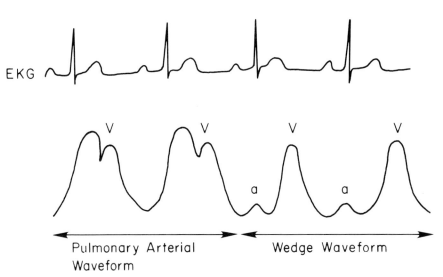

EKG

V   V   V   V

a   a

Pulmonary Arterial Waveform   Wedge Waveform

Figure 5–15. Presence of a large V wave with mitral regurgitation. (From Nadeau S, Noble WH: Misinterpretation of pressure measurements from the pulmonary artery catheter. Can Anaesth Soc J 1986; 33:352. With permission.)

the pulmonary artery catheter by Forrester and associates[101] permits multiple and rapid determinations of cardiac output in the operating room and intensive care unit via the thermodilution technique. The technique employs a known amount of sterile solution of known temperature, usually 2–10 ml of 0°C 5% dextrose. The cold indicator is injected into the right atrium, and the resultant change in blood temperature is measured in the pulmonary artery by the distal thermistor. By integrating the temperature change over time, cardiac output is computed. Care must be taken to assure rapid injection, complete indicator mixing, and no indicator loss. Once cardiac output data are determined, ventricular function curves can be made and used to assess ventricular performance while evaluating therapies. If intracardiac shunts and tricuspid regurgitation are present, the method is not accurate, in which case indicator dilution or other techniques must be used. Refer to the appropriate cardiac output computer manual for specific instructions on the use of thermodilution catheters for cardiac output determination (see also Chapter 7). In addition to cardiac output, systemic and pulmonary vascular resistance are easily calculated from directly measured values provided by the pulmonary artery catheter, intra-arterial catheter, and standard laboratory tests (Table 5–5).

Insertion Technique

Choice of Catheter.

The standard no. 7-F thermodilution pulmonary artery catheter is 110 cm in length and contains four lumina: a distal pulmonary artery port, a

Table 5–5. DERIVED HEMODYNAMIC VARIABLES

Cardiac Index (CI)	CI = CO/BSA
Systemic Vascular Resistance (SVR)	SVR = (MAP − CVP)/CO × 80
Systemic Vascular Resistance Index (SVRI)	SVRI = (MAP − CVP)/CI × 80
Pulmonary Vascular Resistance (PVR)	PVR = (MPAP − PCWP)/CO × 80
Pulmonary Vascular Resistance Index (PVRI)	PVRI = (MPAP − PCWP)/CI × 80
Stroke Index (SI)	SI = CI/HR
Left Ventricular Stroke Work Index (LVSWI)	LVSWI = SI × (MAP − PCWP) × 0.0136
Right Ventricular Stroke Work Index (RVSWI)	RVSWI = SI × (MPAP − CVP) × 0.0136

Key: CO = cardiac output, BSA = body surface area, MAP = mean arterial pressure, CVP = central venous pressure, MPAP = mean pulmonary arterial pressure, PCWP = pulmonary capillary wedge pressure, HR = heart rate

proximal central venous port, a balloon inflation port, and a thermistor connector (Fig. 5–16). It is constructed of flexible, radiopaque polyvinylchloride. Thermodilution catheters with an additional proximal venous infusion port are available and are helpful when managing critically ill patients who are receiving numerous vasoactive infusions or parenteral hyperalimentation.

The quadruple-lumen catheter comes in two sizes: nos. 5 and 7 F. The no. 5-F size is suitable for children under 18 kg, whereas the no. 7 F is used in larger children and adults.[102] Both have proximal and distal ports and an inflatable balloon of 1.5-cc capacity. The fourth lumen supports the wiring to the thermistor located near the tip. Proper use of the 5-F catheter requires an understanding of the differences between the two sizes. The smaller catheter does not allow rapid infusion of fluids, which would falsely elevate pressure readings. Its use in small infants is difficult/because of the distance between the proximal and the distal ports. Although the tip may be placed appropriately in the pulmonary artery, the proximal port may lie outside the internal jugular vein. For such infants, nos. 2.5- and 3.5-F double-lumen thermodilution catheters, consisting of a vascular lumen and thermistor, are available (Fig. 5–17). They can be used in children under 10 kg of weight for the measurement of cardiac output, with the separate insertion of a right atrial catheter for the injection of cold saline.[103, 104] These nonballoon thermodilution catheters are inserted directly into the right atrium and pulmonary artery[105] at the time of cardiac surgery. Such catheters are also used in adults who have disease of tricuspid or pulmonic valves.

Choice of Site

Catheterization of the pulmonary circulation is accomplished from subclavian, internal jugular, external jugular, femoral, or antecubital veins. In general, insertion into the internal jugular vein is preferred because this approach is associated with a lower incidence of pneumothorax than insertion into the subclavian vein.[46, 106–108] The internal jugular vein is readily available to the anesthesiologist, allowing intraoperative manipulation of the catheter if necessary. Pulmonary artery catheters are easier to secure in the neck or subclavian area than in the antecubital fossa and are less likely to

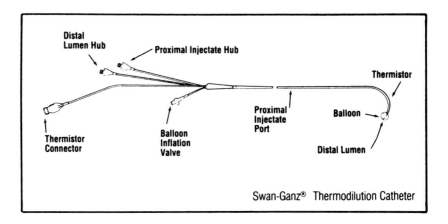

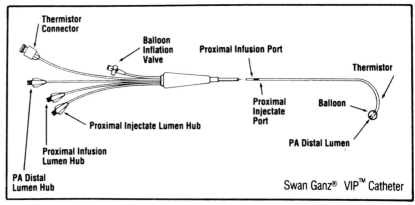

Figure 5–16. Four- and five-lumen balloon-tipped pulmonary artery catheters. (From American Edwards, Santa Ana, CA. With permission.)

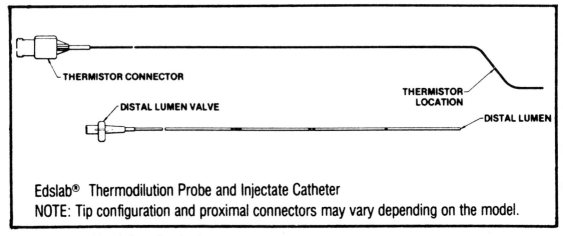

Figure 5–17. Non–balloon-tipped pulmonary artery catheter and separate injectate catheter. (From American Edwards, Santa Ana, CA. With permission.)

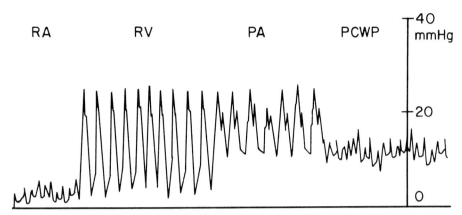

Figure 5–18. Pressure waveforms obtained from a balloon-tipped pulmonary artery catheter during insertion. (From Matthay MA: Invasive hemodynamic monitoring in critically ill patients. Clin Chest Med 1983; 4:234.)

become malpositioned by patient movement. However, in patients with tracheostomies requiring frequent suctioning, antecubital insertion is preferable. The antecubital fossa is a preferred site in patients with a bleeding diathesis in order to avoid hemorrhage associated with accidental carotid or subclavian artery puncture.

Intravascular Placement

Pulmonary artery catheters can be inserted after preparation of the patient as previously described for central venous catheter placement. It is essential to decrease the patient's pain, anxiety, and myocardial stimulation with appropriate sedatives and analgesics. Pressure transducers are zeroed and calibrated. The catheter's injectate and pressure monitoring lumina are debubbled and connected to the flush system and pressure transducers. The patency of the balloon is checked prior to insertion. Continuous electrocardiographic monitoring is used to evaluate any arrhythmias that occur during insertion. Antiarrhythmic drugs, defibrillating equipment, and respiratory-assist equipment should be readily available. Catheters should not be bent, stretched, or wiped excessively (removal of heparin coating) during preparation.

The catheter can be inserted directly into the vein, but it is usually inserted through an introducer sheath that is one size larger than the pulmonary artery catheter being used. Prepackaged trays containing the necessary supplies for venous cannulation and placement of no. 8-F introducers are available. After successful catheterization of the central veins, the pulmonary artery catheter is inserted into the introducer and advanced while the pressure and waveform of the distal port are observed (Fig. 5–18). After it enters the central circulation (usually a distance of 20–30 cm from jugular or subclavian entry), the balloon is fully inflated and advanced into the right atrium. Venous entry at the right arm requires about 40 cm, left arm 50 cm, and femoral vein 60 cm to reach the right atrium. Only the recommended volume of air, never liquid, for balloon inflation should be used. The catheter length necessary to reach the right atrium can be initially measured by noting the length from the insertion site to the sternomanubrial notch.

The catheter floats across the tricuspid valve through the right ventricle, across the pulmonic valve, and into the pulmonary artery, verified by the waveform. The catheter is advanced into the pulmonary artery with the balloon inflated until the pressure waveform appears "damped" and the numeric display records a pressure less than the PADP level. This represents the PCWP. If deflation of the balloon does not restore the pulmonary artery waveform, the catheter has been inserted too far and should be withdrawn slowly until a pulmonary artery waveform returns. The catheter is then secured in place at the insertion site and protected by a sterile dressing. A chest x-ray confirms proper placement of the catheter.

It is important not to use an excessive length of pulmonary artery catheter during insertion. If the right ventricle pressure waveform is still observed after advancing the catheter 15 cm beyond the point that the initial right ventricle pressure was observed, the catheter may be looping in the ventricle, which can result in kinking or knotting of the catheter. If insertion is unsuccessful initially, the catheter should be withdrawn to the right atrial position after balloon deflation and the catheter readvanced. Failure of a balloon-tipped pulmonary artery catheter to enter the right ventricle or pulmonary artery is rare, but it occurs in patients with an enlarged right atrium or ventricle, low cardiac output, tricuspid insufficiency, or pulmonary hypertension. Deep inspiration by the patient during advancement may facilitate passage. Fluoroscopic guidance for placement should only rarely be required. At no time should force be used during insertion, as this may damage the catheter lumina.

Pediatric Pulmonary Artery Catheterization

Flow-directed pulmonary artery catheters are used in critically ill pediatric patients to monitor left and right ventricular preload.[102, 109-111] Measurement of cardiac output by the thermodilution technique is reliable in children over a wide range of flow values.[112, 113]

The indications for the use of pulmonary artery catheters in infants and children include (1) assessment of right ventricular preload and tricuspid valve adequacy by monitoring the CVP, (2) assessment of left ventricular function and adequacy of mitral valve function by monitoring the PADP and PCWP, (3) assessment of pulmonary blood flow and resistance, (4) measurement of cardiac output, (5) assessment of systemic vascular resistance, and (6) measurement of mixed venous oxygen tension.

The degree of difficulty in cannulating the central circulation in infants and children necessitates a high degree of vigilance to maintain catheter position and patency. As in central venous catheters, pulmonary artery catheters require only 1 ml/hour delivery of fluid to maintain patency that should be delivered by syringe or Holter pump. If pulmonary pressures exceed 50 mmHg, a constant infusion of 2 ml/hour maintains patency. If the pulmonary artery pressures are greater than 100 mmHg, an infusion rate of 3 ml/hour is needed.[114]

The same sterile technique and precautions (e.g., continuous electro-cardiogram and pressure monitoring) employed in adult patients are used in children. Common insertion sites include the internal and external jugular veins, subclavian vein, median basilic vein, and femoral vein. After the introducer is inserted, the pulmonary artery catheter is passed. Air is normally used to inflate the balloon, but the risk of air embolism in patients with intracardiac shunts may be reduced by the use of carbon dioxide.

Complications of Pulmonary Artery Catheterization

Since the introduction of the pulmonary artery catheter for continuous monitoring of hemodynamic function, numerous complications related to both catheter insertion and the presence of the catheter in the pulmonary artery have been reported.[106, 108, 115]

Erroneous Data

Equipment. The pressure transducer must be calibrated in the range of PAPs rather than systemic pressures and zeroed at the level of the mid left atrium. If the patient's position changes, the transducer should be repositioned to obtain accurate data.

The discrepancy between automated digital and analog (strip-chart) recording systems may be therapeutically misleading because of the unselective nature of averaging values with digital readout (see Chapter 3).[116] In a patient with respiratory variability (as in asthma, chronic obstructive pulmonary disease, or positive-pressure ventilation with high-peak inspiratory pressures), the pulmonary pressures are subject to considerable alteration. The errors in automated pressure measurement believed to be clinically important vary with the ventilatory mode used.[117] Patients breathing spontaneously have the largest measurement error, with 42% of these patients having a clinically important error in PADP. Patients on assist/control modes have the fewest errors in automated pressure measurements.[117]

Because graphic data can be correlated to changes in intrathoracic pressure and end-expiration can be identified, it is prudent to measure pulmonary vascular pressures with an analog recording system. Pressures are read directly from a calibrated screen or printout rather than from a digital readout.[118] In a patient with rapid respiration, identifying the end-expiratory point may be difficult, and a simultaneous tracing of airway pressures may be helpful.

Overwedging. Serious complications are related to peripheral migration of the catheter tip as a result of cardiac contractions, catheter softening, or cardiac manipulation. The catheter should initially be positioned so that full balloon inflation is required to obtain a wedge waveform. When the pulmonary artery catheter has migrated too far peripherally, a PCWP waveform is obtained spontaneously without inflating the balloon. The permanent wedge position must be recognized and corrected before any attempts are made to inflate the balloon. Other times, a PCWP waveform is obtained without complete inflation of the balloon, and full inflation causes "over-wedging," giving falsely elevated values. These complications of pulmonary artery catheterization can be minimized by meticulous attention to detail. One should anticipate this migration and continuously monitor the waveform as well as obtain daily chest x-rays. Balloon inflation should be performed gradually with constant monitoring and be stopped as soon as the PCWP waveform is seen.

Physical Damage during Insertion of the Catheter

Complications from Passage of the Catheter. Central venous access must be obtained prior to passage of a pulmonary artery catheter. The complications of this procedure—arterial puncture, pneumothorax, air embolization, hematoma formation, and nerve injury—have been discussed previously. Complications reported with passage of the pulmonary artery catheter include dysrhythmias, valvular damage, and knotting of the catheter.[46, 106–108, 115]

Dysrhythmias. Serious ventricular dysrhythmias during pulmonary artery catheterization are common in the critically ill patient and are usually self-limited, but they may be sustained and require therapeutic intervention.[107, 119–125] Premature ventricular contractions usually stop once the tip of the catheter has left the ventricle. If they are sustained, or deteriorate to ventricular tachycardia, the absence of effective cardiac output prevents flotation of the catheter from the ventricle. In such cases, the pulmonary artery catheter should be pulled back to the right atrium until the dysrhythmia ceases.

Administration of lidocaine has been advocated prior to the flotation of the catheter tip through the right side of the heart to electrically stabilize the myocardium.[121, 126] However, in a double-blind comparison, lidocaine, 1 mg/kg, is no more effective than saline solution in suppressing catheter-induced ventricular ectopy.[127]

Dysrhythmias related to catheterization may also occur long after insertion,[128] and they are usually associated with looping of the catheter in the right atrium or ventricle. The catheter tip may also become displaced from the pulmonary artery into the right ventricle. These arrhythmias are highly resistant to antiarrhythmic therapy and require removal or repositioning of the catheter.

The pulmonary artery catheter can affect the cardiac conduction pathways. Up to 5% of patients develop new right bundle-branch block with passage of the catheter through the heart.[107, 120, 124, 129–131] Although it is usually hemodynamically insignificant, the pre-existence of a left bundle-branch block may predispose the patient to complete heart block, and the capability for artificial pacing should be available prior to inserting the catheter. Alternatively, pacemaker pulmonary artery catheters are available, but these may be unreliable pacemakers during insertion attempts.

Valvular Damage and Intracardiac Knotting. Pulmonary artery catheters have also been associated with tricuspid and pulmonary valve damage,[107, 132–134] particularly with prolonged catheterization.

Intracardiac knotting of the catheter has been reported.[135–137] Knots occur during insertion when the catheter coils in the right ventricle. This can be suspected when excessive length is used to float the catheter out of the right ventricle, although it is usually not recognized until a chest x-ray is obtained after placement of the catheter. The coiled catheter can be removed through the introducer, but this approach should be abandoned when resistance is encountered. Sometimes the knot can be resolved by insertion of a suitable guidewire and manipulation of the catheter.[138] More often, it becomes necessary to utilize fluoroscopy to untie the knot. If the knot does not include any intracardiac structures, it can be gently tightened and the catheter withdrawn through the site of entry.[135, 138–140] Occasionally, operative intervention becomes necessary.

Rupture of the Balloon. Rupture of the balloon has been rarely reported.[72] Air should never be used for balloon inflation in any pediatric patient or an adult with suspected right-to-left intracardiac or intrapulmonary shunts.[76] Instead, carbon dioxide (passed through a bacterial filter) should be used because of its rapid absorption. No more than the recommended volume of 1.5 cc of air is used to inflate the balloon. Passive balloon deflation prolongs balloon lifespan.

Complications from Improper Position of the Catheter

Pulmonary Infarction. Thromboembolism in the pulmonary vascular bed does occur with the use of pulmonary artery catheters, resulting in pulmonary infarction.[107, 141–144] In one series, a 7% incidence of infarction occurred secondary to persistent wedging of the catheter in a peripheral artery, obstruction of a more central artery by an inflated balloon, or formation of pulmonary emboli related to thrombosis at the catheter tip.[140] Prolonged balloon inflation while the catheter is in a wedge position should be avoided because it occludes the pulmonary artery and leads to pulmonary infarctions.

Pulmonary Artery Rupture. The most serious of all complications when using pulmonary artery catheters is rupture of the pulmonary artery, leading to massive pulmonary hemorrhage and death.[143–150] Several significant risk factors have been identified. Serious injury to the pulmonary artery is more likely in patients with pulmonary hypertension, hypothermia, and advanced age. Imminent rupture may be preceded by small amounts of hemoptysis. A fatal outcome may be more likely in patients given anticoagulants. Usually the episode of bleeding is associated with distal migration of the catheter and subsequent balloon inflation, although hemoptysis has been reported after flushing a catheter in the wedge position.[151]

Extreme caution should be exercised during the measurement of PCWP in patients with pulmonary hypertension. It is recommended that the period of time during which the balloon remains inflated and wedged in these patients should be limited to two respiratory cycles, of 10–15 seconds. If PADP and PCWP are nearly identical, PADP is substituted for PCWP, obviating the need for repeated balloon inflation.

Long-Term Complications

Local and Systemic Infections. The incidence of catheter-related sepsis is low but averages about 2% in most series.[107, 108, 115, 152, 153] However, an incidence as high as 35% has been reported.[107, 108, 115, 152, 153] Catheter-related infections are probably more likely if catheters are inserted in patients with bacteremia, if they are left in place for more than 72 hours, or if inflammation occurs around the insertion site.[152] The diagnosis of catheter colonization and sepsis is guided by the use of semiquantitative cultures of the pulmonary artery catheter and introducer tips as described by Maki and colleagues.[55] Senagore and coworkers[154] report that pulmonary artery catheters can be changed safely over a guidewire after 72 hours, avoiding further insertion risks without increasing infectious complications. Because of the serious nature of catheter-related septicemia in the critically ill patient, further controlled randomized clinical studies are needed before recommending this as a routine practice.

Endocardial Vegetations. Intravascular catheters traumatize the intimal vascular surface and may produce intramural thrombosis or hemorrhage.[155] Asymptomatic thrombotic complications are frequent with the routine use of pulmonary artery catheters and may be more likely with a diminished cardiac output.[107, 156, 157]

Review of autopsies documented the presence of petechial hemorrhages on the pulmonary valve leaflets and thrombotic vegetations on the endocardial surface of the right atrium as well as on the tricuspid and pulmonic valves.[107, 158–161] Evidence suggests that both septic and aseptic vegetations occur within the right side of the heart and that these vegetations may embolize.[158, 160, 162–164]

Left Atrial Pressure

Normally, left atrial pressure corresponds to the PCWP and PADP. In the presence of increased pulmonary vascular resistance, this relationship is altered, and the information obtained with routine central venous and pulmonary artery catheters is inadequate to estimate LVEDP. In such situations, direct measurement of left atrial pressure with a transthoracic catheter inserted at the time of cardiac surgery is necessary to guide fluid and drug therapy during the postoperative period.

Use in Cardiac Surgery

At the time of cardiothoracic surgery, catheters are inserted directly into the left atrium, through the chest wall. The catheter is inserted through the right superior pulmonary vein and threaded into the left atrium (Fig. 5–19). Left atrial catheters are indicated when the pulmonary circulation cannot be cannulated because of congenital anomalies or pulmonary hypertension. Direct atrial cannulation is also warranted when pulmonary pressures provide inaccurate reflection of left ventricular pressure, as in mitral stenosis. These catheters ensure continuous, accurate assessment of left ventricle filling pressure during the separation of the patient from cardiopulmonary bypass and throughout the postoperative period. Similar catheters are also available for infants and children.[112]

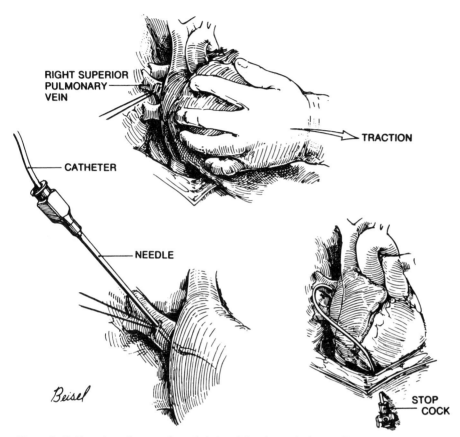

RIGHT SUPERIOR
PULMONARY
VEIN

TRACTION

CATHETER

NEEDLE

STOP
COCK

Beisel

Figure 5–19. Insertion of a transthoracic left atrial catheter during cardiac surgery. (From Waldausen JA, et al: Johnson's Surgery of the Chest, 5th Ed. Chicago: Year Book Medical, 1985; 257. Reproduced with permission.)

Complications

Problems related to transthoracic intracardiac monitoring catheters include bleeding, retained catheter fragments, catheter malposition, and dysrhythmias. In a series of 100 adult patients with transthoracic left atrial catheters undergoing open heart surgery for acquired valvular disease of the heart, no fatal complications occurred, although one patient required reexploration for uncontrolled bleeding after the catheter needle inadvertently damaged the internal mammary artery.[165]

A study of 5666 pediatric patients undergoing cardiac surgical procedures who had 6690 transthoracic intracardiac monitoring catheters inserted in the pulmonary artery, left atrium, and right atrium demonstrates an overall complication rate of 0.59%.[166] A total of 40 children suffered complications, and 1 of these died. The complications can be broken down into two general types. The first group included patients with catheters that could not be removed at the time desired. These patients required various procedures, including surgical exploration, to remove the retained catheter fragments.

The second group was composed of patients in whom intrapericardial bleeding occurred after catheter removal. Patients should be monitored closely for bleeding after catheter removal, and the physician should be prepared to rapidly resuscitate and re-explore the patient if hemodynamic compromise occurs.

Most complications of transthoracic intracardiac monitoring catheters can be safely managed if recognized early and treated aggressively. The hemodynamic information obtained with the use of these catheters is highly valued, and their use is a routine practice for many cardiac surgeons performing valve replacement and congenital heart surgery.

DETERMINATION OF BLOOD VOLUME

The end result of an inadequate blood volume is organ failure leading to immediate or delayed patient death. The normal blood volume of an adult human is about 5000 ml, about 3000 ml of which is plasma and the remaining 2000 ml is erythrocytes. However, age, sex, weight, antidiuretic hormone, atrial stretch receptors, sympathetic nervous system activity, and other factors affect blood volume. Plasma volume is determined by dilution techniques using Evans blue dye or radiolabeled albumin (^{131}I albumin). Alternatively, labeled erythrocytes (^{51}Cr) are used to determine blood volume by a dilution technique. Because the greater the blood volume, the less concentrated the labeled erythrocytes are after dissemination in the circulation, blood volume is calculated as

$$\text{Blood volume (ml)} = \frac{\text{Quantity of radiolabeled test substance}}{\text{Concentration of radiolabel/ml blood}}$$

The treatment of hypovolemia is directed toward restoring cellular and organ perfusion with adequately oxygenated blood. During the initial assessment of blood volume, monitoring vital signs, urinary output, level of consciousness, and CVP is important. If hypovolemia is suggested by the history and physical examination, initially fluid therapy is started. Further therapeutic and diagnostic decisions are based on the observed response. In general, return of blood pressure, pulse pressure, and pulse rate toward normal is a positive sign and indicates stabilization of the circulation. However, these observations give no information regarding organ perfusion. Improvements in the neurologic status and skin circulation are important evidence of enhanced perfusion but are difficult to quantitate. The urinary output can quantitate the renal response to restoration of perfusion and is reasonably sensitive (if not modified by diuretics). Adequate blood volume should produce a urinary output of approximately 1 ml/kg/hour. Inability to obtain a urinary output at this level suggests an inadequate blood volume. This situation should stimulate further fluid replacement and diagnostic endeavors.

Changes in CVP can provide useful information in the more complex patient. CVP monitoring is used as a guide to the ability of the right side of the heart to accept a fluid load. Properly interpreted, the response of the CVP to fluid administration is helpful in evaluating volume replacement. CVP and the actual blood volume are not necessarily related. The initial CVP is sometimes increased, even with a significant volume deficit, especially in patients with generalized vasoconstriction and rapid fluid replacement. A minimal increase in an initially low CVP with fluid therapy suggests the need for further volume expansion. A declining CVP suggests ongoing fluid loss and the need for additional fluid or blood replacement. An abrupt or persistent elevation in the CVP suggests that volume replacement has been adequate or is too rapid or that compromised cardiac function is present. The use of a flow-directed pulmonary artery catheter is then indicated to monitor the PADP and PCWP and to assess cardiac output.

References

1. Alderman EL, Glantz SA: Acute hemodynamic interventions shift the diastolic pressure-volume curve in man. Circulation 1976; 54:662–671.
2. Risk C, Rudo N, Falltrick R, et al: Comparison of right atrial and pulmonary capillary wedge pressures. Crit Care Med 1978; 6:172–175.
3. Mangano DT: Monitoring pulmonary arterial presssure in coronary-artery disease. Anesthesiology 1981; 53:364–370.
4. Coyle JP, Teplick RS, Long MC, et al: Respiratory variations in systemic arterial pressure as an indicator of volume status. (Abstract.) Anesthesiology 1983; 59:A53.
5. Seldinger SI: Catheter replacement of the needle in percutaneous arteriography. Acta Radiol 1953; 39:368–376.
6. Otto CW: Central venous pressure monitoring. *In* Blitt, CD (ed): Monitoring in Anesthesia and Critical Care Medicine. New York: Churchill Livingstone, 1985; 121–166.
7. Horrow JC, Metz S, Thickman D, Frederic MW: Prior carotid surgery does not affect the reliability of landmarks for location of internal jugular vein. Anesth Analg 1987; 66:452–456.
8. Jobes DR, Schwartz AJ, Greenhow DE, et al: Safer jugular vein cannulation: Recognition of arterial puncture and preferential use of the external jugular route. Anesthesiology 1983; 59:353–355.
9. Blitt CD: Catheterization Techniques for Invasive Cardiovascular Monitoring. Springfield, IL: CC Thomas, 1981.
10. Aubaniac R: Une novelle voie d'injection ou de ponction veineuse: La voie sous-claviculaire (veins sous-clavière, tronc brachio-céphalique). Semaine Hop Paris 1952; 28:3445.
11. Aubaniac R: L'injection intraveineuse sous-claviculaire. Avantages et technique. Presse Med 1952; 60:1456.
12. Yoffa D: Supraclavicular subclavian venipuncture and catheterization. Lancet 1965; 2:614–617.
13. Parsa MH, Ferrer JM, Habif DV, et al: Experience with central venous nutrition: problems and their prevention. Scientific exhibition presented at 57th Annual Clinical Congress, American College of Surgeons, October 1971.
14. Blitt CD, Carlson GL, Wright WA, et al: J-wire versus straight wire for central venous system cannulation via the external jugular vein. Anesth Analg 1982; 61:536–537.

15. Blitt CD, Wright WA, Petty WC, et al: Central venous catheterization via the external jugular vein: A technique employing the J-wire. JAMA 1974; 229:817–818.

16. Belani KG, Buckley JJ, Gordon JR, Castenada W: Percutaneous cervical central venous line placement: A comparison of the internal and external jugular vein routes. Anesth Analg 1980; 59:40–44.

17. Burri C, Ahnefeld FW: The Caval Catheter. Berlin: Springer-Verlag, 1978.

18. Duffy B: The clinical use of polyethylene tubing for intravenous therapy. Ann Surg 1949; 130:929–936.

19. Bonner CD: Experience with plastic tubing in prolonged intravenous therapy. N Engl J Med 1951; 245:97–98.

20. Bansmer G, Keith D, Tesluk H: Complications following use of indwelling catheters of inferior vena cava. JAMA 1958; 167:1606–1611.

21. Webre DR, Arens JF: Use of cephalic and basilic veins for introduction of central venous catheters. Anesthesiology 1973; 38:389–392.

22. Burgess GE, Marino RJ, Peuler MJ: Effect of head position in the location of venous catheters inserted via basilic veins. Anesthesiology 1977; 46:212–213.

23. Dietel M, McIntyre JA: Radiographic confirmation of site of central venous pressure catheters. Can J Surg 1971; 14:42–52.

24. Langston CS: The aberrant central venous catheter and its complications. Radiology 1971; 100:55–59.

25. Cobb LM, Vinocur CD, Wagner CW, Weintraub WH: The central venous anatomy in infants. Surg Gynecol Obstet 1987; 165:230–234.

26. Cote CJ, Jobes DR, Schwartz AJ, Ellison N: Two approaches to cannulation of a child's internal jugular vein. Anesthesiology 1979; 50:371–373.

27. Rao TLK, Wong AYU, Salem MR: A new approach to percutaneous catheterization of the internal jugular vein. Anesthesiology 1977; 46:362–364.

28. Prince SR, Sullivan RL, Hackel A: Percutaneous catheterization of the internal jugular vein in infants and children. Anesthesiology 1976; 44:170–174.

29. Humphrey MJ, Blitt CD: Central venous access in children via the external jugular vein. Anesthesiology 1982; 57:50–51.

30. Sweeney MF, Nicolson SC, Moore RA: Approaches to central venous catheterization in the pediatric patient. (Abstract.) Society of Cardiovascular Anesthesiologists, 5th Annual Meeting 1983; 197.

31. Groff DB, Ahmed N: Subclavian vein catheterization in the infant. J Pediatr Surg 1974; 9:171–174.

32. Poole JL: Subclavian vein catheterization for cardiac surgery in children. Anaesth Intensive Care 1980; 8:81–83.

33. Eichelberger MR, Rous PG, Hoelzer DJ, et al: Percutaneous subclavian venous catheters in neonates and children. J Pediatr Surg 1981; 16:547–553.

34. Pybus DA, Poole JL, Crawford MC: Subclavian venous catheterization in small children using the Seldinger technique. Anaesthesia 1982; 37:451–453.

35. Kron IL, Rheuban K, Miller ED, et al: Subclavian vein catheterization for central line placement in children under 2 years of age. Am Surg 1985; 51:272–273.

36. Verweij J, Kester A, Stroes W, et al: Comparison of three methods for measuring central venous pressure. Crit Care Med 1986; 14:288–290.

37. Constant J: The bedside recognition of abnormal jugular contours. Resident and Staff Physician 1987; 33:51–58.

38. Qvist J, Pontoppidan H, Wilson RS, et al: Hemodynamic responses to mechanical ventilation with PEEP: The effect of hypervolemia. Anesthesiology 1975; 42:54–55.

39. Shah KB, Rao TLK, Laughlin S, El-Etr AA: A review of pulmonary artery catheterization in 6245 patients. Anesthesiology 1984; 61:271–275.

40. Paskin DL, Hoffman WS, Tuddenham WJ: A new complication of subclavian vein catheterization. Ann Surg 1974; 179:266–268.
41. Steiner ML, Bartley TD, Byers FM, Krovetz LJ: Polyethylene catheter in the heart. Report of a case with successful removal. JAMA 1965; 193:1054–1056.
42. Doering RB, Stemmer EA, Connolly JE: Complications of indwelling venous catheters. With particular reference to catheter embolus. Am J Surg 1967; 114:259–266.
43. Massumi RA, Ross AM: Atraumatic, nonsurgical technique for removal of broken catheters from cardiac cavities. N Engl J Med 1967; 277:195–196.
44. McSweeney WJ, Schwartz DC: Retrieval of a catheter foreign body from the right heart using a guide wire deflector system. Radiology 1971; 100:61–62.
45. Edelstein J: Atraumatic removal of a polyethylene catheter from the superior vena cava. Chest 1970; 57:381–383.
46. Feliciano DV, Mattox KL, Graham JM, et al: Major complications of percutaneous subclavian vein catheters. Am J Surg 1979; 138:869–874.
47. Smyth NPD, Rogers JB: Transvenous removal of catheter emboli from the heart and great veins by endoscopic forceps. Ann Thorac Surg 1971; 11:403–408.
48. Lillehei CW, Bonnabeau RC Jr, Grossling S: Removal of iatrogenic foreign bodies within cardiac chambers and great vessels. Circulation 1965; 32:782–787.
49. Block PC: Transvenous retrieval of foreign bodies in the cardiac circulation. JAMA 1973; 224:241–242.
50. Brown CA, Kent A: Perforation of right ventricle by polyethylene catheter. South Med J 1956; 49:466–467.
51. Johnson CE: Perforation of right atrium by a polyethylene catheter. JAMA 1966; 195:584–586.
52. Friedman BA, Jurgeleit HC: Perforation of atrium by polyethylene central venous catheter. JAMA 1968; 203:1141–1142.
53. Green HL, Nemir P Jr: Air embolism as a complication during parenteral alimentation. Am J Surg 1971; 121:614–616.
54. Brady RE, Weinberg PM: Atrioventricular conduction disturbance during total parenteral nutrition. J Pediatr 1976; 88:113–114.
55. Maki DG, Weise CE, Sarafin HW: A semiquantitative culture method for identifying intravenous-catheter-related infection. N Engl J Med 1977; 296:1305–1309.
56. Cooper GL, Hopkins CC: Rapid diagnosis of intravascular catheter-associated infection by direct Gram staining of catheter segments. N Engl J Med 1985; 312:1142–1147.
57. Collignon P, Chan R, Munro R: Rapid diagnosis of intravascular catheter-related sepsis. Arch Intern Med 1987; 147:1609–1612.
58. Passerini L, Phang PT, Jackson FL, et al: Biofilms of right heart flow-directed catheters. Chest 1987; 92:440–446.
59. Maki DG: Infections associated with intravascular lines. *In* Swartz M, Remington J (eds): Current Topics in Clinical Infectious Disease. New York: McGraw-Hill, 1982; 309–363.
60. Maki DG, Goll M, Hassemer C, Alvarado C: Safety and cost-effectiveness of 4 dressing regimens for peripheral IV catheters including indefinite gauze and a povidone-iodine impregnated transparent dressing. (Abstract.) Clin Res 1985; 33:845A.
61. Snydman DR, Pober BR, Murray SA, et al: Predictive value of surveillance skin cultures in total-parenteral nutrition-related infection. Lancet 1982; 2:1385–1388.
62. Bjornson HS, Colley R, Bower RH, et al: Association between microorganism

growth at the catheter insertion site and colonization of the catheter in patients receiving total parenteral nutrition. Surgery 1982; 92:720–727.

63. Becker AE, Becker MJ, Martin FH, et al: Bland thrombosis and infection in relation to intracardiac catheter. Circulation 1972; 46:200–203.

64. Hoshal VL Jr, Ause RG, Hoskins PA: Fibrin sleeve formation on indwelling subclavian central venous catheters. Arch Surg 1971; 102:353–358.

65. Firor HV: Pulmonary embolization complicating total intravenous alimentation. J Pediatr Surg 1972; 7:81.

66. Peters WR, Bush HW Jr, McIntyre RD, Hill LD: The development of fibrin sheath on indwelling venous catheters. Surg Gynecol Obstet 1973; 137:43–47.

67. Ryan JA Jr, Abel RM, Abbott WM, et al: Catheter complications in total parenteral nutrition: A prospective study of 200 consecutive patients. N Engl J Med 1974; 290:757–761.

68. Bouchard RJ, Gault JH, Ross J Jr: Evaluation of pulmonary arterial end-diastolic pressure as an estimate of left ventricular end-diastolic pressure in patients with normal and abnormal left ventricular performance. Circulation 1971; 44:1072–1079.

69. Falicov RE, Resnekov L: Relationship of the pulmonary artery end-diastolic pressure to the left ventricular end-diastolic and mean filling pressures in patients with and without left ventricular dysfunction. Circulation 1970; 42:65–73.

70. Lappas D, Lell WA, Gabel JC, et al: Indirect measurement of left-atrial pressure in surgical patients—pulmonary capillary wedge and pulmonary artery diastolic pressures compared with left atrial pressure. Anesthesiology 1973; 38:394–397.

71. Forrester JS, Diamond G, McHugh TJ, Swan HJC: Filling pressures in the right and left sides of the heart in acute myocardial infarction: A reappraisal of central-venous-pressure monitoring. N Engl J Med 1971; 285: 190–193.

72. Archer G, Cobb LA: Long-term pulmonary artery pressure monitoring in the management of the critically ill. Ann Surg 1974; 180:747–752.

73. Forrester J, Diamond G, Ganz W, et al: Right and left heart pressures in the acutely ill patient. Clin Res 1970; 18:306.

74. Rahimtoola SH, Loeb HS, Ehsani A, et al: Relationship of pulmonary artery to left ventricular diastolic pressures in acute myocardial infarction. Circulation 1972; 46:283–290.

75. West JB, Dollery CT, Naimark A: Distribution of blood flow in isolated lung: Relation to vascular and alveolar pressures. J Appl Physiol 1964; 19:713–724.

76. Goldenheim PD, Kazemi H: Cardiopulmonary monitoring of critically ill patients, part 2. N Engl J Med 1984; 311:776–778.

77. Todd TR, Baile EM, Hogg JC: Pulmonary arterial wedge pressure in hemorrhagic shock. Am Rev Respir Dis 1978; 118:613–616.

78. Tooker J, Huseby J, Butler J: The effect of Swan-Ganz catheter height on the wedge pressure–left atrial pressure relationship in edema during positive-pressure ventilation. Am Rev Respir Dis 1978; 117:721–725.

79. Shasby DM, Daube IM, Pfister S, et al: Swan-Ganz catheter location and left atrial pressure determine the accuracy of the wedge pressure when positive end-expiratory pressure is used. Chest 1981; 80:666–670.

80. Roy R, Powers SR Jr, Feustel PJ, Dutton RE: Pulmonary wedge catheterization during positive end-expiratory pressure ventilation in the dog. Anesthesiology 1977; 46:385–390.

81. Zapol WM, Snider MT: Pulmonary hypertension in severe acute respiratory failure. N Engl J Med 1977; 296:476–480.

82. Downs JB: A technique for direct measurement of intrapleural pressure. Crit Care Med 1976; 4:207–210.

83. McCans JL, Parker JO: Left ventricular pressure-volume relationship during myocardial ischemia in man. Circulation 1973; 48:775–785.

84. Mirsky I: Assessment of passive elastic stiffness of cardiac muscle. Mathematical concepts, physiological and clinical considerations. Direction in future research. Prog Cardiovasc Dis 1976; 18:277–308.

85. Levine HJ, Gaasch WH: Diastolic compliance of the left ventricle. Mod Concepts Cardiovasc Dis 1978; 47:95–98.

86. Mann T, Mann R, Goldberg S, et al: Factors contributing to altered left ventricular diastolic properties during angina pectoris. Circulation 1979; 59:14–20.

87. Calvin JE, Driedger AA, Sibbald WJ: Does the pulmonary capillary wedge pressure predict left ventricular preload in critically ill patients? Crit Care Med 1981; 9:437–443.

88. Alyono D, Ring WS, Anderson RW: The effects of hemorrhagic shock on the diastolic properties of the left ventricle in the conscious dog. Surgery 1978; 83:691–698.

89. Jenkins BS, Bradley RD, Branthwaite MA: Evaluation of pulmonary arterial end-diastolic as an indirect estimate of left atrial mean pressure. Circulation 1970; 42:75–90.

90. Scheinman M, Evans GT, Weiss A, et al: Relationship between pulmonary artery end-diastolic pressure and left ventricular filling pressure in patients in shock. Circulation 1973; 47:317–324.

91. Kohanna FH, Cunningham JN: Monitoring of cardiac output by thermodilution after open-heart surgery. J Thorac Cardiovasc Surg 1977; 73:451–457.

92. Attia RR, Murphy JD, Snider M, et al: Myocardial ischemia due to infrarenal aortic cross-clamping during aortic surgery in patients with severe coronary artery disease. Circulation 1976; 53:961–965.

93. Chatterjee K, Parmley WW, Ganz W, et al: Hemodynamic and metabolic responses to vasodilator therapy in acute myocardial infarction. Circulation 1973; 48:1183–1193.

94. Dalen JE: Bedside hemodynamic monitoring. N Engl J Med 1979; 301:1176–1178.

95. Chatterjee K, Swan HJ, Kaushik VS, et al: Effects of vasodilator therapy for severe pump failure in acute myocardial infarction on short-term and long-term prognosis. Circulation 1976; 53:797–802.

96. Gore JM, Goldberg RJ, Spodick DH, et al: A community-wide assessment of the use of pulmonary artery catheters in patients with acute myocardial infarction. Chest 1987; 92:721–731.

97. Danek SJ, Lynch JP, Weg JG, Dantzker DR: The dependence of oxygen uptake on oxygen delivery in the adult respiratory distress syndrome. Am Rev Respir Dis 1980; 122:387–395.

98. Keefer JR, Barash PG: Pulmonary artery catheterization. *In* Blitt CD (ed): Monitoring in Anesthesia and Critical Care Medicine. New York: Churchill Livingstone, 1985; 177–228.

99. Danek SJ, Lynch JP, Weg JG, Dantsker DR: The dependence of oxygen uptake on oxygen delivery in the adult respiratory distress syndrome. Am Rev Respir Dis 1980; 122:387–395.

100. Goldman RH, Klughaupt M, Metcalf T, et al: Measurement of central venous oxygen saturation in patients with myocardial infarction. Circulation 1968; 38:941–946.

101. Forrester JS, Ganz W, Diamond G, et al: Thermodilution cardiac output determination with a single flow-directed catheter. Am Heart J 1972; 83:306–311.

102. Katz RW, Pollack M, Weibley R: Pulmonary artery catheterization in pediatric intensive care. Adv Pediatr 1983; 30:169–190.

103. Alfieri O, Agosti J, Subramanian S: Thermodilution cardiac output measurement in infants and small children following intracardiac surgery. J Pediatr Surg 1975; 10:649–656.

104. Mathur M, Harris EA, Yarrow S, Baratt-Boyes BG: Measurement of cardiac output by thermodilution in infants and children after open-heart operations. J Thorac Cardiovasc Surg 1976; 72:221–225.

105. Rah KH, Dunwiddle WC, Lower RR: A method of continuous postoperative monitoring of mixing venous oxygen saturation in infants and children after open heart procedures. Anesth Analg 1984; 63:873–881.

106. Jernigan WR, Gardner WC, Mahr MM, Milburn JL: Use of the internal jugular vein for placement of central venous catheter. Surg Gynecol Obstet 1970; 130:520–524.

107. Elliot CG, Zimmerman GA, Clemmer TP: Complications of pulmonary artery catheterization in the care of critically ill patients. Chest 1979; 76:647–652.

108. Puri VK, Carlson RW, Bander JJ, Weil MH: Complications of vascular catheterization in the critically ill: A prospective study. Crit Care Med 1980; 8:495–499.

109. Freed MD, Keane JF: Cardiac output measured by thermodilution in infants and children. J Pediatr 1978; 92:39–42.

110. Pollack MM, Reed TP, Holbrook PR, et al: Bedside pulmonary artery catheterization in pediatrics. J Pediatr 1980; 96:274–276.

111. Swan HJ, Ganz W: Measurement of right atrial and pulmonary arterial pressures and cardiac output: Clinical application of hemodynamic monitoring. Adv Intern Med 1982; 27:453–473.

112. Wyse SD, Pfitzner J, Rees A, et al: Measurement of cardiac output by thermodilution in infants and children. Thorax 1975; 30:262–265.

113. Moodie DS, Feldt RH, Kaye MP, et al: Measurement of cardiac output by thermodilution: Development of accurate measurement at flow applicable to the pediatric patient. J Surg Res 1978; 25:305–311.

114. Webster H: Hemodynamic monitoring in children. *In* Daily EK, Schroeder JS (eds): Techniques of Hemodynamic Monitoring. St Louis: CV Mosby, 1985; 138–179.

115. Pinilla JC, Ross DF, Martin T, Crump H: Study of the incidence of intravascular catheter infection and associated septicemia in critically ill patients. Crit Care Med 1983; 11:21–25.

116. Maran AG: Variables in pulmonary capillary wedge pressure: Variation with intrathoracic pressure, graphic and digital recorders. Crit Care Med 1980; 8:102–105.

117. Cengiz M, Crapo RO, Gardner RM: The effect of ventilation on the accuracy of pulmonary artery and wedge pressure measurements. Crit Care Med 1983; 11:502–507.

118. Berryhill RE, Benumof JL, Rauscher LA: Pulmonary vascular pressure reading at the end of exhalation. Anesthesiology 1978; 49:365–368.

119. Steele P, Davies H: The Swan-Ganz catheter in the cardiac laboratory. Br Heart J 1973; 35:647–650.

120. Cairnes JA, Holder D: Ventricular fibrillation due to passage of a Swan-Ganz catheter. (Letter.) Am J Cardiol 1975; 35:589.

121. Swan HJC, Ganz W, Forrester J, et al: Catheterization of the heart in man with use of a flow-directed balloon-tipped catheter. N Engl J Med 1979; 283:447–451.

122. Shaw TJI: The Swan-Ganz pulmonary artery catheter. Incidence of complications, with particular reference to ventricular dysrythmias and their prevention. Anaesthesia 1979; 34:651–656.

123. Sprung CL, Jacobs LJ, Caralis PV, et al: Ventricular arrhythmias during Swan-Ganz catheterization of the critically ill. Chest 1981; 79:413–415.

124. Sprung CL, Poizen RG, Rozanski JJ, et al: Advanced ventricular arrhythmias during bedside pulmonary artery catheterization. Am J Med 1982; 72:203–208.

125. Geha DG, Davis NJ, Lappas DG: Persistent atrial arrhythmias associated with placement of a Swan-Ganz catheter. Anesthesiology 1973; 39:651–653.

126. Clark JL, Dedrick DF, Lebowitz PW: Preparation prior to induction. *In* Lebowitz PW (ed): Clinical Anesthesia Procedures of the Massachusetts General Hospital. Boston: Little, Brown, 1978; 10–29.

127. Salmenpera M, Peltola K, Rosenberg P: Does prophylactic lidocaine control cardiac arrhythmias associated with pulmonary artery catheterization? Anesthesiology 1982; 56:210–212.

128. Voukydis PC, Cohen SI: Catheter-induced arrhythmias. Am Heart J 1974; 88:588–592.

129. Abernathy WS: Complete heart block caused by the Swan-Ganz catheter. Chest 1974; 65:349.

130. Luck JC, Engel TR: Transient right bundle branch block with "Swan-Ganz" catheterization. Am Heart J 1976; 92:263–264.

131. Thomson IR, Dalton BC, Lappas DG, Lowenstein E: Right bundle branch block and complete heart block caused by the Swan-Ganz catheter. Anesthesiology 1979; 51:359–362.

132. O'Toole JD, Wurtzbacher JJ, Wearer NE, et al: Pulmonary valve injury and insufficiency during pulmonary-artery catheterization. N Engl J Med 1979; 301:1167–1168.

133. Boscoe MJ, Delange S: Damage of the tricuspid valve with a Swan-Ganz catheter. Br Med J 1981; 283:346–347.

134. Smith WR, Glauser FL, Jemison P: Ruptured chordae of the tricuspid valve: The consequence of flow directed Swan-Ganz catheterization. Chest 1976; 70:790–792.

135. Lipp H, O'Donoghue K, Resnekov L: Intracardiac knotting of a flow-directed balloon catheter. N Engl J Med 1971; 284:220.

136. Thijs LG, Van-Heukelem HA, Bronsveld W, et al: Double intracardiac knotting of a Swan-Ganz catheter. (Letter.) Br J Anaesth 1981; 53:672.

137. Iberti TJ, Jayagopal SG: Knotting of a Swan-Ganz catheter in pulmonary artery. (Letter.) Chest 1983; 83:711.

138. Mond HG, Dwight WC, Nesbitt SJ, et al: A technique for unknotting an intracardiac flow-directed balloon. Chest 1975; 67:731–732.

139. Dach JL, Galbut DL, Lepage JR: The knotted Swan-Ganz catheter: New solution to a vexing problem. AJR 1981; 137:1274–1275.

140. Thomas HA: The knotted Swan-Ganz catheter: A safer solution. (Letter.) AJR 1982; 183:986–987.

141. Foote GA, Schabel SI, Hodges M: Pulmonary complications of the flow-directed balloon-tipped catheter. N Engl J Med 1974; 290:927–931.

142. McLoud TC, Putman CE: Radiology of the Swan-Ganz catheter and associated pulmonary complications. Radiology 1975; 116:19–22.

143. Pape LA, Haffajee CI, Markis JE, et al: Fatal pulmonary hemorrhage after use of the flow-directed balloon-tipped catheter. Ann Intern Med 1979; 90:344–347.

144. Krantz EM, Viljoen JF: Haemoptysis following insertion of a Swan-Ganz catheter. Br J Anaesth 1979; 51:457–459.

145. Forman MB, Obel IW: Pulmonary hemorrhage following Swan-Ganz catheterization in a patient without severe pulmonary hypertension. S Afr Med J 1980; 58:329–331.

146. Rosenbaum L, Rosenbaum SH, Askanazi J, Hyman AI: Small amounts of he-

moptysis as an early warning sign of pulmonary artery rupture by a pulmonary arterial catheter. Crit Care Med 1981; 9:319–320.

147. Barash PG, Nardi D, Hammond G, et al: Catheter-induced pulmonary artery perforation. Mechanisms, management, and modifications. J Thorac Cardiovasc Surg 1981; 82:5–12.

148. Hart U, Ward DR, Gillilian R, Brawley RK: Fatal pulmonary hemorrhage complicating Swan-Ganz catheterization. Surgery 1982; 91:24–27.

149. Chun GMH, Ellestad MH: Perforation of the pulmonary artery by Swan-Ganz catheter. N Engl J Med 1971; 295:1356–1362.

150. Golden MS, Pinder T Jr, Anderson WT, et al: Fatal pulmonary hemorrhage complicating use of a flow-directed balloon-tipped catheter in a patient receiving anticoagulant therapy. Am J Cardiol 1973; 32:865–867.

151. Meltzer R, Kint PP, Simmons M: Hemoptysis after flushing Swan-Ganz catheters in the wedge position. (Letter.) N Engl J Med 1981; 304:1171.

152. Applefeld JJ, Caruthers TE, Reno DJ, Civetta JM: Assessment of the sterility of long-term cardiac catheterization using the thermodilution Swan-Ganz catheter. Chest 1978; 74:377–380.

153. Lange HW, Galliani CA, Edwards JE: Local complications associated with indwelling Swan-Ganz catheters. Am J Cardiol 1983; 52:1108–1111.

154. Senagore A, Waller JD, Bonnell BW, et al: Pulmonary artery catheterization: A prospective study of internal jugular and subclavian approaches. Crit Care Med 1987; 15:35–37.

155. Lapin ES, Murray JA: Hemoptysis with flow-directed cardiac catheterization. (Letter.) JAMA 1972; 220:1246.

156. Chastre J, Cornud F, Bouchama A, et al: Thrombosis as a complication of pulmonary-artery catheterization via the internal jugular vein: Prospective evaluation by phlebography. N Engl J Med 1982; 306:278–281.

157. Becker RC, Martin RG, Underwood DA: Right-sided endocardial lesions and flow-directed pulmonary artery catheters. Cleve Clin J Med 1987; 54:384–388.

158. Greene JF Jr, Cummings KC: Aseptic thrombotic endocardial vegetations: A complication of indwelling pulmonary artery catheters. JAMA 1973; 225:1525–1526.

159. Pace NL, Horton W: Indwelling pulmonary artery catheters: Their relationship to aseptic thrombotic endocardial vegetations. JAMA 1974; 233:893–894.

160. Greene JF Jr, Fitzwater JE, Clemmer TP: Septic endocarditis and indwelling pulmonary artery catheters. JAMA 1976; 233:891–938.

161. Katz JD, Cronau LH, Barash PG, et al: Pulmonary artery flow-guided catheters in the perioperative period. JAMA 1977; 237:2832–2834.

162. Ehrie M, Morgan AP, Moore FP, O'Connor NE: Endocarditis with the indwelling balloon-tipped pulmonary artery catheter in burn patients. J Trauma 1978; 18:664–666.

163. Ford SE, Manley PN: Indwelling cardiac catheters: An autopsy study of associated endocardial lesions. Arch Pathol Lab Med 1982; 106:314–317.

164. Rowley KM, Clubb KS, Smith GJW, Cabin HS: Right-sided infective endocarditis as a consequence of flow-directed pulmonary-artery catheterization. N Engl J Med 1984; 311:1152–1156.

165. Sarin CL, Yalav E, Clement AJ, Braimbridge MV: The necessity for measurement of left atrial pressure after cardiac valve surgery. Thorax 1970; 25:185–189.

166. Gold JP, Jonas RA, Lang P, et al: Transthoracic intracardiac monitoring lines in pediatric surgical patients: A ten year experience. Ann Thorac Surg 1986; 42:185–191.

chapter six

Intraoperative Echocardiography

DANIEL M. THYS, M.D. ■ STEVEN KONSTADT, M.D.
■ ZAHARIA HILLEL, M.D., Ph.D.

Hemodynamic monitoring is conventionally performed by measuring various intravascular and intracardiac pressures as well as cardiac output. Although the results of these measurements undoubtedly greatly facilitate the management of patients with compromised cardiovascular function, the measurements also have limitations, which recently have been better recognized.

With the introduction of intraoperative echocardiography, a new dimension has been added to hemodynamic monitoring. Not only can cardiac structures and function be directly visualized but flow within the structures can also be measured.

The purpose of this chapter is to briefly describe the basic principles of echocardiography, to review the different techniques of cardiac imaging and flow determination, and to describe some current applications of intraoperative echocardiography. The reader is referred to other sources for extensive discussions on each of these topics.[1-4]

BASIC PRINCIPLES

Echocardiography utilizes sound waves with a frequency beyond the human audible range (> 1 MHz) to penetrate living tissues.[4] These waves

197

Table 6–1. HALF-POWER
DISTANCES FOR TISSUES AND
SUBSTANCES IMPORTANT IN
ECHOCARDIOGRAPHY

Material	Half-Power Distance (cm)
Water	380
Blood	15
Soft tissue*	5–1
Muscle	1–0.6
Bone	0.7–0.2
Air	0.08
Lung	0.05

* Except muscle

are emitted in a narrow beam by ultrasound transducers that contain pie-zoelectric crystals. A high-frequency electrical signal stimulates the piezo-electric crystal, which vibrates and emits the ultrasound. Conversely, re-flected ultrasound echoes, striking the crystal's surface, generate vibrations that are converted to electrical impulses, amplified, and processed. The portion of the ultrasound waves that is reflected by cardiac tissues contains information on the distance, density, and velocity of the examined tissues. Electronic circuits measure the time delay between the emitted sound and the received echo and, using the known speed of ultrasound in tissue, convert this time delay into the precise *distance* between transducer and tissue. The intensity of the reflected echoes is proportional to the *density* of the reflecting tissue, whereas an analysis of the frequency shift between the emitted and the reflected ultrasound waves provides information on *velocity*. The dis-tance and density information are used to generate unidimensional or two-dimensional (2D) images of the tissue. Velocity data are used to study flow within the cardiac structures.

Commonly used transducers spend a small amount of time, typically on the order of 1 μsec (10^{-6} seconds), emitting a pulse of ultrasound waves. They then "listen" for the returning echoes for about 0.25 msec and pause for 0.75 msec or less before repeating the cycle. Ultrasound takes about 0.1 msec to travel through 10 cm of human tissue and to be reflected or echoed back to the transducer. There is no time lost in the reflection process. Any ultrasound beam traveling through tissues is weakened or attenuated as it progresses. Table 6–1 gives the distance in various tissues at which the intensity of amplitude of an ultrasound wave of 2 MHz is halved (the half-power distance). Clearly, echo studies across lung or other gas-containing tissues are not feasible. Nor are these studies feasible across dense structures such as bone or strongly scattering tissues such as thick muscle. The ultra-sound waves are harmless to humans unless excessive power (amount of ultrasound waves or energy applied per unit of time) is employed.

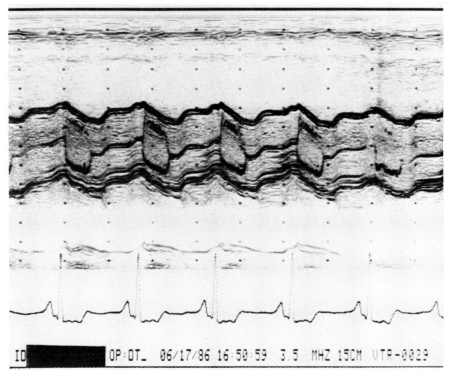

Figure 6–1. M-mode recording obtained at the root of the aorta. The timing of the aortic valve opening and closing can easily be determined as well as the aortic cross-sectional diameter, delineated by the two solid wavelike tracings.

TECHNIQUES AND INSTRUMENTATION

Imaging Echocardiography

M-Mode Echocardiography

In M-mode echocardiography, a unidimensional image is obtained that displays cardiac structures as they would be encountered by a long needle piercing the heart. In its usual presentation on a television screen, M-mode echocardiography displays a graph in which the density (image brightness) of tissues and their position along a single stablike line are plotted on the vertical axis, while the time history of the image sweeps horizontally across the screen. Timed motion of cardiac structures is displayed from right to left (the M in M-mode stands for motion). Using a strip-chart recorder, this moving display can be inscribed on a permanent record (Fig. 6–1).

For the diagnosis of cardiac lesions, M-mode echocardiography has to a great extent been surpassed by 2D echocardiography. However, by virtue of the simplicity and high image quality of M-mode echocardiography, it retains a certain advantage over 2D echocardiography for the determination of hemodynamic performance. Indeed, M-mode measurements can easily be quantitated with calipers, a pencil, and a ruler, whereas 2D measurements often require sophisticated computer analysis. Since most modern echo scanners combine 2D and M-mode capabilities, M-mode measurements are best obtained under 2D guidance. After a selected tomographic plane has been displayed on a 2D screen, the M-mode cursor is directed toward the desired tissue section.

The major disadvantage of M-mode measurements is their unidimensional nature. Single dimensions are not always representative of an entire cardiac chamber. This is particularly true in patients whose hearts have ischemic regional dysfunction or who have dilated hearts with atypical geometry.[5]

Two-Dimensional Echocardiography

Although the M-mode display contains time information, it is essentially unidimensional. By moving the narrow ultrasound beam across the target field (scanning), information can be obtained on position and motion in a second dimension, perpendicular to the ultrasound beam. During scanning, the ultrasound beam examines an entire plane or cross-section of the target object. The image that is generated consists of a series of adjacent M-mode line displays in which the bright dots and lines are fused by the observer's eye to form an integrated picture. Since emitted and reflected echoes take little time to cross distances of clinical interest, the beam scans the field so rapidly that very few changes can occur in the field during a single scanning period. This scanning technique is called real-time, B-mode, cross-sectional scanning of the heart, or, more commonly, 2D echocardiography. Once a cross-sectional view of the heart has been obtained, changes within the cross-section can be followed by repeating the scan, often as frequently as every 17 msec.

To scan the target field, either mechanical or electronic 2D sector scanners are utilized. The former employ oscillating or rotating transducer heads, whereas the latter steer or aim the beam electronically. Electronic scanners use linear phased-array transducers, which can contain as many as 64 piezoelectric elements.

A significant advantage of the electronic phased-array scanner is that it can simultaneously display 2D and M-mode images on two separate television screens. In addition, it is more flexible in its Doppler or combined 2D-Doppler capabilities. The mechanical scanner requires a smaller electronic analysis section but has a bulkier transducer. It can also perform M-mode and 2D examinations but only in a sequential manner. The techniques used to generate 2D images have been extensively discussed by Thys and coworkers.[4]

A different type of transducer uses an annular phased array. Annular phased-array transducers were introduced a few years ago but were unpopular because they required very large scanners. With the advent of electronic miniaturization, the potential benefits of annular array geometry are again being explored. A transesophageal probe of this type is actually under development. By using elements of circular shape, the annular array allows focusing of the ultrasound beam in both the x and y directions of the scanning plane. This leads to improved lateral spatial resolution in the 2D scan. The signal-to-noise ratio is larger than that obtained with other transducers, because the same ultrasound energy can be focused in a smaller tissue element. Improved tissue penetration allows the use of higher frequency waves, which improves the axial image resolution.

Doppler Echocardiography

For the ultrasonic examination of the heart and great vessels, 2D and Doppler echocardiography are complementary techniques. Whereas the cardiac structures and their motion are visualized with 2D echocardiography, Doppler echocardiography studies the flow of blood within these structures. In the clinical applications of the Doppler principle, ultrasound is emitted by a stationary transducer, the red blood cells act as moving reflectors, and the reflected ultrasound is recorded by the same or a different transducer. Blood flow velocity, v, is obtained from the Doppler equation

$$v = \frac{c}{2f_o} \times \frac{f_d}{\cos \theta} \qquad \textbf{6-1}$$

where f_d represents the observed frequency shift between the emitted and reflected signals, f_o equals the frequency of the emitted ultrasound signal, c equals the velocity of sound in tissues (1540 m/second), and θ represents the angle of incidence between the direction of the blood flow and the direction of the ultrasonic signal.[6]

Because the Doppler equation incorporates the cosine function of the angle between the ultrasound beam and the blood flow, the most accurate velocity measurements are obtained when the beam and flow are parallel. The angle is then 0° and its cosine equals 1.[7]

In clinical practice, velocity measurements are not considered accurate when the angle exceeds 25°.[8] A spectral analysis of the velocity signals can be displayed, as a function of time, on rectangular coordinates. By convention, flow toward the transducer is above an arbitrary baseline, whereas flow away is below the line. In modern echo scanners, both imaging and Doppler measurement capabilities are often combined. There are two basic Doppler measuring techniques: pulsed and continuous wave.

Pulsed Wave Doppler

In pulsed wave Doppler, a short burst of ultrasound is transmitted at a fixed pulse-repetition frequency and sampled at an identical sampling frequency. The distance at which the velocities are measured defines the *sampling volume* and is determined by the time delay between the emission of the ultrasound signal burst and the sampling of the reflected signal. The major advantage of pulsed wave Doppler is its ability to measure velocities at selected locations within the circulation. It also has a major disadvantage, however, since it is limited in its ability to measure moderate to high velocities. When velocities exceed the sampling, or Nyquist, limit, a phenomenon known as aliasing occurs. In aliasing, blood flow velocities are displayed in a direction opposite to the conventional one.

Continuous Wave Doppler

In continuous wave Doppler, separate crystals are used to transmit and receive the ultrasound. The transmitting element continuously sends ultrasound, and the other element continuously receives it. As a result of the continuous sampling technique, depth determination is not available, but analysis of flow at high velocities is possible. This ability is of particular importance in the evaluation of patients with valvular and congenital heart disease, since high-velocity flows are frequently detected in these disorders. Continuous wave Doppler is also the preferred method for the measurement of continuous flows.

Real-Time Doppler Color Flow Mapping

To obtain better spatial orientation of flow within the cardiovascular system, real-time Doppler color flow mapping, a technique that combines 2D echocardiography and pulsed wave Doppler, has been developed.[9] Doppler color flow imaging systems use the three primary colors, red, blue, and green, to encode flow information. Most Doppler flow imaging systems encode flow toward the transducer in red and flow away from the transducer in blue. In the absence of flow or when flow is perpendicular to the transducer, no signal is generated. In the simplest color flow map, the higher the velocity in a given sample volume, the more intense or brighter the color at the corresponding picture element or pixel (Fig. 6-2a).

This color encoding scheme is often modified by assigning brighter hues in addition to more color intensity to higher velocities.[10] This is achieved by adding varying intensities of white to the reds or blues to produce a so-called enhanced color map (Fig. 6-2b). The color, or exact shade of color, seen in any pixel (smallest image element) is determined by the time average of the velocity of the blood cells that have passed through that unit of space over the brief sampling time interval. A minimum of three (typically six to eight) ultrasound pulse trains are used to determine blood flow velocities at each of several hundred gates along each scan line. The narrower the sector scan (e.g., 30° vs 90°), the more pulse trains or the fewer the number of gates per scan line, the better the estimate of velocity at any point.

Although anatomic 2D image information can currently be updated as often as 120 times each second, color flow information cannot be updated more than about 30 times each second, because it undergoes more electronic processing. Thus, blood flow maps may change less smoothly with time than do the conventional 2D components of the image. An example of normal intracardiac blood flow in the left side of the heart is shown in Figure 6-3 (note that dynamic changes cannot be represented in static photographs).

Abnormal intracardiac blood flow, as in valvular regurgitation or

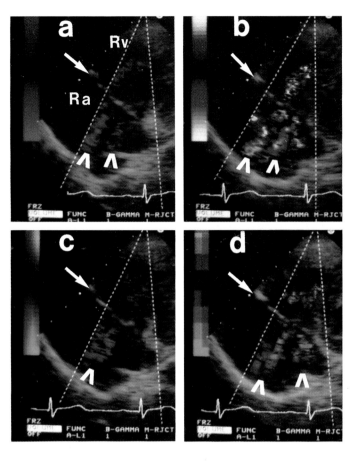

Figure 6–2. Tricuspid valve regurgitation imaged with four different color flow maps on an ATL Ultramark-6 device. A 90° sector scan of a modified apical four-chamber view was imaged with standard two-dimensional (2D) echo, whereas the 45° sector between the dashed lines was also imaged for blood flow. The right ventricle (Rv), the right atrium (Ra), and the closed tricuspid valve (*closed arrow*) are identified. Two jets of tricuspid valve regurgitation (*open arrows*) map in shades of cyan and blue since they move away from the closed valve. The left upper corner of each panel shows the legend used for color encoding of blood flow. Flow toward the transducer (situated at the apex of the sector) is imaged in shades of orange or red, whereas flow away is imaged in shades of cyan or blue. *a*, The faster the flow the higher the intensity of the blue or the red colors. *b*, In the enhanced map, the faster flows are mapped in lighter shades of blue or red generated by adding increasing amounts of white. Aliasing is seen in the regurgitant jet (red-white colors). *c*, A variance map in which, in addition to changes in blue-red intensity associated with faster flows, greater intensities of green are added for increasing flow variance (from left to right in the color legend). *d*, A different variance flow map in which a constant intensity of green was added to the blue-red color map whenever the variance exceeded a set value.

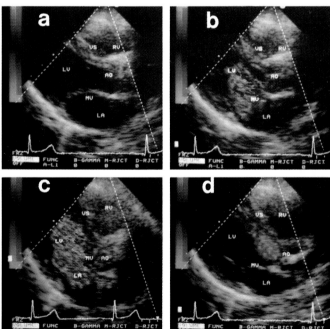

Figure 6–3. Color Doppler flow map of normal blood flow in the left side of the heart. (RV = right ventricle, VS = intraventricular septum, LV = left ventricle, MV = mitral valve, LA = left atrium, AO = aortic valve.) A 60° sector was scanned for flow using a variance map. *a*, The standard 2D left parasternal long-axis view. *b*, An early diastolic view in which blood flowing from LA into LV, toward the transducer, is shown in shades of orange-red. *c*, A later diastolic frame in which blood from the LA continues to fill the LV (shown in orange-red) while some blood inside the LV moving in the opposite direction (away from the transducer) in the outflow tract is imaged in shades of blue. *d*, A systolic frame in which blood from the LV exiting through the AO is shown in blue because the general direction of flow is away from the transducer.

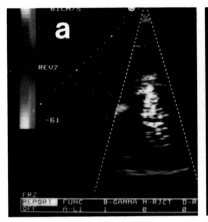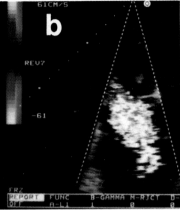

Figure 6–4. Tricuspid valve regurgitation (TR) with significant flow turbulence. *a*, Flow jet variance is mapped mostly in white within a red-blue envelope. *b*, A different view of the TR jet in the same patient. The jet has higher variance than that seen in *a* as indicated by the brighter white and the occasional green mapped areas.

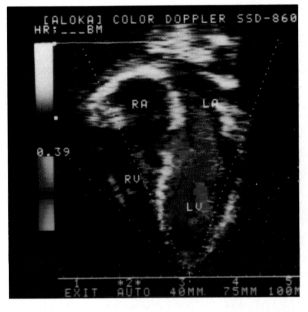

Figure 6–5. An example of blood flow aliasing associated with left ventricular filling in diastole. This is an apical four-chamber view with the transducer situated at the apex of the 45° flow sector. (RA = right atrium, LA = left atrium, RV = right ventricle, LV = left ventricle.) At the front of the orange-red blood column in the area marked LV the red surrounds an area mapped in blue. This blue represents blood flow toward the transducer in excess of the Nyquist limit, which in this map is 0.39 m/second.

through a stenotic valve, is usually turbulent. To image these flows more clearly, the variance of the velocities in each sample volume is used to modify the color display. Variance reflects the degree to which the lowest and the highest velocities recorded at any one gate during a single sampling interval differ from their mean value. Variance increases with more turbulent blood flow, because turbulent fluid changes direction and velocity often and rapidly during a sampling interval. In a variance flow map, green is added to the different hues of red or blue with an intensity proportional to the velocity variance at that location. The typical variance map of turbulent blood flow is a mosaic pattern composed of red, blue, white, and occasionally some green pixels (Fig. 6–4). Thus, white regions inside a color map usually represent highly turbulent flow rather than cardiac tissue, as in standard 2D echocardiography.

The exact composition of the color mix, in enhanced and variance mapping, varies from device to device and is often a matter of esthetics. As a result, the color representation of blood flow varies slightly in different systems. More important, however, the size of a region, imaged as turbulent flow (which depends in part on transducer orientation), also depends on the device used and the particular settings of the variance display. This is a matter of clinical importance that should be kept in mind.

An example of how different color maps depict the same cardiac flow abnormality is shown in Figure 6–2. In this examination, an attempt was made to obtain very comparable views of a heart with tricuspid valve regurgitation. In all four modified four-chamber apical views, two narrow, pencil-like jets of flow away from the transducer are visualized in blue-cyan hues in the right atrium at end-systole (note the closed tricuspid valve leaflets). In Figure 6–2*a*, where a simple red/blue color map has been used (see the one-dimensional, vertical color legend at left), the two jets are visible but faint. In Figure 6–2*b*, an enhanced color map has been used in which increasing amounts of white have been added to both the "toward" and the "away" higher flow velocities. In this map, the two tricuspid regurgitation jets appear brighter at their center and are easier to identify. Figure 6–2*c* depicts a variance map representation of tricuspid regurgitation. The 2D color legend shows green color added incrementally from left to right for increasing turbulence to the standard red/blue map of average velocities. Figure 6–2*d* is a different variance map in which a fixed intensity of green was added (for variance exceeding a set value) to an enhanced red/blue map. Figures 6–2*b* and *d*, both mapped in enhanced color displays, provide a clearer image of the tricuspid regurgitation jets. Thus, color enhancement in a Doppler flow map appears to increase the eye's sensitivity for abnormal flows. A closer examination of the same figure reveals that the areas of the tricuspid regurgitation jets appear larger in the enhanced color maps, demonstrating that with any technique, images are, in part, determined by the settings of the measuring device.

The problem of aliasing, seen with conventional Doppler measurements of velocity, has a unique presentation in color flow imaging. In a color coding system in which red is used to display flow toward the transducer, the "toward" flow is imaged in the bright blue colors assigned to the fastest receding ("away") flow velocities whenever the flow velocity exceeds the Nyquist limit (Fig. 6–5). At sites of very fast blood flow, as for example in jets seen across normal or diseased heart valves, multiple rounds of aliasing can occur, producing a pattern of adjacent bright red and bright blue colors. Turbulent flow, or neighboring streamlines of blood flowing in opposite directions, images in shades of magenta (the eye's perception of a mixture of red and blue light) when mapped without variance or enhancement. Because of the 2D nature of color flow Doppler, aliasing is less of a problem than in conventional Doppler echocardiography, and it can be helpful in identifying pathologic blood flow. However, owing to the low pulse-repetition frequency mentioned previously, the Nyquist limit may be reached at fairly low velocities, obscuring the difference between normal and pathologic flows.

A recent publication has addressed the accuracy of color flow Doppler for the intraoperative determination of mitral regurgitation.[11] Using a scanner with variance mapping and an epicardial transducer, Czer and associates demonstrated that color flow Doppler had 94% sensitivity and 93% specificity for detecting the presence or absence of mitral regurgitation diagnosed by left ventriculography (Fig. 6–6).[11] The false-positive and false-negative results were mostly due to rhythm disturbances during measurements. In the same study, a semiquantitative comparison of the grading of mitral regurgitation by color flow Doppler and angiography in 68 patients revealed complete agreement between grades in 49 patients, a difference of one grade in 17, and a difference of two grades in 2 patients. The angiographic and Doppler color flow gradings of mitral regurgitation (0, 1+, 2+, 3+, and 4+) were based on the length of the regurgitant jet relative to the size of the atrial cavity. This establishes the usefulness of the Doppler color flow technique for intraoperative detection of mitral regurgitation and points to its potential as an aid in surgical decision making in patients with residual mitral regurgitation after valve repair or myocardial revascularization. Current problems with intraoperative color flow Doppler are the high cost of the devices and the limited availability of transesophageal transducers.

Esophageal Echocardiography

Because fat, bone, and air-containing lung interfere with sound wave penetration, clear transthoracic echocardiographic views are particularly difficult to obtain in patients with obesity, emphysema, or abnormal chest wall anatomy. To avoid these problems, esophageal echo transducers have been developed.[12–14] Sound waves emitted from an esophageal transducer only have to pass through the esophageal wall and the pericardium before reaching the heart; thus, there is less likelihood of image distortion. Other advantages of transesophageal echocardiography (TEE) include the stability of the transducer position and the possibility of obtaining continuous recordings of cardiac activity for extended periods of time. Because of these advantages, the potential for continuous intraoperative echocardiographic examinations has been recognized and has led to the evaluation of TEE as a monitoring tool (Table 6–2).[15]

Although initially only M-mode instruments were available for esophageal echocardiography, current equipment provides a combination of

PREPUMP COLOR DOPPLER

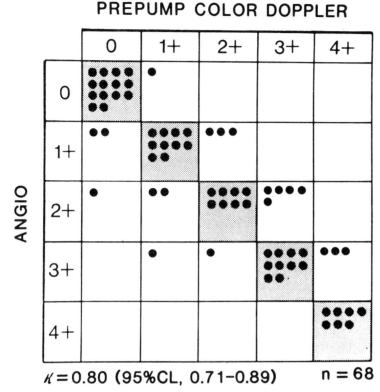

$\kappa = 0.80$ (95%CL, 0.71–0.89)   n = 68

Figure 6–6. Comparison of mitral regurgitation grading by intraoperative Doppler color flow mapping and left ventricular angiography. (For details of the grading see the text.) A kappa (κ) value of 1.0 indicates perfect agreement; a value of 0.75 is considered very good agreement. (CL = confidence limits of the κ value.) (From Czer LSC, Maurer G, Bolger AF, et al: Intraoperative evaluation of mitral regurgitation by Doppler color flow mapping. Circulation 1987; 76[suppl 3]:III111. By permission of the American Heart Association, Inc.)

M-mode, 2D, and color flow capabilities. The transducer is usually mounted on a standard gastroscope. In anesthetized patients, the transducer is introduced after tracheal intubation into the esophagus, either blindly or with the aid of a laryngoscope. Once it is in the esophagus, the scope can be manipulated under image observation for optimal placement. Passage of the TEE probe in awake patients and volunteers has also been described, after intravenous sedation and topical anesthesia of the oropharynx with viscous lidocaine.[14] An 80% success rate has been reported, and all examinations provided adequate images.

With TEE, the two most commonly used views are the short-axis view at midpapillary level and the four-chamber view. The four-chamber view is used to assess chamber size, mitral and tricuspid valve function, septal thickness, regional wall motion, and the presence of air emboli (Fig. 6–7). The short-axis left ventricular view is used to determine global ventricular func-

TABLE 6–2. TRANSESOPHAGEAL ECHOCARDIOGRAPHY

Indications	Contraindications
Assessment	*Absolute*
Chamber size	Esophageal pathology: stricture, varices,
Valvular function	scleroderma esophagitis, or a history of
Septal thickness	esophageal surgery
Intracardiac shunts	
Intracardiac masses	
Thoracic aorta	
Myocardial perfusion	
Monitoring	*Relative*
Global ventricular function	Coagulopathy or anticoagulation
Regional ventricular function	Left atrial myxoma with history of
Intracardiac contrast	embolization

tion (Fig. 6–8). Since myocardium perfused by the three major coronary arteries is represented at this level, this view is also useful for monitoring changes in regional wall function due to myocardial ischemia. TEE can also be used to image the entire thoracic aorta, including the aortic root and the descending thoracic aorta. The large coronary arteries are often well visualized.

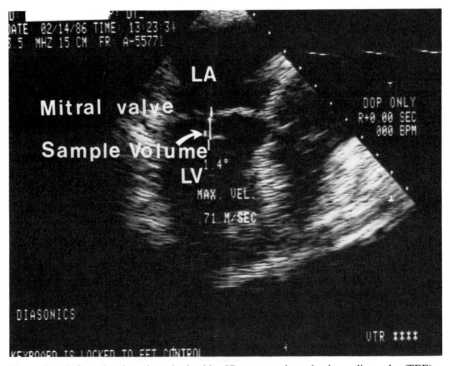

Figure 6–7. A four-chamber view obtained by 2D transesophageal echocardiography (TEE). The left atrium (LA), left ventricle (LV), and mitral valve are clearly visualized. A pulsed-Doppler sample volume is located on the ventricular side of the mitral valve (*arrow*). The right atrium, right ventricle, and tricuspid valve are on the right side of the sector.

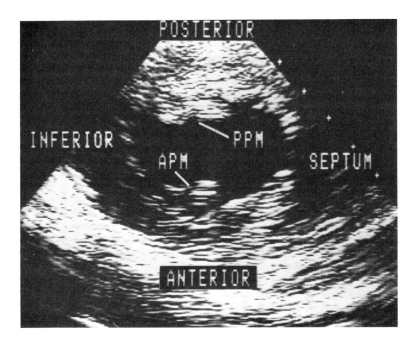

Figure 6–8. A short-axis view at the level of the papillary muscles obtained by 2D TEE. The posterior papillary muscle (PPM) is closest to the transducer, whereas the anterior papillary muscle (APM) is farther away from the top of the sector.

Available TEE Systems

Diasonics. Several 2D TEE systems are available in the United States. The instrument that first became commercially available and is still widely used is manufactured by Diasonics. It consists of a specially designed phased-array probe that can be connected to a number of standard echo scanners (Diasonics Cardiovue 3400 and 6400). The transducer is 17 mm long, 15 mm wide, and 16 mm thick. To avoid injury to the esophagus, the transducer is embedded in soft plastic with rounded edges. The transducer is attached to a standard gastroscope, consisting of a 110-cm flexible shaft and a 7-cm deflection section. Deflection controls permit 180° angulation of the probe in two planes. The use of the controls and the rotation of the entire unit make it possible to obtain many echocardiographic views. Internally, the probe consists of 32 linearly arranged elements with a center frequency of 3.5 MHz, corresponding to a wavelength of 0.43 mm. The array has a 9-mm total aperture, and, with the appropriate phasing of the single elements, an 84° section angle is obtained for real-time imaging. The spheric acoustic lens gives an anatomically appropriate depth of field of 2–10 cm in front of the array.

Hewlett-Packard. Hewlett-Packard has recently introduced a 5 MHz phased-array 2D TEE system. This probe is slightly smaller than the Diasonics probe (probe size: 26 × 13 × 10 mm; active transducer area: 10 × 12 mm). The focal zone depth is similar (1.5–8.0 cm), and although it is smaller, the probe contains twice as many elements (64). In addition to 2D imaging and pulsed wave Doppler capabilities, the Hewlett-Packard system also performs Doppler color flow mapping.

Other TEE Systems. Other systems include those of Toshiba, Corometrics, and Hoffrel. In the Toshiba system, the optical elements of the gastroscope have been maintained, so that the operator can combine echocardiographic imaging with visual examination of the esophagus and stomach. The Hoffrel probe is unique in that it employs a mechanical transducer rather than a phased-array system. This should, theoretically, allow the manufacturer to produce a very compact echo scanner. The design of the transducer heads varies from one manufacturer to the other, and whereas the shape of the transducer head may be of importance for image quality, this question has not been systematically studied.

APPLICATIONS

Global Ventricular Function

In clinical cardiology, echocardiography plays a major role in the hemodynamic evaluation of patients with heart disease. Because anatomic structures are easily recognized on a 2D image, rapid qualitative assessment of cardiac function can often be performed by simple visual analysis of the echo images. Continuous monitoring of the short-axis left ventricular view yields information on ventricular size, function, systolic wall motion, and wall thickening. Left ventricular function is estimated by observing the extent of ventricular emptying. In systole, all segments of the normal myocardium move toward the geometric center of the cavity. In a poorly functioning ventricle, this motion is significantly decreased for most segments of the ventricular wall.

Quantitative echo measurements can be performed on-line on still images or later from videotape recordings. They usually require the determination of left ventricular cavity size, measured as a single dimension, an area, or a volume. End-diastolic and end-systolic sizes are used to calculate global performance indices.

M-mode measurements of left ventricular cavity size are performed at a level between the mitral valve and the papillary muscles, using the interventricular septum and posterior left ventricular wall endocardium as markers. According to the American Society of Echocardiography guidelines, the left ventricular end-diastolic internal diameter (LVIDd) coincides with the Q wave on the electrocardiogram, whereas the left ventricular end-systolic internal diameter (LVIDs) is measured at the peak of downward motion of the interventricular septum.[16] If abnormal septal motion is observed, the measurement should be obtained at the time of peak upward motion of the posterior endocardium. As considerable beat-to-beat variation occurs, measurements should be made for several consecutive beats and the results averaged.[17]

For the quantitative evaluation of 2D echocardiographic views, the endocardial, and sometimes epicardial, borders need to be delineated. Because 2D echocardiography provides tomographic cuts of the heart, the major questions concerning the determination of global ventricular function evolve around the choice and number of cuts required to accurately characterize the whole ventricle. One method uses Simpson's rule,[18] which divides the ventricle into slices of known thickness. The volume of each slice is calculated by multiplying the surface area by the thickness. The volume of the ventricle is obtained from the sum of the volumes of all slices. The number of slices required to accurately define the volume of the ventricle depends on the shape of the ventricle. The more irregular the shape, the more slices that are required.

Since in clinical practice it is often difficult to obtain a sufficient number of slices, it is common to utilize modifications of Simpson's rule. One such modification utilizes two perpendicular tomographic views of the ventricle to calculate the volume.[19] An apical two-chamber view and a short-axis view at the level of the papillary muscles are traced at the endocardial border, and a computer utilizes a modification of Simpson's rule to calculate the left ventricular volume.

In simpler derivations of left ventricular volume, a single short-axis area or a single internal ventricular dimension is used to calculate volume. It is not totally clear whether, in clinical practice, the more complicated models, such as Simpson's rule, yield more accurate volumes than those volumes calculated from a single M-mode dimension.

In some studies, end-diastolic volumes obtained by 2D echocardiography correlated significantly better with cineangiographic volumes than did the end-diastolic volumes obtained by M-mode.[20] However, no statistically significant differences were observed for the correlations between M-mode or 2D echocardiographic end-systolic volumes and cineangiographic end-systolic volume. Opposite findings were obtained by other investigators.[19, 21] Schiller and colleagues observed that 2D echo end-systolic volume correlated significantly better with cineangiographic end-systolic volume than did M-mode end-systolic volume, but they observed no differences for end-diastolic volume.[19] In a third study, the correlations between 2D echocardiographic end-diastolic or end-systolic volume and the same cineangiographic volumes were not significantly better than those between the M-mode end-diastolic or end-systolic volume and the corresponding cineangiographic volumes.[21] Comparisons between correlations of 2D echocardiography or M-mode ejection fractions and cineangiographic or radionuclide ejection fractions are similarly inconclusive. The reasons for the ambiguous conclusions of these various studies are often to be found in the small numbers of observations.

Another quantitative analysis question is more specifically related to TEE. Because TEE examines the heart from a retrocardiac position with a different orientation and somewhat more oblique angulation than does routine echocardiography, it is possible that the images and the measurements derived by TEE may be relatively inaccurate. Matsumoto and coworkers compared standard parasternal M-mode echocardiography, prior to induction of anesthesia, with M-mode TEE after induction with enflurane.[12] They observed a close correlation for the end-diastolic dimensions ($r = 0.96$) and end-systolic dimensions ($r = 0.93$). Matsuzaki and colleagues validated M-mode TEE for the evaluation of left ventricular anterior wall motion by comparing transthoracic echocardiography (TTE) and TEE recordings to left ventriculographic findings.[22] TEE not only obtained adequate images in more patients but it also had a higher correlation with measured left ventricular anterior wall motion than did TTE.

Left ventricular diameters can also be accurately measured by TEE. Kremer and associates demonstrated a good correlation (r = 0.84) between preinduction transthoracic 2D left ventricular diameter measurements and postinduction 2D TEE–derived measurements.[15] To eliminate the possible effects of time differences and induction of anesthesia in these comparisons, Konstadt and coworkers compared measurements of end-diastolic area and ejection fraction area obtained by TEE with those obtained by almost simultaneous on-heart echocardiography under identical hemodynamic conditions.[23] They found a close correlation between the two techniques for each of the three measurements (end-systolic area, r = 0.94; end-diastolic area, r = 0.88; ejection fraction area, r = 0.92). Furthermore, they found minimal interobserver variability (r = 0.91). TEE is therefore an accurate tool with which to measure ventricular dimensions in anesthetized patients.

Preload

Preload can be assessed by estimating left ventricular cavity size on the echocardiogram. In M-mode echocardiography, preload is represented by a single ventricular dimension: the diastolic left ventricular internal diameter (LVIDd). This single dimension, however, is not always representative of the global ventricle, particularly in the presence of ischemic regional dysfunction or atypical geometry in dilated hearts. The LVIDd can also be converted to a diastolic volume dimension with the equation

$$V = \frac{7D^3}{2.4 + D} \qquad\qquad 6\text{--}2$$

where V = volume and D = internal diameter.[5]

Using M-mode TEE, Terai and coworkers have shown that LVIDd (and RVIDd) decrease with the application of positive end-expiratory pressure (PEEP).[24] These findings suggest that a reduction in preload is the mechanism for PEEP-induced decrease in cardiac output.

With 2D echocardiography, a short-axis area obtained at end-diastole is indicative of preload. Since echocardiography provides a measure of diastolic left ventricular cavity size, it seems reasonable that it would provide information on left ventricular preload. It has, in fact, been proposed that left ventricular end-diastolic area may be a better index of left ventricular preload than the pulmonary capillary wedge pressure (PCWP). Cahalan and colleagues reported an intraoperative episode of hypotension in a patient with normal PCWP in which TEE measurements of end-diastolic area established that hypovolemia was the cause.[25] Thys and associates converted left ventricular end-diastolic area measurements into volume measurements and compared those with PCWP[26] in patients undergoing coronary revascularization. They found no relationship between these two variables but demonstrated good correlation between end-diastolic volume and cardiac output. The effects of PEEP on left ventricular preload have also been studied with 2D TEE, and the results were similar to those obtained by

M-mode.[27] Konstadt and colleagues have assessed the influence of pericardiotomy on left ventricular preload as well as on other indexes of left ventricular function.[28] They did not observe any significant changes after opening the pericardium. In patients anesthetized for coronary artery bypass, the same investigators observed PCWP elevation without changes in the left ventricular end-diastolic area 1 and 3 minutes after passive leg raising or use of the Trendelenburg position.[29]

Contractility

In general, the determination of contractility is difficult, as indicated by the large number of contractility indexes. Contractility can be measured during isovolumic contraction, in ejection phase, or at end-systole. Although contractility has been measured by echocardiography during each of these phases, the most commonly utilized echocardiographic indexes of contractility are obtained during the ejection phase.

Ejection Phase Indexes. After the systolic and diastolic internal dimensions are measured, a variety of ejection phase indexes can be calculated. These indexes were initially described for the angiographic evaluation of ventricular function and were later adapted for use in echocardiography. In numerous studies, the values of ejection phase indexes obtained by echocardiography have been compared with the angiographic values. Some of the studies showed a good correlation between echocardiographic and angiographic results; in others, the correlation was poor.[30-32]

Fractional shortening (FS) is the simplest of the ejection phase indexes, since no assumptions are made about the shape or the volume of the left ventricle in this calculation.[33] FS is calculated using the following equation and is expressed as a percentage:

$$\text{FS}(\%) = \frac{\text{LVIDd} - \text{LVIDs}}{\text{LVIDd}} \times 100 \qquad \textbf{6-3}$$

Circumferential fiber shortening (CFS) is a similar ejection phase index. In the measurement of CFS, it is assumed that the ventricle is composed of a series of concentric circles and that the M-mode dimensions are the diameters of these circles. CFS is then calculated as the difference between the diastolic and the systolic circumferences divided by the diastolic circumference, using the equation:[34]

$$\text{CFS} = \frac{\pi\text{LVIDd} - \pi\text{LVIDs}}{\pi\text{LVIDd}} \qquad \textbf{6-4}$$

If the circumference of the ventricle and its contractility are symmetric, the values of FS and CFS are identical, because the M-mode slices are representative of the entire ventricle.

When the left ventricular ejection time (LVET) is known, another ejection phase index, the mean rate of circumferential fiber shortening (Vcf), can be computed by the formula

$$\text{Mean Vcf} = \frac{\text{LVIDd} - \text{LVIDs}}{\text{LVIDd} \times \text{LVET}} \qquad \textbf{6-5}$$

In a number of studies, the addition of LVET enhanced the ability of M-mode echocardiography to separate subjects with normal and abnormal ventricular function.[35, 36]

The M-mode–derived ejection phase index most closely related to the angiographic indexes is the ejection fraction (EF). The computation of EF requires conversion from a linear to a volume dimension. Although numerous formulas have been suggested for this conversion, the results are often erroneous and unreliable.[37] It is generally accepted that the best equation for these conversions is that described by Teichholz and coworkers (see Equation 6–2).[5, 38] After the left ventricular end-diastolic volume (LVEDV) and end-systolic volume (LVESV) have been calculated, the EF is obtained with the following formula:

$$EF(\%) = \frac{LVEDV - LVESV}{LVEDV} \times 100 \qquad \textbf{6–6}$$

A number of these ejection phase indexes have been utilized intraoperatively to assess the effects of cardiac valve replacement or the administration of anesthetic agents on ventricular function. Wong and Spotnitz demonstrated that in patients with chronic mitral regurgitation, valve replacement resulted in a marked decrease in FS.[39]

Effects of Anesthesia. Barash and colleagues studied the effects of halothane on ventricular function in healthy children.[40] Data were obtained prior to the induction of anesthesia and at halothane concentrations ranging from 0.5% to 2.0%. At 2.0% halothane, they noted a 26% reduction in EF and a 36% decrease in the mean Vcf. No significant change in LVEDV was noted. Gerson and Gianaris performed a comparable study on healthy adult patients and observed similar results regarding the depressant effects of halothane on left ventricular performance.[41]

Rathod and colleagues studied 20 healthy patients scheduled for minor surgical procedures.[42] They compared the effects of halothane and enflurane on ventricular performance and found that 0.93% end-tidal concentration of halothane caused a significant decrease in LVIDd and a significant increase in LVIDs. The calculation of FS showed a highly significant decrease. Vcf and the percentage of systolic thickening of the left ventricular posterior wall also decreased significantly. Enflurane, at 2.4% end-tidal concentration, caused a significant reduction in both end-systolic and end-diastolic dimensions. However, enflurane did not produce significant changes in FS, Vcf, or the percentage of systolic thickening of the left ventricular posterior wall.

In children who were not premedicated, Wolf and coworkers found that, at equipotent doses, halothane and isoflurane had different effects on myocardial performance. Halothane significantly decreased left ventricular FS, whereas isoflurane did not.[43]

In addition to these studies of anesthetic effects on myocardial performance, M-mode echocardiography also has been utilized in recent investigations of the effects of narcotics on ventricular function. Schieber and associates used M-mode echocardiography and invasive hemodynamic monitoring to assess the cardiovascular effects of high-dose fentanyl in newborn piglets.[44] No significant change in FS was observed. Moore and colleagues, studying the cardiovascular effects of sufentanil as the sole anesthetic for pediatric cardiac surgery, reported no significant change in EF after induction with 5, 10, or 20 μg/kg of sufentanil.[45]

In 2D echocardiography, the ejection fraction area (EFA), a measure of left ventricular performance, is obtained by the formula

$$EFA(\%) = \frac{EDA - ESA}{EDA} \times 100 \qquad\qquad \textbf{6-7}$$

where ESA represents end-systolic area and EDA end-diastolic area.

Roizen and colleagues were able to demonstrate that EFA was a more sensitive indicator of left ventricular performance than was cardiac output alone. Indeed, in some patients undergoing abdominal aortic cross-clamping, the authors observed marked reductions in EFA with minimal changes in cardiac output.[46]

Murray and coworkers used 2D echocardiography to compare the effects of halothane and isoflurane on contractility in infants and small children. They observed that at equipotent doses both drugs decreased EF to a similar extent.[47]

Information on left ventricular contractility can also be derived from the combined analysis of 2D short-axis echocardiograms and peak systolic arterial pressure. In recent experiments, Hillel and coworkers demonstrated a linear correlation between the end-systolic volume, derived from a 2D short-axis area, and the systolic arterial pressure during preload manipulations.[48] In patients undergoing coronary artery bypass surgery, the authors further showed that the method was sufficiently sensitive to detect changes in contractility after administration of dopamine or halothane.[49, 50] Left ventricular volume calculations in these experiments were based on a modified ellipsoid model for single-plane data, using the following equation:

$$V = SA^{3/2} \frac{SA + 36}{SA + 12} \qquad\qquad \textbf{6-8}$$

where V stands for volume and SA for a short-axis area at the papillary muscle level.[51]

Effects of Ischemia. Doppler velocity signals can also be utilized to measure ventricular performance. In 1966, Noble and associates first demonstrated in dogs that positive inotropic drugs consistently increased maximum aortic flow acceleration, whereas myocardial ischemia produced an early, large decrease in maximum acceleration.[52] Subsequently, similar findings were reported in humans, using either catheters with tip-mounted velocity transducers or conventional Doppler transducers.[53-55] Sabbah and colleagues reported good correlation (r = 0.9) between EF at angiography and maximum aortic acceleration.[56] In normal subjects, maximum acceleration doubles during exercise, whereas in patients with ischemic heart disease, it fails to do so, even in patients with normal resting EFs.[57] Blood flow acceleration measured in the descending aorta also reflects ventricular performance, and esophageal Doppler probes can thus be utilized to continuously monitor left ventricular performance intraoperatively.[58]

Cardiac Output

Cardiac output can be determined by M-mode, 2D, and Doppler echocardiography. For M-mode and 2D echocardiographic determinations, linear or area measurements are converted to volumes, and cardiac output is computed as the product of heart rate and stroke volume (end-diastolic volume − end-systolic volume). When M-mode TEE has been used to measure the left ventricular systolic and diastolic volumes, correlations between cardiac output measured by dye or thermodilution and by echocardiography varied markedly (r = 0.72 to r = 0.97).[12, 24] A good correlation between thermodilution and echo-derived cardiac output was observed when 2D echocardiography was used to determine left ventricular size (r = 0.8).[26]

The determination of stroke volume by Doppler echocardiography is based on the measurement of blood flow velocities across cardiac valves or in the aorta.[59] To calculate stroke volume, the duration of flow, the flow velocity integral, and the cross-sectional area of the conduit through which flow occurs need to be known. The ascending aorta is frequently selected for Doppler velocity measurements, because parallel alignment of the ultrasound beam and the aortic flow can readily be obtained by placement of a transducer in the suprasternal notch. Although the best location for the measurement of aortic cross-sectional area is still being debated, it is commonly accepted that the aortic root is nearly circular and that its size changes minimally during ventricular ejection.

Numerous investigators found good correlation between the cardiac output measured by combined Doppler echocardiography and that measured by thermodilution or Fick cardiac output.[60–63] Recently, a dedicated continuous wave Doppler device has been introduced for the intraoperative measurement of cardiac output. The Doppler transducers are mounted on a no. 24-F esophageal stethoscope, which continuously measures blood flow velocities in the descending aorta. A single measurement of ascending aortic flow is obtained by suprasternal sampling, after the aortic diameter has been measured by echocardiography or calculated by an algorithm. The relationship between ascending and descending aortic flow is assumed to be constant. In two recent studies, a fairly good correlation was observed between esophageal Doppler and thermodilution cardiac output determinations.[64, 65]

Although the shape of the mitral valve changes during diastolic flow, velocity measurements across the mitral valve have also been utilized for cardiac output determinations (Fig. 6–9). Using a transesophageal pulsed Doppler probe, Roewer and coworkers found that thermodilution and mitral valve cardiac output figures correlated well (r = 0.95).[66] They also observed good correlation between thermodilution cardiac output and pulmonary artery blood flow velocity.

Afterload

Afterload is usually determined by the calculation of systemic vascular resistance, but it can also be determined from arterial pressure, left ven-

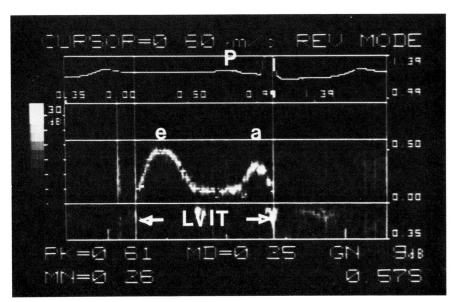

Figure 6–9. Velocity profile across the mitral valve during diastole. Inflow time (LVIT) is displayed on the horizontal axis, and the spectrum of blood velocities is shown on the vertical axis. An early (e) and atrial (a) inflow peak are recognizable. For stroke volume calculation the area under the velocity profile is multiplied by the LVIT and mitral valve area.

tricular wall thickness, and left ventricular cavity dimensions through a relationship called end-systolic wall stress.

$$\text{Wall stress} = \frac{1.33 \times P \times LVIDd}{4 \times WT \times (1 + WT/LVIDd)} \qquad \textbf{6–9}$$

where P = systolic blood pressure, WT = wall thickness, and LVIDd = internal diameter at end-diastole. WT is calculated from M-mode or 2D echocardiography as the average of diastolic interventricular and posterior wall thickness.[67] The cavity dimension is measured echocardiographically in diastole, because it is assumed that peak-systolic wall stress occurs during isovolumic ventricular contraction while the ventricle still possesses its diastolic anatomic configuration. A useful simplification of the above formula is

$$\text{Wall stress} = \frac{P \times LVIDd}{WT} \qquad \textbf{6–10}$$

Patients with left ventricular enlargement (systemic hypertension, aortic stenosis, or regurgitation) show increased wall stress when compared with patients with normal left ventricles.[68] Wall stress certainly provides a better index of left ventricular afterload than does systemic vascular resistance, when forward stroke volume is not equal to the total ventricular ejection (mitral regurgitation, ventricular septal defect). During pharmacologic interventions, systemic vascular resistance and wall stress vary in opposite directions and correlate poorly.[69] It remains to be determined whether systemic vascular resistance or wall stress is more useful for assessing ventricular function intraoperatively.

Regional Ventricular Function

In 1935, Tennant and Wiggers first demonstrated that left ventricular contractile function was impaired shortly after coronary artery ligation.[70] Subsequently, Herman and colleagues described four patterns of abnormal regional ventricular wall motion: asynchrony, or disturbed temporal sequence of contraction; asyneresis, or local hypokinesis; akinesis; and dyskinesis, or paradoxical systolic expansion.[71] Although the areas of these localized disturbances of wall motion were in close anatomic relation to regions of known ischemic heart disease, no specific causal relationship between the ischemic heart disease and the contractile abnormalities was established.

Recently, the correlation between myocardial blood flow and ventricular function has become clearer. Forrester and coworkers demonstrated that stepwise reductions in perfusion pressure produce a predictable progression of segmental contractile abnormalities from asynchrony to hypokinesis to akinesis and finally to dyskinesis.[72] Similarly, coronary blood flow correlates closely with ventricular function.[73]

Echocardiography is an ideal method with which to detect regional wall motion abnormalities in clinical practice. In patients with ventricular aneurysms and localized ventricular dysfunction, Weyman and colleagues observed an excellent correlation between echocardiographic and ventriculographic patterns of regional wall motion abnormalities.[74] In a more quantitative fashion, Kisslo and coworkers compared 2D echocardiography and cineangiography for the detection of regional wall motion abnormalities.[75] In 430 of the 525 analyzed segments (82%), the echocardiographic images of the examined regions were adequate. In a double-blind analysis of the two techniques, there was agreement in detection of regional wall motion abnormalities in 365 of 430 segments examined. Retrospective analysis of the 55 discrepancies revealed that 34 were due to echocardiographic error, 6 were indeterminant, and 15 were due to angiographic error. Kisslo and coworkers concluded that echocardiography was useful for assessing left ventricular asynergy.[75]

The diagnosis of acute myocardial ischemia can be made by evaluating endocardial motion or systolic wall thickening. Intraoperatively, one is usually limited to the study of endocardial motion, because the reproducibility of wall thickness measurements by TEE is poor.[76] To measure endocardial motion, it is necessary to first identify the endocardial borders of a diastolic frame. An approximate center of the cavity is then assigned, and an end-systolic frame is superimposed. In a fixed-reference system, the center of the cavity is assumed to remain unchanged between diastole and systole. In a floating-axis system, a small correction is applied to compensate for the rotational and translational motion of the heart during systole.

Whether the fixed-reference or floating-axis system provides the most

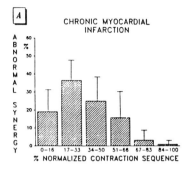

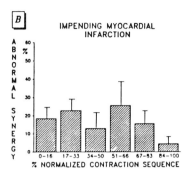

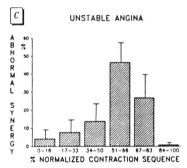

Figure 6–10. Histogram displaying the mean relative frequency distribution (± 1 standard deviation) of the temporal occurrence of abnormal synergy during the normalized contraction sequence in the chronic infarction group (*A*), in the impending infarction group (*B*), and during unstable angina (*C*). (From Zeiher AM, Wollschlarger H, Bonzel T, et al: Hierarchy of levels of ischemia-induced impairment in regional left ventricular systolic function in man. Circulation 1987; 76:773. By permission of the American Heart Association, Inc.)

accurate results is, as yet, unresolved.[77] Numerous other problems related to the analysis of regional function also need further clarification. They are related to the pattern of contraction in normal ventricles, to the influence of inotropism and loading conditions on regional function, and to the specificity of regional wall motion abnormalities.[78] In a recent study by Zeiher and colleagues, it was shown that various levels of ischemia-induced impairment in left ventricular systolic function are characterized by specific patterns of regional contraction.[79] In humans, ischemic injury first manifests itself as asynchronous polyphasic wall motion rather than as changes in the amplitude of the contraction. The exact pattern of abnormal synergy varies for different types of ischemia (Fig. 6–10).

Despite these limitations, echocardiography has been found to be useful for diagnosing intraoperative ischemia and for assessing the immediate results of coronary artery bypass grafting. Using M-mode TTE, Elliott and associates detected significant changes in wall motion in 10 of 24 patients studied with M-mode echocardiography during the induction of anesthesia for coronary artery bypass surgery, whereas only one patient developed corresponding electrocardiogram changes.[80] Two-dimensional TEE detects myocardial ischemia prior to the appearance of electrocardiogram changes. Smith and coworkers, using TEE to detect altered endocardial motion and myocardial thickening, found that 24 of 50 patients developed regional wall motion abnormalities consistent with intraoperative myocardial ischemia.[81] During this period, electrocardiographic monitoring detected only six episodes of myocardial ischemia, and no patient had ST segment changes without corresponding regional wall motion abnormalities. Echocardiographic monitoring also predicts the likelihood of progression of ischemia to myocardial infarction better than the electrocardiogram.

In 30 patients who underwent coronary artery bypass grafting, Koolen and colleagues, using TEE, demonstrated that dysfunctional myocardium frequently improved immediately after revascularization.[82] Similar findings were reported by Topol and coworkers.[83]

Other Applications

Intraoperative Assessment of Valvular Function and Surgical Repair

Mitral Valve Disease. Goldman and associates first applied intraoperative contrast echocardiography to the assessment of mitral valve surgery.[84] Imaging of the valvular and subvalvular apparatus allows the surgeon to assess the extent of fibrous or calcific involvement and to determine whether a conservative repair is feasible.

The presence and severity of both left- and right-sided valvular regurgitation can be determined from the "contrast" pattern generated by the injection of 5 ml of agitated saline solution or 5% dextrose in water through a long needle placed into the left or right ventricle. The needle and syringe generate microbubbles by creating surface agitation and microcavitation within the fluid, even after all visible air bubbles have been removed.[85, 86]

Goldman and associates reported more than 175 echocardiographic left ventriculograms with contrast agent successfully performed for the evaluation of mitral regurgitation in native and prosthetic valves. During surgery, the ultrasound method of mitral valve evaluation proved superior to the standard methods, such as digital palpation and hemodynamic measurement of V wave size. Recently, Equaras and colleagues reported similar success using intraoperative contrast echocardiography to evaluate 15 patients with mitral regurgitation.[87]

Color flow Doppler can also be utilized to assess mitral regurgitation intraoperatively. In 96 patients undergoing cardiac surgery, Czer and associates[11] demonstrated that Doppler color flow mapping had a sensitivity of 94% and a specificity of 93% for the detection of the presence or absence of mitral regurgitation. Interestingly, they also observed that pulmonary capillary wedge V wave pressure correlated poorly with the simultaneously obtained mitral regurgitation grade by color Doppler.[11]

Aortic Valve Disease. Intraoperative echocardiography can adequately visualize all three cusps of the aortic valve (in the short-axis view) and valve mobility (in the long-axis view). Aortic regurgitation can be demonstrated

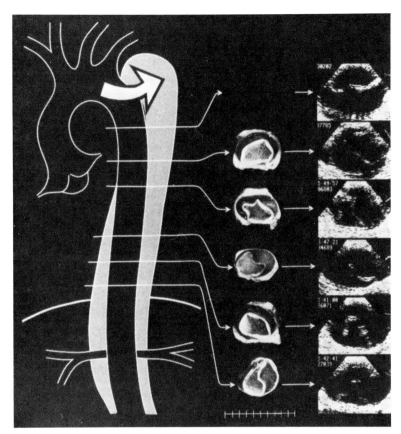

Figure 6–11. Cross-sectional images of the thoracic aorta obtained by TEE and computed tomography scan. This example demonstrates a type III dissection according to DeBakey. (From Mohr-Kahaly S, Erbel R, Steller D, et al: Aortic dissection detected by transesophageal echocardiography. Int J Card Imaging 1987; 2:32. Copyright © 1986 by Martinus Nijhoff Publishers. Reprinted by permission of Kluwer Academic Publishers. February 17, 1988.)

by injecting saline solution or dextrose in water into the proximal aortic root and visualizing diastolic reflux of microbubbles into the left ventricle. The degree of aortic regurgitation is assessed in a manner similar to that used to assess mitral regurgitation, from the degree of filling of the left ventricle during diastole and the time for clearing of the contrast material. After aortic valve repair or prosthesis insertion, a postoperative contrast agent injection can determine the possible presence or severity of regurgitation. This is extremely valuable in congenital aortic valve anomalies, when surgical treatment is reparative and residual or new aortic regurgitation may be present. In 75 aortic root echocardiographic contrast medium injections performed, there was excellent correlation with severity of aortic regurgitation determined by catheterization.[88] Equaras and colleagues reported similar results in 14 patients.[87] Color flow Doppler can also be utilized for the diagnosis of aortic regurgitation.

Aortic Disease. Because of its posterior location, the thoracic aorta is difficult to image by TTE. Numerous investigators have reported that TEE is superior to conventional echocardiography for the diagnosis of thoracic aortic aneurysms and dissections (Fig. 6–11).[89–91] Hashimoto and coworkers found that when it was compared with angiography transesophageal color flow Doppler had a sensitivity of 85% and 80% for the localization of flow entry into the false lumen for type 1 and type 3 aneurysms, respectively.[92]

Congenital Heart Disease. Echocardiography is indispensible today in the management of newborns with congenital cardiac abnormalities, especially cyanotic lesions. With the use of 2D echocardiography, the heart can be examined for chamber size, intactness of the various septa, origins of the great vessels, valvular anatomy, and ventricular function. Doppler echocardiography locates and quantitates shunt flows. This is especially important when the anatomy causing the shunt is too small to be visualized by 2D echocardiography. Color flow Doppler enhances the display of congenital cardiac abnormalities. It allows simultaneous examination of chamber walls, valvular movement, and blood flow. Since the Doppler beam interrogates a major part of the 2D image, even some of the smallest flow abnormalities, as in multiple "shower head" muscular ventricular septal defects, can be detected. This, of course, is of great help to the surgeon. In some patients, such as those with septal defects, 2D echocardiographic diagnosis avoids the added morbidity of cardiac catheterization.[93] Intraoperative contrast echocardiography has also been used to evaluate intracardiac shunts.[94, 95] It is particularly helpful in the assessment of surgical repairs by detecting residual shunts due to suture dehiscence or inadequate repair.

The use of intraoperative echocardiography in pediatric patients increases steadily. The combined experience from over 100 cases, which included neonates, shows that it provides immediate information about closure of intracardiac shunts, relief of obstruction, redirection of blood flow, quality of valve repair, and abnormalities that escaped detection on initial examination.[96, 97]

Color flow Doppler also gives the anesthesiologist new means by which to study the effects of anesthetic agents on shunts. Hillel and coworkers demonstrated changes in the shunt flow pattern of a pediatric patient with tetralogy of Fallot during induction of halothane anesthesia using transthoracic color flow Doppler.[98]

A new development is the use of intraoperative TEE in the pediatric population. The obvious concern is the potential morbidity related to transducer size, mobility, and heat dissipation characteristics. A brief report from the Children's Hospital in Cincinnati, Ohio, established the safety and reliability of intraoperative TEE in the pediatric patient.[99] Twelve children, ages 9–16 years, undergoing surgery for various congenital heart defects were studied. Standard 2D imaging, color flow Doppler, and contrast medium 2D imaging were performed, using a Hewlett-Packard system with a 5-MHz TEE probe. Intraoperative wall motion abnormalities were detected in three patients. Color flow Doppler and contrast medium imaging confirmed correction of intracardiac blood flow abnormalities in all patients. Most significantly, fiberoptic endoscopic examination in 9 of the 12 patients within 24 hours after surgery revealed no significant postoperative esophageal abnormalities. In the near future, technologic advances may provide transeophageal transducers safe for use in neonates.

Intracardiac Air. The ability of echocardiography to demonstrate intracardiac air (bubbles) was realized early in its application. Oka and associates studied patients undergoing cardiac surgery with cardiopulmonary bypass using M-mode TEE and reported evidence of intracardiac air in 79% of patients who had open cardiotomy and in 11% of those who did not.[100] Topol and colleagues used 2D echocardiography and observed intracardiac micro-bubbles in 74% of a similar group of patients.[101] No patient revealed new focal neurologic deficits postoperatively, but there was evidence of intra-cardiac air in three of seven patients with generalized postoperative en-cephalopathy.

Two different studies in dogs by Furuya and coworkers and Glenski and associates determined that the sensitivity of 2D TEE to detect a bolus injection of air was about 0.02 ml/kg.[102, 103] This is somewhat higher than the sensitivity of a nonimaging transthoracic Doppler ultrasound device. In a parallel study in patients undergoing craniotomy in the sitting position, Furuya's group showed that TEE, transthoracic Doppler, pulmonary artery catheter monitoring, and end-tidal CO_2 analysis detected venous air em-bolism equally well. In a different study, Cucchiara and colleagues reported that they were able to detect air embolism convincingly in 9 of 15 neuro-surgical patients using TEE but in only 7 patients using transthoracic Dop-pler.[104] Furthermore, the authors reported detection of paradoxical air em-bolism to the left side of the heart using TEE. Thus, TEE appears superior to all other techniques for the detection of intracardiac air emboli, especially to the left side of the heart. During cardiac surgery, TEE is the only practical ultrasound modality to monitor for intracardiac air.

Medical Diagnosis. Because TEE generates high-resolution images and allows certain unique tomographic cuts, its use as a diagnostic tool has been explored by a number of investigators. In adult patients with congenital heart disease, TEE was used to diagnose cor triatriatum when TTE failed.[105] Using a combination of 2D TEE and color flow Doppler, others have been able to measure the anatomic size of atrial septal defects and the shunt volumes.[106] TEE is also useful in the diagnosis of valvular vegetations. Two studies have compared the incidence of detection by TEE and TTE. Both studies have shown that TEE is more sensitive.[107, 108] Similar results have been ob-tained in the detection of both intracardiac and extracardiac masses (Fig. 6–12).[109, 110]

Another potential benefit of TEE is that the probe is internal and can easily be fixed in the same position. These properties led one group of in-vestigators to use TEE for stress echocardiography.[111] In conclusion, it ap-pears that TEE is a useful diagnostic tool, particularly in patients whose TTE images are of poor quality and in patients with pathology of the atria or the thoracic aorta.

FUTURE DEVELOPMENTS

Quantitation

The ultrasound system of the future should, ideally, perform objective, on-line quantitation using feedback to improve video data acquisition while yielding detailed three-dimensional anatomic and flow information. New de-velopments in video data analysis will lead to the integration of multiple

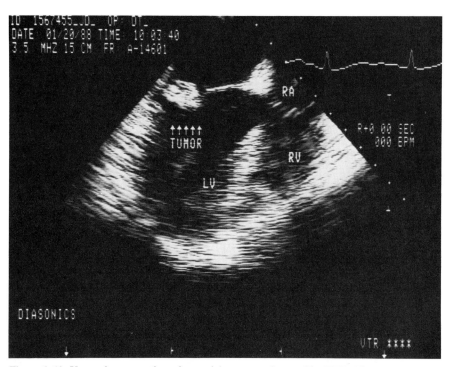

Figure 6–12. Unusual presentation of an atrial myxoma detected by TEE. The tumor was located at the free edge of the anterior mitral valve leaflet and was easily removed at surgery.

advanced automated features.[112] The video data will be stored on laser-generated, optical digital storage media, since ultrasound devices generate video data at amazing rates. The current digital output of 4 megabytes each second exceeds the capacity of most conventional data storage devices. The existing digital processors will have to yield to more powerful array processors capable of performing iconic-symbolic mapping of preprocessed data. This will reduce the information flow rate to a more manageable size of hundreds of features (with their x-y coordinates) per second. A sophisticated host computer will then be able to interpret in real-time the changing information as a contour or a border. Currently, one state-of-the-art preprocessing algorithm, spatiotemporal Fourier noise filtration (electronic noise reduction in both time and the three dimensions of space), can be performed in milliseconds. In the future, this technique is expected to facilitate automatic border localization, which, in turn, will lead to better quantitation of left ventricular wall motion.[113]

Color Flow Echocardiography

The clinical significance of color Doppler echocardiography as a quantitative tool is still being actively defined. Helmcke and coworkers modified the current methods to assess mitral regurgitation with 2D color Doppler by using multiple echocardiography planes.[114] The three orthogonal planes were the parasternal long axis and short axis and the apical four-chamber views. Of the several parameters studied, the best correlation with angiography was obtained when the maximum (or average) regurgitant jet area obtained from three orthogonal planes, expressed as a percentage of the left atrial area, was used.

A bench-top device (a left-sided heart pulse duplicator) has been used to study blood flow through several incompetent prosthetic aortic valves during different hemodynamic states (aortic insufficiency simulation).[115] The purpose was to define the limits of resolution of aortic regurgitation by color Doppler imaging and to determine which of the color jet features reliably predicts the size of the defect and the regurgitant fraction during extreme hemodynamic conditions. Aortic regurgitation could be detected from a valve defect as small as a 1-mm pinhole, provided the net forward flow exceeded 1.5 L/minute and the mean arterial pressure was more than 75 mmHg. The only reliable independent predictor of both defect size and regurgitant fraction was the width of the color jet immediately below the valve plane. Neither the jet length nor width nor the duration of the color variance was useful in grading the degree of incompetence without knowledge of the pressure gradient.

Bench-top devices have also been used to model mitral valve regurgitation by bolusing known volumes of fluid, with fixed velocities, through orifices of known size.[116] When Doppler color flow images were compared with the actual fluid flow parameters, single-frame color jet area and volume (area$^{3/2}$) were shown to correlate well with flow rate. The color jet volume, however, overestimated the actual regurgitant volume. This discrepancy was assigned in part to the different time course of the Doppler-imaged flow and the actual fluid flow.

It has become increasingly clear that true regurgitant volume and regurgitant jet volume measured with color flow Doppler are not necessarily related quantities.[117] Jet volume often overestimates true regurgitant volume. This is not surprising, considering that flow currents persist for some time in a fluid mass after a fluid bolus is introduced rapidly. This leads to mistaking persistent currents for new flow when no additional fluid is being introduced into the chamber.

Some investigators have turned to back-extracting actual flow velocities and calculating fluid jet momentum from the color flow maps, hoping that these better reflect regurgitant flow. In fact, the laws of momentum, conservation, and dissipation of kinetic energy by entrainment (viscous interaction), which govern the behavior of fluid dynamic systems, must also apply to regurgitant blood flow. These lines of analysis may provide a better approach to the quantitation of valvular regurgitation.

Three-Dimensional Echocardiography

By reconstructing planar projections of the heart, a computer linked to an echocardiographic scanner generates what is termed three-dimensional imaging.[118] In fact, since only planar or 2D imaging modalities exist today, no real three-dimensional image can be generated. The computer merely acquires a sufficient number of 2D views from the ultrasound scanner to be able to mathematically generate any desired projection. ''Wire frame'' representation of such superimposed 2D projections gives the impression of three-dimensionality. Data required for three-dimensional reconstructions are synchronous 2D views of the epicardium or endocardium, or both, at different levels through the heart. They must be obtained at exactly the same time point in consecutive cardiac cycles. As few as five to ten of these views may be sufficient. The relative location of these images in real space needs to be known, and the more images used, the more accurate the three-dimensional reconstruction.

There are three different ways to track the position and orientation of the transducer in space in order to orient the 2D image data sets: electronic potentiometry, ultrasonic signals, and optical laser light. The first method, using electronic potentiometers at the elbows of an articulated mechanical arm, is accurate to several millimeters. The ultrasonic signal emitted by the transducer and received by three remote receivers is accurate to 2–3 mm and allows unrestricted motion of the transducer, but it limits the number of accessible transducer orientations. The optical laser light reflected by reflectors mounted on the transducer has an accuracy of about 3 mm but, like the ultrasonic signal, limits the number of possible transducer orientations.

Three-dimensional echocardiographic reconstructions yield more precise cardiac chamber volumes than 2D echocardiography, since data from multiple different views are used, and fewer geometric assumptions are made. Practical applications of the method are limited by the long time required for data collection, during which breathing, motion of the heart, and beat-by-beat variations in hemodynamics cause artifacts. Thus, real-time three-dimensional echocardiography at present is only a research tool with exciting potential for the future.

Tissue Characterization

The analysis of ultrasonic backscatter provides information on tissue characteristics. The amplitude and frequency of an ultrasonic signal are altered as the signal traverses tissue. Abnormal tissue alters the signal in a different fashion from normal tissue. For example, fibrotic or scarred tissues increase the magnitude of integrated ultrasonic backscatter. Hoyt and coworkers, studying the relationship between ultrasonic backscatter and collagen deposition in 10 excised human hearts with old myocardial infarctions, found a linear correlation ($r = 0.78$) between the magnitude of integrated backscatter and the collagen content of the myocardium.[119]

Ischemic tissue becomes edematous and reflects ultrasound in a different fashion from normal tissue. Schnittger and colleagues, studying the effects of acute myocardial ischemia on the ultrasonic signal, found that the baseline mean amplitude over the standard deviation of the amplitude was significantly elevated after 30 minutes of acute ischemia.[120] Thus, statistical analysis of the ultrasonic signal helps to recognize ischemic and infarcted myocardium.

To understand the possible differences in reflected ultrasonic energy from normal, ischemic, and infarcted myocardium, Fitzgerald and associates, comparing endocardial wall motion and cyclic ultrasonic backscatter power in dogs, noted a phase difference between endocardial wall motion and cyclic backscatter power.[121] They concluded that the combined study of cyclic backscatter power and the phase difference between endocardial wall motion and cyclic backscatter power provides a noninvasive tool to differentiate among normal, ischemic, and infarcted myocardium. In humans, Vered and colleagues demonstrated that quantitative ultrasonic tissue characterization allowed quantitative differentiation between normal and myopathic myocardium.[122]

Contrast Perfusion

Computer processing of the echocardiographic signal has led to additional applications of contrast echocardiography. One such application is the assessment of global ventricular function. In a dog model, it was shown that time-intensity curves of the washout phase of contrast medium from the left ventricle conform to a monoexponential function and that analysis of these curves can be used to obtain an ejection fraction that correlates well (r = 0.87) with ejection fractions obtained by angiography.[123] This contrast washout estimate of ejection fraction is totally free of geometric assumptions.

Other investigators attempted to use contrast echocardiography to quantitate myocardial perfusion. In this technique a baseline echocardiogram is first obtained, followed by injection of contrast material into the aortic root or coronary arteries during echocardiographic interrogation. Subsequently, the signals are digitized and analyzed by a computer. The baseline image is subtracted from the postinjection image and a digital subtraction echocardiogram is obtained (Fig. 6–13).[124] The myocardium can be divided into endocardial, epicardial, and radial segments. This digital subtraction echocardiogram can be analyzed in different ways. Time to peak intensity and washout half-life have both been shown to be sensitive indicators of myocardial perfusion.[125, 126] These contrast medium decay half-lives appear more sensitive for the detection of changes in perfusion during rapid atrial pacing than do changes in regional wall thickening.[127] One potential problem with these contrast material measurements is that they may actually assess regional myocardial blood volume and not regional myocardial perfusion.[128] Although these two parameters usually change in a similar fashion, occasionally they do not.

Digital subtraction echocardiography has other potentially important uses. Currently, TEE is not useful in the measurement of regional wall thickening. The better definition of the endo- and epicardial borders by digital subtraction echocardiography may allow for the reproducible calculation of regional wall thickening. Regional wall thickening is more specific than wall motion in the diagnosis of myocardial ischemia. The enhanced definition of the borders may also help reduce the variability in measurements of global ventricular function. Perhaps most important, digital subtraction echocardiography may permit automatic edge detection and allow on-line analysis

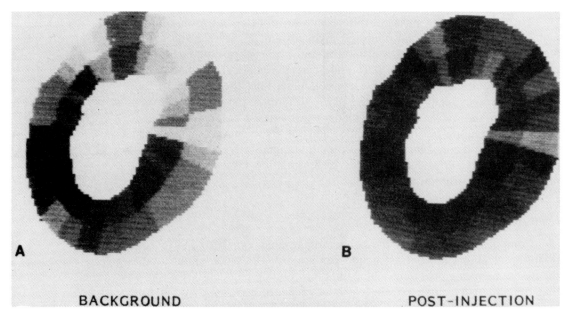

Figure 6–13. Baseline (*A*) and postinjection (*B*) digital subtraction echocardiograms. Note the chan and the clearly defined endocardial and epicardial borders after injection. (From Gewertz B, Krem al: Transesophageal echocardiographic monitoring of myocardial ischemia during vascular surgery. 5:610. With permission.)

of regional wall thickening. The addition of digital subtraction echocardiography would greatly increase the value of TEE as a clinical tool.

References

1. Weyman AE: Cross-sectional Echocardiography. Philadelphia: Lea & Febiger, 1982.
2. Feigenbaum H: Echocardiography, 4th Ed. Philadelphia: Lea & Febiger, 1986.
3. Krembau FW: Diagnostic Ultrasound: Principles, Instrumentation, and Exercises, 2nd Ed. New York: Grune & Stratton, 1984.
4. Thys D, Hillel Z, Konstadt S, Goldman ME: Intraoperative echocardiography. *In* Kaplan J (ed): Cardiac Anesthesia, 2nd Ed. New York: Grune & Stratton, 1987; 255–318.
5. Teichholz LE, Kreulen T, Herman MV, et al: Problems in echocardiographic volume determinations: Echocardiographic angiographic correlations in the presence or absence of asynergy. Am J Cardiol 1976; 37:7–11.
6, Hatle L, Angelsen B: Blood velocity measurements using the Doppler effect of backscattered ultrasound. *In* Hatle L, Angelsen B (eds): Doppler Ultrasound in Cardiology. Philadelphia: Lea & Febiger, 1985.
7. Schuster AH, Nanda NC: Doppler examination of the heart, great vessels and coronary arteries. *In* Nanda NC (ed): Doppler Echocardiography. New York: Igaku-Shoin, 1985.
8. Goldberg SJ, Allen HD, Marx GR, et al: Doppler physics. *In* Goldberg SJ, Allen HD, Marx GR, et al (eds): Doppler Echocardiography. Philadelphia: Lea & Febiger, 1985.

9. Sahn DJ: Real-time two-dimensional Doppler echocardiographic flow mapping. Circulation 1985; 71:849–853.

10. Kisslo J, Adams DB, Belkin RN: Doppler Color Flow Imaging. New York: Churchill Livingstone, 1988.

11. Czer LSC, Maurer G, Bolger AF, et al: Intraoperative evaluation of mitral regurgitation by Doppler color flow mapping. Circulation 1987; 76 (supp 3):III108–III116.

12. Matsumoto M, Oka Y, Strom J, et al: Application of transesophageal echocardiography to continuous intraoperative monitoring of left ventricular performance. Am J Cardiol 1980; 46:95–105.

13. Hisanaga K, Hisanaga A, Nagata K, Ichie Y: Transesophageal cross-sectional echocardiography. Am Heart J 1980; 100:605–609.

14. Schluter M, Langenstein B, Polster J, et al: Transesophageal cross-sectional echocardiography with a phased array transducer system. Technique and initial clinical results. Br Heart J 1982; 48:68–72.

15. Kremer P, Schwartz L, Cahalan M, et al: Intraoperative monitoring of left ventricular performance by transesophageal M-mode and 2-D echocardiography. (Abstract.) Am J Cardiol 1982; 49:956.

16. Sahn DJ, DeMaria A, Kisslo J, et al: Recommendations regarding quantitation in M-mode echocardiography: Results of a survey of echocardiographic measurements. Circulation 1978; 58:1072–1083.

17. Bett JHN, Dryburgh LG: Beat-beat variation in echocardiographic measurements of left ventricular dimensions and function. JCU 1981; 9:119–125.

18. Rogers EW, Feigenbaum H, Weyman AE: Echocardiography for quantitation of cardiac chambers. *In* Yu PN, Goodwin JF (eds): Progress in Cardiology, Vol 8. Philadelphia: Lea & Febiger, 1979.

19. Schiller NB, Acquatella H, Ports TA, et al: Left ventricular volume from paired biplane two-dimensional echocardiography. Circulation 1979; 60:547–555.

20. Mercier JC, Disessa TG, Jarmakani JM, et al: Two-dimensional echocardiographic assessment of left ventricular volumes and ejection fraction in children. Circulation 1982; 65:962–969.

21. Folland ED, Parisi AF, Moynihan PF, et al: Assessment of left ventricular ejection fraction and volumes by real-time, two-dimensional echocardiography: A comparison of cine-angiographic and radionuclide techniques. Circulation 1979; 60:760–766.

22. Matsuzaki M, Matsuda Y, Ikee Y, et al: Esophageal echocardiographic left ventricular anterolateral wall motion in normal subjects and patients with coronary artery disease. Circulation 1981; 63:1085–1092.

23. Konstadt S, Thys D, Mindich B, et al: Validation of quantitative intraoperative transesophageal echocardiography. Anesthesiology 1986; 65:418–421.

24. Terai C, Venishi M, Sugimoto H, et al: Transesophageal echocardiographic dimensional analysis of four cardiac chambers during positive end-expiratory pressure. Anesthesiology 1985; 63:640–666.

25. Cahalan M, Kremer P, Schiller N, et al: Intraoperative monitoring with two-dimensional transesophageal echocardiography. Anesthesiology 1982; 57:A153.

26. Thys DM, Hillel Z, Goldman M, et al: A comparison of hemodynamic indices derived by invasive monitoring and by two-dimensional echocardiography. Anesthesiology 1987; 67:630–634.

27. Koolen J, Visser C, Wever E, et al: Transesophageal two-dimensional echocardiographic evaluation of biventricular dimension on function during positive end-expiratory pressure ventilation after coronary artery bypass grafting. Am J Cardiol 1987; 59:1047–1051.

28. Konstadt S, Thys D, Reich D, et al: The normal pericardium does not affect left ventricular function. J Cardiothorac Anesth 1987; 1:284–288.

230

29. Reich DL, Konstadt SN, Hubbard M, Thys DM: Do Trendelenburg and passive leg raising improve cardiac performance? Anesth Analg 1988; 67:S184.
30. Quinones MA, Gaasch WH, Alexander JK: Echocardiographic assessment of left ventricular function with special reference to normalized velocities. Circulation 1974; 50:42–51.
31. Fortuin NJ, Hood WP Jr, Craige E: Evaluation of left ventricular function by echocardiography. Circulation 1972; 46:26–35.
32. Rosenblatt A, Clark R, Burgess J, et al: Echocardiographic assessment of the level of cardiac compensation in valvular heart disease. Circulation 1976; 54:509–518.
33. Quinones MA, Pickering E, Alexander JK: Percentage of shortening of the echocardiographic left ventricular dimension: Its use in determining ejection fraction and stroke volume. Chest 1978; 74:59–65.
34. Benzing G, Stockert J, Nave E, et al: Evaluation of left ventricular performance: Circumferential fiber shortening and tension. Circulation 1974; 49:925–932.
35. Cooper R, Karliner JS, O'Rourke RA, et al: Ultrasound determinations of mean fiber-shortening rate in man. (Abstract.) Am J Cardiol 1972; 29:257.
36. Cooper RH, O'Rourke RA, Karliner JS, et al: Comparison of ultrasound and cineangiographic measurements of the mean rate of circumferential shortening in man. Circulation 1972; 46:914–923.
37. Feigenbaum H: Echocardiographic examination of the left ventricle. Circulation 1975; 51:1–7.
38. Kronik G, Slany J, Mosslacher H: Comparative value of eight M-mode echocardiographic formulas for determining left ventricular stroke volume. A correlative study with thermodilution and left ventricular single-plane cineangiography. Circulation 1979; 60:1308–1316.
39. Wong CYH, Spotnitz HM: Effect of nitroprusside on end-diastolic pressure-diameter relations of the human left ventricle after pericardiotomy. J Thorac Cardiovasc Surg 1981; 82:350–357.
40. Barash P, Glanz S, Katz J, et al: Ventricular function in children during halothane anesthesia: An echocardiographic evaluation. Anesthesiology 1978; 49:79–85.
41. Gerson J, Gianaris C: Echocardiographic analysis of human left ventricular diastolic volume and cardiac performance during halothane anesthesia. Anesth Analg 1979; 58:23–29.
42. Rathod R, Jacobs H, Kramer N, et al: Echocardiographic assessment of ventricular performance following induction with two anesthetics. Anesthesiology 1978; 49:86–90.
43. Wolf WJ, Neal MB, Peterson MD: The hemodynamic and cardiovascular effects of isoflurane and halothane anesthesia in children. Anesthesiology 1986; 64:328–333.
44. Schieber M, Stiller R, Cook R: Cardiovascular and pharmacodynamic effects of high-dose fentanyl in newborn piglets. Anesthesiology 1985; 63:166–171.
45. Moore R, Yank S, McNicholas K, et al: Hemodynamic and anesthetic effects of sufentanil as the sole anesthetic for pediatric cardiovascular surgery. Anesthesiology 1985; 62:725–731.
46. Roizen M, Beaupre P, Alpert R, et al: Monitoring with two-dimensional transesophageal echocardiography. Comparison of myocardial function in patients undergoing supraceliac, suprarenal-infraceliac, or infrarenal aortic occlusion. J Vasc Surg 1984; 1:300–305.
47. Murray D, Vandewalker G, Matherne GP, Mahoney LT: Pulsed Doppler and two-dimensional echocardiography: Comparison of halothane and isoflurane

on cardiac function in infants and small children. Anesthesiology 1987; 67:211–217.

48. Hillel Z, Thys DM, Mindich BP, et al: A new method for the intraoperative determination of contractility. Anesth Analg 1986; 65:S72.
49. Hillel Z, Thys DM, Mindich BP, et al: Intraoperative measurement of the effects of dopamine on LV contractility. Anesthesiology 1985; 63:A25.
50. Thys DM, Hillel Z, Mindich BP, et al: Halothane is a potent myocardial depressant during fentanyl anesthesia. Anesth Analg 1986; 65:S159.
51. Parisi AF, Moynihan PF, Feldman CL, et al: Approaches to determination of left ventricular volume and ejection fraction by real-time two-dimensional echocardiography. Clin Cardiol 1979; 2:257–263.
52. Noble MIM, Trenchard D, Guz A: Left ventricular ejection in conscious dogs. Part 1. Measurement and significance of the maximum acceleration of blood from the left ventricle. Circ Res 1966; 19:139–147.
53. Bennett ED, Else W, Miller GAH, et al: Maximum acceleration of blood from the left ventricle in patients with ischaemic heart disease. Clin Sci Mol Med 1974; 46:49–59.
54. Bennett ED, Barclay SA, Davis AL, et al: Ascending aortic blood velocity and acceleration using Doppler ultrasound in the assessment of left ventricular function. Cardiovasc Res 1984; 18:632–638.
55. Mehta N, Bennett DE: Impaired left ventricular function in acute myocardial infarction assessed by Doppler measurement of ascending aortic blood velocity and maximum acceleration. Am J Cardiol 1986; 57:1052–1058.
56. Sabbah HN, Khaja F, Brymer JF, et al: Noninvasive evaluation of left ventricular performance based on peak aortic blood acceleration measured with a continuous-wave Doppler velocity meter. Circulation 1986; 74:323–329.
57. Teague SM, Conn C, Sharma M, et al: A comparison of Doppler and radionuclide ejection dynamics during ischemic exercise. Am J Card Imaging 1987; 1:145–151.
58. Thys DM, Hillel Z, Estioko MR: Left-ventricular contractility can be determined by continuous esophageal Doppler. Anesthesiology 1987; 67:A77.
59. Skjaerpe T, Hegrenaes L, Ihlen H: Cardiac output. *In* Hatle L, Angelsen B (eds): Doppler Ultrasound in Cardiology, 2nd Ed. Philadelphia: Lea & Febiger, 1985.
60. Leoppky JA, Greene ER, Hockenga DE, et al: Beat-by-beat stroke volume assessment by pulsed Doppler in upright and supine exercise. J Appl Physiol 1981; 50:1173–1182.
61. Goldberg SJ, Sahn DJ, Allen HD, et al: Evaluation of pulmonary and systemic blood flow by 2-dimensional Doppler echocardiography using fast Fourier transform spectral analysis. Am J Cardiol 1982; 50:1394–1400.
62. Fisher DC, Sahn DJ, Friedman MJ, et al: The effect of variations of pulsed Doppler sampling site on calculation of cardiac output: An experimental study in open-chest dogs. Circulation 1983; 67:370–376.
63. Magnin PA, Stewart JA, Myers S, et al: Combined Doppler and phased-array echocardiographic estimation of cardiac output. Circulation 1981; 63:388–392.
64. Mark JB, Steinbrook RA, Gugino LD, et al: Continuous noninvasive monitoring of cardiac output with esophageal Doppler ultrasound during cardiac surgery. Anesth Analg 1986; 65:1013–1020.
65. Freund PR: Modification in the transesophageal Doppler: Comparison with thermodilution measurement during cardiac output in anesthetized man. (Abstract.) Anesthesiology 1986; 65:A144.
66. Roewer N, Bednarz F, Driadha A, et al: Intraoperative cardiac output determination from transmitral and pulmonary blood flow measurement using transesophageal pulsed Doppler echocardiography. Anesthesiology 1987; 67:A639.

67. Reichek N, Wilson J, St John Sutton M, et al: Noninvasive determination of left ventricular end-systolic stress: Validation of the method and initial application. Circulation 1982; 65:99–108.

68. Hartford M, Wikstand JCM, Wallentin I, et al: Left ventricular wall stress and systolic function in untreated primary hypertension. Hypertension 1985; 7:97–104.

69. Lang RL, Borow KM, Newman A, et al: Systemic vascular resistance: An unreliable index of afterload. Circulation 1986; 74:1114–1123.

70. Tennant R, Wiggers CJ: Effects of coronary occlusion on myocardial contraction. Am J Physiol 1935; 112:351–361.

71. Herman M, Heinle R, Klein M, et al: Localized disorders in myocardial contraction. Asynergy and its role in congestive heart failure. N Engl J Med 1967; 277:222–232.

72. Forrester JS, Wyatt HL, Paluz PL, et al: Functional significance of regional ischemic contraction abnormalities. Circulation 1976; 54:64–70.

73. Vatner SF: Correlation between acute reductions in myocardial blood flow and function in conscious dogs. Circ Res 1980; 47:201–207.

74. Weyman A, Peskoe S, Williams E, et al: Detection of left ventricular aneurysms by cross-sectional echocardiography. Circulation 1976; 54:936–944.

75. Kisslo J, Robertson D, Gilbert B, et al: A comparison of real-time two-dimensional echocardiography and cineangiography in detecting left ventricular asynergy. Circulation 1977; 55:134–141.

76. Abel MD, Nishimura RA, Callahan MJ: Evaluation of intraoperative transesophageal two-dimensional echocardiography. Anesthesiology 1987; 66:64–68.

77. Schnittger I, Fitzgerald PJ, Gordon EP, et al: Computerized quantitative analysis of left ventricular wall motion by two-dimensional echocardiography. Circulation 1984; 70:242–254.

78. Thys DM: The intraoperative assessment of regional myocardial performance: Is the cart before the horse? (Editorial.) J Cardiothorac Anesth 1987; 1:272–275.

79. Zeiher AM, Wollschlarger H, Bonzel T, et al: Hierarchy of levels of ischemia-induced impairment in regional left ventricular systolic function in man. Circulation 1987; 76:768–776.

80. Elliott PL, Schauble JF, Weiss J, et al: Echocardiography and LV function during anesthesia. Anesthesiology 1980; 53:S105.

81. Smith J, Cahalan M, Benefield D, et al: Intraoperative detection of myocardial ischemia in high-risk patients: Echocardiography versus two-dimensional transesophageal echocardiography. Circulation 1985; 72:1015–1021.

82. Koolen JJ, Visser CA, Van Wezel MB, et al: Influence of coronary artery bypass surgery on regional left ventricular wall motion: An intraoperative two-dimensional transesophageal echocardiography study. J Cardiothorac Anesth 1987; 1:276–283.

83. Topol EJ, Weiss JL, Gazman PA, et al: Immediate improvement of dysfunction segments after coronary revascularization: Detection by intraoperative transesophageal echocardiography. J Am Coll Cardiol 1984; 4:1123–1134.

84. Goldman ME, Mindich BP, Stavile K, et al: Intraoperative contrast two-dimensional echocardiography to assess mitral valve operations. J Am Coll Cardiol 1984; 4:1035–1040.

85. Feinstein SB, Folkert JTC, Zwehl W, et al: Two-dimensional contrast echocardiography: Development and quantificative analysis of echocardiographic contrast agents. J Am Coll Cardiol 1984; 3:14–20.

86. Austen SG, Houry DH: Ultrasound as a method to detect bubbles of particulate matter in the arterial line during cardiopulmonary bypass. J Surg Res 1965; 51:273–284.

87. Equaras BG, Pasalodos J, Gonzalez V, et al: Intraoperative contrast two-dimensional echocardiography: Evaluation of the presence and severity of aortic and mitral regurgitation during cardiac operations. J Thorac Cardiovasc Surg 1985; 89:573–579.

88. Goldman ME, Mindich BP: Intraoperative two-dimensional echocardiography: New application of an old technique. J Am Coll Cardiol 1986; 7:374–382.

89. Mohr-Kahaly S, Erbel R, Steller D, et al: Aortic dissection detected by transesophageal echocardiography. Int J Card Imaging 1987; 2:31–35.

90. Borner N, Erbel R, Braun B, et al: Diagnosis of aortic dissection by transesophageal echocardiography. Am J Cardiol 1984; 54:1157–1158.

91. Mohr-Kahaly S, Rennollet H, Wittlich N, et al: Follow-up of aortic dissection by transesophageal color Doppler echocardiography. Circulation 1987; 76 (supp 4):IV37.

92. Hashimoto S, Kumada T, Osakada G, et al: Detection of the entry by color Doppler in dissecting aortic aneurysm: Clinical significance of the transesophageal color Doppler. Circulation 1987; 76 (supp 4):IV37.

93. Macartney FJ: Cross-sectional echocardiography diagnosis of congenital heart disease. Br Heart J 1983; 50:501–505.

94. Valdes-Cruz L, Pieroni D, Roland J, et al: Recognition of residual postoperative shunts by contrast echocardiographic techniques. Circulation 1977; 55:148–152.

95. Fraker T, Harris P, Behar V, et al: Detection and exclusion of interatrial shunts by two-dimensional echocardiography and peripheral venous injection. Circulation 1979; 59:379–384.

96. Maurer G, Czer L, Bolger A, et al: Intraoperative color Doppler flow mapping for repair of congenital heart disease. Circulation 1986; 74 (supp 2):II37.

97. Hagler DJ, Seward JB, Tajik J, et al: Intraoperative two-dimensional color flow imaging. Circulation 1986; 74 (supp 2):II36.

98. Hillel Z, Thys D, Ritter S, et al: Two-dimensional color flow Doppler echocardiography for the intraoperative monitoring of cardiac shunt flows in patients with congenital heart disease. J Cardiothorac Anesth 1987; 1:42–47.

99. Cyran SE, Meyer RA, Bailey WW, et al: Intraoperative transesophageal echocardiographic assessment of congenital heart disease in children. Circulation 1987; 76 (supp 4):IV172.

100. Oka Y, Boriwaki K, Hong Y, et al: Detection of air emboli in the left heart by M-mode transesophageal echocardiography following cardiopulmonary bypass. Anesthesiology 1985; 63:109–113.

101. Topol EH, Humphrey LS, Basham M, et al: Value of intraoperative left ventricular microbubbles detected by transesophageal two-dimensional echocardiography in predicting neurologic outcome after cardiac operations. Am J Cardiol 1985; 56:773–775.

102. Furuya H, Suzuki T, Okumura F, et al: Detection of air embolism by transesophageal echocardiography. Anesthesiology 1983; 58:124–129.

103. Glenski FA, Cucchiara RF, Michenfelder JD: Transesophageal echocardiography and transcutaneous O_2 and CO_2 monitoring for detection of venous air embolism. Anesthesiology 1986; 64:541–545.

104. Cucchiara R, Nugent M, Seward J, et al: Air embolism in upright neurosurgical patients: Detection and localization by two-dimensional transesophageal echocardiography. Anesthesiology 1984; 60:353–355.

105. Schlüter M, Langenstein B, Thier W, et al: Transesophageal two-dimensional echocardiography in the diagnosis of cor triatriatum in the adult. J Am Coll Cardiol 1983; 2:1011–1015.

106. Morimoto K, Matsuzaki M, Toham Y, et al: Diagnosis and quantitative evaluation of atrial septal defect by transesophageal 2-D color Doppler echocardiography. Circulation 1987; 76 (supp 4):IV39.

107. Gussenhoven E, Taams M, Roelandt J, et al: Transesophageal two-dimensional echocardiography: Its role in solving clinical problems. J Am Coll Cardiol 1986; 8:975–979.

108. Geibel A, Hofmann T, Behroz A, et al: Echocardiographic diagnosis of infective endocarditis: Additional information by transesophageal echocardiography? (Abstract.) Circulation 1987; 76 (supp 4):IV38.

109. Thier W, Schlüter M, Krebber H, et al: Cysts in left atrial myxomas identified by transesophageal cross-sectional echocardiography. Am J Cardiol 1983; 51:1793–1795.

110. Daniel W, Schroder E, Nellessen U, Hausmann D: Diagnosis of intra- and extracardiac masses by echocardiography: Comparison between the transthoracic and transesophageal approach. (Abstract.) Circulation 1987; 76 (supp 4):IV38.

111. Matsumoto M, Hanrath P, Kremer P, et al: The evaluation of left ventricular function by transesophageal M-mode exercise echocardiography. *In* Hanrath P, Bleifeld W, Souquet J (eds): Cardiovascular Diagnosis by Ultrasound. The Hague: Martinus Nijhoff, 1981; 227–236.

112. Thomas JD: On-line digital data acquisition and real-time array processing: What are they? What are their potential clinical applications? Update in Echocardiography. Boston: Massachusetts General Hospital, 1987.

113. Thomas JD: Can Fourier analysis improve our ability to assess regional wall motion? Update in Echocardiography. Boston: Massachusetts General Hospital, 1987.

114. Helmcke F, Nanda NC, Hsiung MC, et al: Color Doppler assessment of mitral regurgitation with orthogonal planes. Circulation 1987; 75:175–183.

115. Switzer DF, Yoganathan AP, Nanda NC, et al: Calibration of color Doppler flow mapping during extreme hemodynamic conditions in vitro: A foundation for a reliable quantitative grading system for aortic incompetence. Circulation 1987; 75:837–846.

116. Davidoff R, Wilkins GT, Thomas JD, et al: Regurgitant volumes by color flow overestimate injected volumes in an in vitro flow model. J Am Coll Cardiol 1987; 9:110A.

117. Yoganathan AP, Cape E: The fundamental difference between regurgitant volume and jet volume. Update in Echocardiography. Boston: Massachusetts General Hospital, 1987.

118. Skorton DJ, Collins SM, Garcia E, et al: Digital signal and image processing in echocardiography. The American Society of Echocardiography. Am Heart J 1985; 110:1268–1283.

119. Hoyt R, Collins S, Skorton D, et al: Assessment of fibrosis in infarcted human hearts by analysis of ultrasonic backscatter. Circulation 1985; 71:740–744.

120. Schnittger I, Vieli A, Heiserman J, et al: Ultrasonic tissue characterization: Detection of acute myocardial ischemia in dogs. Circulation 1985; 72:193–199.

121. Fitzgerald PJ, McDaniel MM, Rolett EL, et al: Two-dimensional ultrasonic tissue characterization: Backscatter power, endocardial wall motion, and their phase relationship for normal, ischemic and infarcted myocardium. Circulation 1987; 76:850–859.

122. Vered Z, Barzilai B, Moh GA, et al: Quantitative ultrasonic tissue characterization with real-time integrated backscatter imaging in normal human subjects and in patients with dilated cardiomyopathy. Circulation 1987; 76:1067–1073.

123. Rovai D, Nissen S, Elion J, et al: Contrast echo washout curves from the left ventricle: Application of basic principles of indicator-dilution theory and calculation of ejection fraction. J Am Coll Cardiol 1987; 10:125–134.

124. Gewertz B, Kremser P, Zarins C, et al: Transesophageal echocardiographic

monitoring of myocardial ischemia during vascular surgery. J Vasc Surg 1987; 5:607–613.

125. Rovai D, Lombardi M, Ferdeghini E, et al: Color-coded functional imaging of myocardial perfusion by contrast echocardiography. (Abstract.) Circulation 1987; 76 (supp 4):IV504.

126. Zotz R, Kann B, Brennecke R: Evaluation of PTCA by video-intensitometric analysis of contrast echocardiograms. (Abstract.) Circulation 1987; 76 (supp 4):IV505.

127. Berwing K, Schlepper M, Kremer P, Bahawar H: Comparison of myocardial perfusion determined by contrast echocardiography with left ventricular regional function in patients. (Abstract.) Circulation 1987; 76:IV–506.

128. Segil L, Dick C, Feinstein S, Silverman P: Contrast echocardiography: Experimental coronary blood volume. (Abstract.) Circulation 1987; 76 (supp 4):IV504.

chapter seven

Monitoring of Ventricular Function

■ CAROL L. LAKE, M.D.

Ventricular function includes both the performance of the heart as a pump and the intrinsic inotropic state of the myocardium. Both components are assessed by invasive and noninvasive means. Ideally, a measure of contractility should be sensitive to changing inotropy, reproducible, easily measured, insensitive to preload or afterload, and correctable for body size, ventricular dimensions, and thickness. None of the methods described in this chapter, however, achieves this ideal.

Accurate assessment of cardiac performance requires measurement of both pressure and flow, using several methods.[1] Cardiac work describes ventricular function by the load that is carried and the distance it is moved. Advantages of using cardiac work instead of cardiac output or stroke volume to describe ventricular function follow. (1) The stroke work index defines the area of the pressure-volume loop (described later). (2) Stroke work index measures both systolic and diastolic performance. (3) Calculation of cardiac work includes the major variables affecting cardiac function: heart rate, preload, and afterload. Changes in stroke work indicate a change in either contractility or afterload. Cardiac output is often the best clinical index of cardiac performance, despite its lack of a statistically significant relationship to total hemodynamic power.[1] Experimental determinations of ventricular power index using angiography are independent of preload.[2]

Cardiac output, the volume of blood pumped by the heart each minute, is the product of heart rate and stroke volume. It varies slightly with body

237

position. During exercise, stroke volume increases in the upright position but is unchanged in the supine position. Intracardiac pressures also vary with position, but there are conflicting reports regarding whether the right or left lateral decubitus position has a greater effect. Lange and coworkers noted that right ventricular peak systolic and end-diastolic pressures and left ventricular end-diastolic pressure are greater in the left lateral decubitus than in the supine position.[3] Other investigators noted greater increases in right ventricular pressures in the right lateral decubitus position than in the left lateral decubitus position due to changes in hydrostatic pressure secondary to the height of the right ventricle relative to the inferior vena cava.[4] The increases in ventricular pressures may result from extrinsic compression from lungs, intra-abdominal organs, pericardium, or a combination.[3]

A newer approach to the assessment of cardiovascular function is the use of oxygen uptake kinetics. This method is based on the concept that a primary function of the circulatory system is oxygen transport between the cells and the lungs. Wasserman reviews four methods for assessing adequacy of oxygen delivery: anaerobic threshold, rate of rise of oxygen uptake related to work rate increase, magnitude of phase I oxygen uptake (first 20 seconds of exercise) compared with phase II oxygen uptake (increase in cellular respiration), and the slope of carbon dioxide production compared with oxygen consumption.[5]

PHYSIOLOGY OF THE HEART

Myocardial Loading Conditions

Preload is the end-diastolic stress on the ventricle (end-diastolic fiber length or end-diastolic volume). End-diastolic volume is not linearly related to, or synonymous with, end-diastolic pressure. It is determined by blood volume, ventricular compliance, ventricular afterload, venous tone, and myocardial contractility. Increased preload increases wall tension, end-diastolic volume, and work performed by the ventricle. The clinical substitution of pulmonary wedge pressure for preload is predicated on the observation that within the clinical range of ventricular volume, ventricular pressure increases almost linearly with increased volume.

Ventricular contraction occurs against the resistance of the peripheral vasculature or afterload. Although often used clinically to estimate afterload, systemic vascular resistance is a poor index of left ventricular afterload. Systemic vascular resistance reflects peripheral arteriolar tone, whereas ventricular afterload is the ventricular fiber load (force opposing ventricular fiber shortening) during systole. The ventricular fiber load or wall stress is inversely related to wall thickness and directly related to chamber dimensions (shape, size, and radius). Left ventricular afterload peaks during the first one third of systole and declines throughout the rest of systole. Reductions in afterload cause the ventricle to shorten more completely and quickly. Increased afterload decreases the velocity and extent of shortening, but it increases the active tension and the time to peak tension.

Cardiac Muscle Mechanics

Myocardial muscle contraction occurs in three phases: resting phase, isometric contraction, and isotonic contraction. The resting phase exists prior to intrinsic or extrinsic stimulation when the muscle length depends upon its preload. Myocardial contraction begins with passage of an action potential through the tubular system of the sarcoplasmic reticulum, which stimulates calcium release.

Cellular sarcolemma controls calcium influx and efflux. Beat-to-beat regulation of contractility occurs by sequestration and release of intracellular calcium from the sarcoplasmic reticulum, the intracellular tubular membranes. Myoplasmic calcium ion concentrations probably control myocardial contractility. Occupation of the calcium-binding site (by calcium) on the troponin-calcium–binding subunit results in cessation of tropomyosin's interference with actin-myosin binding.

Generation of myocardial contractile force requires splitting of adenosine triphosphate (ATP) by a calcium-stimulated, magnesium adenosine triphosphatase (ATPase) in the cross-bridging regions of the thick myosin filaments in order to release energy for sliding the myosin and actin filaments in relation to one another. ATP bound to the myosin head causes loose binding of actin to myosin and hydrolysis of ATP. Strong binding of the actin-myosin cross-bridge occurs in response to ATP hydrolysis products. Initial contraction is isometric (tension development without a change in muscle length). Isotonic contraction follows with shortening of the muscle dependent upon preload and afterload. Mechanical function in isotonic contraction is defined by shortening velocity, time after activation, force or tension, and instantaneous muscle length.

During relaxation, the regulatory protein tropomyosin covers the actin-binding sites. Reuptake or binding of calcium by the sarcoplasmic reticulum occurs in conjunction with cyclic adenosine monophosphate. Troponin, another regulatory protein, alters the configuration of tropomyosin to expose the actin-binding sites. At myoplasmic calcium concentrations below 10^{-7} relaxation occurs, whereas contractile activation is maximum at concentrations of 10^{-5}. Changes in contractile proteins also modify developed force.

Myocardial contractile force depends upon two factors: myocardial contractile state and initial myocardial fiber stretch. Greater stretch of the fibers occurs at high filling volumes or pressures, i.e., increased preload. This relationship is the Frank-Starling law (Fig. 7–1*A*). The primary determinant of active tension development in the ventricle is sarcomere length, not muscle length *per se*. Normal hearts operate on the ascending limb of the curve, with peak output occurring at filling pressures of 10 mmHg. Both atrial and ventricular muscles obey Starling's law. However, the Starling curve for the right ventricle is upward and to the left of the left ventricular curve, indicating the sensitivity of the right ventricle to preload.

A descending limb of Starling's curve is questionable, since sarcomere length in mammalian myocardium never exceeds 2.3 μm.[6] Rather than on a descending limb for cardiac decompensation, the heart probably operates on a different curve. Starling's curves are affected by both preload and

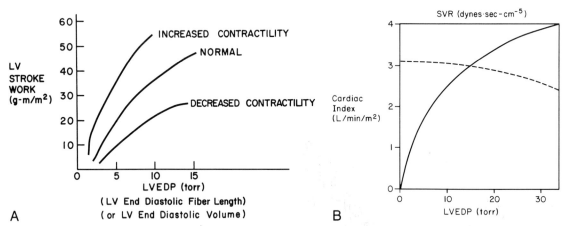

Figure 7–1. *A,* The Frank-Starling relationship, in which ventricular work is determined by end-diastolic fiber length (*solid lines*). (From Lake CL: Cardiovascular Anesthesia. New York: Springer-Verlag, 1985; 9. With permission.) *B,* The normal heart is affected more by preload (*solid line*—LVEDP) than by afterload (*dotted line*—systemic vascular resistance [SVR]). (From Lake CL: Cardiovascular anatomy and physiology. *In* Barash PG, Cullen BF, Stoelting RK [eds]: Clinical Anesthesia. Philadelphia: JB Lippincott, 1989; 965. With permission.)

afterload, which must be controlled for changes in contractility to be verified (Fig. 7–1*B*).

EVALUATION OF VENTRICULAR INOTROPY

Ventricular inotropy is studied using either ejection phase indexes or isovolemic phase indexes. The ejection phase indexes are mean and peak velocity of circumferential fiber shortening at peak wall stress (Vcf), mean systolic ejection rate, ejection fraction (EF), and percent fractional shortening (FS). The isovolemic phase indexes are measurements made prior to the opening of the aortic valve, and they include peak rate of left ventricular pressure development (peak dP/dt), max dP/dt, peak velocity of shortening of the contractile element (Vpm), velocity of shortening of the unloaded contractile element (Vce or Vmax), and dP/dt at a ventricular pressure of 40 mmHg (dP/dt40). Such isovolemic phase indexes are sensitive to acutely increased afterload. Vce and Vmax, the extrapolation of Vce to zero pressure, are least sensitive to mild degrees of ventricular dysfunction.[7] Vpm is less sensitive to preload, but it underestimates contractility if compliance is decreased. A comprehensive theoretic analysis of the contractility indexes is beyond the scope of this chapter. The interested reader should consult the paper by Kass and coworkers for details (Table 7–1).[8]

Isovolemic Phase Indexes

Rate of Rise of Left Ventricular Pressure (dP/dt)

The rate of rise of interventricular pressure during the isometric phase of ventricular contraction is dP/dt. Maximal force of tension developed dur-

Table 7–1. EVALUATION OF VENTRICULAR
FUNCTION

Ejection Phase Indexes
Mean velocity of circumferential fiber shortening
Peak velocity of circumferential fiber shortening
Mean systolic ejection rate
Mean normalized systolic ejection rate
Ejection fraction
Fractional shortening
Cardiac output
Left ventricular ejection time
Pressure-length loops
Pressure-volume loops
End-systolic pressure-volume relation

Isovolemic Phase Indexes
Peak dP/dt
Max dP/dt
dP/dt40
Peak velocity of shortening of contractile element
Velocity of shortening of the unloaded contractile element
Force-velocity curves
Pre-ejection period

Miscellaneous Methods
Ventricular pressures and volumes
Pulse pressure and contour

ing contraction is max dP/dt. Factors affecting dP/dt are contractile state, preload, afterload, and muscle mass. It is underestimated when aortic regurgitation is present, because aortic diastolic pressure is below normal and max dP/dt occurs early during ventricular ejection. Using the quotient (max dP/dt)/P, the max dP/dt at a specific ventricular pressure, obviates the preload dependence. Normal dP/dt values are 800–1700 mmHg/second, but these are affected by interpatient variation and complicated recording equipment.

EVALUATION OF VENTRICULAR FUNCTION

Ventricular function is measured noninvasively by transthoracic echocardiography, cardiokymography, systolic time intervals, and bioimpedance cardiography. Invasive methods include radionuclide, Fick, indicator-dilution, transesophageal echocardiographic, flowmeter, and strain gauge arch techniques. Highly invasive methods such as flowmeters and strain gauge arches are used only in experimental animals. Cardiac output, ejection fraction, and ventricular volumes are commonly measured.

Ejection Fraction

Radionuclide Methods

Technique. Ejection fraction is the ratio of the blood ejected by the ventricle (stroke volume) to the blood in the ventricle at the end of diastole.

Two techniques are commonly used to assess ejection fraction from either ventricular volumes or radioactivity counts at end-systole and end-diastole: gated blood pool imaging and first-pass studies. First-pass techniques usually give slightly lower ejection fractions than gated blood pool images do. Ejection fractions determined by radionuclide methods correlate well with those determined by angiography.[9] Radionuclide determinations of ejection fraction are relatively independent of ventricular geometry. A major limitation with radionuclide measurements is the inability to precisely determine onset and end of systole and diastole.

Intraoperative Use. A portable nuclear cardiac probe or "nuclear stethoscope" has been used during anesthesia to quantitate ejection fraction, end-systolic and end-diastolic ventricular volumes, filling velocities, and other parameters of ventricular performance.[10] Technetium-labeled human serum albumin or erythrocytes are injected intravenously. In nonportable devices, electrocardiogram-synchronized, computer-processed recording of cardiac radioactivity images the cardiac blood pool, providing views of ventricular wall motion throughout the cardiac cycle. In portable devices, only regional and global ventricular time-activity curves are generated. Elimination of the capability to visualize ventricular wall motion in these devices permits global ventricular function to be determined on a beat-to-beat basis.

However, even the portable computer-camera device is expensive and cumbersome and requires operator practice for accurate positioning over the left ventricle. A 40° left anterior oblique projection with a 10–20-degree caudal tilt is used in supine, spontaneously breathing patients. The probe is slowly moved over the chest wall until the region of maximal counts is located. Background radioactivity is similarly determined and stored in the computer.

Variability of measurements with these instruments is about 6% in humans.[10] There is good correlation (r = 0.9) between ejection fractions measured with the nuclear stethoscope and those measured with the nonportable Anger scintillation camera-computer devices.[11] Positive pressure ventilation changes the measured ejection fractions by about 3%.[10]

Using technetium-labeled erythrocytes and the nuclear probe, Giles and colleagues demonstrated decreased ejection fraction associated with hypertension and tachycardia due to laryngoscopy in patients with coronary artery disease.[10] Serial radionuclide monitoring also rapidly evaluates the effects of pharmacologic intervention in patients with poor ventricular function.[12]

Angiographic Methods

Ejection fraction (EF) is commonly measured by angiography using biplane views. However, this technique is generally not applicable intraoperatively and is limited by the patient's exposure to radiation and contrast material. Dependence on preload, afterload, and heart rate causes EF to reflect mechanical ventricular performance but not actual myocardial contractility. Increased preload increases EF, whereas increased heart rate and afterload reduce it. Reduced EF is present if EF is less than 0.64 ± 0.08.

Left ventricular angiograms are also used to determine the mean normalized systolic ejection rate (MNSER) and the mean velocity of circumferential fiber shortening (Vcf).

$$\text{MNSER} = \text{EF/ET} \qquad\qquad \textbf{7-1}$$

$$\text{Mean Vcf} = \frac{\text{Med} - \text{Mes}}{\text{ET}} \times \text{Med} \qquad\qquad \textbf{7-2}$$

where ET = ejection time and Med and Mes = the ventricular short axes at end-diastole and end-systole in the right anterior oblique angiogram. MNSER and Vcf are affected by ET but generally provide information similar to EF.

Cardiokymography

Cardiokymography is a noninvasive method used to determine regional wall motion in the closed chest without radiation or radioisotopes. The cardiokymograph consists of a transducer that has a flat capacitive plate and a high-frequency oscillator. The transducer is strapped to the patient's chest, separated only by an air gap. Activation of the capacitive plate causes emission of a low-energy electromagnetic field, which penetrates the chest. Motion within the electromagnetic field alters the capacitance and changes the frequency of oscillation. The change in frequency is converted to voltage proportional to the original motion, amplified, and recorded. Only motion directly beneath the transducer is recorded.

Normal cardiokymograms (Fig. 7-2) include an I point that occurs shortly after the beginning of ejection and a long period of inward motion during systole. Near the end of systole is the O point where outward movement begins. In ventricular dyssynergy or dyskinesis, outward motion occurs during systole. Bellows and associates noted a 4% incidence of abnormal cardiokymograms indicative of ischemia during anesthesia induction.[13] These findings were confirmed with scintigraphy[10] and M-mode echocardiography.[14]

Systolic Time Intervals

Systolic time intervals are measured by simultaneously recording the electrocardiogram, phonocardiogram, and systemic arterial pressure. Total electromechanical systole is QS_2, the time from the onset of the Q wave to the first deflection of the second heart sound. The pre-ejection period (PEP) includes electromechanical delay and isovolemic contraction time. Noninvasive evaluation of systolic function is easily made using left ventricular ejection time (LVET), the time from the arterial upstroke to the dicrotic notch. LVET is measured from the carotid pulse or M-mode echocardiography of the aortic valve opening or with pulsed or continuous wave Doppler. Doppler measurement of ejection time results in a shorter value than when ejection time is determined by carotid pulse or M-mode echocardiography,

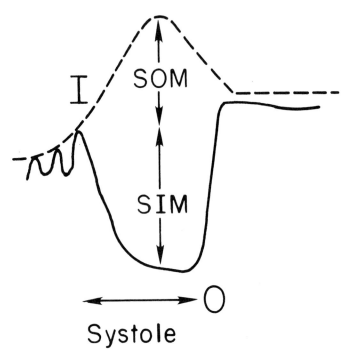

Systole

Figure 7–2. A normal cardiokymogram (*solid line*) has an I point indicating initial outward motion at the onset of ventricular ejection due to changes in the contour of the heart and an O point near the end of ejection. The majority of ventricular wall motion is inward during systole (SIM) with normal function. The *dashed line* indicates the alterations seen with ventricular dyskinesis, in which much of the ventricular wall motion during systole is outward (SOM).

possibly because flow velocity is shorter than mechanical valvular movements.[15] Another variable determined from systolic time intervals is the ratio PEP/LVET, which increases with ventricular dysfunction because of an increase in PEP and a decrease in LVET. Systolic time intervals reflect alterations in ventricular performance before changes are visible on chest radiograph or physical examination. They are also sensitive to changes in performance caused by ischemia, vasodilators, and alterations in load. Lack of standardization of recording methods and normalization of values for age, sex, or body build confound the clinical use of systolic time intervals.

Echocardiographic Doppler Methods

Pulsed Doppler echocardiography assesses left ventricular filling dynamics and diastolic function by determining the percentage of left ventricular filling due to atrial systole or the percentage of atrial contribution and the one-third filling fraction. Left ventricular systolic function (wall motion, chamber size, and cardiac output) is assessed by echocardiography, as was detailed in Chapter 6.

Theory

The Doppler principle is that ultrasound waves are reflected by moving objects with a change in their frequency. The interrogating Doppler sound beam is produced when an electrical potential is applied to a piezoelectric crystal, changing its dimension. This process causes the crystal to emit and transmit sound through an acoustically coupled medium as a beam. Sound reflected from an object returns to the crystal and is transduced as an electrical signal. Processing of the electrical signal produces either an auditory or a visual indication of the frequency shift. The change in frequency between the transmitted and the reflected sound waves, the Doppler shift, is directly proportional to the velocity of the moving object and the angle at which the ultrasound wave strikes the object.

Two techniques, continuous wave and pulsed wave Doppler, are used in equipment for measurement of ventricular function. Only the velocity of flow and its relative direction are determined with continuous wave Doppler. Continuous wave Doppler transducers have two crystals, one continuously transmitting and one continuously receiving sound waves. The Doppler shift occurs only when blood moves relative to the transducer, so that angle correction must be applied. Angle correction refers to the process of dividing the detected flow by the cosine of the angle between the blood flow and the beam. A disadvantage of continuous wave Doppler is the inability to locate the detected flow spatially, because of a lack of range resolution.

Pulsed wave Doppler has only a single crystal responsible for both transmission and reception of sound. Sound is transmitted intermittently at a specific number of sound pulses/second, the pulse-repetition frequency. Because of the spatial localization of the source of sound reflection, pulsed wave Doppler is more informative.

Doppler output techniques measure blood flow in meters or centimeters per second rather than the traditional liters/minute. Flow is measured across a heart valve (mitral) or great vessel such as the aorta using either pulsed or continuous wave techniques. The product of the area under the flow velocity curve and the cross-sectional area of the structure where the flow velocity is measured is the stroke volume.

Clinical Applications

Transesophageal and Transthoracic Devices. Doppler methods measure ascending and descending aortic flow using a suprasternal probe (noninvasive) or an esophageal (semi-invasive) probe. In clinically available systems, the esophageal probe is a no. 24-F esophageal stethoscope with a 2.5-MHz continuous wave Doppler (Fig. 7–3). The esophageal transducer is placed to a depth of 25–35 cm from the lip in a left lateral posterior position. Optimal position is achieved by slow rotation, insertion, and withdrawal until a clear, intense signal is present. The cardiac outputs measured with the suprasternal probe are then used to calibrate the esophageal probe. The proportionality constant, K, relates the suprasternal to the esophageal velocity signal. Reproducibility of the K factor has been problematic in some patients. Alternatively, the initial value obtained with the esophageal probe is used to indicate subsequent trends. Calibration against cardiac output obtained by another method such as thermodilution is also feasible.

In clinical applications, the cross-sectional aortic area is determined by two-dimensional echocardiogram. Stroke volume is estimated from the product of mean aortic-root flow velocity, aortic cross-sectional area, and the

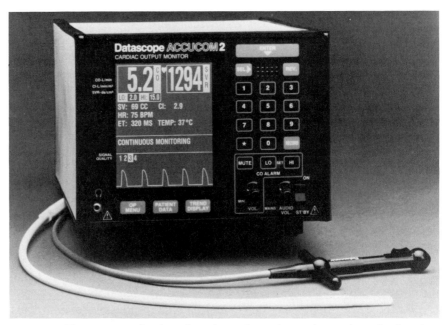

Figure 7–3. The suprasternal and esophageal transducers for continuous determination of cardiac output by continuous wave echo Doppler. (From Datascope, Paramus, NJ. With permission.)

R-R interval divided by the cosine θ, the angle between the ultrasound beam and the direction of blood flow summarized by the equation

$$SV = v \times ET \times CSA \qquad\qquad 7\text{--}3$$

where CSA = aortic cross-sectional area, ET = systolic ejection time, and v = average aortic systolic blood velocity.[16] Figure 7–4 demonstrates the velocity of blood in the aorta over time indicating the maximum systolic blood flow velocity, the time from upstroke of systolic blood flow to maximum velocity, and the maximum systolic acceleration of blood flow. The velocity sensitivity ranges of these devices are 10–300 cm/second with maximum radiating power of 100 mW/cm².[17]

Practical Problems. Most clinical devices incorporate a nomogram into the monitor software in order to estimate aortic dimensions based upon age, sex, height, and weight, rather than measuring these by echocardiographic techniques. Another problem is the assumption that ascending and descending aortic velocities are constant. Only blood flowing beyond the great vessels is included in the cardiac output measured by the esophageal probe. Accurate velocity determinations also depend upon knowledge of the angle between the blood flow and the ultrasound beam. With these devices, the angle is assumed to be less than 20° and to remain constant during measurements. Reported values for maximum linear acceleration range from 8 to 12 m/second, varying with ejection fraction.[17, 18] Nicolosi and colleagues studied the variability of six methods for determining Doppler flow and aortic

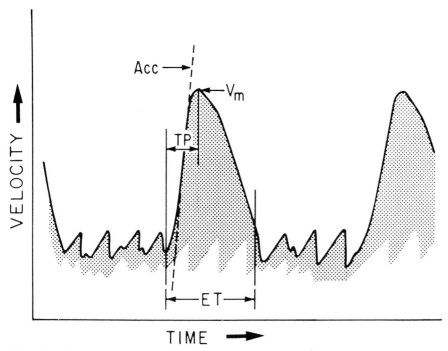

Figure 7–4. Doppler devices for continuous measurement of cardiac output determine the blood flow velocity in the ascending or descending aorta. Other variables that can be determined from the Doppler signal are maximum systolic acceleration of blood flow (Acc), ejection time (ET), maximum systolic blood flow velocity (V_m), and time from onset of systolic blood flow velocity to maximum velocity (TP). (From Thys DM, Hillel Z: Left ventricular performance indices by transesophageal Doppler. Anesthesiology 1988; 69:728–737. With permission.)

cross-sectional area and found the greatest variability with measurement of flow across the mitral and tricuspid valves rather than with measurement across the aorta or pulmonary trunk.[19] More error is introduced during recording of the Doppler flows and the cross-sectional echocardiograms than during subsequent analysis.[20] Perfect alignment of the transducer beam across the axis of flow is probably never achieved clinically. Thus, the correlation of echocardiographic measurement of aortic diameter with actual diameter is poor (r = 0.31).[21]

Systematic evaluation of the esophageal Doppler devices has been reported by Thys and Hillel.[17] In addition to the usual output measurements, they measured maximum blood flow velocity, maximum blood flow acceleration, and maximum linear blood flow acceleration in order to evaluate left ventricular performance (Fig. 7–4). Ascending aortic blood flow correlated well with descending aortic blood flow (r = 0.91). However, maximum linear acceleration and maximum flow velocity were greater in the ascending than in the descending aorta. Additional parameters studied were the product of mean arterial pressure and linear blood flow acceleration and the product of systemic vascular resistance and linear blood flow acceleration. The latter parameters changed appropriately in response to increasing minimum alveolar concentrations (MAC) of halothane as well as to an acute increase in mean arterial pressure during halothane anesthesia.

Accuracy. The echocardiographic Doppler method correlates well with cardiac outputs measured by the Fick technique in infants and small children.[21] In adults, Doppler velocimeter measurements of cardiac output correlate well with both electromagnetic flow probes and thermodilution measurements.[22, 23] Crobson and coworkers reported a coefficient of variation of 8.8% for Doppler echocardiographic determination of cardiac output, with coefficients of variation of 4.1%, 6.4%, and 5.0% for aortic annular diameter, aortic velocity integral, and heart rate.[20] Differences of Doppler measurements of 0.41–0.9 L/minute from thermodilution measurements have been reported.[22, 24, 25] Correlation coefficients of esophageal Doppler outputs with thermodilution measurements are about 0.68.[24, 25] It must be noted that Doppler outputs do not include coronary blood flow, are inaccurate in the presence of turbulent aortic blood flow (aortic stenosis), and may be less reliable in the presence of left-to-right shunt through a patent ductus or in low-flow states.[16]

Limitations. Limitations of the Doppler output technique include esophageal pathology, abnormalities in the thoracic aorta, and inadequate acoustic windows in occasional patients. Averaging techniques create an additional source of error in patients with atrial fibrillation or frequent ventricular extrasystoles. Alterations in descending aortic flow secondary to aortic clamping also limit use of this technique. However, the usefulness of echocardiographic Doppler cardiac output determinations for monitoring trends in the perioperative period has been amply demonstrated.[23]

Other Echocardiographic Doppler Devices. Doppler devices have also been attached to pulmonary artery catheters or endotracheal tubes[26] or have been placed directly on the aorta. Advantages of the intratracheal position are measurements of the ascending aortic flow proximal to the great vessels, more constant anatomic position between aorta and trachea than between aorta and esophagus, and, in patients requiring intubation, the capability of cardiac output determination without additional invasive instrumentation.[26] The device is a 5-mm, 5-mHz transducer attached to an endotracheal tube beyond the tracheal cuff. The transducer itself is surrounded by a cuff to assure acoustic contact with the anterolateral tracheal wall. Essential requirements for satisfactory use include intratracheal positioning below the aortic arch but above the carina (suitable anatomy), adequate acoustic contact so the ultrasound beam intersects the ascending aorta, and measurements of ascending aortic dimensions and blood velocity. The correlation of outputs measured by transtracheal pulsed Doppler and thermodilution was 0.82 in a prototype device studied in dogs. As is found with the esophageal devices, measurement of aortic diameter is a major source of error.

Miniaturized Doppler flow probes have been anchored on the aorta by two small metal tines at the time of cardiac surgery, passed through the chest wall, and removed by gentle traction in the postoperative period.[27, 28] Although these probes permit accurate assessment of cardiac output in patients with congenital heart disease (r = 0.9, compared with electromagnetic flow probe), their use in pediatric cardiac surgery has been limited.

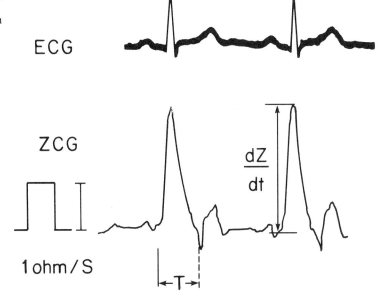

Figure 7–5. An impedance cardiogram (ZCG) is similar to an arterial pressure waveform. (T = the ejection time in seconds, dZ/dt = the first derivative of the maximal rate of change of thoracic impedance, ECG = electrocardiogram.)

Bioimpedance Cardiography

Technique

Bioimpedance cardiography is a noninvasive technique measuring stroke volume on a beat-to-beat basis. A constant sinusoidal alternating current of 2.5–4 mA at 70–100 kHz is passed through the chest to sensing electrodes that detect the change in voltage due to transcardiac passage of the current. A total of eight electrodes is used, two sensing and two transmitting electrodes at the base of the neck and a similar set at the xiphoid process. The electrical conductivity of blood, varying in volume and velocity in the descending thoracic aorta, is the major source of the impedance change. The impedance, based on Ohm's law, is calculated from the current applied and the voltage produced. Stroke volume is determined from analysis of the impedance change over the cardiac cycle. An impedance cardiogram (Fig. 7–5) is similar to an arterial pressure waveform. It is used to calculate stroke volume using the relationship

$$\text{SV (ml)} = (p) (L/Z_o)^2 (dZ/dt \text{ max}) (T) \qquad 7\text{--}4$$

where T = left ventricular ejection time in seconds, L = distance between electrodes, e.g., the length of the thorax from the root of the neck to the xiphoid, dZ/dt max = first derivative of the maximum rate of change of thoracic impedance in ohms/second, Z_o = total thoracic impedance in ohms, and p = resistivity of blood, 110–200 ohm·cm. The small, usually negative, wave preceding the main systolic wave is probably atrial in origin. Heart rate is simultaneously determined and multiplied by stroke volume to give the cardiac output. Other parameters determined with this technique are ejection velocity index, thoracic fluid index, and ventricular ejection time.

Accuracy

In adults, impedance cardiographic measurements of cardiac output correlate well with the Fick method ($\leq 5\%$ difference).[29, 30] Correlation with Fick is further improved by comparison with stroke volume or stroke index rather than with cardiac output.[30, 31] Salandin and associates note excellent repeatability of bioimpedance measurements in adults.[29] The accuracy of bioimpedance measurements corresponding to that of dye-dilution outputs has also been confirmed.

Good correlation of cardiac output measured by bioimpedance in children was noted by Introna and colleagues and Miles and coworkers.[32, 33] However, in their studies thoracic length (L) was adjusted until the measured bioimpedance output was within 10% of thermodilution outputs rather than using a nomogram or measured thoracic length. An error of 1 cm in thoracic length causes a 20% error in measured output. The assumption that thoracic length is 17% of patient height (as in adults) is inaccurate in children.[32] In children with systemic shunts (atrial septal defect, ventricular septal defect, or extracardiac shunts), Fick outputs were greater than systemic flow measured by bioimpedance.[33]

Practical Problems

Repetition of measurements is easily performed without discomfort or risk to patients. However, the premise of the measurement, that the thorax is a homogeneous cylinder of blood during the cardiac cycle, is an extreme simplification. In children, the thorax more closely resembles a cylinder, whereas in adults, it is a truncated cone. Weber and associates, Siegel and coworkers, and other investigators found poor correlation of impedance measurements with thermodilution (r = 0.43,[24] r = 0.41[34]) or between individual measurements using the Fick method.[30] Other problems occur in the presence of pulmonary edema or when hematocrit level varies during major cardiac surgery. The bioimpedance method is also difficult to apply without infringing on the surgical field during many procedures and is unreliable for following trends in cardiac function in the perioperative period,[24, 34] during dysrhythmias with widely variable R-R intervals, in aortic regurgitation, and in hyperdynamic septic shock.[29]

Walton-Brodie Strain Gauge

A strain gauge sutured to the myocardium was developed by Walton and Brodie to directly measure contractile force of the right or left ventricle. It has been used extensively in anesthesia research on dogs, cats, rats, and rabbits.[35] The Walton-Brodie device consists of a strain element, bonded to an arch with feet, which is sutured to the myocardium. Myocardial sutures are placed about 2 cm apart, penetrating nearly the full thickness of the myocardium.[35] After the arch is in place, the muscle segment beneath is stretched about 40% by separation of the feet, so that the muscle segment is functioning at or near the top of the Starling curve. Because the strain gauge is one limb of a Wheatstone bridge, deformation of the arch by muscle contraction changes its resistance and alters the current of the bridge. The change in current is sensed by an amplifier and recorded. Increased heart rate increases contractile force as measured by the arch, whereas increases in preload decrease contractile force. Changes in afterload have little effect on arch performance. However, the use of the Walton-Brodie arch has not been systematically compared with other methods of measuring ventricular contractility.[35] Other limitations include limited lifespan (about 7–10 days) and sensitivity to temperature changes.[35]

Pressure-Volume Loops

The end-systolic pressure-volume relation is a clinically useful index of ventricular function, because it is independent of load and sensitive to changes in contractility. The slope of the end-systolic pressure-volume relation separates normal from abnormal ventricles better than ejection fraction or end-systolic volume does. A ventricular pressure-volume loop is constructed by relating intracavitary pressure on the y axis to the ventricular volume on the x axis over the entire cardiac cycle, providing information on both systolic and diastolic function. The height of the loop is determined by ventricular systolic pressure, and the width of the loop is determined by stroke volume. End-systolic pressure and volume are determined by afterload and ventricular inotropy. End-diastolic pressure and volume reflect preload and ventricular lusitropy (relaxation).[36] An ideal loop for the left ventricle has four phases: phase I is the lower horizontal limb representing diastolic filling; phase II is the vertical limb of isovolemic contraction; phase III is the upper horizontal limb of systolic ejection; and phase IV is the phase of isovolemic relaxation. The loop begins at the bottom left with opening of the mitral valve and initiation of ventricular filling. At the lower right portion of the loop is end-diastole, when the mitral valve closes and isovolemic contraction begins. At the upper right, aortic valvular opening and ejection begin, causing the loop to turn to the left. As the aortic valve closes at the upper left of the loop (the end-systolic pressure-volume relation) (Fig. 7–6), isovolemic relaxation begins. The slope of the end-systolic pressure-volume relation, determined by connecting the upper left-hand corners of pressure-volume loops generated at varying afterloads, is Emax, the maximum value of end-systolic elastance (Fig. 7–7). Calculation of the area within the loop gives stroke work (pressure × volume).

Pressure-volume loops also indicate ventricular compliance. The normal relationship between diastolic pressure and volume is curvilinear. At low end-diastolic pressure the slope is gentle, with little change in pressure for large changes in volume. When end-diastolic pressures are abnormally increased, the curve becomes steeper, and pressure is almost exponentially related to end-diastolic volume.

MONITORING OF VENTRICULAR FUNCTION

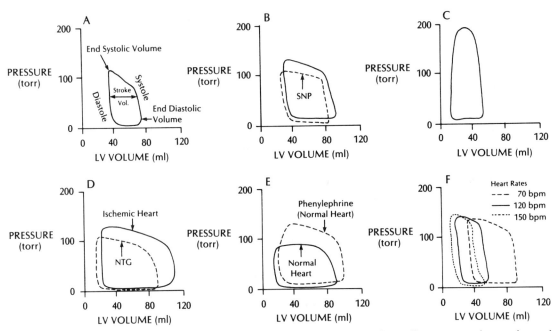

Figure 7–6. The normal pressure-volume loop is in *A*. At the upper left is the end-systolic pressure-volume point, and the lower right is the end-diastolic volume point. Extension of this point gives a diastolic pressure-volume curve. Cardiac work is the area of the pressure-volume loop, and the width of the loop is stroke volume. Alterations in various states are shown in *B–F*. *B*, Afterload reduction with sodium nitroprusside (SNP). *C*, Aortic stenosis. *D*, Ischemia and relief of ischemia with nitroglycerin (NTG). *E*, Increased afterload in a normal heart. *F*, Tachycardia. (From Lake CL: Cardiovascular anatomy and physiology. *In* Barash PG, Cullen BF, Stoelting RK [eds]: Clinical Anesthesia. Philadelphia: JB Lippincott, 1989; 966. With permission.)

Technique

Measurement of ventricular pressure using transducer-tipped catheters is possible, although the presence of a ventricular catheter increases ventricular ectopy. Likewise, ventricular volume can be measured using echocardiography. However, determination of volume changes in real time is not readily available. Another limitation of pressure-volume relationships is that pressure may not accurately measure end-systolic afterload. However, the end-systolic pressure-volume relation is relatively load-independent, and its slope correlates with ejection fraction. It is, nevertheless, sensitive to end-diastolic volume and contractility.

The use of the simple ratio between end-systolic pressure and volume to represent the end-systolic pressure-volume relation is an oversimplification, although it has been used as an index of ventricular contractility. It is more easily measured than the end-systolic pressure-volume relation. However, changes in inotropy have variable effects on the slope of the relationship of peak pressure and end-systolic dimension.[37]

Right ventricular pressure-volume loops are similar to those of the left ventricle. Compared with left ventricular loops, however, right ventricular loops are more triangular in shape, with early peaking of pressure.[38] Right ventricular volume often continues to decrease beyond end-systole. Although the slope of the end-systolic pressure-volume relation Emax reflects

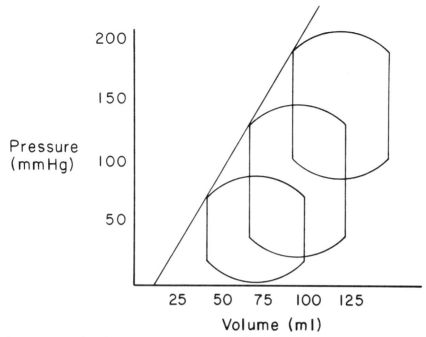

Figure 7-7. A series of pressure-volume loops are created at different preloads and afterloads to define the end-systolic pressure-volume relation. The end-systolic points are connected in order to define the contractile state of the ventricle. A shift to the right of the normal relation indicates decreased contractility and a shift to the left shows increased contractility.

contractile state in the right ventricle, right ventricular Emax has a wide range in normal hearts.[38]

Pathophysiologic Changes

Alterations in pressure-volume loops occur in response to drugs and disease (Fig. 7-6). The end-systolic point is determined by contractility and afterload. End-systolic elastance is altered by chamber volume and mass. Positive inotropic interventions shift the end-systolic pressure-volume relation upward and leftward, and negative inotropic interventions cause shifts downward and to the right. Decreased venous return reduces end-diastolic pressure and volume. Increased preload moves the point of end-diastole to the right and upward along the end-diastolic pressure-volume relation. Positive lusitropic interventions (e.g., relief of ischemia) enhance ventricular filling, so that the loop begins at a higher end-diastolic volume and a lower end-diastolic pressure. Patients with primarily systolic heart failure demonstrate increased ventricular volume at end-diastole and reduced extent of shortening but normal developed systolic pressure. With primary diastolic dysfunction, a decrease in diastolic distensibility occurs, so that a higher diastolic pressure is required to achieve the same diastolic volume.

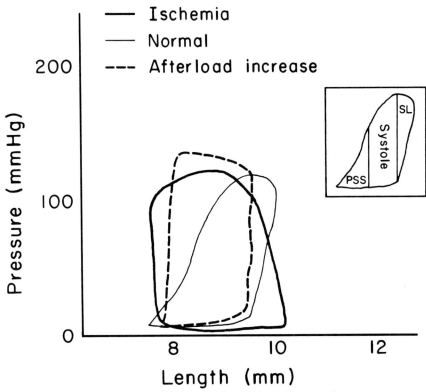

Figure 7–8. The normal pressure-length loop and alterations caused by ischemia and increased afterload are similar to those seen in pressure-volume loops. The inset demonstrates specific alterations during ischemia, including development of postsystolic shortening (PSS) and systolic lengthening (SL). Only during systole does ventricular segment shortening contribute to effective cardiac work.

Pressure-Length Loops

Measurement of pressure-length loops requires placement of a length gauge directly on the myocardium and thus is primarily applicable to animal studies. However, it is a sensitive and reproducible method for assessing total cardiac and regional myocardial function during both systole and diastole.[39] Like the pressure-volume loop, ventricular pressure is plotted on the x axis, and ventricular segment length appears on the y axis. Pressure-length loops have four segments: isovolemic contraction, ejection, isovolemic relaxation, and ventricular filling. The end-systolic pressure-length relation is the point at the upper left of the loop. Pressure-length loops are usually rectangular (Fig. 7–8). A series of pressure-length loops at different preloads or afterloads permits determination of the slope of the end-systolic pressure-length relation.[40]

Pressure-length loops are indexes of regional ventricular work. They lean to the right when contraction is asynchronous, as in the presence of ischemia. Ischemia of a small portion of the ventricle may not be visible on a pressure-length loop, if the remaining ventricle compensates to maintain

Figure 7–9. Force-velocity curve for cardiac muscle. Point A is Vmax, the point of maximum velocity of shortening with no load. Point B is Po, where tension development is maximum but no shortening occurs. The effect of increased preload is seen in curve C; on any curve, afterload increases from left to right. Curve D demonstrates the effect of increased contractility. (From Lake CL: Cardiovascular Anesthesia. New York: Springer-Verlag, 1985; 10. With permission.)

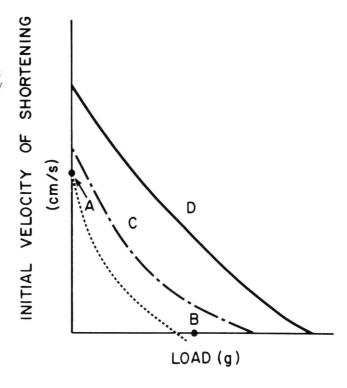

function. Increased preload increases the area of the loop. As afterload increases, the loop becomes taller at a similar preload. With ischemia, ventricular segment lengthening occurs after the end of diastole. Postsystolic shortening is ventricular contraction occurring after aortic valve closure, which does not effectively contribute to the work of the heart. Placement of markers directly on the myocardium is an inherent disadvantage of this method.

Force-Velocity Curves

Force-velocity curves evaluate the velocity of shortening at a constant fiber length in a preloaded (passively stretched) muscle that is stimulated to contract against either no load or an afterload. A Walton-Brodie strain gauge is used to measure the muscle contraction. As afterload is increased, the initial rate of shortening follows a hyperbolic relationship (Fig. 7–9). The point at which no shortening occurs, although the muscle is developing maximal force, is Po. Vmax is the maximum velocity of shortening at zero pressure, determined by extrapolation of the curve back to zero load. It is sensitive to preload, although less so than dP/dt. Increased myocardial contractility shifts the force-velocity curve upward and to the right, increasing both the developed tension and the maximum velocity of shortening.

Cardiac Output

Fick Method

The Fick principle uses the following relation to determine cardiac output:

$$\text{Cardiac output (ml/minute)} = \frac{\dot{V}_{O_2}}{C_{aO_2} - C_{vO_2}} \times 100 \qquad \textbf{7-5}$$

because the size of a fluid stream can be calculated if the amount of a substance entering or leaving the stream and the concentration difference resulting from entry and removal are known. Oxygen is the traditional indicator substance in clinical determinations of cardiac output by the Fick method. Oxygen uptake or consumption is $\dot{V}_{O_2}$ (milliliters per minute), which is the product of the volume of expired air and the difference between the oxygen content in the inspired and the expired air (determined by gas analysis). Arterial and venous oxygen content differences ($C_{aO_2} - C_{vO_2}$) are determined from blood samples. Oxygen content is calculated as the solubility of oxygen in whole blood (0.0031 ml/100 ml/mmHg) plus 1.34 hemoglobin (gm/100 ml) times percentage of oxyhemoglobin saturation.

Although the Fick technique is often referred to as the gold standard, cardiac output measurement by this method has numerous inherent difficulties.[41] The Fick equation assumes that pulmonary oxygen consumption is negligible and that the rate of oxygen removal from the blood (tissue oxygen uptake) equals the rate of oxygen uptake at the mouth (lung oxygen uptake). The major disadvantage of the Fick technique is the necessity for maintaining steady state conditions (unchanged right and left ventricular outputs, constant oxygen saturation and arterial P_{O_2}) for several minutes during the measurement. Values are inaccurate if cardiac, pulmonary, or hepatopulmonary shunts are present. Inaccuracy also results from errors in sampling of mixed venous blood or inspired/expired gases, and other measurements as detailed by Taylor and Silke.[41] Recent widespread use of mass spectrometry has rekindled interest in the perioperative measurement of cardiac output using the Fick method.

Rebreathing Fick Method

Morton recently described a rebreathing maneuver to estimate the oxygenated mixed venous P_{CO_2}. This value, when combined with end-tidal P_{CO_2} and CO_2 production, allows noninvasive assessment of cardiac output by the Fick method.[42] Carbon dioxide production was determined using the Siemens 930 carbon dioxide analyzer by integrating the product of instantaneous expiratory flow and instantaneous expired P_{CO_2}. Mixed venous P_{CO_2} was determined by allowing the patient to rebreathe a test mixture of 6-9% carbon dioxide in oxygen with the rate and volume of the ventilator approximated manually. Expired P_{CO_2} is recorded after the second, third, and fourth breaths. The rebreathing maneuver is repeated three or four times with different test gases, and a plot of inspired P_{CO_2} against the difference of expired and inspired P_{CO_2} is created. The x intercept (where expired P_{CO_2} equals inspired P_{CO_2}) is mixed venous carbon dioxide. Arteriovenous oxygen content difference is then determined as

$$11.02 \ (P_{VCO_2}^{0.396} - P_{aCO_2}^{0.396}) -$$

$$0.015 \ (P_{VCO_2} - P_{aCO_2}) \ (15 - Hb) -$$

$$0.064 \ (95 - S_{aO_2}) \qquad\qquad \textbf{7–6}$$

and used in the classic Fick equation. This method has good correlation with dye-dilution methods (r = 0.9).[42]

Continuous Fick Method

A continuous method for determination of cardiac output by the Fick technique is described by Davies and coworkers.[43] The components of the Fick equation were measured using a gas exchange analyzer to determine inspired/expired gas content and volumes with pulse and mixed venous cathNeter oximetry to determine oxygen contents. A computer calculated the output from these parameters every 20 seconds. Correlation between this method and thermodilution outputs was 0.86, but outputs were always lower than those measured by thermodilution. Advantages of the continuous Fick method over the thermodilution method are its rapid repetition, recognition of the contribution of each of the individual components to the patient's overall cardiorespiratory status, and the validity of the Fick principle for measuring cardiac output.

Indicator-Dilution Method

The major difference between the indicator-dilution and the Fick methods is that the concentration gradient of a nontoxic dye, rather than oxygen, is measured. The usual indicator is indocyanine green dye, which is rapidly mixed with blood, is bound to plasma protein, is rapidly metabolized in the liver, is nondiffusible in the lungs, and is easily measured with a photodensitometer. A bolus of dye is injected into the central venous or peripheral circulation. Blood is withdrawn from an artery continuously into a photo-electrical cuvette densitometer where the concentration of the dye is measured. As blood is drawn through the light pathway of the densitometer, its electrical output is proportional to the dye concentration. The curve relating the dye concentration to elapsed time is plotted. Figure 7–10 shows the normal indicator-dilution curve in which there is an uninterrupted build-up slope, a sharp concentration, a steep disappearance slope, and a prominent recirculation peak. The area under a dye-dilution curve is rapidly estimated using the fore-'n-aft triangle method of Bradley and Barr.[44] Total curve area does not indicate the total concentration of dye for the measured time interval, because some dye recirculates early and is measured twice. For this reason, the downslope of the curve is extrapolated to near zero to eliminate recirculation effects.

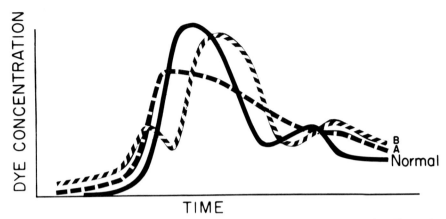

Figure 7–10. A normal indicator (dye)–dilution curve. Curve A demonstrates the effects of LR shunting, whereas curve B shows RL shunting. (From Lake CL: Cardiovascular Anesthesia. New York: Springer-Verlag, 1985; 70. With permission.)

The following equation (termed the Stewart-Hamilton equation for the two investigators who described it) indicates the relationship between dye concentration and cardiac output (L/minute):

$$\frac{60 \times \text{indicator dose (mg)}}{\text{average concentration} \times \text{time (second)}} \qquad 7\text{–}7$$

Cardiac output equals the amount of indicator injected divided by the area under the curve.

The efficacy of the dye-dilution method in the evaluation and management of infants and children during and after cardiac surgery was demonstrated by Truccone and coworkers.[45] In the presence of right-to-left shunting, there is an abnormal early-appearing hump in the build-up slope, because the dye reaches the arterial circulation early. With left-to-right shunts, there is a decreased peak concentration of dye, disappearance of dye is prolonged, and recirculation is absent (Fig. 7–10). In patients in shock, recirculation may occur so early that its recognition is impossible.

Limitations of the indicator-dilution method include the need to withdraw 50 ml of blood (which can be returned to the patient if it is drawn into sterile tubing), the necessity for arterial catheterization, the measurement of only mean flow, and the need for a steady state for 30–40 seconds. As little as 4–5 ml of arterial blood can be withdrawn in children without decreasing the accuracy of measurement.[45] Cardiopulmonary bypass significantly decreases clearance of indocyanine green owing to decreased hepatic blood flow.[46]

Because of these limitations, dye dilution has been refined to use a thermal indicator in the popular thermodilution method. Common to both dye dilution and thermal dilution are the need for constant flow, constant blood volume, absence of recirculation, constant indicator distribution times, and measured flow representative of total flow.[47]

Thermodilution Method

The use of a thermal indicator was introduced by Fegler in 1954.[48] However, Ganz and colleagues introduced the thermodilution technique for cardiac output determination in 1971.[49] Advantages of the thermodilution technique are simplicity, reproducibility, lack of recirculation, rapid repetition, safe indicator, rapid indicator mixing with blood, and no need for blood withdrawal.

Technique

Thermodilution is a modification of the indicator-dilution technique in which cooled dextrose is injected into the right atrium or central veins through the proximal lumen of a pulmonary artery catheter or a central venous pressure catheter. A thermistor, balanced through a Wheatstone bridge, in the pulmonary artery records the decrease in temperature as a resistance change. The current in the thermistor is small and does not significantly heat the blood. Theoretically, if a known amount of cold indicator (i.e., "negative" heat) is injected into the circulation, calculation of the cardiac output from the resultant cooling curve recorded downstream of the injection is possible. Passage through two cardiac valves (tricuspid and pulmonic) and one cardiac chamber (right ventricle) allows adequate mixing of injectate with blood.

The equation for calculation of cardiac output by thermodilution is

$$\text{Cardiac output} = \frac{V_I \times (T_b - T_I) \times S_I \times C_I \times 60}{S_B \times C_B \int_0^\infty \Delta T_B(t) dt} \qquad 7\text{-}8$$

where T_b = initial blood temperature, T_I = time from start to termination of percent integration at 30% of peak of thermodilution curve, S_I and S_B = the specific gravity of indicator and blood, respectively, C_I and C_B = the specific heat of indicator and blood, respectively, V_1 = volume of injectate in liters, and $\int_0^\infty \Delta T_B(t) dt$ = the area under the blood temperature change curve in degrees Celsius multiplied by time in seconds. Correction factors for the increase in injectate temperature during passage through the catheter, injectate volume, the area lost by cutoff of the curve at 30% of peak, and 60 are often entered as a constant ("computation constant") into commercially available thermodilution computers (Fig. 7–11). An operator's manual for the specific computer should be consulted for details.

Equipment

Thermodilution cardiac output determinations in adults are performed using a multilumen pulmonary artery catheter, with injectate administered through a proximal lumen placed in the right atrium or central vein and the thermistor located in the pulmonary artery. Alternatively, in patients undergoing surgery of the tricuspid or pulmonic valves or those in whom

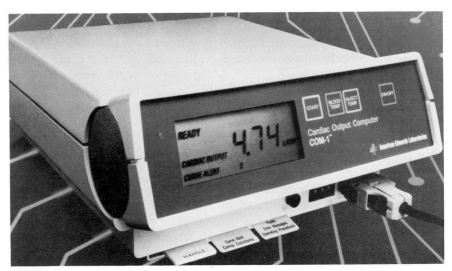

Figure 7–11. The American Edwards Laboratories COM-1 thermodilution cardiac output computer. The "computation" constant, a factor used to correct for the increase in injectate temperature during passage through the catheter, injectate volume, and other factors, is entered at the bottom right. (1988 Baxter Healthcare Corporation. All rights reserved.)

size precludes accurate placement of the injection site and thermistor (pediatric patients), separate central venous and pulmonary artery thermistors can be placed (Figs. 7–12 and 7–13).[50, 51] The thermistor is placed through a purse-string suture in the right ventricular outflow tract and threaded into the main pulmonary artery; its position is verified by palpation. The central venous catheter is placed either directly or percutaneously. The injectate catheter must be accurately calibrated for the thermal exchange occurring between the catheter and the tissue during injection.[52] Either a precalibrated catheter supplied with the thermistor or any central venous catheter may be used.

Cardiac Output Curves

The thermal curve should be inspected before accepting the computed/calculated cardiac output. Many computers have integrated strip-chart recorders or can be connected to multichannel recording devices in order to record the curves. Planimetry of the area under the recorded curve in square millimeters, multiplication by the calibration factor, temperature in degrees Celsius per millimeter for the temperature deflection, and the recorder paper speed in seconds per millimeter permit manual calculation of the cardiac output. A normal cardiac output curve (Fig. 7–14A) is smooth, with a rapid rise to peak and a slow return to baseline.

Accuracy

Close correlation (r = 0.94) of thermodilution with Fick and dye dilution is demonstrable (Fig. 7–15).[53, 54] In adult patients, cardiac outputs deter-

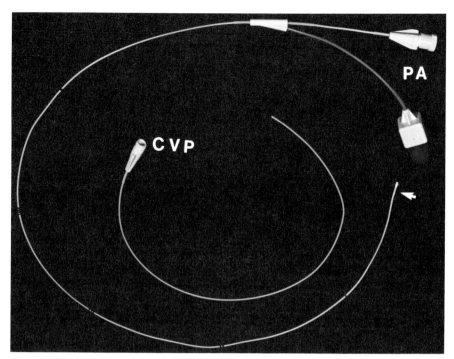

Figure 7–12. Separate central venous (CVP) and pulmonary artery (PA) thermistor (*arrow*) catheters allow direct intravascular placement in patients undergoing cardiac surgery. Such catheters obviate the inability to cross stenotic or prosthetic valves and permit accurate placement of injection site and thermistor in children of varying sizes. (From Lake CL [ed]: Pediatric Cardiac Anesthesia. East Norwalk, CT: Appleton & Lange, 1988; 97. With permission.)

mined with separate thermistor probes and standard pulmonary artery catheters are almost identical.[55] McCormick and coworkers used two identical computers to compute values for cardiac outputs from a single injection sensed by both the separate and the catheter-mounted thermistor.[55] Variation of the position of the injection catheter in the vena cava did not influence measurement.

Similar excellent correlations between thermistors and pediatric pulmonary artery catheters are reported in pediatric patients.[52, 56, 57] Kohanna and Cunningham compared 125 thermodilution and dye-dilution outputs in 10 postoperative patients.[56] Except in extremely low-output states in which dye-dilution outputs were always smaller, results were similar with both techniques. Thermodilution outputs always exceeded dye-dilution measurements by 1.6%, even in normal circulatory states. Reproducibility of the dye-dilution outputs was always less than that of thermodilution. Maruschak and colleagues recommended prefilling of the central venous injectate catheter with 1 ml of injectate-temperature fluid 20 seconds prior to bolus injection in order to prevent thermal injectate loss and overestimation of cardiac output.[58]

Standard errors of the mean of thermodilution determinations vary from 2–5% for three measurements per determination to 3–8% for single mea-

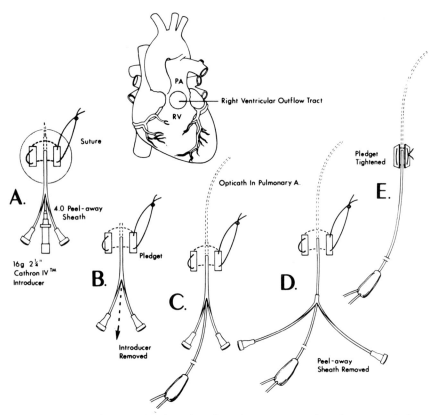

Figure 7–13. *A–E,* Direct surgical insertion of a pulmonary artery thermistor through the right ventricular outflow tract permits thermodilution cardiac output determinations in pediatric patients and patients with disease of tricuspid or pulmonic valves. A central venous catheter must be inserted either directly or percutaneously. (Reprinted with permission from the International Anesthesia Research Society from A method of continuous postoperative measurement of mixed venous oxygen saturation in infants and children after open heart procedures, by Rah KH, Dunwiddie WC, Lower RR, Anesthesia and Analgesia 1984; 63:873–881.)

surements.[59, 60] Thus, clinical significance should not be attributed to differences in values of less than 12–15%.[60]

Sources of Inaccuracy

There are numerous sources of inaccuracy in the thermodilution technique. Variation between cardiac outputs performed in the clinical setting results from inconsistent technical performance, catheter or computer malfunction, respiratory effects on right ventricular filling, cardiac shunting or valvular regurgitation, and hemodynamic instability. Specific factors causing inaccuracy are rewarming of injectate, improper constants, inaccurate measurement of patient or injectate temperature, inadequate temperature difference between patient and injectate, improper thermistor position (against vessel wall or in ventricle), wrong type or volume of injectate, intracatheter septal defects, and insufficient mixing of injectate and blood. Indicator in-

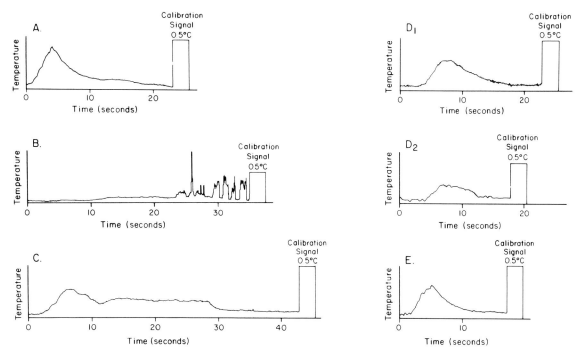

Figure 7–14. Types of cardiac output curves. *A*, Normal thermodilution cardiac output curve. The 0.5°C calibration signal appears after the termination of the curve. *B*, The thermodilution curve is delayed and of low amplitude when injectate is administered slowly over 15 seconds. *C*, The thermistor is against the vessel wall in a wedge position, causing an irregular, low-amplitude curve. *D₁*, The type of curve resulting from injection of 10 ml of injectate; *D₂*, the curve in the same patient when only 5 ml of injectate is given, erroneously increasing the measured output. *E*, An irregular curve with an unsteady baseline results from patient motion during injection.

jection during use of the electrocautery or rapid fluid infusion also causes incorrect values (Table 7–2).

Some computers contain internal verification systems that give error messages when baseline drift is present, when the thermistor is against a vessel wall, or when the catheter is too distal in the pulmonary artery. Figure 7–14B–E demonstrates common types of anomalous curves.[53] Both respiratory and cardiac cycles alter baselines. The thermal curve rises slowly when the thermistor is positioned too distally in the pulmonary artery.[53, 61] Irregularities in thermal curves result from rapid changes in heart rate or blood pressure, patient movement, inadequate indicator mixing with blood, or contact between vessel wall and thermistor.[53, 61] Low-amplitude curves occur when the injectate volume is too small, the thermistor is too distal or is within the right ventricle, or the temperature differential between injectate and patient is too small.[61]

Injectate. Both room temperature and iced injectates are used. Variability among outputs is about 5.5% with room temperature injectate.[53] However, the signal of temperature change is two to three times smaller with room temperature injectates than with iced injectates. Several investigators have demonstrated similar results with either room temperature or iced injectates (Fig. 7–16).[62–64] Although the temperature differential between room temperature injectate and blood temperature in a hypothermic (31–

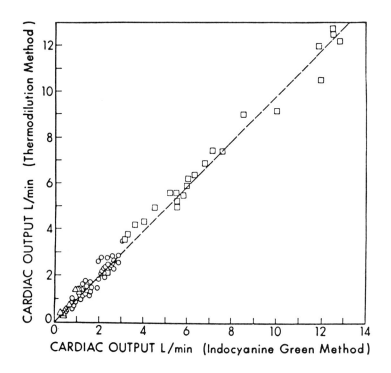

Figure 7–15. There is excellent correlation between cardiac output measured by dye dilution and that measured by thermodilution in monkeys (*triangles*), dogs (*circles*), and humans (*squares*). (From Weisel RD, Berger RL, Hechtman HB: Current concepts: Measurement of cardiac output by thermodilution. 1975; 292:682–684. Reprinted with permission from the New England Journal of Medicine.)

33°C) patient is small, correlation coefficients of 0.951 for 10-ml volumes and 0.925 for 5-ml volumes of injectate were demonstrated in mechanically ventilated adults by Shellock and associates and Merrick and coleagues.[63, 65] Volume of injectate is an important factor in accuracy since volumes of 5 ml or less caused significant variability (as much as 1.5 L/minute) in outputs.[64]

Table 7–2. THERMODILUTION METHOD: SOURCES OF ERROR

Patient Variables
Motion (shivering, extremity movement)
Respiration (panting, Valsalva maneuver, sighing)
Alterations in ventricular performance/dysrhythmias
Valvular regurgitation
Intracardiac shunts

Injectate Factors
Wrong substance
Wrong temperature
Wrong volume
Rapid repetition of measurements

Thermistor Factors
Thermistor malposition
Thermistor thrombus
Intracatheter shunts
Rapid volume infusion
Concurrent electrocautery use

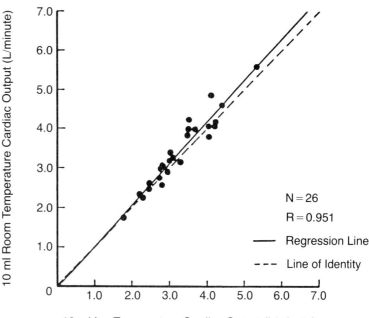

Figure 7–16. Thermodilution cardiac output determinations using either room temperature or iced injectate yield similar results. (From Shellock FG, Riedinger MS, Bateman TM, Gray RJ: Thermodilution cardiac output determination in hypothermic postcardiac surgery patients: Room vs ice temperature injectate. Crit Care Med 11(8):668–670, © by Williams & Wilkins, 1983.)

Closed injectate systems obviate the need to prepare individual syringes for injectate, minimizing infection risk[66] and equilibration time.[61] Repeated aspiration of injectate from a rubber-stoppered intravenous bottle immersed in an ice bath and connection/disconnection from the injection port of the pulmonary artery catheter are sources of bacterial contamination.[66]

However, if the tubing of such systems is not maintained at the same temperature as that of the injectate or the injectate temperature as it enters the catheter, measured cardiac output is inaccurate.[67] Prefilled refrigerated syringes offer an alternative to closed injectate systems. Rewarming of iced injectate begins within 30 seconds of its removal from an iced bath, particularly with application of firm manual pressure on the syringe by the person making the injection.[61, 68] A 1°C error in injectate temperature causes an error in measured output of 2.7% with iced injectate and a 7.7% error with room temperature injectate in a normothermic patient.[61] Measurement of the injectate temperature as it enters the circulation is optimal.[68]

Timing of Injection. Measurement of pulmonary artery diastolic pressures is timed to the apneic period at the end of expiration because of the respiratory effects on the right side of the heart and pulmonary pressures. Performance of thermodilution outputs at random times in the respiratory cycle causes marked variability in results, because pulmonary artery temperature decreases during inspiration, particularly in mechanically ventilated patients (Fig. 7–17).[53, 69–71] Maximum variability in outputs was 70% for the right side of the heart and 40% for the left side of the heart during random measurements during the respiratory cycle.[71] Pulmonary artery temperature variation with the phase of the respiratory cycle results from right ventricular surface cooling from overlying lung and changes in vena caval flows.[61] Mea-

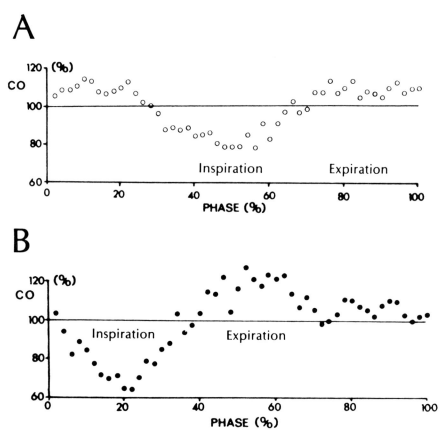

Figure 7–17. Alterations in left side of the heart output (*A*) and right side of the heart output (*B*) during a single respiratory cycle. Flow decreases during inspiration and increases and reaches a plateau during expiration. For this reason, thermodilution outputs should be determined at end-expiration. (From Jansen JRC, Schreuder JJ, Bogaard JM, et al: Thermodilution technique for measurement of cardiac output during artificial ventilation. J Appl Physiol 1981; 51:584–591. With permission.)

surements at peak inspiration or end-expiration have less variability and smaller standard deviations.[72] For convenience, end-expiration is often used, because cessation of respirator noise and chest wall movement permits easy detection of the optimal time.

Marked variation in pulmonary artery temperatures may preclude the use of room temperature injectate for thermodilution output determinations. Such changes occur with panting, shivering, deep spontaneous respiration, the Valsalva maneuver, or elevation of the extremities.[61]

Disease Process. Structural cardiac disease impairs or prevents measurement of cardiac output by thermodilution. Tricuspid regurgitation produces such significant recirculation of blood in the right side of the heart that accurate output measurements are impossible because of effects on the downslope of the curve. Broad, low-amplitude curves result from tricuspid regurgitation. However, in patients with regurgitant lesions on the left side of the heart, the thermodilution technique produces curves with less recirculation-induced distortion than does the dye-dilution method with right-sided injection and left-sided sampling.[54]

The downslope of the curve is also affected to an unknown extent by recirculation of indicator through a ventricular septal defect.[53, 61] Morady and coworkers reported a method for determining the magnitude of left-to-right shunt by extrapolation of the curve to baseline just before early recirculation.[73] The area under the extrapolated portion and the entire curve are measured by planimetry. Shunt size is the ratio of the total area to the area prior to recirculation ([A + B]/A), which correlated well with shunt ratios determined using the Fick equation.[73] Erroneously high outputs were measured in a patient in cardiogenic shock with an aortopulmonary fistula.[74]

The thermodilution method can be satisfactorily used to measure cardiac output in patients with residual left-to-right shunts.[75] Placement of right and left atrial catheters and a pulmonary artery thermistor allows measurement of output to be made after injection through either catheter. When a computer that stops integrating the thermal curve at 30% of baseline is used to avoid recirculation, systemic flow (Qs) is determined by the equation

$$Qs = Drai\ (1\ -\ Drai/Dlai) \qquad\qquad 7\text{--}9$$

where rai and lai = thermodilution outputs determined after right and left atrial injections, respectively.[75]

Finally, during moderate exercise at outputs between 2 and 13 L/minute, both thermodilution and Fick methods accurately measure cardiac output.[76] However, during maximum exercise, thermodilution cardiac outputs are lower than those measured using the Fick technique.[77] At outputs of 15–23 L, thermodilution and Fick methods correlate well, but they may be subject to inaccuracy owing to alterations in mixed venous oxygen saturation, hematocrit level, fluctuation in pulmonary artery temperature during hyperventilation, and increased heat exchange.

Injectate Factors. Dextrose, 5% in water, is the recommended injectate. However, because the specific gravity and specific heat of dextrose and saline are similar (specific gravity, 1.018 for dextrose versus 1.005 for saline; specific heat, 0.965 for dextrose and 0.997 for saline), the product of the specific heat and specific gravity for either substance is similar. The volume of injectate varies according to the type of syringe used, but the error is small. However, if the syringe volume is less than the value entered into the computer, the area under the thermal curve is proportionately smaller, causing overestimation of cardiac output.[78] Recirculation of the cold injectate causes the thermal curve to have a diminished peak and longer tail than in dye-dilution curves. The cold ''radiates'' from the catheter after injection and arrives at the thermistor about 5–35 seconds after the bolus injection.

Repetition of injections must be delayed at least 90 seconds to permit resumption of steady blood temperature. Mechanical automatic injectors are helpful for maintaining consistency of injection rate.[79] Speed of injection affects the constants in the thermodilution equation that are based on a rate of 10 ml injected within 4 seconds or less in most computer systems.[80] The increase in injectate temperature (injectate at 0–1°C) during passage through a catheter inserted to 45 cm is 6–7°C.[59]

Mixing and Thermistor Factors. A distance of 20 cm or more is necessary for adequate mixing of the injectate with blood. The thermistor must also be located in the center of the flowing blood, at least 2 mm from the vessel wall for reproducibility of the outputs, because a thermal gradient exists between the central and the lateral portions of a flowing stream.[81] An undamped pulmonary artery waveform usually assures acceptable thermistor position.

Bjoraker and Ketcham reported that the presence of thrombus on the catheter prolongs warming and cooling of the thermistor after the cool bolus, leading to overestimation of the area under the curve and decreased values for cardiac output.[82] The error is proportional to the size of the thrombus, with underestimation of flow as thrombus size increases.

The presence of a defect in the septum of the catheter between the proximal and the distal lumina decreases measured cardiac output. Such defects cause a greater decrease in temperature at the thermistor, because the injectate is channeled into the distal lumen and emerges close to the thermistor.[83-85] Rapid volume infusions during determinations also artifactually reduce measured outputs.[86]

Complications

The major complication, cardiac dysrhythmias, relates to the temperature of the injectate. Iced injectate has been associated with atrial fibrillation,[87] bradycardia,[88] and other transient dysrhythmias such as slowing of the intrinsic sinus rhythm,[89] resulting from cooling of the sinoatrial node.[90] Ventricular fibrillation after injection of room temperature injectate was reported by Katz and coworkers.[91]

Saline-Indicator Method

A related method, the saline-indicator method, which uses a catheter-mounted resistivity indicator, has been studied in animals.[92, 93] The indicator is 5 ml of 3% saline, which is detected by the resistivity sensor in the pulmonary artery. Correlation with measurements by electromagnetic flowmeter was 0.965. Advantages of this technique include the lack of effect from injectate handling, catheter length within the animal, or injection rate, and no loss of indicator between the sites of injection and detection.[93]

Pulse Contour and Pressure Methods

The area under the arterial waveform is indicative of cardiac output. Numerous techniques for the determination of stroke volume from central aortic pressure waveform have been described. Common to all methods is the equation

$$\text{Stroke volume} = K \int \{P(t) - PED\}dt \qquad \textbf{7-10}$$

where K = a constant, {P(t) − PED}dt = the difference between the actual pressure (P[t]) and the end-diastolic pressure (PED) over time (dt).[94]

In the Warner method, pressure waveforms from a central aortic catheter are sampled by computer at 200 samples/second for 45 seconds. Computer analysis of the waveform using the following equation allows determination of stroke volume:

$$\text{Stroke volume} = K \, (\text{pmd}) \, (1 + \text{Sa/Da}) \qquad \textbf{7–11}$$

where K = a calibration constant equal to F(1 + Ts/Td), F = the factor relating calculated stroke volume to stroke volume measured with another technique (thermodilution, dye dilution), Ts = duration of systolic ejection, Td = duration of diastole, pmd = the difference between average aortic pressures during the last 80 msec of systole and diastole, Sa = the systolic area of the curve, and Da = the diastolic area. K is representative of arterial compliance. The calibration constant varies markedly.[95] Despite the variation in calibration constants, English and colleagues found good correlation of cardiac outputs measured by thermodilution, flowmeter, and pulse contour during halothane administration, 0.5–2%, in dogs.[96] However, changes in systemic vascular resistance greater than 30–50% of control reduced the correlation.[96] Cundick and associates noted poor correlation of Warner pressure-pulse cardiac output determinations with those obtained by the Fick method.[95]

Monitoring of Right Ventricular Function

The right ventricle has limited functional significance during normal circulatory states. Although the spiral muscles of the right ventricle contract during systole, the right ventricular free wall is pulled toward the interventricular septum by alignment of septal fibers and the left ventricular pressure. Right ventricular stroke volume is more sensitive to increased afterload than that of the left ventricle. Other factors determining right ventricular function include its contractility, filling volume, sympathetic tone, myocardial structural integrity, and the chemical content of the coronary perfusate.[97] Compliance of the right ventricle is greater than that of the left ventricle.

Evaluation of right ventricular function includes the measurement of both pressure and volume. Central venous or right atrial pressure, discussed in Chapter 5, is most commonly used to assess right ventricular pressure. Normal right ventricular systolic pressures are 30–40 torr, with diastolic pressures of 0–5 torr. Many of the techniques described previously for measurement of left ventricular volume have been applied with limited success to the right ventricle. However, the anatomic shape of the right ventricle is variable, appearing as an ellipse, a tetrahedron, a crescent, or a pyramid, depending upon the viewpoint.

Radionuclide Techniques

Both the first-pass and the equilibrium-gated blood pool scans have been used successfully to determine right ventricular ejection fraction, systolic ejection time, peak filling rates, peak ejection fraction, and rate of contractility. Problems with the first-pass technique include invalidation of results by artifacts such as arrhythmias and the need to inject radioactive tracers for each determination. Equilibrium-gated scans permit repeated measurements with a single bolus injection of radioactive tracer and scanning in the left anterior oblique position.[98] One problem with this technique is the superimposition of the right atrium over the right ventricle.[99] For this reason, first-pass studies are preferred for determination of right ventricular ejection fraction.

Echocardiographic Techniques

Echocardiography of either two-dimensional or M-mode types provides information about right ventricular dimensions, interventricular septal motion, and right ventricular free wall thickness. The apical four-chamber view permits calculation of right ventricular short and long axes and systolic shortening. From the echocardiographic data, Simpson's rule is used to determine right ventricular volume. However, these methods often overestimate right ventricular volume and fail to allow for alterations in right ventricular size and geometry under various clinical conditions.

Thermodilution Techniques

Right ventricular ejection fraction can be measured by the thermodilution technique, using a rapid response thermistor pulmonary artery catheter.[100] Kay and colleagues compared thermodilution measurements of right ventricular ejection fraction with radionuclide studies in both animal models and humans.[101] The rapid-response thermistor has a response time of 50 msec, compared with the usual thermodilution thermistor response of 300–1000 msec. Increased response time permits beat-to-beat variations in pulmonary artery temperature in response to atrial injection (just proximal to the tricuspid valve) through a multiorificed catheter to be observed. The changes in temperature associated with successive diastolic plateaus can be measured (Fig. 7–18). Calculation of the ejection fraction, stroke volume, and right ventricular end-systolic and end-diastolic volumes is possible using the following formulas:

$$EF = 1 - RF \qquad\qquad \textbf{7–12}$$

where EF = ejection fraction and RF = mean residual fraction. RF is determined as

$$RF = \frac{RF_1 + RF_2}{2} \text{ and } RF_1 = \frac{T_2 - T_B}{T_1 - T_B} \text{ and } RF_2 = \frac{T_3 - T_B}{T_2 - T_B} \qquad \textbf{7–13}$$

Normal right ventricular EF is 0.4.

Limitations in this technique arise when evaluating regurgitant lesions of the tricuspid or pulmonic valve and cardiac dysrhythmias.[102] Only forward flow is measured, but placement of a thermistor in the right atrium allows

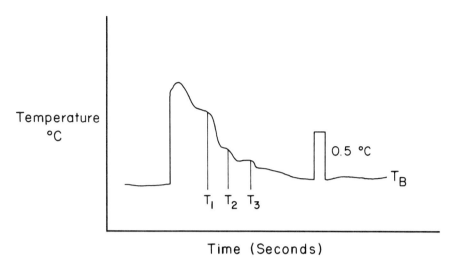

Figure 7–18. A right ventricular thermodilution curve demonstrates the plateaus on the downslope during diastole when temperature change is minimum. The standard 0.5°C is shown after the curve. (T_1, T_2, T_3 = the differences between each diastolic temperature, and T_B = the baseline temperature.

calculation of the regurgitant fraction resulting from tricuspid insufficiency. The problem with dysrhythmias is overcome by averaging the thermal curves obtained over five beats.

Determinations of right ventricular ejection fraction vary by about 12%.[103] Correlations between right ventricular ejection fractions measured by thermodilution and nuclear techniques are 0.8–0.9.[103, 104] Thermodilution underestimates right ventricular ejection fraction more than angiography does.[103] Weaker correlations with two-dimensional echocardiographic measurements (0.74) were noted by Jardin and colleagues.[105]

Changes in right ventricular function occur with ischemia, infarction, application of positive end-expiratory pressure to the airway, chronic obstructive lung disease, and pulmonary vasoconstriction of any etiology. The reader is referred to the review by Hines for the details of pathologic alterations in right ventricular function.[106]

Determination of Derived Parameters

Monitoring of isolated parameters leads to erroneous conclusions about a patient's general status. For this reason, profiles including data on hemodynamic, respiratory, renal, and metabolic functions are often used.[107] Assessment of respiratory, renal, and metabolic functions is discussed in Chapters 9, 17, and 18, respectively. The basis of most of these profiles is calculated hemodynamic variables. Systemic and pulmonary vascular resistance, right and left ventricular stroke volume and work, and cardiac index are calculated from directly measured intravascular pressures and systemic and pulmonary flows (Table 7–3). Cardiac index is calculated by normalizing cardiac output for body surface area (determined from a nomogram of height

Table 7–3. CALCULATION OF HEMODYNAMIC VARIABLES*

Variables	Formula	Normal Values
Cardiac index	$\dfrac{\text{cardiac output (L/minute)}}{\text{body surface area (m}^2)}$	2.8–4.2 L/minute/m^2
Stroke index	$\dfrac{\text{stroke volume (ml/beat)}}{\text{body surface area (m}^2)}$	30–65 ml/beat/m^2
Stroke volume	$\dfrac{\text{cardiac output (L/minute)} \times 1000}{\text{heart rate (beats/minute)}}$	60–90 ml/minute
Right ventricular stroke work index	0.0136 (mean pulmonary artery pressure − central venous pressure) × stroke index	5–10 gm-m/beat/m^2
Left ventricular stroke work index	0.0136 (mean arterial pressure − pulmonary capillary wedge pressure) × stroke index	45–60 gm-m/beat/m^2
Systemic vascular resistance	$\dfrac{\text{mean arterial pressure − central venous pressure}}{\text{cardiac output (L/minute)}} \times 79.9$	1200–1500 dynes-second/cm^{-5}
Pulmonary vascular resistance	$\dfrac{\text{mean pulmonary artery pressure − mean pulmonary capillary wedge pressure}}{\text{cardiac output (L/min)}} \times 79.9$	100–300 dynes-second/cm^{-5}

* All pressures are measured in torr.

and weight). The usefulness of these measures of ventricular performance is enhanced by construction of a ventricular function curve, relating stroke work or stroke power to end-diastolic fiber length (end-diastolic volume or pressure is usually substituted clinically). These curves can be replotted after interventions such as administration of drugs, exercise, diuresis, relief of ischemia, or volume loading.

Values of systemic and pulmonary vascular resistance are expressed in hybrid (Wood's) units or in absolute resistance units (dynes-second/cm^{-5}). Absolute resistance units are converted to Wood's units by dividing by 79.9. Systemic and pulmonary vascular resistance values are also normalized for body surface area by using cardiac index in place of cardiac output in the formula. Mohr and coworkers report a continuous on-line method to measure systemic vascular resistance using the peripheral arterial waveform.[108] Computer solution of the following equation is utilized:

$$ SVR = F \times \frac{P'}{dP/dt} - a \qquad\qquad \textbf{7–14} $$

where dP/dt = the peak dP/dt of the peripheral arterial waveform, P' = the pressure at peak dP/dt, and F and a = calibration constants. This method requires determination of these calibration constants against thermodilution or other independent methods. Because pulmonary vascular resistance varies with pulmonary blood flow, pulmonary tone, and left atrial pressure, the effects of therapeutic intervention should be monitored by pulmonary pressure-flow curves, direct measurement of pulmonary flow, or the pulmonary diastolic–pulmonary wedge pressure gradient.[109]

ALTERATIONS IN VENTRICULAR FUNCTION

Normal Changes

Cardiac output is increased by increased load, either pressure or volume, a process termed heterometric autoregulation. It also increases because of the treppe phenomenon and the Anrep effect. The staircase effect (treppe or Bowditch phenomenon) is a progressive increase in contractile force in response to sudden increases in heart rate. The reverse or negative staircase effect is an increased force of contraction following a long pause between heartbeats.

Abrupt increases in aortic or left ventricular pressure cause the Anrep effect, a response of increased contractility resulting from more rapid activation of the contractile process, increased velocity of shortening, or increased developed force. The Anrep effect is transient, because the initially increased ventricular end-diastolic volume and circumference decrease as stroke work recovers.

Alterations of volume and pressure in one ventricle affect these parameters in the other, because of the phenomenon of ventricular interdependence. Although interdependence is somewhat subject to the presence of the pericardium, it exists after pericardiotomy. The transseptal pressure gradient, septal position and deformability, and ventricular distensibility affect ventricular interdependence. Distention of either ventricle alters the geometry and compliance of the opposite ventricle. Ventricular hypertrophy, particularly of the interventricular septum, limits interdependence by decreasing the transfer of pressure and volume changes. Increased left ventricular pressure decreases right ventricular systolic function and diastolic compliance.

Pathologic Alterations

Ventricular function deteriorates during ischemia. Global ventricular function decreases less severely than regional function in the presence of progressive, single-vessel coronary stenosis. However, using ejection phase indexes, Akaishi and coworkers demonstrated correlation between regional and global dysfunction during ischemia.[110] Cardiac output did not decrease during progressive ischemia in their model. The ratio of left ventricular end-systolic pressure to end-systolic area decreased with progressive ischemia.[110] Ventricular function also deteriorates during acute or chronic pressure or volume overload (hypertension, valvular stenosis, or regurgitation) and in primary myocardial failure of any etiology.

References

1. Wright G, Sum Ping JST, Campbell CS, Tobias MA: Assessment of cardiovascular function in patients undergoing coronary artery bypass grafting. J Thorac Cardiovasc Surg 1988; 96:400–407.
2. Unterberg RH, Korfer R, Politz B, et al: Assessment of left ventricular function by a power index: An intraoperative study. Basic Res Cardiol 1984; 79:423–431.
3. Lange RA, Katz J, McBride W, et al: Effects of supine and lateral positions on cardiac output and intracardiac pressures. Am J Cardiol 1988; 62:330–333.
4. Nakao S, Come PC, Miller MJ, et al: Effects of supine and lateral positions on cardiac output and intracardiac pressures: An experimental study. Circulation 1986; 73:579–585.
5. Wasserman K: New concepts in assessing cardiovascular function. Circulation 1988; 78:1060–1071.
6. Spotnitz HM, Sonnenblick EH, Spiro D: Relation of ultrastructure to function in the intact heart: Sarcomere structure relative to pressure-volume curves of intact left ventricles of dog and cat. Circ Res 1966; 18:49–66.
7. Kreulen TH, Bove AA, McDonough MT, et al: The evaluation of left ventricular function in man. Circulation 1975; 51:677–688.
8. Kass DA, Maughan WL, Guo ZM, et al: Comparative influence of load versus inotropic states on indexes of ventricular contractility: Experimental and theoretical analysis based on pressure-volume relationships. Circulation 1987; 76:1422–1436.
9. Schelbert HR, Verba JW, Johnson AD, et al: Nontraumatic determination of left ventricular ejection fraction by radionuclide angiography. Circulation 1975; 51:902–909.
10. Giles RW, Berger HJ, Barash PG, et al: Continuous monitoring of left ventricular performance with the computerized nuclear probe during laryngoscopy and intubation before coronary artery bypass surgery. Am J Cardiol 1982; 50:735–741.
11. Wagner HN, Rigo P, Baxter RH, et al: Monitoring ventricular function at rest and during exercise with a nonimaging nuclear detector. Am J Cardiol 1979; 43:975–979.
12. Breisblatt WM, Vita NA, Armuchastegui M, et al: Usefulness of serial radionuclide monitoring during graded nitroglycerin infusion for unstable angina pectoris for determining left ventricular function and individualized therapeutic dose. Am J Cardiol 1988; 61:685–690.
13. Bellows WH, Bode RH, Levy JH, et al: Noninvasive detection of periinduction ischemic ventricular dysfunction by cardiokymography in humans: Preliminary experience. Anesthesiology 1984; 60:155–158.
14. Elliott PL, Schauble JF, Weiss J, et al: Echocardiography and LV function during anesthesia. Anesthesiology 1980; 53:S105.
15. Avgeropoulou CC, Rahko PS: Comparison of five methods for the measurement of left ventricular ejection time. Am J Cardiol 1988; 61:492–494.
16. Alverson DC, Eldridge M, Dillon T, et al: Noninvasive pulsed Doppler determination of cardiac output in neonates and children. J Pediatr 1982; 101:46–50.
17. Thys DM, Hillel Z: Left ventricular performance indices by transesophageal Doppler. Anesthesiology 1988; 69:728–737.
18. Sabbah HN, Lhaja F, Brymer JF, et al: Noninvasive evaluation of left ventricular performance based on peak aortic blood acceleration measured with a continuous-wave Doppler velocity meter. Circulation 1986; 74:323–329.

19. Nicolosi GL, Pungercic E, Cervesato E, et al: Feasibility and variability of six methods for the echocardiographic and Doppler determination of cardiac output. Br Heart J 1988; 59:299–303.

20. Crobson S, Murray A, Peart I, et al: Reproducibility of cardiac output measurement by cross sectional and Doppler echocardiography. Br Heart J 1988; 59:680–684.

21. Lees MH: Cardiac output determination in the neonate. J Pediatr 1983; 102:709–711.

22. Bojanowski LMR, Timmis AD, Najm YC, Gosling RG: Pulsed Doppler ultrasound compared with thermodilution for monitoring cardiac output responses to changing left ventricular function. Cardiovasc Res 1987; 21:260–268.

23. Mark JB, Steinbrook RA, Gugino LD, et al: Continuous noninvasive monitoring of cardiac output with esophageal Doppler ultrasound during cardiac surgery. Anesth Analg 1986; 65:1013–1020.

24. Siegel LC, Shafer SL, Martinez GM, et al: Simultaneous measurements of cardiac output by thermodilution, esophageal Doppler, and electrical impedance in anaesthetized patients. J Cardiothorac Anesth 1988; 2:590–595.

25. Freund PR: Transesophageal Doppler scanning versus thermodilution during general anesthesia. Am J Surg 1987; 153:490–494.

26. Abrams JH, Weber RE, Holman KD: Transtracheal Doppler: A new procedure for continuous cardiac output measurement. Anesthesiology 1989; 70:134–138.

27. Keagy BA, Wilcox BR, Lucas CL, et al: Constant postoperative monitoring of cardiac output after correction of congenital heart defects. J Thorac Cardiovasc Surg 1987; 93:658–664.

28. Van Orden DE, Farley DB, Fastenow C, Brody MJ: A technique for monitoring blood flow changes with miniaturized Doppler flow probes. Am J Physiol 1984; 247:H1005–1009.

29. Salandin V, Zussa C, Risica G, et al: Comparison of cardiac output estimation by thoracic electrical bioimpedance, thermodilution, and Fick methods. Crit Care Med 1988; 16:1157–1158.

30. Smith SA, Russell AE, West MJ, et al: Automated non-invasive measurement of cardiac output: Comparison of electrical bioimpedance and carbon dioxide rebreathing techniques. Br Heart J 1988; 59:292–298.

31. Naggar CZ, Dobnik DB, Flessas AP, et al: Accuracy of the stroke index as determined by the transthoracic electrical impedance method. Anesthesiology 1975; 42:201–205.

32. Miles DS, Gotshall RW, Golden JC, et al: Accuracy of electrical impedance cardiography for measuring cardiac output in children with congenital heart defects. Am J Cardiol 1988; 61:612–616.

33. Introna RPS, Pruett JK, Crumrine RC, Cuadrado AR: Use of transthoracic bioimpedance to determine cardiac output in pediatric patients. Crit Care Med 1988; 16:1101–1105.

34. Weber J, Heidelmeyer CF, Kubatz E, Bruckner JB: Measuring cardiac output under positive end-expiratory pressure with the noninvasive continuous cardiac output monitor "NCCOM 3" by bioimpedance as compared with thermodilution measurements. A study in anaesthetized dogs. Anaesthesist 1986; 35:744–747.

35. Reves JG, Pruett JK: Use of the Walton-Brodie strain gauge arch to measure contractile force during anesthesia. Br J Anaesth 1988; 60:78S–84S.

36. Katz AM: Influence of altered inotropy and lusitropy on ventricular pressure-volume loops. J Am Coll Cardiol 1988; 11:438–445.

37. Fifer MA, Braunwald E: End-systolic pressure-volume and stress-length relations in the assessment of ventricular function in man. Adv Cardiol 1985; 32:36–55.

38. Brown KA, Ditchey RV: Human right ventricular end-systolic pressure-volume relation defined by maximal elastance. Circulation 1988; 78:81–91.

39. Forrester JS, Tyberg JV, Wyatt HL, et al: Pressure-length loop: A new method for simultaneous measurement of segmental and total cardiac function. J Appl Physiol 1974; 37:771–775.

40. Foëx P, Francis CM, Cutfield GR, Leone B: The pressure-length loop. Br J Anaesth 1988; 60:65S–71S.

41. Taylor SH, Silke B: Is the measurement of cardiac output useful in clinical practice? Br J Anaesth 1988; 60:90S–98S.

42. Morton WD: The non-invasive determination of cardiac output in children. Anesthesiology 1988; 69:223–226.

43. Davies GG, Jebson PJR, Glasgow BM, Hess DR: Continuous Fick cardiac output compared to thermodilution cardiac output. Crit Care Med 1986; 14:881–885.

44. Bradley EC, Barr JW: Fore-'n-aft triangle formula for rapid estimation of area. Am Heart J 1969; 78:643–648.

45. Truccone NJ, Spotnitz HM, Gersony WM, et al: Cardiac output in infants and children after open-heart surgery. J Thorac Cardiovasc Surg 1976; 71:410–414.

46. Kramer WG, Romagnoli A: Effect of surgery and cardiopulmonary bypass on indocyanine green pharmacokinetics. Texas Heart Institute J 1986; 13:77–82.

47. Bilfinger TV, Lin CY, Anagnostopoulos CE: In vitro determination of accuracy of cardiac output measurements by thermal dilution. J Surg Res 1982; 33:409–414.

48. Fegler G: Measurement of cardiac output in anesthetized animals by a thermodilution method. Q J Exp Physiol 1954; 39:153–164.

49. Ganz W, Donoso R, Marcus HS, et al: A new technique for measurement of cardiac output by thermodilution in man. Am J Cardiol 1971; 27:392–396.

50. Romano A, Niguidula FN: Technique of intraoperative placement of thermodilution catheter for cardiac output measurement in children. J Cardiovasc Surg 1980; 21:267–270.

51. Rah KH, Dunwiddie WC, Lower RR: A method of continuous postoperative measurement of mixed venous oxygen saturation in infants and children after open heart procedures. Anesth Analg 1984; 63:873–881.

52. Mathur M, Harris EA, Yarrow S, Barratt-Boyes BG: Measurement of cardiac output by thermodilution in infants and children after open-heart operations. J Thorac Cardiovasc Surg 1976; 72:221–225.

53. Fischer AP, Benis AM, Jurado RA, et al: Analysis of errors in measurement of cardiac output by simultaneous dye and thermal dilution in cardiothoracic surgical patients. Cardiovasc Res 1978; 12:190–199.

54. Hillis LD, Firth BG, Winniford MD: Comparison of thermodilution and indocyanine green dye in low cardiac output or left-sided regurgitation. Am J Cardiol 1986; 57:1201–1202.

55. McCormick JR, Dobnik DB, Mieszala JR, Berger RL: Simple method for measurement of cardiac output by thermodilution after cardiac operation. J Thorac Cardiovasc Surg 1979; 78:792–795.

56. Kohanna FH, Cunningham JN: Monitoring of cardiac output by thermodilution after open heart surgery. J Thorac Cardiovasc Surg 1977; 73:451–457.

57. Moodie DS, Feldt RH, Kaye MP, et al: Measurement of postoperative cardiac output by thermodilution in pediatric and adult patients. J Thorac Cardiovasc Surg 1979; 78:796–798.

58. Maruschak GF, Potter AM, Schauble JF, Rogers MC: Overestimating pediatric cardiac output by thermal indicator loss. Circulation 1982; 65:380–383.

59. Forrester JS, Ganz W, Diamond G, et al: Thermodilution cardiac output determination with a single flow-directed catheter. Am Heart J 1972; 83:306–311.

60. Stetz CW, Miller RG, Kelly GE, Raffin TA: Reliability of the thermodilution method in the determination of cardiac output in clinical practice. Am Rev Respir Dis 1982; 126:1001–1004.

61. Levett JM, Replogle RL: Thermodilution cardiac output: A critical analysis and review of the literature. J Surg Res 1979; 27:392–404.

62. Vennix CV, Nelson DH, Pierpoint GL: Thermodilution cardiac output in critically ill patients: Comparison of room-temperature and iced injectate. Heart Lung 1984; 13:574–578.

63. Shellock FG, Riedinger MS, Bateman TM, Gray RJ: Thermodilution cardiac output determination in hypothermic postcardiac surgery patients: Room vs ice temperature injectate. Crit Care Med 1983; 11:668–670.

64. Pearl RG, Rosenthal MH, Nielson L, et al: Effect of injectate volume and temperature on thermodilution cardiac output determination. Anesthesiology 1986; 64:798–801.

65. Merrick SH, Hessel EA, Dillard DH: Determination of cardiac output by thermodilution during hypothermia. Am J Cardiol 1980; 46:419–422.

66. Stiles GM, Imazaki G, Stiles QR: Thermodilution cardiac output studies as a cause of prosthetic valve bacterial endocarditis. J Thorac Cardiovasc Surg 1984; 88:1035–1037.

67. Plachetka JR, Larson DF, Salomon NW, Copeland JG: Comparison of two closed systems for thermodilution cardiac outputs. Crit Care Med 1981; 9:487–489.

68. Meissner H, Glanert G, Stackmeier B, et al: Indicator loss during injection in the thermodilution system. Res Exp Med 1973; 159:183–196.

69. Buchbinder N, Ganz W: Hemodynamic monitoring: Invasive techniques. Anesthesiology 1976; 45:146–155.

70. Woods M, Scott RN, Harken AH: Practical considerations for the use of pulmonary artery thermistor catheter. Surgery 1976; 79:469–475.

71. Jansen JRC, Schreuder JJ, Bogaard JM, et al: Thermodilution technique for measurement of cardiac output during artificial ventilation. J Appl Physiol 1981; 51:584–591.

72. Stevens JH, Raffin TA, Mihm FG, et al: Thermodilution cardiac output measurement. JAMA 1985; 253:2240–2242.

73. Morady F, Brundage BH, Gelberg HJ: Rapid method for determination of shunt ratio using a thermodilution technique. Am Heart J 1983; 106:369–373.

74. Kahan F, Profeta J, Thys DM: High cardiac output measurements in a patient with congestive heart failure. J Cardiothorac Anesth 1987; 1:234–236.

75. Sade RM, Richi AA, Dearing JP: Calculation of systemic blood flow with pulmonary artery thermistor probe. J Thorac Cardiovasc Surg 1979; 78:576–578.

76. Lipkin DP, Poole-Wilson PA: Measurement of cardiac output during exercise by the thermodilution and direct Fick techniques in patients with chronic congestive heart failure. Am J Cardiol 1985; 56:321–324.

77. Kubo SH, Burchenal JEB, Cody RJ: Comparison of direct Fick and thermodilution cardiac output techniques at high flow rates. Am J Cardiol 1987; 59:384–386.

78. Reininger EJ, Troy BL: Error in thermodilution cardiac output measurement caused by variation in syringe volume. Cathet Cardiovasc Diag 1976; 2:415–417.

79. Nelson LD, Houtchens BA: Automatic versus manual injections for thermodilution cardiac output determination. Crit Care Med 1982; 10:190–192.

80. Dizon CT, Gezari WA, Barash PG, Crittenden JF: Hand held thermodilution cardiac output injector. Crit Care Med 1977; 5:210–212.

81. Wessel HU, Paul MH, James GW, Grahn AR: Limitations of thermal dilution curves for cardiac output determination. J Appl Physiol 1971; 30:643–652.

82. Bjoraker DG, Ketcham TR: Catheter thrombus artifactually decreases thermodilution cardiac output measurements. Anesth Analg 1983; 62:1031–1034.

83. Spackman TN: Thermodilution cardiac output due to an intracatheter septal defect. Anesth Analg 1984; 63:962–963.

84. Kiggins CM, Lake CL, Ross WT: The shunting Swan-Ganz catheter. J Cardiothorac Anesth 1989; 3:229–234.

85. Paulsen AW, Valek TR: Artifactually low cardiac outputs resulting from a communication between the proximal and distal lumens of an Edwards pacing thermodilution Swan-Ganz catheter. Anesthesiology 1988; 68:308–309.

86. Wetzel RC, Latson TW: Major errors in thermodilution cardiac output measurement during rapid volume infusion. Anesthesiology 1985; 62:684–687.

87. Todd MM: Atrial fibrillation induced by the right atrial injection of cold fluids during thermodilution cardiac output determination. A case report. Anesthesiology 1983; 59:253–255.

88. Nishikawa T, Dohi S: Slowing of heart rate during cardiac output measurement by thermodilution. Anesthesiology 1982; 57:538–539.

89. Harris AP, Miller CF, Beattie C, et al: The slowing of sinus rhythm during thermodilution cardiac output determination and the effect of altering injectate temperature. Anesthesiology 1985; 63:540–541.

90. Nishikawa T, Namiki A: Mechanisms for slowing of heart rate and associated changes in pulmonary circulation elicited by cold injectate during thermodilution cardiac output determination in dogs. Anesthesiology 1988; 68:221–225.

91. Katz RI, Teller ED, Poppers PJ: Ventricular fibrillation during thermodilution cardiac output determination. Anesthesiology 1985; 62:376–377.

92. Grubbs D, Geddes LA, Voorhees WD III: Right-side cardiac output determined with a newly developed catheter-tip resistivity cell using saline indicator. Jpn Heart J 1984; 25:105–111.

93. Voorhees WD, Bourland JD, Lamp ML, et al: Validation of the saline-dilution method for measuring cardiac output by simultaneous measurement with a perivascular electromagnetic flowprobe. Med Instrum 1985; 19:34–37.

94. Prys-Roberts C: Monitoring of the cardiovascular system. *In* Saidman LJ, Smith NT (eds): Monitoring in Anesthesia. New York: John Wiley, 1978; 62.

95. Cundick RM, Gardner RM: Clinical comparison of pressure-pulse and indicator-dilution cardiac output determination. Circulation 1980; 62:371–376.

96. English JB, Hodges MR, Sentker C, et al: Comparison of aortic pulse-wave contour analysis and thermodilution methods of measuring cardiac output during anesthesia in the dog. Anesthesiology 1980; 52:56–61.

97. Weber KT, Janicki JS, Shroff SG, et al: The right ventricle: Physiologic and pathophysiologic considerations. Crit Care Med 1983; 11:323–328.

98. Maddahi J, Berman DS, Matsuoka DT, et al: Technique for assessing right ventricular ejection fraction using rapid multiple-gated equilibrium cardiac blood pool scintigraphy: Description, validation and finding in coronary artery disease. Circulation 1979; 60:581–589.

99. Dehmer GJ, Firth BG, Hills LO, et al: Nongeometric determination of RV volume from equilibrium blood pool scans. Am J Cardiol 1982; 49:78–84.

100. Bing R, Heimbecker R, Falholt W: An estimation of the residual volume of blood in the right ventricle of normal and diseased human hearts in vivo. Am Heart J 1951; 42:483–502.

101. Kay H, Afshari M, Barash PG, et al: Measurement of ejection fraction by thermal dilution techniques. J Surg Res 1983; 34:337–346.

102. Hines R, Barash PG: Right ventricular function in the perioperative period. Mt Sinai J Med (NY) 1985; 52:529–533.

103. Urban P, Scheidegger D, Gabathuler J, Rutishauser W: Thermodilution deter-

mination of right ventricular volume and ejection fraction: A comparison with biplane angiography. Crit Care Med 1987; 15:652–655.

104. Dhainaut JF, Brunet F, Monsallier JF, et al: Bedside evaluation of right ventricular performance using a rapid computerized thermodilution method. Crit Care Med 1987; 15:148–152.

105. Jardin F, Gueret P, Dubourg O, et al: Right ventricular volumes by thermodilution in ARDS. Chest 1985; 88:34–39.

106. Hines R: Monitoring right ventricular function. *In* Barash PG (ed): Cardiac Monitoring. Philadelphia: WB Saunders, 1988; 851–863.

107. Savino JA, Vo N, Agarwal N, et al: Systemic organ assessment using computerized profiles. Med Instrum 1983; 17:433–436.

108. Mohr R, Meir O, Smolinsky A, Goor DA: A method for continuous on-line monitoring of systemic vascular resistance (COMS) after open heart procedures. J Cardiovasc Surg 1987; 28:558–565.

109. Hilgenberg JC: Pulmonary vascular impedance: Resistance versus pulmonary artery diastolic–pulmonary artery occluded pressure gradient. Anesthesiology 1983; 58:484–485.

110. Akaishi M, Schneider RM, Mercier RJ, et al: Relation between left ventricular global and regional function and extent of myocardial ischemia in the canine heart. J Am Coll Cardiol 1985; 6:104–112.

Monitoring Respiratory Function

chapter eight

Monitoring of Oxygen

KEVIN K. TREMPER, Ph.D., M.D.
■ STEVEN J. BARKER, Ph.D., M.D.

While reading this sentence you are consuming approximately 100 million trillion molecules of oxygen per second. This phenomenal oxygen transport to the tissues is required in order to maintain aerobic metabolism in the average 70-kg adult at rest. As single-celled animals evolved to multicelled organisms and eventually to large mammals, an immense problem of oxygen distribution had to be solved. There are two limitations on oxygen delivery in cellular life in an aqueous environment. First, molecular diffusion of gases in liquids is an extremely slow process. Second, the solubility of oxygen in water is very low. The diffusion constant (diffusivity) of oxygen in water is approximately 10^{-5} cm^2/sec. For single-celled creatures, oxygen can diffuse rapidly from the cell wall to the mitochondria because the diffusion distance is so short. As the number of cells grows and the diffusion distance increases, the rate of oxygen transport limits aerobic metabolism. It would take nearly a day for an oxygen molecule to diffuse 1 cm in water by pure molecular diffusion. Consequently, as multicellular organisms evolved, they developed a more efficient transport system to distribute oxygen by bulk flow to each cell. Since the solubility of oxygen in water is low, the transport system also needed a mechanism to increase the oxygen-carrying capacity of an aqueous medium. The result in vertebrate life is the cardiovascular system and blood, using hemoglobin as a carrier to increase the oxygen capacity of the transport medium.

Over the past several decades, medicine has developed a number of oxygen transport variables to quantitate the effectiveness of the oxygen delivery system. Since the 1970s, both invasive and noninvasive continuous monitoring systems have been developed to assess the adequacy of oxygen transport. These devices monitor oxygenation by different means and at different points in the oxygen transport system. In this chapter, the commonly measured and calculated oxygen transport variables are described, and available oxygen monitoring techniques are reviewed in depth. For each technique, the physics and engineering behind the measurement as well as the physiologic interpretation of the measured variable are discussed. Each technique has its limitations in the detection of hypoxia.

ANALYSIS OF INSPIRED OXYGEN

Monitoring the oxygen concentration in the anesthetic or ventilator circuit is mandatory (see Chapter 13). Although this does not ensure an adequate PaO_2, it assures that hypoxic oxygen concentrations are not delivered to the patient's airway.

Methods of Measurements

Either a mass spectrometer or an analyzer for oxygen gas alone can be used in clinical situations. Mass spectrometers are discussed in Chapter 14. Several types of oxygen analyzers are available: polarographic electrode, paramagnetic, and galvanic cell types.

Polarographic Analyzers

Polarographic analyzers are based on the principle of the Clark electrode (described in Chapters 17 and 18). The breakdown (reduction) of oxygen occurs at a charged metal cathode (a "rest" voltage of 0.5–0.8 V is applied) in the polarographic electrode, and the current produced by the reaction alters the conductivity of an electrolyte solution of potassium chloride. Essential components are a silver anode, a platinum or gold cathode, and a gas-permeable polymeric membrane. The specific "rest" voltage causes only oxygen to react. When a gas sample containing oxygen is present, the current flow is proportional to the partial pressure of oxygen in the electrolyte solution. Response times for these analyzers are about 10–60 seconds.

If accuracy at concentrations of oxygen of less than 50% is desired, these analyzers are calibrated using room air. Accuracy in the 90–100% range requires calibration on 100% oxygen. Several minutes are required for calibration. Because the analyzer depends upon a battery (to operate the meter and to induce a voltage on the electrode) and the electrode has a limited life span, regular preventive maintenance (replacement of electrode membrane and electrolyte gel) is essential to ensure a functional analyzer.

The function switch of the instrument usually has a setting for "battery check."

Paramagnetic Analyzers

Oxygen is a paramagnetic gas, whereas most other gases are diamagnetic. Paramagnetic gases are attracted to the strongest portion of a magnetic field. If two glass spheres (containing nitrogen or another diamagnetic gas) are attached to a dumbbell suspended on a quartz fiber in a chamber between two magnetic poles, introduction of oxygen into the chamber results in displacement of the spheres from between the magnetic poles. A mirror attached to the quartz fiber reflects a beam of light onto a translucent scale to measure the oxygen concentration. The number of oxygen molecules or the partial pressure of oxygen determines the degree of mirror displacement.

Paramagnetic analyzers have inherently long response times owing to the washout time of the sample cell. Of the anesthetic agents, only nitrous oxide has a weak diamagnetic effect. Although these analyzers are highly accurate, their fragile suspension system, sensitivity to water vapor, and long response time have caused them to be replaced by polarographic analyzers in anesthesia practice.

Galvanic Cell Analyzers

These analyzers produce a current flow by the reduction of molecular oxygen, which releases electrons. An electrolyte solution in the galvanic cell is contained by a thin plastic membrane over the cathode through which oxygen diffuses to the anode. The percentage of oxygen is displayed on a scale when a microammeter senses the current produced, which is proportional to the oxygen partial pressure. Because of their limited life span, galvanic analyzers have been largely replaced by polarographic analyzers on anesthesia machines.

Clinical Use

Ideally, an oxygen analyzer should be accurate to $\pm 2\%$ and capable of response within 2–10 seconds. It should be unaffected by the relative humidity within the 30–90% range. Studies have demonstrated that water vapor significantly affects (i.e., gives falsely low readings) the Beckman OM-1 analyzer.[1] Analyzer data should be compensated for both temperature and pressure. Exposure to anesthetic gases should not affect accuracy. Westenskow and coworkers noted that Critikon model 800–021 and Teledyne microfuel cell class C-1 (Harris-Lake) sensors had higher rates of drift in halothane-air mixtures than those noted in air alone.[1] Such effects may result from diffusion of halothane into the oxygen-permeable membrane. Calibration is best performed using dry 100% oxygen. After calibration, accuracy should be maintained for at least 8 hours.

High- and low-pressure alarms are essential features of most oxygen analyzers. Both visual and auditory alarms should be present and functional during use of an anesthesia machine or ventilator. Although oxygen analyzers detect disconnections in fresh gas lines, they are unable to detect disconnection of the patient's endotracheal tube from the anesthetic breathing circuit, unless the sensor is placed in the expiratory limb of the circle system.[2]

QUANTITATIVE OXYGEN TRANSPORT VARIABLES

Oxygen Content

Oxygen content is defined as the volume of oxygen (milliliters) carried in 100 ml of blood. It is a basic variable that is found in all oxygen transport calculations. Although oxygen content can be measured directly by the volumetric method of Van Slyke and Neill,[3] it is usually calculated from this equation:

$$Ca_{O_2} = Hb \times 1.37 \times Sa_{O_2} + 0.0034 \times Pa_{O_2} \qquad \textbf{8–1}$$

where Ca_{O_2} = arterial oxygen content (a denotes an arterial sample) in ml/100 ml (also called vol%), Hb = hemoglobin concentration in gm/dl, 1.37 = the volume of oxygen (ml) carried by 1 gm of fully saturated hemoglobin, Sa_{O_2} = fractional hemoglobin saturation (discussed later), 0.0034 = the solubility coefficient of oxygen in plasma (ml of oxygen/100 ml plasma/mmHg), Pa_{O_2} = the arterial oxygen tension in mmHg.

With a normal hemoglobin of 15 gm and normal arterial Pa_{O_2} and Sa_{O_2} values of 95 mmHg and 95%, respectively, the arterial oxygen content is 20 ml/100 ml. Coincidentally, this is very similar to the oxygen content of room air at sea level. Thus, the cardiovascular system produces the same oxygen content near each cell that would exist if the cells were surrounded by room air. Methods of measuring both hemoglobin saturation and oxygen partial pressure are discussed later.

In Equation 8–1, the oxygen content is very sensitive to the hemoglobin concentration and hemoglobin saturation, whereas it is relatively insensitive to the oxygen tension owing to the small solubility coefficient for oxygen in plasma. However, the oxygen saturation itself depends nonlinearly upon oxygen tension. Since oxygen content is proportional to hemoglobin concentration, if the arterial hemoglobin is fully saturated, the content can be roughly estimated as equaling slightly less than half the hematocrit level. The hematocrit level equals approximately three times the hemoglobin concentration.

Oxygen Delivery

The overall flow rate of oxygen to the tissues is called the oxygen delivery (O_2 del), determined by multiplying the arterial oxygen content by the cardiac output. At a cardiac output of 5 L/minute for a 70-kg adult, normal oxygen delivery is 1 L of oxygen/minute (20 ml of oxygen/100 ml or 200 ml of oxygen/L × 5 L/minute = 1 L of oxygen/minute). Since normal cardiac output is dependent on the size of the patient, cardiac output is indexed to body surface area: cardiac index (CI) = cardiac output/body surface area (m²). A normal cardiac index is 3 L/minute/m²; the normal range is 2.7–3.4 L/minute/m².[4] The oxygen delivery index (Equation 8–2) is defined as the arterial oxygen content times the cardiac index:

$$O_2 \text{ del} = Ca_{O_2} \times CI \text{ (ml oxygen/minute/m}^2\text{)}$$

$$\text{Normal } O_2 \text{ del} = 20 \text{ ml/dl} \times 10 \text{ dl/L} \times 3 \text{ L/minute/m}^2$$

$$= 600 \text{ ml/minute/m}^2 \qquad\qquad \textbf{8–2}$$

The oxygen delivery index is an overall assessment of oxygen transport to the tissues but does not ensure adequate oxygen supply to any specific organ. The oxygen delivery to each organ can be defined as the arterial oxygen content times the blood flow to the specific organ.

Oxygen Consumption

Human tissues consume an average of 5 ml of oxygen from every 100 ml of blood flow. Since the normal arterial oxygen content is 20 ml/100 ml of blood, 75% of the oxygen remains in the venous blood. The oxygen consumption ($\dot{V}_{O_2}$) of the body (Equation 8–3) can be calculated by subtracting the mixed venous blood oxygen content from the arterial oxygen content and multiplying by the cardiac output:

$$\text{Oxygen consumption} = (Ca_{O_2} - Cv_{O_2}) \times \text{cardiac output} \qquad \textbf{8–3}$$

As with oxygen delivery, oxygen consumption is indexed so that the normal value is independent of patient size:

$$\text{Oxygen consumption index} = \dot{V}_{O_2} (Ca_{O_2} - Cv_{O_2}) \times CI$$

$$\dot{V}_{O_2} = (20 \text{ ml/dl} - 15 \text{ ml/dl}) \times 3 \text{ L/minute/m}^2 \times 10 \text{ dl/L}$$

$$\dot{V}_{O_2} = 150 \text{ ml/minute/m}^2$$

The normal range for the oxygen consumption index is 115–165 ml/minute/m². These values are for healthy resting humans and increase severalfold with exercise, shivering, hyperthermia, or sepsis. $\dot{V}_{O_2}$ decreases during anesthesia and hypothermia.

Mixed Venous Oxygen

Mixed venous blood is sampled from the pulmonary artery to ensure proper mixing. A mixed venous sample does not reflect the oxygen returned to the heart from any specific organ. The normal mixed venous oxygen content is 15 ml/dl, which corresponds to a mixed venous saturation of 75% and an oxygen tension of 40 mmHg. Mixed venous blood oxygen tension should reflect tissue oxygen tension. Although there is great variability in tissue oxygen tensions, the mean oxygen tension of interstitial fluid is the same as the mixed venous oxygen tension, i.e., 40 mmHg.[5]

Oxygen Extraction

The oxygen extraction ratio (O_2 ext) (Equation 8–4) is a supply-demand balance for oxygenation:

$$O_2 \text{ ext} = \frac{Ca_{O_2} - Cv_{O_2}}{Ca_{O_2}} \times 100\% \qquad \textbf{8–4}$$

Extraction ratio is actually the ratio of oxygen consumption to oxygen delivery:

$$O_2 \text{ ext} = \frac{(Ca_{O_2} - Cv_{O_2}) \times CI}{Ca_{O_2} \times CI} \times 100\%$$

Since cardiac index appears in both the numerator and the denominator of this equation, it need not be measured to calculate O_2 ext. For this reason O_2 ext was an especially useful variable for assessing oxygen transport prior to the availability of thermodilution catheters. The normal extraction ratio is only 25%, so there appears to be a wide margin of safety for oxygen transport. In fact, the body can easily extract up to 50% of the delivered oxygen without obligatory tissue hypoxia. When the extraction ratio exceeds 50%, there is an increasing incidence of tissue hypoxia because of the low oxygen tension, corresponding to a 50% hemoglobin saturation (P_{50} of adult hemoglobin is normally 26.7 mmHg).

HYPOXIA

Definitions

Hypoxia is defined as inadequate tissue oxygenation owing to either inadequate blood flow or low arterial oxygen content. Hypoxia due to inadequate blood flow is ischemic hypoxia. Hypoxia due to low oxygen content is hypoxemic hypoxia. Arterial oxygen content can be reduced as a result of decreased hemoglobin (anemic hypoxemia), Pa_{O_2} (hypoxemic hypoxemia), or Sa_{O_2} (toxic hypoxemia). Toxic hypoxia (decreased fractional hemoglobin saturation) results from increased methemoglobin or carboxyhemoglobin, which is discussed later.

Figure 8–1. *A,* Schematic of a Clark polarographic oxygen electrode. The circuit consists of a voltage source (battery) and a current meter connecting platinum and silver electrodes. The electrodes are immersed in an electrolyte cell. A membrane permeable to oxygen but not to the electrolyte covers one surface of the cell. Oxygen diffuses through the membrane and reacts with water at the platinum cathode to produce hydroxyl ions. The ammeter measures the current produced at the cathode by the electrons consumed in this reaction. *B,* A plot of current produced as a function of the voltage between the two electrodes (polarizing voltage). This plot is called a polarogram. In the range near 660 mV there is a plateau in the polarogram. The plateau occurs at higher currents as the P_{O_2} in the cell is increased. Most polarographic oxygen electrodes use 600 to 800 mV polarizing voltage to obtain a stable current at each P_{O_2}.

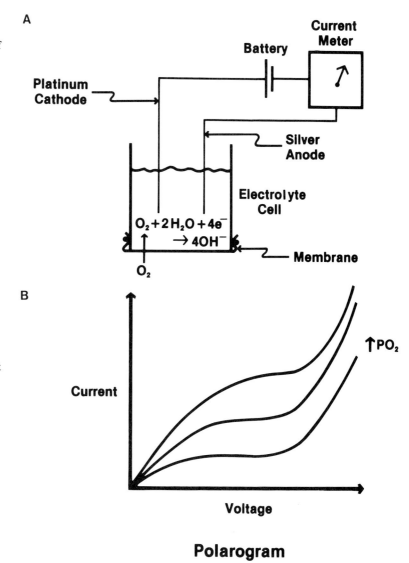

Polarogram

MEASUREMENT OF OXYGEN TENSION

Clark P_{O_2} Electrode

Oxygen partial pressure or tension in a liquid phase is defined as the oxygen partial pressure in the equilibrium gas phase. When several phases are in contact at equilibrium (e.g., lipid, water, and gas), the oxygen tension is equal in all phases, but the oxygen concentration in each phase is proportional to its solubility in that phase. In 1956, Clark developed the polarographic oxygen electrode for measuring oxygen partial pressure.[6] Before this invention, blood oxygen partial pressure was not measured. With the

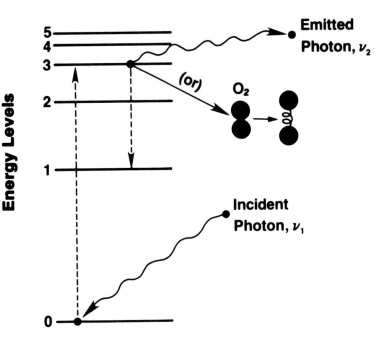

Energy Levels

Emitted Photon, ν_2

(or)

O_2

Incident Photon, ν_1

Figure 8–2. The photo-luminescence-quenching phenomenon. An electron of the luminescent dye is excited to a higher energy level by an incident photon (γ_1). This excited electron can return to a lower energy level either by emitting a photon (γ_2) or by interacting with an oxygen molecule and raising the latter to a higher vibrational energy level. (From Barker SJ, Tremper KK, Hyatt J, et al: Continuous fiberoptic arterial oxygen tension measurements in dogs. J Clin Monit 1987; 3:48–52. With permission.)

addition of the Severinghaus carbon dioxide electrode in 1958, the blood gas machine was developed, and critical patient care was revolutionized.[7]

The Clark electrode is an electrical cell composed of a platinum cathode and a silver anode (Fig. 8–1). As in any resistive circuit, as the voltage increases the current also increases. In this electrochemical cell there is a plateau voltage range over which the current does not increase with voltage but does increase with oxygen tension in the cell. An oxygen-consuming electrochemical reaction takes place at the cathode, and the electrical current in the circuit is directly proportional to the oxygen consumed at the cathode. This cell is covered with a membrane that is freely permeable to oxygen. Clark's polarographic oxygen electrode has been used for 30 years to measure oxygen partial pressure in gases and liquids in both medicine and industry. Other methods to measure oxygen in the gas phase are used clinically to measure inspired and expired oxygen concentration. These methods include mass spectrometry (see Chapter 14), paramagnetic oxygen analysis, and the oxygen fuel cell.[8]

Po$_2$ Optode

Recently, a new technique called photoluminescence quenching has been used experimentally to measure blood oxygen tension.[9, 10] When light shines on a luminescent material, specific light frequencies are absorbed, exciting electrons to a higher energy state (Fig. 8–2). These electrons then fall spontaneously into a lower energy state by emitting a photon of a frequency different from that of the original light. In some luminescent dyes, this light emission is "quenched" by the presence of oxygen. When the

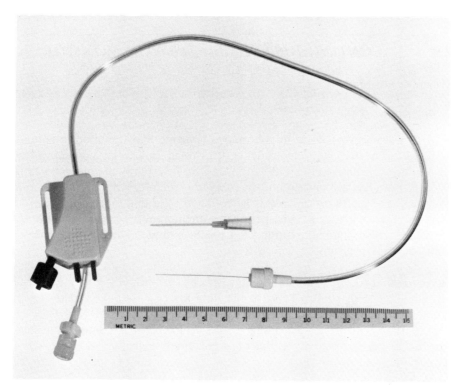

Figure 8–3. An optode probe and the 20-gauge cannula through which it is inserted. (From Barker SJ, Tremper KK, Hyatt J, et al: Continuous fiberoptic arterial oxygen tension measurements in dogs. J Clin Monit 1987; 3:48–52. With permission.)

excited electron falls into a lower energy state, its energy can be either emitted as a photon (luminescence) or absorbed by an oxygen molecule, thereby increasing the vibrational and rotational energy of the latter (Fig. 8–2). For these photoluminescence-quenching dyes, the amount of oxygen present can be related to the luminescent intensity. The empirical relationship governing this phenomenon is known as the Stern-Volmer equation (Equation 8–5).[9]

$$I (P_{O_2}) = \frac{I_0}{(1 + K \times P_{O_2})} \qquad \textbf{8–5}$$

where I = the intensity of the luminescent signal at the P_{O_2} being measured, I_0 = the intensity of the luminescent signal in the absence of oxygen, P_{O_2} = the oxygen partial pressure, K = the quenching constant.

The advantages of the optode as a P_{O_2} measuring device are its simplicity and size. The sensor consists of a small fiberoptic strand with a dye encapsulated at the tip, and it can be easily miniaturized. Figure 8–3 shows an optode that easily fits through a 22-gauge intravenous cannula.[10] Another advantage of optode technology is that pH-sensitive dyes are also available, and therefore, a three-fiber optode sensor can measure P_{O_2}, P_{CO_2}, and pH simultaneously.[11]

CONTINUOUS OXYGEN TENSION MONITORING

Invasive P_{O_2} Monitoring

Clark Electrode

The primary problem in continuous invasive Pa_{O_2} monitoring is miniaturization of the Clark electrode to fit through an arterial cannula. There are two approaches to this problem. One is to insert only the platinum cathode in the arterial cannula and to place the reference anode on the skin surface. The platinum cathode is surrounded by a thin layer of electrolyte and covered with an oxygen-permeable membrane.[12, 13] The second approach involves miniaturization of the entire anode-cathode electrode for intra-arterial insertion.[14, 15]

Several studies of intra-arterial P_{O_2} monitoring using Clark electrodes have yielded conflicting results with respect to accuracy. It is often difficult to compare such studies because the data are usually analyzed by linear regression and correlation coefficients. Altman and Bland describe the inappropriate and often misleading results from methods-comparison studies.[16-18] The correlation coefficient is extremely sensitive to the x and y range over which the data are collected. Furthermore, a high correlation coefficient (r close to 1.0) implies a high degree of association between the methods (i.e., when one goes up the other goes up), but it does not imply that one method can replace the other.

As an alternative, Altman and Bland recommend using the mean and standard deviations of the difference between the two methods of measurement as an assessment of agreement.[16-18] The mean difference is called the "bias," and the standard deviation is referred to as the "precision." The bias indicates a consistent over- or underestimate of one method relative to the other, and the precision represents the scatter or random error.[16-18] Note that a larger precision implies a less precise measurement. As an example, Figure 8–4 is a "scattergram" plot of data from an intra-arterial Clark electrode used in neonatal patients.[15] The abscissa of this plot is Pa_{O_2} determined on arterial samples by a blood gas analyzer, and the ordinate is the intra-arterial electrode Pa_{O_2}. Although these data yield a correlation coefficient of 0.88, there is a large amount of variation of y on x over the entire range of Pa_{O_2}. For example, at a Pa_{O_2} of 40 mmHg, the intra-arterial probe Pa_{O_2} values vary from the mid-20s to 70 mmHg, with one data point as high as 100 mmHg.

Umbilical artery Clark electrodes in neonates have been associated with a number of complications, including thrombus formation, embolism, vascular perforation, infarction, lower extremity ischemia, and infection. The size of the electrode also causes problems with blood pressure monitoring and arterial blood sampling.[13] Probe size has also caused problems in the use of Clark electrodes for radial arterial P_{O_2} monitoring. The early electrodes required a 16-gauge or larger arterial cannula, but difficulties in pressure monitoring and blood sampling still occurred.[19, 20] More recently, the electrodes have been miniaturized to fit through 18- and even 20-gauge ar-

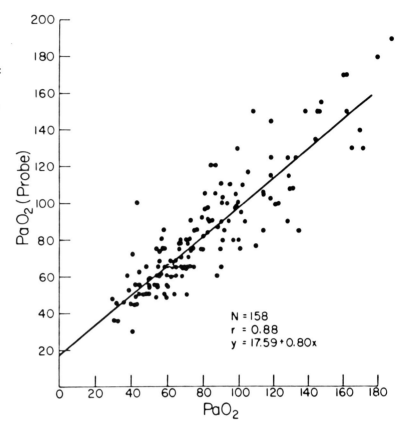

Figure 8–4. Relation between arterial oxygen tension (PaO$_2$) and intravascular oxygen tension (probe) measurements. (From Malalis L, Bhat R, Vidyasagar D: Comparison of intravascular PO$_2$ with transcutaneous and PaO$_2$ values. Crit Care Med 11(2):110–113, © by Williams & Wilkins, 1983.)

terial cannulas.[14, 21] Damping of the arterial pressure waveform and inaccurate blood pressure measurements are commonly reported.[14, 19] It is unclear whether this phenomenon results from the Clark electrode itself or from the formation of clot around the sensor. Other reported problems include calibration drift and systematic underestimation of Pao$_2$. The causes of these errors are not understood, but they may involve decreased blood flow around the electrode tip or clot formation on the electrode surface. The most recently developed electrodes have reportedly reduced these problems, but there are no confirmatory studies.[21]

Because of the difficulties in miniaturizing both the Clark electrode and the glass components required for electrochemical CO$_2$ and pH measurement, it is unlikely that an electrochemical blood gas monitoring system will ever be developed for intra-arterial use. The optode technology is therefore being developed for this application.

Optode

From the previous discussion on optode theory we would predict that the equipment used in this method of measuring oxygen tension can be miniaturized more easily. Several recent studies have examined the accuracy of 0.5-mm diameter Po$_2$ optodes.[22] These fiberoptic sensors fit through a

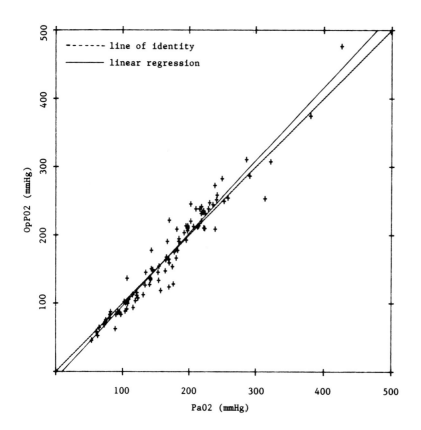

Figure 8–5. Arterial oxygen tension determined by optode (OpPO₂) versus arterial oxygen tension determined by blood gas analysis (PaO₂). There are 96 data points. (From Barker SJ, Tremper KK: Intra-arterial PO₂ monitoring. *In* Tremper KK, Barker SJ [eds]: Advances in Oxygen Monitoring. Int Anesthesiol Clin 1987; 25:206. With permission.)

22-gauge catheter, although the studies cited have reported results only with 20-gauge catheters. Figure 8–5 is a scattergram plot of optode Po_2 versus arterial sampled Pao_2 in 12 patients during surgery. The bias and precision over the range from 0 to 700 mmHg are -1.10 ± 19.0 mmHg, respectively (Table 8–1).[22] For data in the range from 0 to 150 mmHg, the bias and precision are 3.74 ± 11.7 mmHg. Because of the small diameter of these optode sensors, problems with arterial blood pressure monitoring and blood sampling have been reduced. The results of long-duration studies to evaluate drift are yet to be published, but we anticipate that optode sensors will have problems similar to those noted with the Clark electrodes, i.e., thrombus formation and underestimation of Pao_2.

Noninvasive Po_2 Monitoring

Transcutaneous Po_2

In 1972 two European researchers reported that Po_2 values very similar to arterial Po_2 could be obtained by heating a Clark electrode and placing it on the skin surface of a newborn infant.[23, 24] Over the next decade this technique, known as transcutaneous oxygen monitoring, became routine in the care of premature infants at risk of both hypoxia and hyperoxia.[25, 26] In

Table 8–1. STATISTICAL COMPARISON OF
ARTERIAL OXYGEN TENSIONS OBTAINED
BY OPTODE AND BY BLOOD GAS
ANALYSIS IN 12 SURGICAL PATIENTS

Variable	0–700 mmHg	0–150 mmHg
n	96	38
r	0.970	0.923
Linear regression		
Slope	1.07	1.05
Intercept	− 10.6	− 8.5
Bias	− 1.10	3.74
Precision	19.0	11.7

From Barker SJ, Tremper KK: Intra-arterial Po_2 monitoring. *In* Barker SJ, Tremper KK (eds) Advances in Oxygen Monitoring. Int Anesthiol Clin 1987; 25:199–208. With permission.

the late 1970s it was found that transcutaneous Po_2 ($Ptco_2$) values were significantly lower than Pao_2 values during conditions of hemodynamic instability.[27, 28] Although this discovery lessened the usefulness of $Ptco_2$ as an arterial oxygen tension monitor, it did give the user a valuable indicator of peripheral perfusion. This blood flow dependence of $Ptco_2$ has also been illustrated in several animal studies on shock and resuscitation.[29, 30]

$Ptco_2$ is the oxygen tension of heated skin. To obtain a measurable Po_2 at the skin surface with a fast response time, the skin temperature must be heated to higher than 43°C. Heating causes several changes in the various layers of the skin. The stratum corneum, composed of lipid in a protein matrix, is normally a very efficient barrier to gas transport. When heated above 41°C the structural characteristics of this layer change, allowing oxygen to diffuse through it readily.[31, 32] In the epidermis, heating causes vasodilatation of the dermal capillaries that is said to "arterialize" this capillary blood.

The perfusion of this hyperemic epidermal capillary bed is also dependent upon adequate blood flow to the dermal vasculature. Consequently, if the cardiac output decreases, skin blood flow and, hence, oxygen delivery to the transcutaneous sensor decrease. Figure 8–6 illustrates the relation between Pao_2 and $Ptco_2$ during induced hypoxemia (hypoxemic hypoxia) followed by hemorrhagic shock (ischemic hypoxia) in an animal study.[29] During the shock state, $Ptco_2$ decreased with decreasing cardiac output even though Pao_2 was relatively unchanged.

This effect of cardiac output on the $Ptco_2$-Pao_2 relationship can be quantitated in terms of a transcutaneous oxygen index:

$$Ptco_2 \text{ index} = Ptco_2/Pao_2 \qquad \textbf{8–6}$$

$Ptco_2$ index has been used as an indicator of peripheral oxygen delivery, analogous to the alveolar-arterial Po_2 gradient for the assessment of pulmonary function.[33] Table 8–2 lists the ranges of $Ptco_2$ index as a function

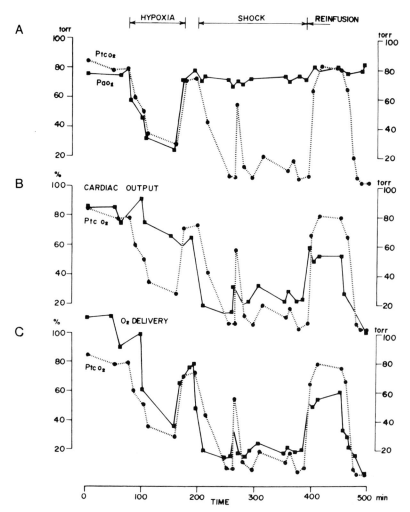

Figure 8–6. Hypoxia and hypovolemic shock study in dogs. *A*, Serial transcutaneous oxygen tension (Ptco$_2$) and arterial oxygen tension (Pao$_2$). *B*, Ptco$_2$ and cardiac output. *C*, Ptco$_2$ and oxygen delivery throughout a representative experiment. Note: Ptco$_2$ values follow the Pao$_2$ values during hypoxia but not during shock; Ptco$_2$ values follow cardiac output during shock but not during hypoxia; however, Ptco$_2$ values most closely follow oxygen delivery throughout the entire experiment. (From Tremper KK, Waxman K, Shoemaker WC: Effects of hypoxia and shock on transcutaneous PO$_2$ values in dogs. Crit Care Med 7(12):529–531, © by Williams & Wilkins, 1979.)

of cardiac index found in adult patients in intensive care units. Under stable hemodynamic conditions, the normal Ptco$_2$ index for adult patients was 0.79, whereas this index fell to 0.49 when the cardiac index decreased below 2.2 L/minute/m^2.[33] In the early work on newborn infants, Ptco$_2$ was found to be similar to Pao$_2$; i.e., the Ptco$_2$ index was approximately 1.0.[23, 24] A review of the published Ptco$_2$ values on hemodynamically stable patients in various age groups reveals that Ptco$_2$ index decreases progressively with age from premature infants to elderly patients (Table 8–2). Glenski and Cucchiara also found that Ptco$_2$ index is relatively independent of probe location as

Table 8–2. CHANGES IN $Ptco_2$ INDEX WITH AGE AND CARDIAC OUTPUT

$Ptco_2$ Index* ($Ptco_2/Pao_2$)	Age Group
1.14	Premature infants
1.0	Newborn
0.84	Pediatric
0.8	Adult
0.7	Older adult (>65 years old)

$Ptco_2$ Index†	Cardiac Index (L/minute/m²)
0.8	>2.2
0.5	1.5–2.2
0.1	<1.5

* All these $Ptco_2$ index values have a standard deviation of approximately 0.1.

† These data are from adult patients.

long as the probe is on the central body rather than on the extremities.[34] $Ptco_2$ index may be slightly higher in adult female patients.[34] $Ptco_2$ is therefore a continuous, noninvasive measure of peripheral tissue oxygen tension. It follows changes in Pao_2 under conditions of hemodynamic stability and decreases relative to Pao_2 as cardiac output falls below the normal range (see Figs. 17–5 to 17–8).

Practical Considerations and Limitations of $Ptco_2$ Monitoring

Probe Temperature and Skin Burn. Since the $Ptco_2$ electrode must be heated above body temperature, there is a possibility of producing small electrode-sized skin burns. Each time a $Ptco_2$ sensor is applied to the skin it produces a red, hyperemic area that usually disappears within 24 hours after electrode removal. No study has reported the incidence of burns from transcutaneous electrodes as a function of probe temperature and duration of application. From the experience of frequent users of the technique, the following guidelines are usually applied. For premature infants, an electrode temperature of 43.5°C is usually used, and the electrode location is changed every 2–4 hours. For older children and adults, an electrode temperature of 44°C is used, and the site is changed every 4–6 hours. As indicated by personal intraoperative experience on adult patients, a 44°C electrode may be left in one location for as long as 8 hours with a very low (less than 1%) incidence of blister formation. Although a 45°C temperature has been used in the past, this higher electrode temperature is unnecessary for adequate function and significantly increases the incidence of skin burns.

Sensor Calibration and Drift. As with any Clark electrode, the $Ptco_2$ sensor must be properly calibrated and maintained. The zero point on the $Ptco_2$ electrode (O_2 tension = 0 mmHg) is usually extremely stable and requires calibration only on a monthly basis. The high Po_2 calibration usually uses room air, and this should be rechecked prior to each application on the skin. Current $Ptco_2$ electrodes have miniaturized electrolyte reservoirs to bathe the electrode and 12–25-μ membranes on the surface. These small electrolyte reservoirs usually carry about one drop (0.02 ml) of electrolyte. Since the electrode is heated to 44°C, the electrolyte evaporates more quickly than that used in the 37°C Clark electrode found in a blood gas machine. The electrolyte reservoir and membrane should therefore be checked daily, and they usually require replacement at least once a week. If the high Po_2 calibration point drifts more than 1%/hour, the membrane should be replaced.

Effects of Anesthetic Agents on $Ptco_2$ Sensors. In 1971, Severinghaus reported that halothane was reduced at the cathode of the Clark electrode, producing a dramatic upward drift of the Po_2 reading.[35] Since halothane exposure to the Clark electrode in a blood gas analyzer is very small, little calibration drift is usually noted during intermittent blood gas analysis. On the other hand, the $Ptco_2$ sensor is applied directly and continuously to the skin surface where there is an opportunity for significant halothane interference. This problem was investigated *in vitro* by Muravchick,[36] who reported that direct exposure of a transcutaneous electrode to 3% halothane caused an upward drift of 50 mmHg. Measurements of the $Ptco_2$ calibration drift after administration of anesthetic agents (involving halothane, enflurane, isoflurane, nitrous oxide, and local anesthesia) revealed a statistically significant drift of 0.7 mmHg/hour in the zero-point calibration in patients receiving halothane anesthesia.[37] This drift is clinically insignificant and within the manufacturer's specifications for the electrode (an electrode covered by a 25-μ polytef [Teflon] membrane). More recent clinical experience with combination transcutaneous O_2 and CO_2 electrodes, in which the membrane is 12.5-μ Teflon, demonstrates that the $Ptco_2$ value exhibits significant upward drift in the presence of halothane anesthesia.

Sensor Location and Warm-up. Most of the clinical $Ptco_2$ data has been collected with sensors on the chest or abdomen. There is a significant site-to-site variation of $Ptco_2$ values; approximately 10% variation occurs even with adjacent locations. Lower values are found on the extremities, even in the absence of peripheral vascular disease. After being placed on the skin surface, a $Ptco_2$ sensor requires at least 8–10 minutes to equilibrate before yielding a steady value. In some circumstances, it takes as long as 20 minutes for complete equilibration, which presents problems during intraoperative monitoring, especially in cases of short duration or when the sensor site must be changed during the procedure. Another limitation in intraoperative use is that the sensor should be placed in a location visible to the user. If the sensor becomes dislodged from the skin surface, it reads room air Po_2 (approximately 159 mmHg at sea level). Furthermore, external pressure on the sensor under the surgical drapes produces falsely low $Ptco_2$ values owing to compression of the dermal capillaries.

In summary, $Ptco_2$ measures peripheral tissue oxygenation continuously and noninvasively. The $Ptco_2$ values follow the trend of Pao_2 under conditions of adequate cardiac output and decrease relative to Pao_2 during low cardiac output states. Thus, $Ptco_2$ aids in the diagnosis and treatment of low-flow shock conditions. The limitations of $Ptco_2$ monitoring include calibration and electrode maintenance, a 10–15-minute warm-up time, the possibility of skin burns, and potential interference by halothane.

Conjunctival Po₂

Equipment. When the eyes are closed, the cornea receives its oxygen supply from the palpebral conjunctiva. Therefore, this inner layer of the eyelid is well vascularized and has few cell layers between the capillaries and the mucous surface. The blood supply to the palpebral conjunctiva is derived from a branch of the ophthalmic artery, which in turn is a branch of the ipsilateral internal carotid artery. To measure Po_2 on this well-perfused surface, miniaturized Clark electrodes have been made to fit inside a polymethyl methacrylate ocular conformer ring. This conformer directly applies the Clark electrode to the inner surface of the palpebral conjunctiva. The electrode is not heated and therefore measures the surface oxygen directly from the tissue. This device is a true tissue oxygen monitor; unlike $Ptco_2$, its values are not perturbed by heating.

Advantages and Limitations. There are several advantages to this technique. First, since the probe is not heated, it requires only 60 seconds to equilibrate with the local tissue Po_2. Second, since the blood supply is from the carotid artery, conjunctival Po_2 ($Pcjo_2$) detects changes in carotid blood flow.[38] Since $Pcjo_2$ is another measure of tissue oxygenation, its values are affected by both Pao_2 and cardiac output in the manner described previously for $Ptco_2$.[39-41] Therefore, its values are also divided by Pao_2 to yield an index analogous to the $Ptco_2$ index. The $Pcjo_2$ index is then a measure of the relative perfusion of conjunctival tissue. The normal $Pcjo_2$ index is reported to be 0.6–0.7, with lower values in elderly patients.[42, 43] The index progressively decreases with decreasing blood volume or cardiac output, again in a manner similar to $Ptco_2$.[39] Clinical studies have demonstrated that a $Pcjo_2$ index of less than 0.5 is associated with a blood volume deficit of at least 15%.[44]

Practical limitations of conjunctival oxygen monitoring are also the same as those of transcutaneous monitoring: electrode maintenance, calibration, and anesthetic (halothane) interference. Unlike $Ptco_2$, the $Pcjo_2$ sensor does not produce burns or require prolonged warm-up, but there is a potential for eye injury. Clinical studies to date have not reported serious eye problems.

MEASUREMENT OF HEMOGLOBIN SATURATION

Hemoglobin Saturation versus Oxygen Saturation

Oxygen saturation is defined as the blood oxygen content divided by the oxygen capacity times 100%. As previously discussed, oxygen content was originally measured volumetrically by the method of Van Slyke and Neill.[3] The oxygen capacity is defined as the oxygen content of the blood after it has been equilibrated with room air (Po_2 = 159 mmHg). At the time of this definition, the maximum blood oxygen content clinically achieved occurred at room air Po_2 because increased inspired oxygen concentrations were not available. From the oxygen content formula (see Equation 8–1), we see that this definition of oxygen saturation includes contributions from both hemoglobin-bound and dissolved oxygen. Adult blood usually contains four types of hemoglobin: oxyhemoglobin (O_2Hb), reduced hemoglobin (Hb), methemoglobin (MetHb), and carboxyhemoglobin (COHb). COHb and MetHb are found in low concentrations except in pathologic states. Because these dyshemoglobins do not transport oxygen, they do not contribute to the oxygen content or to the definition of oxygen saturation given previously. When spectrophotometric methods for measuring the concentration of hemoglobin types became available, hemoglobin saturation could be more easily determined. The term "functional" hemoglobin saturation is defined as

$$\text{Functional Sao}_2 = \frac{O_2Hb}{O_2Hb + Hb} \times 100\% \qquad \text{8--7}$$

This definition of hemoglobin saturation does not include MetHb or COHb because they do not contribute to oxygen transport. Fractional hemoglobin saturation, which is also called oxyhemoglobin fraction, is defined as

$$\text{Fractional Sao}_2 = \frac{O_2Hb}{O_2Hb + Hb + COHb + MetHb} \times 100\% \qquad \text{8--8}$$

This definition of hemoglobin saturation (that is, the ratio of oxyhemoglobin to total hemoglobin) is the saturation used in the calculation of oxygen content and delivery (see Equation 8–2). It is important to remember these definitions when evaluating the clinical utility and limitations of hemoglobin saturation monitors.

Hemoglobin Saturation Measurement: Beer's Law

Spectrophotometry was first used to determine the hemoglobin concentration of blood in the 1930s.[45] This method is based on the Lambert-Beer law (Equation 8–9), which relates the concentration of a solute to the intensity of light transmitted through the solution (Fig. 8–7):

$$I_{trans} = I_{in} \, e^{-DC\alpha_\lambda} \qquad \text{8--9}$$

where I_{trans} = intensity of transmitted light, I_{in} = intensity of incident light, D = distance light is transmitted through the liquid, C = concentration of the solute (hemoglobin), α_λ = extinction coefficient of the solute (a constant for a given solute at a specific light wavelength).* Thus, if a known solute is dissolved in a clear solvent in a cuvette of known dimensions, the solute concentration can be calculated if the incident and transmitted light intensities are measured (Fig. 8–7). The extinction coefficient α_λ is independent of the concentration but is a function of the light wavelength used (Fig. 8–8).

Laboratory oximeters use this principle to determine hemoglobin con-

---

* This law further states that the absorbance from multiple solutes in solution is the sum of the absorbances of the various solutes times their respective concentrations, e.g., $C_{11} + C_{22} + C_{33}$, and so on.

Figure 8–7. The concentration of a solute dissolved in a solvent can be calculated from the logarithmic relationship between the incident and transmitted light intensity and the solute concentration. (From Tremper KK, Barker SJ: Pulse oximetry and oxygen transport. *In* Payne JP, Severinghaus JW [eds]: Pulse Oximetry. Berlin: Springer-Verlag, 1986; 19–27. With permission.)

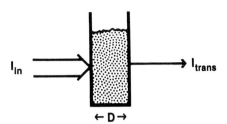

$$I_{trans} = I_{in}e^{-(D \times C \times \alpha_\lambda)}$$

I_{trans} = intensity of light transmitted

I_{in} = intensity of incident light

D = distance light is transmitted through the liquid

C = concentration of solute (oxyhemoglobin)

α_λ = extinction coefficient of the solute (a constant)

centration by measuring the intensity of light transmitted through a hemoglobin dispersion produced from lysed red blood cells.[46] For each wavelength of light used, an independent Lambert-Beer equation can be written. If the number of equations is equal to the number of solutes (i.e., hemoglobin type), then we can solve for the concentration of each type. Therefore, at least four wavelengths of light are required to determine the concentrations of four types of hemoglobin (Fig. 8–9). For the Lambert-Beer law to be valid, both the solvent and the cuvette must be transparent at the light wavelengths used, the light path length must be known exactly, and no other absorbers can be present in the solution. It is difficult to fulfill all these requirements in clinical devices. Consequently, although these devices are theoretically based on the Lambert-Beer law, empirical corrections are required to improve their accuracy.

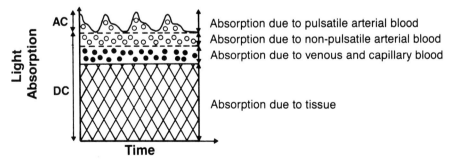

Figure 8–8. Light absorption through living tissue. The alternating current signal is due to the pulsatile component of the arterial blood, and the direct current signal comprises all the nonpulsatile absorbers in the tissue: nonpulsatile arterial blood, nonpulsatile venous and capillary blood, and all other tissues. (Modified from Ohmeda Pulse Oximeter Model 3700 Service Manual, 1986; 22.)

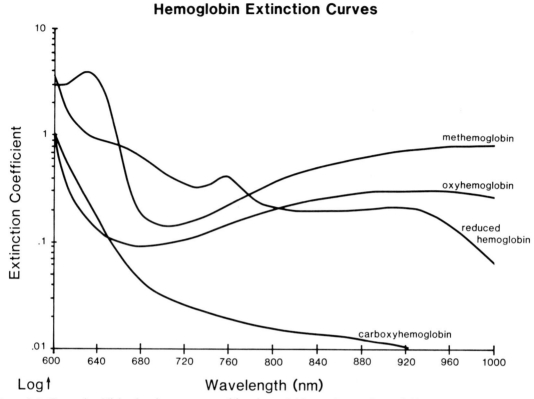

Figure 8–9. Transmitted light absorbance spectra of four hemoglobin species: oxyhemoglobin, reduced hemoglobin, carboxyhemoglobin, and methemoglobin. (From Barker SJ, Tremper KK: Pulse oximetry: Applications and limitations. *In* Barker SJ, Tremper KK [eds]: Advances in Oxygen Monitoring. Int Anesthesiol Clin 1987; 25:155–175. With permission.)

Invasive Hemoglobin Saturation Monitoring

Mixed Venous Hemoglobin Saturation

Mixed venous oxygen tension (Pv_{O_2}) and hemoglobin saturation (Sv_{O_2}) reflect global tissue oxygenation and the ability of the cardiopulmonary system to transport sufficient oxygen to meet the body's oxygen needs. Based on this physiologic argument, continuous mixed venous oxygen monitoring should have great clinical utility. In 1973, a fiberoptic system was reported to accurately measure mixed venous hemoglobin saturation in humans.[47] This device used optical fibers incorporated into a pulmonary artery catheter to estimate the hemoglobin saturation from a reflected light signal. Light at red and infrared wavelengths was transmitted down one set of fiberoptic channels while the reflected signal from intact circulating red cells was transmitted back via other fibers to an external photodetector.[47] Although this first system appeared to work, it was not commercially produced because of the technical problems of inserting a pulmonary artery catheter that was made relatively stiff by the fiberoptic bundles.

In the late 1970s, Oximetrix, Inc. (Division of Abbott Laboratories) developed two fiberoptic reflectance systems for measuring hemoglobin saturation. The first system, introduced in 1977, employed a no. 7-F double-lumen umbilical artery catheter to be used in monitoring critically ill newborn infants.[48] The second system, introduced in 1981, used a no. 7.5-F pulmonary artery catheter with thermodilution capability for cardiac output measurement in addition to continuous mixed venous saturation monitoring.[49] These new systems used three wavelengths of light to calculate saturation. However, a minimum of four wavelengths is required to calculate hemoglobin saturation from Beer's law in the presence of MetHb and COHb. The Oximetrix mixed venous saturation monitor can accurately measure functional hemoglobin saturation in the absence of significant dyshemoglobin concentrations.[49] However, a recent experimental study has shown that methemoglobinemia produces significant errors in the saturation measurement (see Pulse Oximetry).[50]

American Edwards Corporation has also produced a mixed venous saturation pulmonary artery catheter that uses two wavelengths of light. This device requires manual entry of the total hemoglobin content to improve accuracy, whereas the Oximetrix system can accurately measure mixed venous saturation over a wide range of hematocrits.[51, 52]

Continuous Svo_2 monitoring detects acute changes in the relationship of oxygen delivery to oxygen consumption (decreased supply, increased demand, or both). Three causes of reduced oxygen delivery decrease Svo_2: decreased cardiac output and hemoglobin and arterial oxygen saturation. Abnormal hemoglobins also fail to deliver oxygen to tissue. Other factors decreasing Svo_2 in clinical situations are shivering, malignant hyperthermia, exercise, agitation, fever, and thyroid storm. Monitoring Svo_2 has been recommended in cardiac surgery patients and other critically ill patients at risk of acute cardiopulmonary decompensation.[53–55] It is an especially valuable adjunct in the management of ventilator-dependent patients on positive end-expiratory pressure (PEEP). As PEEP increases, arterial saturation improves. Eventually, a point is reached when PEEP decreases venous return and cardiac output, causing a decrease in Svo_2.

Svo_2 monitoring does not determine the source of an imbalance between oxygen delivery and oxygen consumption, nor does it detect regional ischemia. Monitoring of Svo_2 requires the insertion of a pulmonary artery catheter and, hence, is inappropriate in many patients.

Pulse Oximetry

Only a few years after its introduction to the operating room, the pulse oximeter has become an anesthetic standard of care.[56, 57] This technique has been rapidly accepted by the anesthesia community, because it continuously and noninvasively monitors the arterial oxygenation with little user effort. This section discusses the theoretic principles upon which pulse oximetry is based, its technical and physiologic limitations, and its clinical applications.

Technical Development of Pulse Oximetry. The term oximeter was coined by Millikan, who developed a lightweight device for noninvasively monitoring hemoglobin saturation in the 1940s.[58] This device estimated hemoglobin saturation by transilluminating the ear with light of two wavelengths, one in the red range and one in the infrared range. The transmitted light was measured with a photodetector. This device effectively used the earlobe as a cuvette containing hemoglobin (Beer's law) (see Fig. 8–7). The two major technical problems involved estimating arterial hemoglobin saturation in living tissue rather than *in vitro*. First, there are many light absorbers other than hemoglobin in the tissues. Second, the tissues contain not only arterial blood but also venous and capillary blood. Millikan approached these problems by first measuring the absorbance of the ear while it was compressed in order to eliminate the blood. After this bloodless baseline measurement, the ear was heated to "arterialize" the blood. The difference between this absorbent signal and the baseline value was thus related to the arterial blood. This device was demonstrated to accurately detect intraoperative desaturations in the early 1950s, but because of technical difficulties with its use it was never adopted into routine clinical use.[59]

In the mid-1970s, a Japanese engineer named Aoyagi made an ingenious discovery. He noted that the pulsatile components of the absorbances of red and infrared light transmitted through tissue were related to arterial hemoglobin saturation.[58] This eliminated the need to heat the tissue to obtain an arterial estimate. He used two wavelengths of light, one in the red (660 nm) and one in the infrared (940 nm). Such a device relies on the detection of a pulsatile signal and is referred to as a pulse oximeter.

Figure 8–8 schematically illustrates the absorbers in the living tissue. At the top of the figure is the pulsatile or alternating current (AC) component, which is attributed to the pulsating arterial blood. The baseline or direct current (DC) component represents the absorbance of the tissue bed, including venous blood, capillary blood, and nonpulsatile arterial blood. All pulse oximeters assume that the only pulsatile absorbance between the light source and the photodetector is that of arterial blood. The pulse oximeter first determines the AC component of the absorbance at each wavelength and then divides this by the corresponding DC component to obtain a "pulse-added" absorbance that is independent of the incident light intensity. It then calculates the ratio of the pulse-added absorbances at the two wavelengths, which is then empirically related to Sao_2 (Equation 8–10):

$$R = \frac{AC\ red/DC\ red}{AC\ infrared/DC\ infrared} \qquad \textbf{8–10}$$

Figure 8–10 is an example of a pulse oximeter calibration curve. These curves are developed by measuring the pulse oximeter absorbance ratio (R) in human volunteers and simultaneously sampling arterial blood for *in vitro* saturation measurements. R varies from 3.4 to 0.4 over the saturation range of 0 to 100%. Note that an absorbance ratio of 1.0 corresponds to a pulse oximeter saturation (Spo_2) of approximately 85%.

Technical Application of Pulse Oximetry. Although the theory of the pulse oximeter is relatively straightforward, the application of this theory to a clinically useful device engenders technical problems and physiologic limitations. One of the limitations is a consequence of Beer's law and the definitions of functional and fractional hemoglobin saturation. Since it is a

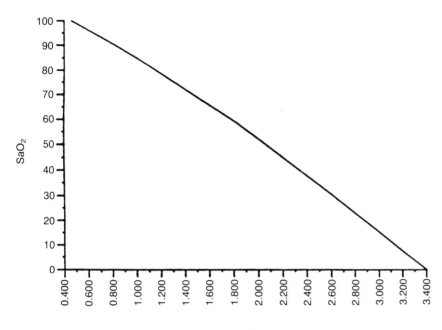

R = A$_{660nm}$/A$_{940nm}$

Figure 8–10. A typical pulse oximeter calibration curve. The Sao$_2$ estimate is determined from the ratio (R) of the pulse-added absorbance at 660 nm to the pulse-added absorbance at 940 nm. The ratios of red to infrared absorbances vary from approximately 0.4 at 100% saturation to 3.4 at 0% saturation. The ratio of red to infrared absorbance is 1.0 at a saturation of approximately 85%. This curve can be approximately determined from theory, but for accurate predictions of Spo$_2$ empirical modifications are required. (From Pologe JA: Pulse oximetry: Technical aspects of machine design. *In* Tremper KK, Barker SJ [eds]: Advances in Oxygen Monitoring. Int Anesthesiol Clin 1987; 25:142. With permission.)

two-wavelength device, the pulse oximeter assumes that there are only two absorbing hemoglobin types in the bloodstream: oxyhemoglobin (O$_2$Hb) and reduced hemoglobin (Hb). If methemoglobin (MetHb) or carboxyhemoglobin (COHb) is present, it contributes to the pulse-added absorbance signal and is interpreted as either O$_2$Hb or Hb, or some combination of the two.

Carboxyhemoglobin. Some insight into the effects of dyshemoglobins on the pulse oximeter is gained by examining the absorbance spectra (see Fig. 8–9). Note that COHb absorbs very little light at 940 nm (infrared light), whereas at 660 nm (red light) it absorbs as much as O$_2$Hb does. This is clinically illustrated by the fact that patients with carboxyhemoglobin toxicity appear red. The effects of COHb on pulse oximeter Spo$_2$ values have been evaluated experimentally.[60] Spo$_2$ can be roughly determined by O$_2$Hb + 0.9 × COHb.

Methemoglobin. In the case of methemoglobin, the absorbance is high at both the red and the infrared wavelengths (see Fig. 8–9). Consequently, MetHb produces a large pulse-added absorbance at both wavelengths used by the pulse oximeter. Adding a large absorbance to both the numerator and the denominator R tends to force this ratio toward unity. On the pulse oximeter calibration curve (Fig. 8–10), a ratio of 1 corresponds to a saturation of 85%, as noted previously. The effects of methemoglobinemia have also been evaluated experimentally, confirming the hypothesis that high MetHb levels force SpO$_2$ toward 85% regardless of the PaO$_2$ and SaO$_2$ values.[50]

Dyes. Any substance that absorbs light at the red and infrared pulse oximeter wavelengths and is present in the pulsatile arterial blood may cause errors. A clinical example of this effect is intravenously injected dyes. Scheller and colleagues evaluated the effects of bolus injections of methylene blue, indigo carmine, and indocyanine green on pulse oximeter SpO$_2$ values in volunteers.[61] They found that methylene blue decreased SpO$_2$ to approximately 65% for 1–2 minutes, whereas indigo carmine produced a very slight decrease. Indocyanine green had an intermediate effect.

Nail polish also adversely affects measurements of arterial oxygen saturation with a pulse oximeter. Blue, black, or green polish significantly decreased saturation. Greater reduction in saturation occurred with blue and green than with purple or red. These findings were unrelated to absorbance by the nail polish at wavelengths used by the oximeter to determine saturation. Red nail polish produces a minimal decrease in arterial oxygen saturation.[62]

Fetal Hemoglobin. With the adoption of pulse oximetry in the neonatal intensive care unit, the accuracy of the pulse oximeter in the presence of fetal hemoglobin (HbF) must be established. Fetal hemoglobin has a greater affinity for oxygen (a lower P$_{50}$) than does adult hemoglobin (HbA); thus it will become fully saturated at a lower PaO$_2$. However, the absorption coefficients for HbF are no different from those for HbA, so the presence of HbF should not cause errors in saturation estimates with pulse oximeters.[63, 64] Since the oxyhemoglobin dissociation curve of HbF is shifted to the left of that of HbA, the PaO$_2$ at a given SaO$_2$ is lower for HbF. Thus, the presence of HbF affects treatment only if one plans to maintain a specific PaO$_2$ as opposed to a specific SaO$_2$.

Technical Limitations. Since the photodiode detectors in the pulse oximeter sensor produce a current from light of any wavelength, ambient light contaminates the light-emitting diode (LED) signal.[65-67] The pulse oximeter designers have reduced this light interference by alternately turning on the red LED and the infrared LED, and then turning both LEDs off. The photodiode sensor first detects a signal from the red LED plus room light, followed by the infrared LED plus room light, and finally the ambient room light signal alone when both LEDs are turned off. This sequence is repeated 480 times/second in an effort to subtract the room light signal, even in a quickly changing light background. Unfortunately, despite this clever design, room light interference causes erroneous SpO$_2$ values or prevents the pulse oximeter from obtaining any SpO$_2$ value. This problem can be alleviated by placing an opaque covering on the sensor.[68]

The most difficult problem in the engineering design of the pulse oximeter is the management of low signal-to-noise ratios. This problem arises from two sources. First, when there is a small absorbance signal owing to a weak pulse, the device automatically increases the signal amplification so that it can analyze the pulse-added absorbance signal. Unfortunately, as the signal is amplified, the background noise is also amplified. In situations of a very weak or nonexistent pulse signal, the noise can be amplified until it is interpreted by the pulse oximeter as a pulse-added absorbance. New pulse oximeters have signal strength limits, below which they display a "low signal strength" error message. Some devices also display a pulse waveform that can be visually observed in order to confirm signal quality.

Because of its automatic gain control, the pulse oximeter can deal with both large and small pulse signals, and it is relatively insensitive to changes in peripheral pulse amplitude and flow. Lawson and coworkers objectively assessed the blood flow limits of pulse oximeter SpO_2 estimation.[69] The peripheral blood flow at the finger was measured by a laser Doppler flow probe that follows changes in red cell flow rate. A pulse oximeter was placed on the finger adjacent to the flow probe while a blood pressure cuff was progressively inflated on the upper arm. The pulse oximeter stopped estimating saturation and gave a "low perfusion" warning when the peripheral blood flow had decreased to 8.6% of the control value. After the blood pressure cuff was slowly deflated from full occlusion, the pulse oximeter again displayed a pulse and saturation estimate when the blood flow was only 4% of baseline. This study demonstrates the ability of the pulse oximeter to estimate saturation over an extreme range of peripheral blood flow. Other clinical experimental studies confirm that the pulse oximeter can estimate saturation over a wide range of cardiac outputs if an adequate pulse is detected.[70-71]

A serious signal-to-noise problem results from patient motion artifacts. For recovery room and intensive care unit applications, this may be the most troublesome design problem of pulse oximeters. Most pulse oximeters employ a variety of signal-averaging modes to minimize motion effects. That is, the device averages multiple pulses to obtain its saturation estimate, thereby diminishing the effect of single spurious motion signals. However, increasing the signal-averaging time has a deleterious effect on the time response of the pulse oximeter to acute changes in saturation. The manufacturers can also incorporate more sophisticated algorithms to discriminate motion signals from arterial pulse signals by using the rate of change of SpO_2. For example, if the calculated SpO_2 changes from 95% to 50% in 0.1 second, this new and presumably spurious saturation estimate is either dropped from the averaging or given a lower weighting factor. As with amplified background noise, motion artifact is probably most reliably detected by direct observation of the plethysmograph waveform.

Another limitation on pulse oximeter accuracy involves the variability of the wavelengths of light emitted by the LEDs. Although these diodes nominally radiate at either 660 nm or 940 nm, in reality each diode emits a slightly different wavelength. The peak or center wavelength of light from the LED can vary ±10 nm from the specified value. As we see from the extinction coefficients in Figure 8–9, shifts in the LED wavelength change the measured absorbance coefficient. Since the oximeter software assumes an extinction coefficient at a specified wavelength, an unknown change in that wavelength causes an error in the saturation estimate. Therefore, in reality there is a probe-to-probe variability in accuracy. Some manufacturers attempt to minimize this error by narrowing the wavelength tolerance on the LEDs used in their sensors. Others compensate for this error by designing the sensor to identify its specific wavelengths to the pulse oximeter monitor, which then electronically corrects for shifted center wavelengths.

Accuracy and Response. Most clinical pulse oximeters have a specified accuracy of ±2% from 100% saturation down to 70%, ±3% from 70% saturation to 50%, and no unspecified accuracy below 50% saturation.[72] This implies that the Sp_{O_2} is within 2% above or below the actual Sa_{O_2} 67% of the time (±1 standard deviation around the mean). This corresponds to a 99% confidence interval of ±6% (i.e., ±3 standard deviations) from 100% to 70% saturation, and ±9% from 70% to 50% saturation. Although these manufacturers' specifications are based on data collected from volunteers under optimal conditions, the accuracies found in clinical studies are comparable. It is often difficult to compare clinical studies with manufacturers' specifications, because the studies usually report correlation coefficients and linear regression analyses rather than the more appropriate bias and precision. From the available studies on adult, pediatric, and neonatal patients, it appears that under steady state conditions the pulse oximeter Sp_{O_2} value is within ±2–3 saturation points (±1 standard deviation).[73–78]

Two recent experimental studies in adult volunteers evaluated the response time of pulse oximeters to sudden desaturation and resaturation.[77, 78] Kagle and colleagues measured the 50% recovery time for resaturation from a hypoxic state. They used a fast (3 second) time averaging mode and found a 50% recovery time ($T\frac{1}{2}$) of 6 seconds for the ear probe and 24 seconds for the finger probe.[77] Severinghaus and Naifeh also found that the ear probe responds more quickly than the finger probe during desaturation and resaturation.[78] Their $T\frac{1}{2}$ values for ear probes ranged from 9.6 to 19.8 seconds, whereas the $T\frac{1}{2}$ values for finger probes ranged from 24 to 35.1 seconds.

However, the hemoglobin saturation provides limited information on the oxygen transport status. Hemoglobin saturation does not imply oxygen content unless the total hemoglobin is known. Furthermore, saturation values do not provide information on the directional change of arterial oxygen tension until the latter drops below 75–80 mmHg. Intraoperatively, there may be large changes in Pa_{O_2} that are thus not detected by pulse oximetry. Finally, the pulse oximeter measures a pulse but not peripheral perfusion. The pulse oximeter is designed to be insensitive to perfusion via its automatic gain control. The presence or absence of a pulse is quickly detected, but the presence of a pulse does not ensure adequate blood flow.

Considering all the sources of possible error, pulse oximeters are impressively accurate clinical devices. Since the manufacturers' specified accuracy at ±2–3% is for a confidence interval of only 68%, it is surprising that clinical studies have found accuracies similar to these.

Monitoring Oxygen Saturation by Pulse Oximetry. In 1947, Comroe and Botelho published a classic study that revealed the unreliability of direct observation for the detection of cyanosis.[79] This finding was confirmed intraoperatively for patients under general anesthesia in 1951.[59] With the advent of pulse oximetry, several perioperative studies have again confirmed this fact during even routine anesthetic procedures in healthy patients.[80–85] Coté and coworkers conducted a randomized, controlled study with pediatric patients under anesthesia.[80] One hundred fifty-two surgical patients were continuously monitored with pulse oximeters. In half of these patients, the pulse oximeter data were unavailable to the anesthesia team. In this study, a major desaturation event was defined to be an SpO_2 ≤85% for 30 seconds or longer. The study revealed 24 major desaturation events in the patients for whom the pulse oximeter data were unavailable, and only 11 in the patients for whom the pulse oximeter data were available. Most of these major events occurred in patients of age 2 years or less.[80] Raemer and colleagues conducted a similar study on healthy outpatients during gynecologic surgery.[81] They noted severe desaturations (pulse oximeter values less than 85%) in 5% of their patients.

Two studies have evaluated oxygenation by pulse oximeter during transport from the operating room to the recovery room.[82, 83] Pullerits and coworkers monitored 71 healthy pediatric patients during transport and found that 28.1% had SpO_2 values equal to or less than 90%, whereas cyanosis was clinically observed in only 45% of these patients.[82] In a similar study on adults, Tyler and colleagues found that in 12% of the patients, saturation values decreased to 85% or less during transport.[83] Both studies concluded that all patients should probably receive supplemental oxygen during transport to the recovery room.

Two studies conducted on recovery room patients have again emphasized the fact that our clinical abilities to detect cyanosis are poor. Soliman and coworkers compared pulse oximeter SpO_2 values to postanesthesia recovery scores in children.[84] These postanesthesia recovery scores are based on motor activity, respiratory effort, blood pressure, level of consciousness, and skin color. They found no correlation between postanesthesia recovery scores and SpO_2 values in these healthy pediatric patients. Morris and colleagues evaluated adult patients in the recovery room by measuring SpO_2 on admission to the recovery room, 5 minutes after admission, 30 minutes after admission, and finally just before discharge.[85] Of the 149 patients studied, 14% had episodes of desaturation (SpO_2 <90%). Curiously, the highest incidence of desaturation was at the time of discharge from the recovery room. Both of these studies concluded that patients in the recovery room should either be continuously monitored with pulse oximeters or at least be tested as part of the routine discharge criteria.

Pulse oximeters are now being adopted as routine recovery room and intensive care unit monitors. SpO_2 monitoring is becoming routine in most settings where supplemental oxygen is required or the possibility of cardiopulmonary compromise is significant. Since pulse oximeters are so easy to use and give data continuously and noninvasively, it is difficult to find an argument not to use them in an acute care setting. Sensors can be placed on fingers, toes, nose, ears, or tongue to assure continuous SpO_2 values.[86]

References

1. Westenskow DR, Jordan WS, Jordan R, Gillmor ST: Evaluation of oxygen monitors for use during anesthesia. Anesth Analg 1981; 60:53–56.
2. McGarrigle R, White S: Oxygen analyzers can detect disconnections. Anesth Analg 1985; 63:464–465.

3. Van Slyke DD, Neill JM: The determination of gases in blood and other solutions by vacuum extraction and manometric measurement. Int J Biol Chem 1924; 61:523–557.

4. Shoemaker WC, Appel PL, Bland R, et al: Clinical trial of an algorithm for outcome prediction in acute circulatory failure. Crit Care Med 1982; 10:390–397.

5. Guyton AC: Transport of oxygen and carbon dioxide in the blood and body fluids. *In* Textbook of Medical Physiology, 6th Ed. Philadelphia: WB Saunders, 1981; Chap 41.

6. Clark LC: Monitor and control of tissue O_2 tensions. Trans Am Soc Artif Intern Organs 1956; 2:41–48.

7. Severinghaus JW, Bradley AF: Electrodes for blood PO_2 and PCO_2 determination. J Appl Physiol 1958; 13:515–520.

8. Parbrook GD, Davis PD, Parbrook EO: Basic Physics and Measurement in Anesthesia, 2nd Ed. East Norwalk: Appleton & Lange, 1986.

9. Gehrich JL, Lubbers DW, Opitz N, et al: Optical fluorescence and its application to an intravascular blood gas monitoring system. IEEE Trans Biomed Eng 1986; 33:117–132.

10. Barker SJ, Tremper KK, Hyatt J, et al: Continuous fiberoptic arterial oxygen tension measurements in dogs. J Clin Monit 1987; 3:48–52.

11. Shapiro BA, Cane RD, Chomka CM, et al: Evaluation of a new intraarterial blood gas system in dogs. (Abstract.) Crit Care Med 1987; 15:361.

12. Kollmeyer KR, Tsang RC: Complications of umbilical oxygen electrodes. J Pediatr 1974; 84:894–897.

13. Harris, TR, Nugent M: Continuous arterial oxygen tension monitoring in the newborn infant. J Pediatr 1973; 82:929–939.

14. Bratanow N, Polk K, Bland R, et al: Continuous polarographic monitoring of intra-arterial oxygen in the perioperative period. Crit Care Med 1985; 13:859–860.

15. Malalis L, Bhat R, Vidyasagar D: Comparison of intravascular PO_2 with transcutaneous and PaO_2 values. Crit Care Med 1983; 11:110–113.

16. Altman DG, Bland JM: Measurement in medicine: The analysis of method comparison studies. Statistician 1983; 32:307–317.

17. Bland JM, Altman DG: Statistical methods for assessing agreement between two methods of clinical measurement. Lancet 1986; 1:307–310.

18. Altman DG: Statistics and ethics in medical research. Vol 6, Presentation of results. Br Med J 1980; 2:1542–1544.

19. Rithalia SVS, Bennett PJ, Tinker J: The performance characteristics of an intraarterial oxygen electrode. Intensive Care Med 1981; 7:305–307.

20. Arai T, Hatano Y, Komatsu K, et al: Real-time analysis of the change in arterial oxygen tension during endotracheal suction with a fiberoptic bronchoscope. Crit Care Med 1985; 13:855–858.

21. Stanley Frank, Ph.D., personal communication. Biomedical Sensors, Inc., Kansas City, MO.

22. Barker SJ, Tremper KK: Intra-arterial PO_2 monitoring. *In* Tremper KK, Barker ST (eds): Advances in Oxygen Monitoring. Int Anesthesiol Clin 1987; 3:199–208.

23. Eberhard P, Hammacher K, Mindt W: Perkutane messung des sauerstoffpartialdruckes: Methodik und anwendungen. (Abstract.) Stuttgart Proc Medizin-Technik 1972; 26.

24. Huch A, Huch R, Meinzer K, et al: Eine schuelle, behitze Ptoberflachenelektrode zur kontinuierlichen Uberwachung des PO_2 beim Menschen: Elektrodenaufbau und Eigenschaften. (Abstract.) Stuttgart Proc Medizin-Technik 1972; 26.

25. Huch R, Huch A, Albani M, et al: Transcutaneous PO$_2$ monitoring in routine management of infants and children with cardiorespiratory problems. Pediatrics 1976; 57:681–688.

26. Peabody JL, Willis MM, Gregory GA, et al: Clinical limitations and advantages of transcutaneous oxygen electrodes. Acta Anaesthesiol Scand [Suppl] 1978; 68:76–81.

27. Marshall TA, Kattwinkel J, Berry FA, Shaw A: Transcutaneous oxygen monitoring of neonates during surgery. J Pediatr Surg 1980; 15:797–803.

28. Versmold HT, Linderkamp O, Holzman M, et al: Transcutaneous monitoring of PO$_2$ in newborn infants. Where are the limits? Influences of blood pressure, blood volume, blood flow, viscosity, and acid base state. Birth Defects 1979; 4:286–294.

29. Tremper KK, Waxman K, Shoemaker WC: Effects of hypoxia and shock on transcutaneous PO$_2$ values in dogs. Crit Care Med 1979; 7:526–531.

30. Rowe MI, Weinberg G: Transcutaneous oxygen monitoring in shock and resuscitation. J Pediatr Surg 1979; 14:773–778.

31. Baumgardner JE, Graves DJ, Newfeld GR, Quinn JA: Gas flux through human skin: Effects of temperature, stripping and inspired tension. J Appl Physiol 1985; 5:1536–1545.

32. Van Duzee BF: Thermal analysis of human stratum corneum. J Invest Dermatol 1975; 65:404–408.

33. Tremper KK, Shoemaker WC: Transcutaneous oxygen monitoring of critically ill adults, with and without low flow shock. Crit Care Med 1981; 9:706–709.

34. Glenski JA, Cucchiara RF: Transcutaneous O$_2$ and CO$_2$ monitoring of neurosurgical patients: Detection of air embolism. Anesthesiology 1986; 64:546–550.

35. Severinghaus JW, Weiskopf RB, Nishimura M, Bradley AF: Oxygen electrode errors due to polarographic reduction of halothane. J Appl Physiol 1971; 31:640–642.

36. Muravchick S: Teflon membranes do not eliminate halothane interference with transcutaneous oxygen electrodes. Anesthesiology 1982; 57:A168.

37. Tremper KK, Barker SJ, Blatt DH, Wender RH: Effects of anesthetic agents on the drift of a transcutaneous PO$_2$ sensor. J Clin Monit 1986; 2:234–236.

38. Shoemaker WC, Lawner P: Method for continuous conjunctival oxygen monitoring during carotid artery surgery. Crit Care Med 1983; 11:946–949.

39. Smith M, Abraham E: Conjunctival oxygen monitoring during hemorrhage. J Trauma 1986; 26:217–224.

40. Abraham E, Fink S: Conjunctival and cardiorespiratory monitoring during resuscitation from hemorrhage. Crit Care Med 1986; 12:1004–1009.

41. Abraham E: Continuous conjunctival and transcutaneous oxygen tension monitoring during resuscitation in a patient. Resuscitation 1984; 12:207–211.

42. Hess D, Evans C, Thomas K, et al: The relationship between conjunctival PO$_2$ and arterial PO$_2$ in 16 normal persons. Respir Care 1986; 31:191–198.

43. Chapman KR, Liu FLW, Watson RM, Rebuck AS: Conjunctival oxygen tension and its relationship to arterial oxygen tension. J Clin Monit 1986; 2:100–104.

44. Abraham E, Oye RK, Smith M: Detection of blood volume deficits through conjunctival oxygen tension monitoring. Crit Care Med 1985; 12:931–934.

45. Severinghaus JW: Historical development of oxygenation monitoring. *In* Payne JP, Severinghaus JW (eds): Pulse Oximetry. Berlin: Springer-Verlag, 1986.

46. Brown LJ: A new instrument for the simultaneous measurement of total hemoglobin, % oxyhemoglobin, % carboxyhemoglobin, % methemoglobin, and oxygen content in whole blood. IEEE Trans Biomed Eng 1980; 27:132–138.

47. Martin WE, Cheung PW, Johnson CC, Wong KC: Continuous monitoring of mixed venous oxygen saturation in man. Anesth Analg 1973; 52:784–793.

48. Wilkinson AR, Phibbs RH, Gregory GA: Continuous measurement of oxygen saturation in sick newborn infants. J Pediatr 1978; 93:1016–1019.

49. Beale PL, McMichan JC, Marsh HM, et al: Continuous monitoring of mixed venous oxygen saturation in critically ill patients. Anesth Analg 1982; 61:513–517.

50. Barker SJ, Tremper KK, Hyatt J, Zaccari J: Effects of methemoglobinemia on pulse oximetry and mixed venous oximetry. (Abstract.) Anesthesiology 1987; 67:A170.

51. Gettinger A, Detraglia MC, Glass DD: In vivo comparison of two mixed venous saturation catheters. Anesthesiology 1987; 66:373–375.

52. Lee SE, Tremper KK, Barker SJ: Effects of anemia on pulse oximetry and continuous mixed venous oxygen saturation monitoring in dogs. Anesth Analg 1988; 67:S130.

53. Jamieson WRE, Turnbull KW, Larrieu AJ, et al: Continuous monitoring of mixed venous oxygen saturation in cardiac surgery. Can J Surg 1982; 25:538–543.

54. Schmidt CR, Frank LP, Forsythe MJ, Estafanous FG: Continuous SvO_2 measurement and oxygen transport patterns in cardiac surgery patients. Crit Care Med 1984; 12:523–557.

55. Waller JL, Kaplan JA, Bauman DI, Craver JM: Clinical evaluation of a new fiberoptic catheter oximeter during cardiac surgery. Anesth Analg (Cleve) 1982; 61:676–679.

56. Eichorn JH, Cooper JB, Cullen BF, et al: Standards for patient monitoring during anesthesia at Harvard Medical School. JAMA 1986; 256:1017–1020.

57. American Society of Anesthesiologists: Standards for basic intra-operative monitoring. Anesthesia Patient Safety Foundation 1987; March 3.

58. Severinghaus JW, Astrup PB: History of blood gas analysis. Int Anesth Clin 1987; 25:1–215.

59. Stephen CR, Slater HM, Johnson AL, Sekelj P: The oximeter—A technical aid for the anesthesiologist. Anesthesiology 1951; 12:541–555.

60. Barker SJ, Tremper KK: The effect of carbon monoxide inhalation on pulse oximeter signal detection. Anesthesiology 1987; 66:677–679.

61. Scheller MS, Unger RJ, Kelner MJ: Effects of intravenously administered dyes on pulse oximetry readings. Anesthesiology 1986; 65:550–552.

62. Coté CJ, Goldstein A, Fuchsman WH, Hoaglin DC: The effect of nail polish on pulse oximetry. Anesth Analg 1988; 67:683–686.

63. Pologe JA, Raley DM: Effects of fetal hemoglobin on pulse oximetry. J Perinatol 1987; 7:324–326.

64. Anderson JV: The accuracy of pulse oximetry in neonates. Effects of fetal hemoglobin and bilirubin. J Perinatol 1987; 7:323.

65. Brooks TD, Paulus DA, Winkle WE: Infrared heat lamps interfere with pulse oximeters. (Letter.) Anesthesiology 1984; 61:630.

66. Costarino AT, Davis DA, Keon TP: Falsely normal saturation reading with the pulse oximeter. Anesthesiology 1987; 67:830–831.

67. Eisele JH, Downs D: Ambient light affects pulse oximeters. Anesthesiology 1987; 67:864–865.

68. Siegel MN, Gravenstein N: Preventing ambient light from affecting pulse oximetry. (Letter.) Anesthesiology 1987; 67:280.

69. Lawson D, Norley I, Korbon G, et al: Blood flow limits and pulse oximeter signal detection. Anesthesiology 1987; 67:599–603.

70. Tremper KK, Hufstedler S, Zaccari J, et al: Pulse oximetry and transcutaneous PO_2 during hemorrhagic and normotensive shock in dogs. (Abstract.) Anesthesiology 1984; 61:A163.

71. Tremper KK, Hufstedler S, Barker SJ, et al: Accuracy of a pulse oximeter in the critically ill adult: Effect of temperature and hemodynamics. (Abstract.) Anesthesiology 1985; 63:A175.
72. Nellcor N100 Technical Manual. Nellcor Corp, Hayward, CA.
73. Mihm EG, Halperin DH: Noninvasive detection of profound arterial desaturations using pulse oximetry device. Anesthesiology 1985; 62:85–87.
74. Cecil WT, Thorpe JK, Fibuch EE, Tuohy GF: A clinical evaluation of the accuracy of the Nellcor N100 and the Ohmeda 3700 pulse oximeters. J Clin Monit 1988; 4:31–36.
75. Boxer RA, Gottesfeld I, Singh S, et al: Noninvasive pulse oximetry in children with cyanotic congenital heart disease. Crit Care Med 1987; 15:1062–1064.
76. Fait CD, Wetzel RC, Dean JM, et al: Pulse oximetry in critically ill children. J Clin Monit 1985; 1:232–235.
77. Kagle DM, Alexander CM, Berko RS, et al: Evaluation of the Ohmeda 3700 pulse oximeter: Steady-state and transient response characteristics. Anesthesiology 1987; 66:376–380.
78. Severinghaus JW, Naifeh KH: Accuracy of response of six pulse oximeters to profound hypoxia. Anesthesiology 1987; 67:551–558.
79. Comroe JH Jr, Botelho S: Unreliability of cyanosis in the recognition of arterial anoxemia. Am J M Sc 1947; 214:1–6.
80. Coté CJ, Goldstein EA, Coté MA, et al: A single blind study of pulse oximetry in children. Anesthesiology 1988; 68:184–188.
81. Raemer DB, Warren DL, Morris R, et al: Hypoxemia during ambulatory gynecologic surgery as evaluated by the pulse oximeter. J Clin Monit 1987; 3:244–248.
82. Pullerits J, Burrows FA, Roy WL: Arterial desaturation in healthy children during transfer to the recovery room. Can J Anesth 1987; 34:470–473.
83. Tyler IL, Tantisira B, Winter PM, Motoyama EK: Continuous monitoring of arterial oxygen saturation with pulse oximetry during transfer to the recovery room. Anesth Analg 1985; 64:1108–1112.
84. Soliman IE, Patel RI, Ehrenpreis MB, Hannallah RS: Recovery scores do not correlate with post-operative hypoxemia in children. Anesth Analg 1988; 67:53–56.
85. Morris RW, Buschman A, Warren DL, et al: The prevalence of hypoxemia detected by pulse oximetry during recovery from anesthesia. J Clin Monit 1988; 4:16–20.
86. Jobes DR, Nicolson SC: Monitoring of arterial hemoglobin oxygen saturation using a tongue sensor. Anesth Analg 1988; 67:186–188.

chapter nine

Monitoring the Function of the Respiratory System

■ THOMAS J. GAL, M.D.

Monitoring the function of the respiratory system is of great importance to the anesthesiologist, because the problems associated with inadequate ventilation, if unrecognized, contribute significantly to anesthetic morbidity. Some monitoring techniques are sophisticated and invasive, whereas others rely on more simple clinical observation. This chapter considers the wide range of techniques available for monitoring respiratory function and ventilation with an emphasis on the physiologic principles that form the basis of the measurements. The goal is to enhance the clinician's understanding of the indications, interpretations, and limitations of such respiratory measurements.

RESPIRATORY MECHANICS

Respiratory mechanics concerns the study of the respiratory system's function as an air pump. It involves the analysis of the means whereby forces are generated to move air and thus physically transport the air into and back out of the alveoli. Contraction of the respiratory muscles produces the force necessary to move air into and out of the lungs. This force must, in turn, overcome three basic opposing forces: inertance, elastance, and resistance.

Respiratory Muscles

Contraction of the inspiratory muscles produces expansion of the chest and fills the lungs with air. The principal muscle of inspiration, the diaphragm, contracts and descends to expand the chest longitudinally and to elevate the lower ribs. This action is responsible for more than two thirds of the air movement during quiet inspiration. The remaining volume is due to contraction of the external intercostals to further elevate the ribs and enlarge both the transverse and the anteroposterior chest dimensions. Expiration during quiet breathing results essentially from the passive recoil of the lungs and chest wall. Only during higher levels of ventilation or when air movement is impeded do the internal intercostals and abdominal muscles contract to depress the ribs and compress the abdominal contents to provide active expiratory effort. The expiratory muscles, however, play important roles in other breathing-related activities, such as talking, singing, and coughing.

All measurements of pulmonary function that require the patient's effort are influenced by respiratory muscle strength. This can be evaluated specifically by measurements of maximum static respiratory pressures. These pressures are generated against an occluded airway during a maximum forced effort and can be measured with simple aneroid gauges.[1] The inspiratory muscles are at their optimal length near residual volume (RV). Thus, maximum inspiratory pressure (PImax) is usually measured after a forced exhalation. Similarly, maximum expiratory pressure (PEmax) is measured at total lung capacity when expiratory muscles are stretched to their optimal length by a full inspiration. Typical values for PImax in healthy young males are about -125 cmH$_2$O, whereas PEmax may be as high as $+200$ cmH$_2$O (Table 9–1).

Values for PEmax less than $+40$ cmH$_2$O suggest impaired coughing ability,[2] whereas PImax values of -25 cmH$_2$O or less indicate severe inability to take a deep breath. The latter value is often utilized as a criterion for extubation; however, observations in healthy volunteers during partial curarization suggest that this level of ventilatory ability is too low to ensure adequate airway integrity.[3]

FORCES OPPOSING AIRFLOW

The movement of air into and out of the lungs is opposed by these basic forces—inertance, elastance, and resistance—that must be overcome. During most breathing activities, inertance, which is the impedance to acceleration of gas and tissue, is negligible. Elastance and its reciprocal force, compliance, are reflections of the relationship of pressure to volume when

Table 9–1. PULMONARY FUNCTION TESTS*

Forced vital capacity (FVC)	5000 ml
Forced vital capacity in 1 second (FEV_1)	4000 ml
FEV_1/FVC	>75%
Functional residual capacity (FRC)	3000 ml
Slow vital capacity (VC)	5000 ml
Inspiratory capacity (IC)	3000 ml
Total lung capacity (TLC)	6000 ml
Expiratory reserve volume (ERV)	1500 ml
Residual volume (RV)	1500 ml
Dead space (VD)	150 ml
Dead space/tidal volume (VD/VT)	$\leq$0.33
Maximum voluntary ventilation (MVV)	170 L/minute
Lung compliance (CL)	0.2 L/cm H_2O
Airway resistance (Raw)	1.5 cm H_2O/L/second
Diffusing capacity (DL) (single breath, carbon monoxide)	31 ml CO/minute/mmHg
Inspiratory pressure (PImax)	-125 cm H_2O
Expiratory pressure (PEmax)	$+200$ cm H_2O
Peak expiratory flow rate (PEFR)	500 L/minute

* Typical values for a young, healthy, 70-kg male.

there is no airflow. Hence, such measurements are referred to as static. Resistance, on the other hand, is highly dependent on the rate of change of lung volume, i.e., flow. Such measurements during active breathing are referred to as dynamic.

Statics

The respiratory system and its component lungs and chest wall are elastic. That is, they tend to regain their original size and configuration following deformation, when the deforming forces are removed. Both lungs and chest wall have positions of equilibrium. These are the volumes that they tend to assume in the absence of external forces acting upon them and the volumes to which they continuously attempt to return when displaced. The equilibrium position of the lung is at RV. To sustain any volume in the lung above RV, force must be applied to the lung, and it recoils with an equal and opposite force. At all volumes above RV, the lung recoils inward. The equilibrium position of the chest wall is at a relatively large volume, about 60% of total lung capacity. To sustain any volume in the chest wall below this point, the wall must be contracted, and it tends to recoil outward, opposite in direction from the lung. To sustain volume in the chest wall above its equilibrium point, the wall must be actively enlarged and it recoils inward, the same direction as the lung.

In the intact respiratory system, the lungs and chest wall are coupled and work together. Behavior of the respiratory system is determined by the individual properties of the lungs and chest wall. The equilibrium position of the respiratory system is that volume at which the tendency of the lung to recoil inward is balanced by the tendency of the wall to recoil outward

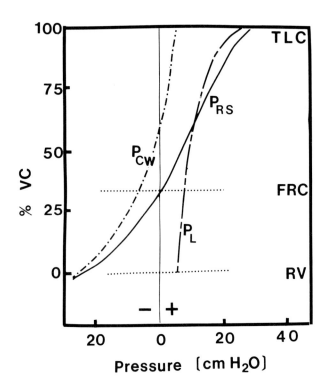

Figure 9–1. Recoil pressures for lung (P_L), chest wall (P_{CW}), and total respiratory system (P_{RS}) are plotted as a function of lung volume, in this case vital capacity (VC). (FRC = functional residual capacity, RV = residual volume, TLC = total lung capacity.)

(Fig. 9–1). To sustain any volume in the respiratory system other than this resting volume, which is the functional residual capacity (FRC), a force must be applied to displace both lungs and chest wall. The recoil pressure of the respiratory system (Prs) that develops is the algebraic sum of the individual recoil pressures of the lung (PL) and the chest wall (Pcw). Thus,

$$PRS = PL + Pcw; \text{ at FRC } PRS = 0 \qquad \textbf{9–1}$$

The lung is a distensible elastic body enclosed in an elastic container, the thoracic cavity. Just as a spring is described by the force required to stretch it to a certain length, so the respiratory system can be described by the static pressure required to change its volume. This relation between changes in volume and changes in pressure is termed compliance ($\Delta V / \Delta P$). For the various components of the respiratory system, compliance is determined by relating the change in volume to a given distending pressure. These various pressures are

1. Transpulmonary pressure (PL) or pressure across lung:

$$PL = Palv - Ppl \qquad \textbf{9–2}$$

where Palv = alveolar pressure. It is the same as mouth pressure under condition of zero flow. Ppl = esophageal pressure.

2. Pressure across chest wall (Pcw):

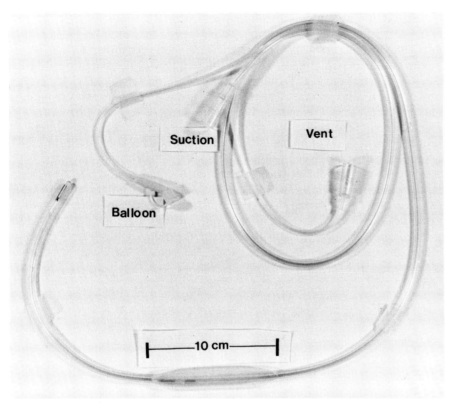

Figure 9–2. Commercially available nasogastric tube incorporating the 10-cm esophageal balloon used to measure pleural pressures. (Courtesy of NCC Division, Mallinckrodt, Argyle, NY.)

$$Pcw = Ppl - Pbs \qquad\qquad \textbf{9–3}$$

where Pbs = pressure at body surface (atmospheric).
3. Transthoracic or pressure across respiratory system (Prs)

$$Prs = Palv - Pbs \qquad\qquad \textbf{9–4}$$

Because the pressure volume curves for the respiratory system are curvilinear (see Fig. 9–1), compliance varies from one portion of the curve to another, depending on the range of lung volume. Values, therefore, are usually obtained in the range of 1 L above FRC, when the P-V relationships are most linear.

The measurement of Ppl has long been estimated by a special thin-walled balloon placed in the midesophagus. The balloon was 10 cm long and usually filled with 0.5 cc of air.[4] More recently, a 127-cm-long nasogastric tube incorporating a similar balloon has become available commercially[5] and has made the measurement more accessible to the clinician (Fig. 9–2). PL is thus measured by connecting the balloon to one port of a differential pressure transducer while the other port senses mouth pressure.

It is important to make the distinction between the terms static and dynamic compliance. When no gas flow occurs and pressure and volume are kept constant, the measurement is termed static compliance. Such would be the case if the patient's lung were inflated and kept inflated by a device such as a giant syringe. Dynamic compliance, on the other hand, relates pressure and tidal volume at the moment inspiration changes to expiration and flow ceases only momentarily. Ideally, these two compliance measurements are similar. However, if flow is impeded for some reason, e.g., by bronchoconstriction or a kink in the endotracheal tube, dynamic compliance is influenced by resistance to flow and does not reflect the true static compliance. The compliance figures differ by an amount related to flow resistance at end-inspiration. The difference in pressures (peak versus plateau) can be readily appreciated in circuits utilizing a ventilator equipped with an inspiratory hold or pause with no flow or by merely clamping the expiratory tubing. The relationship between delivered volume and plateau pressure during this pause is often referred to as the quasi-static or effective compliance (Fig. 9–3).

Dynamics

Resistance

Resistance deals with conditions of airflow and describes the relationships between pressure and flow in the respiratory system. Resistance therefore is computed from pressure differences responsible for flow and the simultaneous measurement of airflow ($R = \Delta P/V$).

Various components of the respiratory system contribute to the total resistance to airflow. These include an elastic component, the chest wall, and a nonelastic component, termed pulmonary resistance, which for practical purposes is synonymous with airway resistance. Approximately 60% of total respiratory resistance is airway resistance (Raw), with the remaining 40% accounted for by the chest wall. It is important to note that the "chest wall" in physiologic terms includes not only the bony thorax but the diaphragm and abdominal contents as well. Therefore, changes in muscle tone may affect measurements of total respiratory system resistance without actually altering Raw.

One other important factor to consider about Raw is that resistance to airflow is determined by the size of the airways. Airways are largest at high lung volumes and smallest at low volumes, such as RV. Passive changes in Raw can thus occur with changes in lung volume in the absence of bronchodilation or constriction. Since the relationship of Raw to lung volume is not linear, the reciprocal of Raw, conductance (Gaw), is related to lung volume in linear fashion and is utilized to identify the presence of bronchoconstriction or bronchodilation. Such determinants of Raw are, by convention, made at FRC.

Methods of Measuring Resistance

Flow-Pressure-Volume Method. Simultaneous recordings of the three variables—flow, pressure, and tidal volume (Fig. 9–4)—provide the basis

Figure 9–3. Flow (L/second), pressure (P), and tidal volume (V) typical of a cycle of mechanical ventilation incorporating an inspiratory pause (area enclosed between dotted lines).

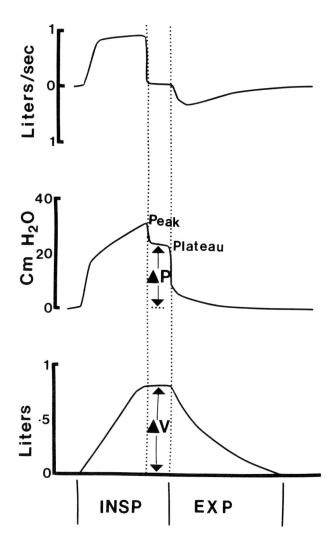

for this analysis. The change in pressure (ΔP) and change in flow (ΔV) between two points at which volume is identical are used to calculate resistance. This method of analysis is termed the isovolume technique. Another, more complex technique relating pressure, flow, and volume is the Comroe-Nissel-Nims technique.[6] With this method, static compliance is first calculated by dividing the total inspired volume by the pressure measured immediately prior to exhalation. Next, the point on the flow trace at which the expiratory flow is 0.5 L/second is noted, and the volume of gas remaining in the lungs at this point is also measured. Dividing this volume by the compliance value gives a pressure that is associated with a flow of 0.5 L/second and thus provides the calculation of resistance. In either of these cases, the use of airway or mouth pressure yields total respiratory system resistance, whereas the use of PL yields pulmonary or essentially airway resistance.

Passive Exhalation Method. The time it takes for the volume of the res-

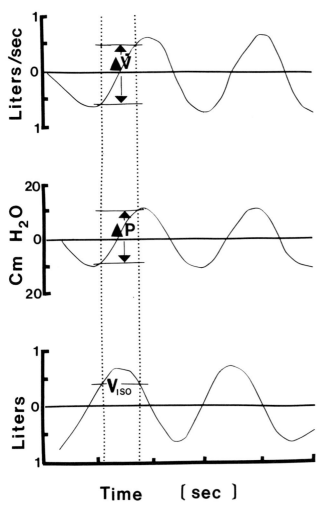

Figure 9–4. Simultaneous record of flow (V̇), pressure (P), and volume (V) for determination of resistance by the isovolume technique. Change in pressure (ΔP) and change in flow (ΔV̇) between two points where volume is identical (V_{iso}) provide an estimate of resistance.

piratory system to decrease to 37% of its initial pre-expiratory value is termed the time constant. This time constant (t) is essentially equal to the product of resistance and compliance. In this method, compliance is determined in similar fashion to the Comroe-Nissel-Nims technique, by relating ΔV to ΔP prior to exhalation. If the time interval to exhale to 370 ml (Fig. 9–5) is then measured and divided by this compliance value, another calculation of total respiratory system resistance is provided.

Forced Oscillation. Total respiratory resistance can be measured during quiet breathing by imposing rapid small sine wave oscillations at the mouth and recording the resultant sine wave flows and pressures. Such oscillations are produced by a loudspeaker or valveless pump. To measure the pressure change due to resistance, the components caused by compliance and inertance must be eliminated. This is done by choosing the resonant frequency of the respiratory system (3–8 Hz) when compliance and inertance are 180° out of phase (i.e., equal magnitude and opposite sign) and cancel out. The oscillating pressure wave is then due to resistance alone.[7] One of the major

Figure 9–5. The passive exhalation method for estimating resistance. Compliance (C) is calculated as V/ΔP prior to exhalation. (t = time required to exhale to 37% of pre-expiratory volume [i.e., 370 ml].) Resistance (R) is calculated from the equation R × C = t.

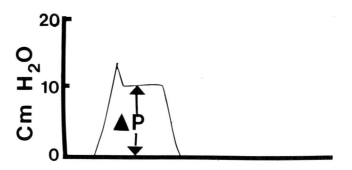

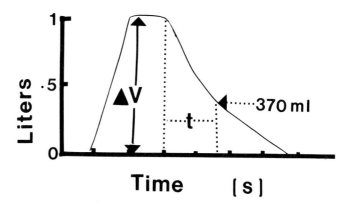

advantages of this technique is that it requires very little cooperation from the patient. However, for this method to reflect changes in airway tone, lung volume changes must be taken into account.

Body Plethysmography. This technique, first described by DuBois and colleagues,[8] has the advantage of specifically determining Raw and simultaneously providing a measurement of thoracic gas volume. The patient sits in a closed box and breathes via a mouthpiece. During pantinglike breaths (2–3 breaths/second), flow at the mouth measured by a pneumotachograph is displayed on the y axis of an oscilloscope while box pressure is displayed on the x axis. The slope of this loop is usually measured between 0 and 5 L/second to compute resistance (Fig. 9–6A). When the airway is occluded during such panting, pressure at the mouth is displayed on the y axis and related to box pressure in order to estimate thoracic gas volume, which in most cases is the FRC (Fig. 9–6B).

MEASUREMENT OF LUNG VOLUMES

In a clinical setting, there are only a few volumes that are worthwhile to monitor. The simplest of these is resting tidal volume. In patients con-

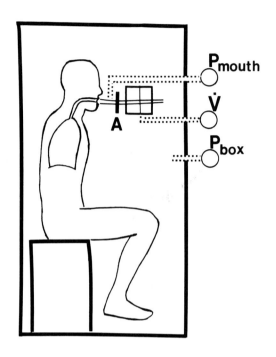

Figure 9–6. Constant volume body plethysmograph used to determine airway resistance (R_{aw}) and thoracic gas volume (FRC) by utilizing relationships of flow ($\dot{V}$), box pressure (P_{box}), and mouth pressure (P_{mouth}) during panting with shutter (*A*) open and (*B*) closed. ($\dot{V}_I$ = inspiratory flow, $\dot{V}_E$ = expiratory flow.)

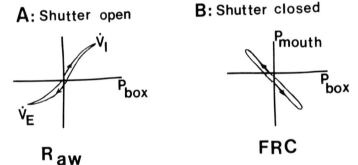

nected to a ventilator or anesthesia circuit, it is necessary to place the measuring device (to be discussed later) on the expiratory side of the circuit and as close to the patient as possible. The latter is important in order to minimize the effects of added gas flow from continuous positive pressure circuits or from an anesthesia machine.

Vital Capacity

The vital capacity in the normal adult is basically a measure of stature; i.e., it strongly correlates with height. The volume represents the difference between the limits of maximum voluntary inspiration (total lung capacity) and voluntary expiration (RV) (see Table 9–1). Devices for measuring this volume are discussed later.

Normally, vital capacity is more than ten times the resting tidal volume. The relationship between the two is often used to estimate ventilatory reserve. In patients with disease, the vital capacity is reduced by abnormalities of the bony thorax, increased lung stiffness, abdominal distention, muscle weakness, and a loss of functional alveoli. Other factors such as pain, fatigue, and poor effort may prevent the maximum full inspiratory and expiratory effort required for normal measured volumes.

Functional Residual Capacity

FRC refers to the gas remaining in the lungs at the end of a normal expiration or, more precisely, the volume at which the recoil pressures of the lung and thorax oppose each other equally (see Fig. 9–1). In most clinical situations, a reduction in FRC is associated with increased lung recoil, i.e., decreased compliance.[9] Thus there appears to be little advantage to measuring FRC in the usual clinical setting of the operating room or intensive care unit.

The techniques available for determining FRC are also somewhat difficult to apply in these areas. The most accurate technique utilizes the body plethysmograph, as during airway resistance determinations. This is virtually impossible in the unconscious, artificially ventilated patient, because of the requirements for confinement in an air-tight box. Lung volume in this case is estimated by using Boyle's law to relate changes in box pressure to changes in mouth pressure during panting against a closed airway (see Fig. 9–6B).

Multiple Breath N_2 Washout

Multiple breath N_2 washout is an open circuit technique that measures the washout of nitrogen (N_2) from the lungs after a switch from breathing air to breathing 100% O_2. Although the volume of the lungs (FRC) is unknown, the gas content is 80% N_2. Thus, if the total volume of N_2 in the lungs could be measured, the volume of the alveolar gas (FRC) could be calculated. The expired gas can be collected in a large spirometer and its final N_2 content determined, or, as is now more common, N_2 concentration and volume are continuously measured until expired N_2 concentration is 1.5% or less. This can be achieved in 2–3 minutes in some healthy subjects, but in patients with obstructive lung disease, it may take 7–10 minutes or even longer. As a consequence of the slower N_2 washout, FRC is usually underestimated in such patients, in contrast to values obtained for the true thoracic gas volume with the body plethysmograph.

Helium Dilution

Helium dilution is a closed circuit technique that has been used most frequently during anesthesia and in other clinical settings. Essentially, the patient's alveolar gas is allowed to equilibrate with a closed circuit (e.g., a bag) containing a known amount of helium (He_1). At the beginning of rebreathing there is no helium in the lung ($He_I = 0$). All helium is in the circuit or bag. At the end of a period of rebreathing, helium concentration is equal in both. Since initial (He_I) and final (He_F) helium concentrations are measured and the volume of the bag or circuit is known, the volume of the lungs (FRC) can be calculated.

$$FRC (He_I) + bag\ vol\ (He_I) = He_F (FRC + bag\ vol) \qquad \textbf{9–5}$$

Much like with N_2 washout, the completeness of helium dilution requires communication of all lung areas with the circuit. In patients with disease, particularly when there is airway obstruction, the technique again underestimates the true FRC.

EFFECTS OF GENERAL ANESTHESIA ON RESPIRATORY MECHANICS

This section briefly discusses the effects of general anesthesia on lung volumes, FRC, pressure volume, and pressure-flow behavior of the respiratory system. In normal recumbent humans, FRC is reduced by about 500 ml after the induction of general anesthesia. The changes occur within a minute and are not further affected by muscle paralysis. Although the exact mechanism is uncertain, simultaneous determinations by N_2 washout and body plethysmography agree and suggest that the changes are not due to gas trapped in closed distal airways.[10] The degree of change appears related to body habitus and shape of the chest wall, which allow for differing degrees of diaphragmatic displacement.

The pressure-volume curve of the respiratory system tends to shift to the right 20–30 minutes after induction of anesthesia. Thus, compliance is decreased. The decrease in lung compliance is due to the decreased FRC. In a sense, the changes can be likened to tightly strapping the chest. The altered function of the chest wall, therefore, secondarily affects the mechanical properties of the lungs.

The changes in pressure-flow relationships of the respiratory system with the patient under anesthesia are much less understood. Pulmonary resistance increases, owing largely to placement of the endotracheal tube, reflex changes in airway smooth muscle tone, airway secretions, and increased lung recoil.

MEASUREMENTS OF VENTILATION

Flow and Volume

Peak Flow Meter. A measurement widely used in the management of variable airflow limitation is the peak expiratory flow rate (PEFR). PEFR

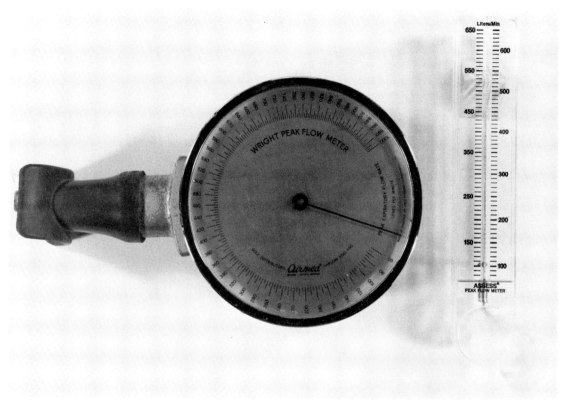

Figure 9–7. Hand-held peak flowmeters for bedside measurement. The original Wright meter is on the left, and an inexpensive model is pictured on the right. (Courtesy of Health Scan Products, Cedar Grove, NJ.)

is the maximum flow generated during a forced expiration begun from a position of full inspiration. This flow can be measured conveniently with hand-held flowmeters (Fig. 9–7) and is markedly affected by changes in the caliber of large airways. Since repeat measurements are relatively easy to obtain, PEFRs are often used to monitor responses to bronchodilator therapy in patients with asthma.[11]

The original instrument, the Wright Peak Flow Meter, and all subsequent devices essentially measure a pressure drop that is directly related to flow in the presence of a fixed resistance. Normal peak flow values in young healthy males are greater than 500 L/minute.[12] Values less than 200 L/minute in the surgical candidate suggest impaired cough efficiency and the increased likelihood of postoperative complications.[13] The test is much less unpleasant and exhausting than the full forced vital capacity maneuver; therefore, it provides the clinician with a valuable tool for identifying gross pulmonary disability at the bedside. It is important to understand, however, that the measurement is dependent on effort and thus can be influenced by the patient's cooperation and other factors such as muscle weakness.

Pneumotachography. Of the devices available to measure flow, the pneumotachograph is perhaps the best known. A low mechanical resistance, usually in the form of a screen, is placed directly in the stream of gas flow. The pressure gradient across this resistance is sensed by a differential pressure transducer and is linearly related to flow if flow is laminar. To assure such linearity, it is important to select the pneumotachograph that is linear in the flow rates likely to be experienced (e.g., for forced expiration, 6–10 L/second; for quiet adult tidal volumes, 0–1 L/second).

The pressure gradient is dependent not only on the flow rate but also on the density and viscosity of the gas mixture as well as its temperature. Furthermore, condensation of moisture increases screen resistance and may cause turbulence. The latter is usually eliminated by electrically heating the screen. Despite these limitations, the rapid response, small dead space, and low resistance of the pneumotachograph render it useful for flow measurement in many situations. Also, when this flow is integrated electronically with respect to time, a measurement of volume can be derived.

Hot Wire Spirometers. A heated wire or thermistor is cooled by a gas stream to an extent dependent on the flow rate and thermal conductivity of the gas. Such devices tend to be robust and easily sterilized, and they are suitable for applications not requiring a high degree of accuracy. They do, however, rapidly diminish in sensitivity if coated with foreign debris such as airway secretions.

Ultrasonic Flowmeters. The velocity of gas flow can be measured by utilizing ultrasound. The basis for such ultrasonic flowmeters is the measurement of the change in the speed of sound. Two piezoelectric crystals aligned at angles to the gas flow alternately transmit and receive bursts of oscillations at a frequency of 100 KHz. Such flowmeters have advantages over pneumotachographs in certain situations because of their low resistance. They also do not have problems with moisture, positive pressure, or motion artifact, and they tend to be more stable, i.e., exhibit less drift over long periods of use.

Thoracoabdominal Movement. Konno and Mead have measured movements of the chest wall and abdomen and demonstrated their relationship to tidal volume during unobstructed respiration.[14] Various transducers and devices have measured the changes in physical shape and, hence, electrical properties of the chest and abdomen during respiration. These devices have consisted of mercury in rubber strain gauges, magnetometers, impedance electrodes, and, most recently, the inductance plethysmography (Respitrace, Ambulatory Monitoring, Ardsley, NY).[15] This device consists of two insulated coils, one of which encircles the abdomen and the other the rib cage. The coils are contained within a netlike garment and are excited by a high-frequency oscillation. The inductance of the coils changes with respiration as a function of changes in the cross-sectional area of the compartment enclosed within. The instrument is useful for detecting apnea and eliminates the need for mouthpieces or masks. For measurement of volumes, however, devices such as the Respitrace must be regarded as semiquantitative, unless rigorous calibrations with a spirometer are repeatedly carried out.

Collection Devices

Gas Meters. Dry gas meters (Parkinson-Cowan) have been utilized to measure minute ventilation for extended periods. The meters have large internal volumes and a large amount of dead space to allow rebreath-ing. Rather, gas must be collected via a one-way valve on the expiratory limb or in a Douglas bag, which is then emptied into the meters. The gas volumes are collected at ambient temperature and pressure saturated with H_2O vapor (ATPS); but for precision, respiratory volumes are expressed at body temperature and pressure saturated with H_2O vapor (BTPS). Many tables are available for such conversion factors, which are calculated as follows:

$$\text{BTPS vol} = \text{ATPS vol} \times \frac{(273 \times Tb°C)}{(273 \times Tatm°C)} \times \frac{(Patm - PH_2O \, Tb)}{(Patm - PH_2O \, Tatm)} \quad \textbf{9-6}$$

where Tb = body temperature, Tatm = atmospheric temperature, PH_2O = vapor pressure of H_2O at Tb or Tatm, Patm = atmospheric or barometric pressure.

Spirometers. The classic Collins water seal spirometers are reliable and accurate, and they serve as the reference standard for volume measure-ments. However, they are cumbersome and poorly suited for use in the operating room or intensive care unit. Dry spirometers, such as the rolling seal or wedge types, have similar problems of bulk but have better frequency responses that render them more useful for forced respiratory maneuvers. In addition, they often have electrical circuitry capable of differentiating the volume signal in order to obtain flow. The principal shortcoming of such spirometers lies in the difficulty of applying them to systems in which re-breathing takes place or additional fresh gas is added to the volume inspired.

Mechanical Respirometers. In contrast to the limitations of conventional spirometers, mechanical respirometers provide less expensive, more con-venient access to the breathing circuit. Such devices estimate volume from rotation of a low-friction inertia vane. The widely used Wright respirometer contains a geared system that converts rotation of the vane into movements of hands on a dial. Tangential slots around the vane ensure that flow is recorded in only one direction. Thus, the vane may be inserted between the endotracheal tube and the breathing circuit. The small dead space (20–25 ml) and relatively low resistance render it suitable for patients who are breathing spontaneously. The instrument is most accurate at flows of about 20 L/minute. These flows are typical of quiet expiration in adults. Because of the inertia, resistance, and momentum of the vane, the Wright respi-rometer tends to overread at higher flows and underread at lower flows. Although changes in gas composition have relatively little effect, water con-densation is often a problem after extended use, as is accumulation of foreign material.

These problems of the Wright respirometer are shared by a number of similar devices. Such is the case with the larger, widely used Drager res-pirometer. This equipment senses flow in either direction and must, of ne-cessity, be placed in an area of unidirectional flow—hence, its conventional location on the expiratory limb of an anesthesia circuit system. Such place-ment of the respirometer renders it prone to overreading, because of in-creases in fresh gas delivery to the system, particularly when such delivered flows are large (e.g., 10 L/minute).[16]

Pressure Monitoring

Airway pressures (Paw) may be simply measured with the aneroid gauges present in anesthesia or ventilator circuits. These simple measurements are usually sufficiently accurate to make some assessment of patient or system mechanics. However, for the most accurate assessment of patient mechanics, pressures should be sensed as close to the patient as possible and ideally at the inlet to an endotracheal tube. Automated measurement of Paw from the same sites can be obtained with simple strain gauge transducers, such as those used to measure blood pressure. If an esophageal balloon is used to measure intrapleural pressure, a differential pressure transducer, i.e., one with two ports, is needed. The negative or subambient intrapleural pressure (Ppl) must be referenced to mouth pressure (Pm) to derive the transpulmonary (PL) pressure. Thus,

$$P_L = Pm - Ppl \qquad\qquad 9-7$$

Pressure-Volume Relationships

The effects of circuit distensibility or compliance on reducing the actual amount of delivered volume are well recognized. This distention of tubing can be minimized by the use of stiffer circuit material. However, another factor, compression of gases within the tubing, is not prevented. The latter is a function of circuit size (including humidifier) and pressure at end-inspiration. The discrepancies due to gas compression become important when small tidal volumes are used, particularly in the face of high inflation pressures. The gas compressed during inspiration is added to the measured expired volume, overestimating volume. The gas composition is also diluted by the same added gas, resulting in decreased tensions from expired gases such as CO_2.

Figure 9–3 illustrates typical flow, volume, and pressure relationships that might exist in the patient circuit during cycling of a mechanical ventilator. Maximum (peak) airway pressure and plateau or static pressures can be readily measured, and, in conjunction with tidal volume (VT) measurements, can be used to estimate dynamic compliance (Cdyn) and static compliance (Cst).

$$Cdyn = VT/peak\ pressure \qquad\qquad 9-8$$

$$Cst = V/plateau\ pressure \qquad\qquad 9-9$$

Plateau pressure can be estimated during the period of no flow, i.e., inspiratory pause available on most ventilators. If this is unavailable, the expiratory limb of the circuit may be clamped. The value is often referred to as quasi-static, since it is not truly a static measurement such as might be obtained by inflation with a giant syringe or passive deflation against an occlusion.

Another useful form of quasi-static compliance measurement applicable to ventilator patients receiving constant inspiratory flow is a pulse method, based on the pressure rise per unit time during such flow.[17] It is based on the principle that when a constant flow is introduced to the respiratory system, the rate of increase in pressure is inversely related to the compliance of the system.[18]

$$\text{Compliance} = \frac{\text{flow}}{\Delta \text{ pressure/time}} \qquad \textbf{9–10}$$

Since flow = Δ volume/time,

$$\text{Compliance} = \frac{\Delta \text{ volume}}{\Delta \text{ pressure}} \qquad \textbf{9–11}$$

Values for compliance estimated by this method in all patients were nearly identical to those obtained by relating delivered VT to the plateau pressure, and they are considered quasi-static. The estimation of compliance by the pulse method is illustrated in Figure 9–8.

MONITORING GAS EXCHANGE

Capnometry and Capnography

Analysis of CO_2 in the respired gases has become commonplace in the operating room setting. The actual measurement of CO_2 concentration is termed capnometry. Capnography, on the other hand, refers to the display of this concentration on a screen or recording chart, usually as a function of time. The ability to visualize CO_2 waveforms enhances their interpretations in contrast to the simple digital readout of CO_2 concentrations (capnometry).

Methods of Analysis

The most common systems available for breath-by-breath CO_2 analysis utilize the infrared absorption of gases. Infrared light of a certain wavelength (2600 or 4300 nm) passes through a reference gas sample containing either no CO_2 or a known amount. The light also passes through the gas sample to be analyzed. The CO_2 absorbs the infrared energy in proportion to its concentration. Photocells sense a difference in intensity between the light transmitted through the reference chamber and that passed through the sample gas, which is related to the CO_2 concentration in the sample chamber.

Instruments monitor CO_2 by direct in-line measurement at the sample site, by a flow-through device, or by aspiration of the gas sample into a separate monitor. The in-line sensors, such as are available from Siemens Corporation and Hewlett-Packard, are placed directly in the breathing system with a special adapter and are ideally as close to the patient as possible. Such sensors are fragile, expensive, and somewhat cumbersome, and they have relatively large dead space. On the other hand, moisture is not a prob-

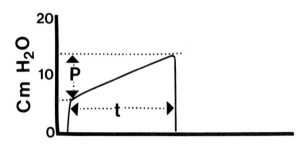

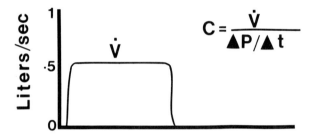

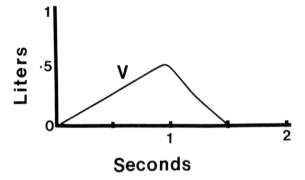

Figure 9–8. The pulse method for estimating compliance (C) by dividing the constant flow ($\dot{V}$) by the rate of rise of pressure ($\Delta P/\Delta t$).

$$C = \frac{\dot{V}}{\Delta P/\Delta t}$$

lem, and there is no limitation to where the actual monitor console is placed. Such monitors also do not require standard gases for calibration.

Analyzers that continually withdraw gas samples are more common. It is important to realize that this sampled gas (usually 250 ml/minute) must be returned to the anesthesia system or scavenger in order to avoid polluting the environment with anesthetic gases. Such analyzers are plagued by excess moisture and require that the small diameter sampling tube be as short as possible in order to improve response time. The response time is inherently shorter with in-line sensors that analyze gas directly in the airway and thus lack the delay and mixing of gases associated with suction and transport to a remote infrared analyzer.

Capnogram

Normally, CO_2 concentrations are displayed with respect to time (Fig. 9–9). However, the expired volume may also substitute for time on the

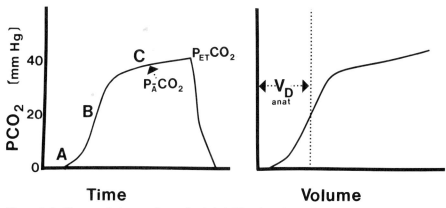

Figure 9–9. Characteristic waveform of exhaled CO_2 plotted as a function of time and volume. ($P\bar{A}CO_2$ = mean alveolar CO_2 tension, $P_{ET}CO_2$ = end-tidal CO_2 tension, $V_D$anat = anatomic dead space.) See the text for an explanation.

abscissa. Such curves require more effort and equipment but may yield more information regarding respiratory dead space.[19]

During each breath, gases emerge sequentially from the conducting airways that compose the anatomic dead space and finally from the alveoli. The characteristic CO_2 waveform displayed in Figure 9–9 exhibits three basic phases during expiration that are followed by an abrupt decrease in CO_2 concentration during inspiration. During the initial phase A, CO_2 remains near the previous inspiratory concentration and reflects gas cleared from the anatomic dead space. In phase B, there is an admixture of residual dead space gas and alveolar gas that is beginning to emerge from lung areas with short conducting airways. CO_2 increases rapidly in phase B to approach alveolar levels. The final phase C is often referred to as the alveolar plateau, since it represents gas washed out of the alveoli. The slope of this phase is increased when there is nonhomogeneous mixing of gas, such as with airway obstruction. It also increases with exercise and hypermetabolic states. Because of this upward slope of the alveolar plateau, end-tidal CO_2 tension (PET_{CO_2}) exceeds the mean alveolar CO_2 (PA_{CO_2}). Normally, however, there is sufficient mixing with dead space gas such that PET_{CO_2} is usually somewhat less than arterial CO_2 tension (Pa_{CO_2}).

Sources of Inaccuracy

Clinically, PET_{CO_2} is used to provide a noninvasive estimate of Pa_{CO_2}. Under ideal conditions, even in the presence of general anesthesia, the difference between them is negligible.[20] The most significant determinant of a gradient between Pa_{CO_2} and PET_{CO_2} is the presence of lung disease characterized by the extremes of high relationships between ventilation and blood flow ($\dot{V}/\dot{Q}$). These lung units behave functionally as dead space areas. These poorly or nonperfused areas have a PA_{CO_2} of nearly zero. Thus, the weighted average of all lung units yields a low PET_{CO_2}.

The other major sources of abnormally low PET_{CO_2} values involve sampling errors. The most obvious is a system leak in which some of the exhaled volume is lost and not subject to sampling. Most leaks are obvious but some, such as that caused by a poorly sealed endotracheal tube cuff, may require more intense scrutiny. The other sampling problem relates solely to aspirating devices and the relationship of sampling volume to the patient's VT. In adults, the expired VTs are usually sufficient to supply the aspirated sample. Dilution of this sample with fresh gas (free of CO_2) occurs if the sample site is far from the patient's airway or exhaled volumes decrease (shallow breathing). The implications of this problem in pediatric patients with high fresh gas flows are obvious.

Dead Space

Respiratory dead space is most often considered in physiologic terms, i.e., the volume of inspired and expired gas that does not partake of gas exchange in the alveoli. This physiologic dead space (VDphys) has two components: the conducting airways or anatomic dead space (VDanat) and the alveolar dead space (VDalv). In most instances, VDanat is of less importance, because it is relatively small and fairly constant in a given individual, since much of its volume is in the rigid airways. The variations of VDanat among different individuals relate to factors affecting lung volume and airway size, such as posture, tracheal intubation, bronchodilators, and pneumonectomy.

The capnograph allows estimation of VDanat (see Fig. 9–9) by what is often referred to as the equal area method, first described by Aitken and Clark Kennedy.[21] Essentially, VDanat is identified by the vertical line that subdivides phase B into two equal portions by assuming this volume represents the abrupt transition between the conducting dead space and the alveolar gas component. Unfortunately, this technique tends to overestimate VDanat in situations in which the slope of the alveolar phase C is increased (i.e., hypermetabolic states and asynchronous alveolar emptying with lung diseases).

The alveolar component of physiologic dead space is not measured directly, but rather it is determined from simultaneous measurements of VDanat and VDphys. The latter, which exceeds VDanat by including VDalv, is now usually defined by the mixing equation originally devised by Bohr but later modified by Enghoff, who substituted arterial CO_2 tension (Pa_{CO_2}) for alveolar CO_2 (PA_{CO_2}) in the equation:

$$\text{VDphys} = \text{VT} \times \frac{(Pa_{CO_2} - PE_{CO_2})}{(Pa_{CO_2} - PI_{CO_2})} \qquad \textbf{9–12}$$

Clinical measurement of VDphys requires a sample of arterial blood for Pa_{CO_2}. Mixed expired gases are collected over several minutes in a large bag or spirometer in order to measure mixed expired CO_2 tension (PE_{CO_2}). VT can be conveniently measured with a Wright respirometer. Since there is usually no rebreathing involved, inspired CO_2 tension (PI_{CO_2}) is usually assumed to be zero. It is also important to subtract apparatus dead space (face mask, valves, tubing) in order to obtain accurate measurements of VDphys.

In normal patients, this VD accounts for less than one third of VT (i.e., VD/VT $\leq$ 0.33). The calculation of VD/VT helps to estimate the relationship between alveolar ventilation and minute ventilation, or more specifically, the efficiency of ventilation. Such information can be very useful in determining whether to institute or discontinue mechanical ventilation.

Clinical Applications and Limitations

The useful information presented by capnography provides particular insight into the mechanical and gas exchange functions of the patient's lung. However, changes in metabolic and cardiovascular function are also detectable. For example, increased CO_2 production in malignant hyperthermia increases PETCO_2 and causes a more prominent slope of the alveolar plateau early in its course. Capnography can also indicate the quality of the circulation. A sudden decrease in PETCO_2 may result from decreased blood flow to the lungs secondary to hypovolemia, embolism, or myocardial dysfunction.

Perhaps the greatest advantage of capnography concerns its potential use for identifying malfunctions of breathing systems such as the anesthesia circuit. For example, incompetent unidirectional valves, exhausted or bypassed CO_2 absorbers, or inadequate fresh gas flows may all result in increased PETCO_2. This is usually due to rebreathing and, therefore, is accompanied by increased inspired CO_2 (i.e., above zero). The same rise in CO_2 without rebreathing may be due to either addition of exogenous or endogenous CO_2 or hypoventilation caused by leaks in the system.

Sudden drops in PETCO_2 to near zero generally signal major problems. These include extubation, esophageal intubation, total airway obstruction, or complete disconnection. Numerous reports have emphasized the utility of capnography in detecting these phenomena (Fig. 9-10). However, it is important to recognize that the capnogram associated with any of these events is nonspecific and provides no clue to diagnosis. It simply indicates that there is a major problem. This may be due to instrument malfunction (e.g., clogged sample tube) and may provide false information or may divert attention from the patient. It is prudent at this point to rule out any of the above problems before trouble-shooting the CO_2 analyzer. Although capnography is invaluable in the detection of circulatory and respiratory problems, its limitations as an early warning device must be recognized.

Assessing Adequacy of Oxygenation

Techniques for measuring and sampling delivered oxygen concentrations are discussed elsewhere (Chapter 8). The end result, the arterial O_2 tension (PaO_2), requires, of course, analysis of arterial blood (Chapter 17).

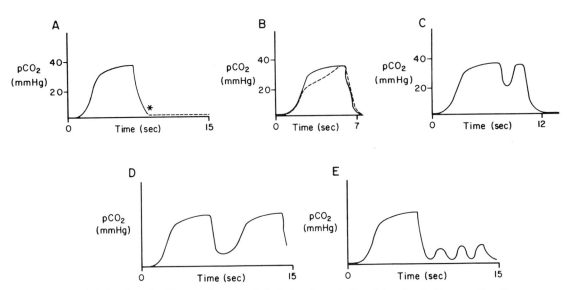

Figure 9–10. Exhaled carbon dioxide waveforms in clinical situations. *A,* Breathing circuit disconnection (*) or esophageal intubation that produces no carbon dioxide at sampling site. Specific cause can be differentiated by clinical findings. *B,* The normal waveform is compared with that occurring during airway obstruction (endotracheal tube kinking or obstructive lung disease). The expiratory ascent to the alveolar plateau is slowed, and the inspiratory portion is unaffected. *C,* Spontaneous ventilation during controlled mechanical ventilation. *D,* Rebreathing within a breathing circuit causes elevation of the baseline of the capnogram owing to inspiration of exhaled CO_2. *E,* Normal breath followed by panting. The sine waves present do not reflect alveolar gas because of the rapid respiratory rate with limited inspiratory time.

Estimation of Shunt ($\dot{Q}s/\dot{Q}t$)

The most common causes of arterial hypoxemia are low or decreased ventilation-perfusion relationships (V/Q) in numerous regional lung units. As these regional units are underventilated and normally perfused, there is a low PA_{O_2} and also a decreased Pa_{O_2} in the blood leaving the lung to enter the systemic circulation. If increasing the fractional inspired concentration of O_2 (FI_{O_2}) has little or no effect in increasing Pa_{O_2}, right-to-left shunting is assumed to be the cause of the low Pa_{O_2}. A regional lung unit is the site of shunting when it has zero ventilation and relatively persistent perfusion, such that V/Q is essentially zero. Blood flows past such an alveolus whose PA_{O_2} is zero and retains its low venous O_2 tension prior to entering the systemic circulation.

The calculation of this shunt ($\dot{Q}s/\dot{Q}t$) has been utilized as an indicator of the ability of the lungs to oxygenate blood. To calculate shunt, one must know barometric pressure, PA_{O_2}, Pa_{CO_2}, hemoglobin concentration, and mixed venous O_2 tension ($P\bar{v}_{O_2}$). Thus, equipment consists of a barometer, blood gas analyzer, blood sampling devices, and either a pulmonary artery or a central venous catheter to obtain $P\bar{v}_{O_2}$. It is also necessary to ensure that the patient is breathing 100% O_2 for at least 20 minutes.

The formula used to calculate shunt is

$$\dot{Q}s/\dot{Q}t = \frac{Cc_{O_2} - Ca_{O_2}}{Cc_{O_2} - C\bar{v}_{O_2}} \qquad \textbf{9–13}$$

where Cc_{O_2} = O_2 content of ventilated and perfused pulmonary capillaries, Ca_{O_2} = O_2 content of arterial blood, $C\bar{v}_{O_2}$ = O_2 content of mixed venous blood.

Since perfused capillaries ventilated with O_2 are exposed to the PA_{O_2}, the latter must be calculated from the alveolar air equation. The PA_{O_2} is multiplied by the solubility coefficient (0.003) to calculate dissolved O_2. Since each gram of hemoglobin also holds 1.39 ml of O_2 when fully saturated,

$$Ca_{O_2} = (Hb \times 1.39) + (PA_{O_2} \times 0.003) \qquad \textbf{9-14}$$

Arterial Hb is not fully saturated; therefore,

$$Ca_{O_2} = (Hb \times 1.39 \times \%Sa_{O_2}) + (Pa_{O_2} \times 0.003) \qquad \textbf{9-15}$$

$C\bar{v}_{O_2}$ is calculated in similar fashion except that Pv_{O_2} is multiplied by 0.003 to estimate dissolved O_2. Thus,

$$C\bar{v}_{O_2} = (Hb \times 1.39 \times \%S\bar{v}_{O_2}) + (Pv_{O_2} \times 0.003) \qquad \textbf{9-16}$$

The accuracy of $\dot{Q}s/\dot{Q}t$ calculations depends on many variables, such as cardiac output, respiratory quotient, the quality of the mixed venous sample, or an assumed arterial venous O_2 content difference. Thus, many clinicians prefer the simpler use of A-a$_{O_2}$ difference rather than shunt to assess the adequacy of oxygenation. Others have proposed short-cut methods for calculating % shunt, assuming unchanged cardiac output and FI_{O_2} of 1.0.[22]

$$\% \text{ shunt} = \frac{\text{A-a}_{O_2} \text{ difference}}{10} \qquad \textbf{9-17}$$

The importance of cardiac output must be emphasized in patients with acute respiratory failure who often experience reduction in cardiac output secondary to continuous positive pressure breathing. Cardiac output profoundly affects Pa_{O_2} for a given level of shunting. Wide variation in Pa_{O_2} can occur because of changes in cardiac output without an actual change in pulmonary status. The same increases and decreases in cardiac output can raise or lower the calculated $\dot{Q}s/\dot{Q}t$ values. Thus, neither $\dot{Q}s/\dot{Q}t$ nor A-a$_{O_2}$ differences can be meaningfully interpreted unless cardiac output changes are considered.

Diffusion

The role of diffusion in producing abnormalities in gas exchange is of little importance and for practical purposes can be ignored under resting conditions, because the oxygen diffusion gradient is normally zero.[23] Diffusion is limited if there is an oxygen gradient between alveolar and end-capillary O_2 tensions. Only if cardiac output is increased and FI_{O_2} decreased does such a gradient develop. Examples of such situations would be vigorous exercise and breathing at altitudes above 10,000 feet.

Diffusing capacity of the lungs (DL) is defined as the rate at which a gas enters the blood divided by its driving pressure. The latter again is the gradient between alveolar and end-capillary tensions. DL is expressed in milliliters per minute per millimeter of Hg (see Table 9–1). Measurement of DL provides information about the amount of functioning capillaries in contact with ventilated air spaces, such as may occur in certain pulmonary vascular parenchymal disease states. The brief inhalation of nontoxic low concentrations of carbon monoxide (CO) has become standard for this purpose in most pulmonary function laboratories. The equipment requirements and the large variations in normal values for each of the techniques (single breath, steady state, rebreathing) render the measurement well outside the usual clinical realm and well beyond the scope of this discussion. For a comprehensive discussion of the interpretation and significance of such testing, the reader is referred to an excellent review.[24]

CO has several features that make it useful for measuring DL. It has 200 times the affinity for hemoglobin that oxygen does. Thus, CO does not build up rapidly in plasma. Most important, however, is the low CO concentration in the blood under normal conditions, such that pulmonary capillary tension can be assumed to be zero. Of the techniques utilizing CO, the rebreathing method is least influenced by changes in V/Q distributions, but it is the least reproducible and requires the greatest amount of the patient's effort. Therefore, for the purpose of this discussion, only the single, breath and steady state methods are briefly outlined.

To measure DL with CO, three values must be obtained. These are the milliliters of CO transferred from alveoli to blood per minute, the mean alveolar CO tension ($P\bar{A}co$), and the pulmonary capillary CO tension ($Pcco$).

$$DLco = \frac{CO\ ml/minute/mmHg}{P\bar{A}co - Pcco} \qquad \textbf{9–18}$$

In the *single breath method*, the patient inspires a dilute mixture of CO and holds her or his breath for 10 seconds. During this period, CO leaves alveolar gas to enter the blood in proportion to the diffusing capacity. The milliliters of CO transferred is calculated by infrared analysis from the percentage of CO in alveolar gas at the beginning and end of the breath hold. To do this, FRC must be calculated from helium dilution and then added to the inspiratory volume. The $P\bar{c}CO$ is essentially zero and can be ignored. However, $P\bar{A}co$ is not the simple average of Pco at the beginning and end of the breath holding; rather, it must be calculated by a special equation that considers alveolar volume as reflected by the ratio of inspired to expired helium concentrations.[25] The single breath method requires little patient cooperation and no blood samples, but it may not be feasible in dyspneic or exercising subjects.

The *steady state method* is therefore regarded as more physiologic than the single breath test, since it can be measured in such patients. The patient breathes a low (0.1%) concentration of CO for about 30 seconds, or until a steady state is established. The rate of CO disappearance from alveoli to blood is measured along with $P\bar{A}co$. Unfortunately, with steady state methods, $P\bar{A}co$ is again difficult to measure and must be estimated using an assumed value for dead space. In general, however, steady state and single breath techniques give similar results. Normal values, depending on individual laboratories, range from 20 to 30 ml/minute/mmHg. Increases in DLco occur with body size, age, lung volume, exercise, body position, and alveolar CO_2 and O_2 tensions. Therefore, changes in these variables must be considered when interpreting DLco values.

SIMPLE MONITORING OF VENTILATION WITHOUT INSTRUMENTATION

In the early days of anesthesia with diethyl ether, most patients breathed spontaneously, and ventilation was monitored by simple inspection of the neck, chest, and abdomen. The data were correlated with gas movement by observing the rebreathing bag. Normal quiet breathing in the supine position is primarily abdominal, i.e., consisting of diaphragmatic descent. Rib cage movement is nonexistent until higher levels of breathing occur or when mechanical ventilation is utilized. In the presence of respiratory obstruction, diaphragmatic power overcomes the action of the rib cage and the rib cage may be drawn in paradoxically. This phenomenon is particularly evident in an infant or child whose thorax is far more flexible than that of an adult. The same paradoxical chest movement occurs with respiratory muscle weakness and is most evident in high levels of spinal cord injury.

In addition to simple observation of the patient, the adequacy of ventilation can be estimated by listening to breath sounds through esophageal or precordial stethoscopes. When placed on the precordium, the stethoscope can provide adequate transmission of heart sounds, but breath sounds may be inaudible, especially during spontaneous breathing. In this case, the relatively low flow rates (<0.2 L/second) are difficult to hear. When the stethoscope is placed over the jugular notch, however, the turbulent flows around the larynx are easily heard and can provide clear evidence of even mild laryngeal spasm. Without question, the simplest and most reliable of the respiratory monitors is the esophageal stethoscope, which conveys both heart and breath sounds clearly. Wheezing, leaks, and accumulation of secretions can readily be identified. In addition, the absence of breath sounds is a simple, reliable monitor of a disconnect in the presence of mechanical ventilation. This should trigger a response to check other components of the breathing circuit, such as ventilator bellows and pressure gauges.

Monitoring movement of the breathing bag has been a mainstay of simple monitoring practice during spontaneous or manually controlled ventilation. One must not be deceived by errors produced by excessively high fresh gas flows or aspiration of gas from the circuit either for analysis or by the scavenging system. Thus, regardless of how simple such respiratory monitoring methods are, each has the potential for misinterpretation. A sound understanding of physiologic and mechanical concepts is equally important for simple monitors of respiration and for more sophisticated techniques.

References

1. Black LF, Hyatt RE: Maximal static respiratory pressures in generalized neuromuscular disease. Am Rev Respir Dis 1971; 103:641–650.
2. O'Donoghue WJ, Baker JP, Bell F, et al: Respiratory failure in neuromuscular disease management in a respiratory intensive care unit. JAMA 1971; 235:733–735.
3. Pavlin EG, Holle RH, Schoene R: Recovery of airway protection compared to ventilation in humans after paralysis with curare. Anesthesiology 1989; 70:381–385.
4. Milic-Emili J, Mead J, Turner JM, et al: Improved technique for estimating pleural pressure for esophageal balloons. J Appl Physiol 1964; 19:207–211.
5. Leatherman NE: An improved balloon system for monitoring intraesophageal pressure in acutely ill patients. Crit Care Med 1978; 6:189–192.
6. Comroe JH, Nissel OL, Nims RG: A simple method for concurrent measurement of compliance and resistance to breathing in anesthetized animals and man. J Appl Physiol 1954; 7:225–228.
7. Fisher AB, DuBois AB, Hyde RW: Evaluation of the oscillation technique for the determination of resistance to breathing. J Clin Invest 1968; 47:2045–2057.
8. DuBois AB, Botelho SY, Comroe JH: A new method for measuring airway resistance in man using a body plethysmograph: Values in normal subjects and in patients with respiratory disease. J Clin Invest 1956; 35:326–335.
9. Katz JA, Zinn SE, Ozanne GM, Fairley HB: Pulmonary chest wall and lung-thorax elastance in acute respiratory failure. Chest 1981; 80:304–311.
10. Westbrook PR, Stubbs SE, Sessler AD, et al: Effects of anesthesia and muscle paralysis on respiratory mechanics in normal man. J Appl Physiol 1973; 34:81–86.
11. Banner AS, Shah RS, Addington WW: Rapid prediction of need for hospitalization in acute asthma. JAMA 1976; 235:1337–1338.
12. Leiner GC, Abramowitz S, Small MJ, et al: Expiratory peak flow rate, standard values for normal subjects, use as a clinical test of ventilatory function. Am Rev Respir Dis 1963; 88:644–651.
13. Stein M, Koota GM, Simon M, et al: Pulmonary evaluation of surgical patients. JAMA 1962; 181:765–770.
14. Konno K, Mead J: Measurement of the separate volume changes of the rib cage and abdomen during breathing. J Appl Physiol 1967; 22:407–422.
15. Cohn MA, Rao ASV, Broudy M, et al: The respiratory inductive plethysmograph: A new noninvasive monitor of respiration. Bull Eur Physiopathol Respir 1982; 18:643–658.
16. Mapleson WW: Physical aspects of automatic ventilators: Some application of basic principles. *In* Mushin MA, Rendell-Baker L, Thompson PW, Mapleson WW (eds): Automatic Ventilation of the Lungs, 3rd Ed. Oxford: Blackwell Scientific, 1980; 132–151.
17. Surratt PM, Owens O: A pulse method of measuring respiratory system compliance in ventilated patients. Chest 1981; 80:34–38.
18. Rattenborg CC, Holaday DA: Constant flow inflation of the lungs, theoretical analysis. Acta Anaesthesiol Scand 1967; 23:211–223.
19. Fletcher R: Deadspace, invasive and noninvasive. Br J Anaesth 1985; 57:245–249.
20. Whitesall R, Assidao C, Gollman D, Jablonski J: Relationship between arterial and peak expired carbon dioxide pressure during anesthesia and factors influencing the difference. Anesth Analg 1981; 60:508–512.
21. Aitken RS, Clark Kennedy AE: On the fluctuation in the composition of the

alveolar air during the respiratory cycle in muscular exercise. J Physiol (Lond) 1928; 65:289–411.

22. Chiang ST: A nomogram for venous shunt (Qs/Qt) calculation. Thorax 1968; 23:563–565.

23. Staub NC: Alveolar-arterial oxygen tension gradient due to diffusion. J Appl Physiol 1963; 18:673–680.

24. Davies NJH: Does the lung work? 4. What does the transfer of carbon monoxide mean? Br J Dis Chest 1982; 76:105–124.

25. Forster RE, DuBois AB, Briscoe WE, Fisher AB: The Lung, Physiologic Basis of Pulmonary Function Tests, 3rd Ed. Chicago: Year Book Medical, 1986; 295.

Maternal-Fetal Monitoring in Obstetrics

chapter ten

Maternal-Fetal Monitoring in Obstetrics

ANDREW M. WOODS, M.D.
■ COSMO A. DIFAZIO, M.D., PH.D.

Obstetric monitoring frequently begins with a very inexpensive device, an oral thermometer. By monitoring body temperature for the specific pattern associated with ovulation, a woman is able to identify the narrow time frame when conception may be possible. Once conception has occurred, obstetric monitoring takes on a unique duality because there are at least two patients with separate, but interdependent, physiologic systems to be assessed. The ideal of maternal-fetal monitoring is the early detection of physiologic abnormalities that, in the absence of intervention, might progress to serious organ injury. Pregnancy is associated with a wide range of physiologic alterations, which are reviewed in order to establish a reference for possible abnormal variations.

MATERNAL PHYSIOLOGY IN NORMAL PREGNANCY

Pregnancy is associated with a number of physiologic changes, most of which subserve the increased metabolic burden imposed by the fetus or alter

345

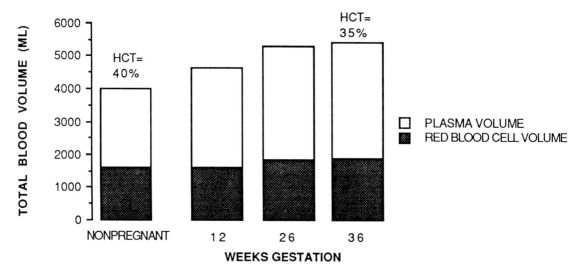

Figure 10–1. Blood volume, plasma volume, and red cell volume over the course of normal pregnancy. Most of the increase in blood volume is accounted for by an increase in plasma volume, producing a modest dilutional "anemia of pregnancy." (HCT = hematocrit.) (Compiled from Blekta, Hlavatý, Trnková, et al, Am J Obstet Gynecol 1970; Davison, Scand J Clin Lab Invest [Suppl] 1984; Goodlin, Quaife, Dirksen, Semin Perinatol 1981; Hayes, Cruikshank, Dunn, Am J Obstet Gynecol 1985; Gallery, Clin Exper Hypertens 1982.)

the maternal physiology to accommodate the mechanical burden of the fetus during pregnancy and delivery. One objective of antepartum maternal monitoring is to determine whether the alterations fall within expected norms and to document the normal progression of these changes.

Cardiovascular Physiology in Normal Pregnancy

Blood Volume and Oxygen Transport

Maternal blood volume increases by 30–40% over the course of normal pregnancy (Fig. 10–1). Red cell volume increases 15%, and plasma volume increases 40–50%, resulting in a dilutional decrease in the hematocrit level from a nonpregnant value of 39–41% to 34–35% during pregnancy.[1] Despite the reduced oxygen-carrying capacity associated with a lower hemoglobin concentration, oxygen transport during pregnancy is actually increased, particularly to organs such as the kidneys and the uterus. This is caused by several factors: (1) Cardiac output increases 40–50% (Fig. 10–2), as a combined result of a 30% increase in stroke volume and a 15% increase in heart rate. (2) An increase in 2,3-diphosphoglycerate causes a rightward shift in the maternal oxyhemoglobin dissociation curve, with P_{50} increasing from 26.7 mmHg to 30.4 mmHg (Table 10–1). This increases the availability of oxygen at the tissue level by decreasing the affinity of hemoglobin for oxygen.

Arterial Pressure

There is a modest decrease in blood pressure during normal pregnancy, although the diastolic pressure tends to return toward nonpregnant levels as

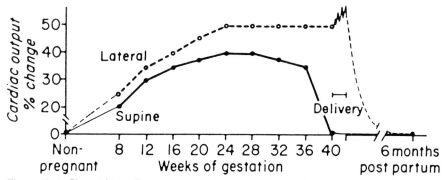

Figure 10–2. Change in cardiac output over the course of normal pregnancy, in the supine and lateral positions. (From Bonica JJ: Obstetric Analgesia and Anesthesia, 2nd Ed. Amsterdam: World Federation of Societies of Anesthesiologists, 1980; 5. With permission.)

term approaches (Fig. 10–3).[2] Blood pressure in the left lateral recumbent position is consistently lower (about 15 mmHg) than it is in the supine position, in both the nonpregnant and the pregnant states. However, this difference is not found when central pressures are measured, indicating that it is due to the elevated position of the brachial artery relative to the heart. This positional difference should be considered when evaluating blood pressure in a recumbent patient, as after epidural block.

The supine position has profound effects on cardiovascular function as the parturient approaches term, as the gravid uterus impairs blood return to the right side of the heart from the lower body. Stroke volume and, hence, cardiac output decrease (Fig. 10–2), and some patients develop symptoms of shock (nausea, vomiting, pallor, sweating, decreased level of consciousness) if the obstruction is not relieved. This obstruction to vena cava flow by the gravid uterus is referred to as the supine hypotensive syndrome, and it is usually effectively treated by turning the patient to the left lateral decubitus position.

Table 10–1. P_{50} VALUES IN PREGNANCY

Subjects		P_{50} (mmHg)	
Status	*n*	*Mean*	*SEM**
Nonpregnant	10	26.7	0.11
Pregnant			
1st trimester	10	27.8	0.08
2nd trimester	10	28.8	0.17
At or near term	24	30.4	0.20

* Standard error of the mean.
From Kambam JR, Handte RE, Brown WU, Smith BE: Effect of normal and preeclamptic pregnancies on the oxyhemoglobin dissociation curve. Anesthesiology 1986; 65:427. With permission.

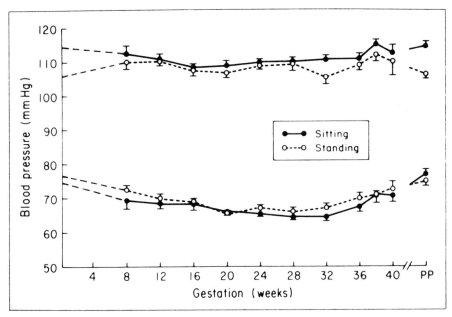

Figure 10–3. Sequential systolic and diastolic blood pressure changes throughout normal pregnancy, in both the sitting and the standing positions ($\pm$ standard error, n = 69). Postpartum (PP) values are used as a baseline, and the dotted lines represent the presumed changes during the first 8 weeks. (From Wilson M, Morganti AA, Zervoudakis I, et al: Blood pressure, the renin-aldosterone system and sex steroids throughout normal pregnancy. Am J Med 1980; 68:97–104. With permission.)

Venous Pressure

Venous pressures in the lower extremities increase sharply after the first trimester, reflecting in part the increased hydrostatic load imposed by the expanded blood volume and also the obstruction to venous return caused by the enlarging uterus (Fig. 10–4). To the degree that these conditions promote venous stasis, they place the mother at risk for embolic complications; pulmonary embolism now ranks as a leading cause of maternal mortality.[3]

Other Cardiovascular Changes

The increased volume of blood flow during pregnancy coupled with decreased maternal blood pressure is accommodated by decreased systemic vascular resistance (SVR). The major component of the decrease in SVR is the low-resistance placental circulation, which receives a large proportion of the increase in cardiac output.

Normal pregnancy is characterized by decreased sensitivity to endogenous vasopressors such as norepinephrine and angiotensin II.[4] Figure 10–5 depicts graphically the dose of angiotensin II required to increase diastolic blood pressure by 20 mmHg over the course of normal pregnancy. At the end of the second trimester, approximately twice the dose of angiotensin II is required compared with nonpregnant controls. The decrease in vaso-

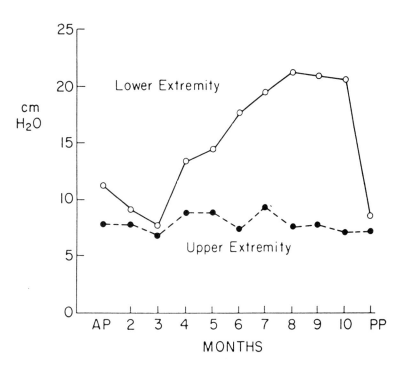

Figure 10–4. Comparison of venous pressures in the upper and lower extremities before (AP), during, and after (PP) pregnancy. (From Brinkman CR: Biologic adaptations to pregnancy. *In* Creasy R, Resnik R [eds]: Maternal-Fetal Medicine. Philadelphia: WB Saunders, 1984; 686.)

pressor sensitivity parallels an increase in plasma renin activity[2] and is important in preventing a hypertensive response to the state of increased vascular volume and plasma renin activity. This decreased sensitivity to pressors is lost in patients with preeclampsia.

Almost all pregnant women develop a grade 2/4 systolic murmur, which is best heard along either the left or the right upper sternal border. Such murmurs are almost always related to increased flow across the pulmonic or aortic outflow tracts or through the mammary vessels.

Total body water increases by 7.5 L during pregnancy, with the increase distributed as described in Table 10–2.[5] Sodium plays a key role in body water balance. Total body sodium increases almost 1000 mmol by increased renal reabsorption of sodium. A balanced increase in both salt and water leaves plasma sodium concentration unchanged.

Colloid osmotic pressure (COP) decreases from a range of 25–28 mmHg in the nonpregnant patient to 21–23 mmHg at term.[6] COP decreases still further following delivery, falling to 13–18 mmHg. Pulmonary capillary wedge pressure (PCWP) is unchanged during normal pregnancy. The net result is a modest decrease in the COP-PCWP gradient and a narrowing of the margin of safety against the development of pulmonary edema.

Cardiovascular Changes during Labor and Delivery

During active labor, cardiac output increases 30–45% over prelabor values as a result of catecholamine-mediated increases in heart rate and stroke volume (see Fig. 10–2). An autotransfusion effect accompanies each

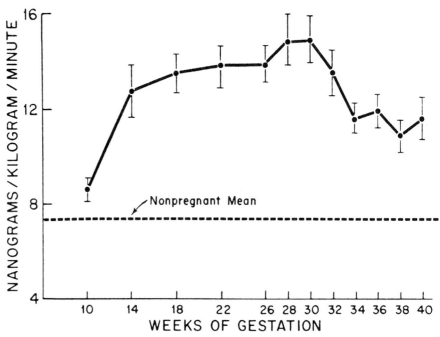

Figure 10–5. Decreased angiotensin II sensitivity over the course of normal pregnancy. The closed circles represent the mean dose of angiotensin II (± standard error of the mean) required to elicit a pressor response of 20 mmHg in diastolic blood pressure in normotensive pregnant patients. The broken line represents the mean for nonpregnant patients. (From Gant NF, Galey GL, Chand S, et al: A study of angiotensin II pressor response throughout primigravid pregnancy. Reproduced from *The Journal of Clinical Investigation*, 1973; 52:2682–2689, by copyright permission of the American Society for Clinical Investigation.)

uterine contraction and results in an additional 10–25% increase in cardiac output as uterine blood (500 ml) is forced into the central circulation. The peak increase in cardiac output occurs immediately after delivery, as uterine involution relieves the obstruction to venous return and also displaces a large volume of uterine blood into the maternal circulation. Since the uterus is now removed as a parallel circuit in the maternal vascular bed, additional maternal vasodilatation is necessary in order to maintain low peripheral

Table 10–2. DISTRIBUTION OF INCREASED TOTAL BODY WATER IN PREGNANCY

Tissue	Volume (L)
Interstitial fluid	1.7
Plasma	1.2
Fetus	2.0
Amniotic fluid	1.2
Uterus, placenta, and breasts	1.4

Modified from Davison JM: Renal hemodynamics and volume homeostasis in pregnancy. Scand J Clin Lab Invest [Suppl] 1984; 169:15–27. With permission of Blackwell Scientific Publications.

vascular resistance and avoid hypertension. Potent vasoconstrictors such as phenylephrine hydrochloride and ergonovine maleate, an oxytocic, can produce severe systemic pulmonary hypertension if administered in the immediate postpartum period. Increases in endogenous catecholamines, as often accompany tracheal suctioning and extubation, can produce similar results. Such hypertension places the patient at risk for both pulmonary edema and cerebral vascular injury, particularly in the presence of underlying disease.

Respiratory Physiology in Normal Pregnancy

Minute ventilation increases 50% during pregnancy to accommodate increased maternal-fetal oxygen consumption and carbon dioxide production. The increase in minute ventilation is due almost entirely to increased tidal volume. Carbon dioxide tension in the blood decreases 30–32 mmHg; the mechanism for this hyperventilation is thought to be related to the effects of increased progesterone upon the respiratory centers in the central nervous system. Serum bicarbonate decreases to about 22 mEq/L, such that arterial pH remains normal.

During labor, hyperventilation accompanying painful contractions may result in pronounced hypocapnia (Pa_{CO_2} less than 20 mmHg) and respiratory alkalemia. Although such acid-base abnormalities have not been shown to directly affect uterine blood flow or fetal oxygenation, the hypoventilation that may occur between contractions when the mother is extremely alkalotic can cause maternal and fetal hypoxia.[7] These ventilatory abnormalities are not seen if effective epidural analgesia is employed during parturition.

Lung volumes and lung capacities show little change with pregnancy, except for a 15–20% decrease in functional residual capacity, which results from cephalad displacement of the diaphragm by the enlarging uterus. Expiratory reserve volume decreases as a result of the expanded tidal volume (Fig. 10–6). There is no change in airway resistance during pregnancy. Forced expiratory volume in 1 second and peak expiratory flow rate are unaffected.

Closing volume refers to the lung volume at which airway closure begins to occur in dependent zones of the lungs, resulting in areas that are perfused but not ventilated. If the lung volume at end-expiration is less than the closing volume, closure occurs and favors an increased alveolar-arterial (A-aD_{O_2}) oxygen gradient. Although there is some controversy in this area, it appears that as many as one half of all pregnant women develop airway closure in the supine position.[8]

The decreased functional residual capacity and the tendency toward airway closure in the supine position have particular significance for the gravida during anesthesia. Both conditions effectively decrease the time to hypoxia in the event of an interruption of oxygen delivery to the alveoli, as might result from airway obstruction associated with induction of general anesthesia. Thus, adequate preoxygenation prior to induction is mandatory. Also, the decrease in functional residual capacity and the increase in minute ventilation accelerate induction of anesthesia with inhalation agents.

Capillary engorgement during pregnancy affects both the nasal and the

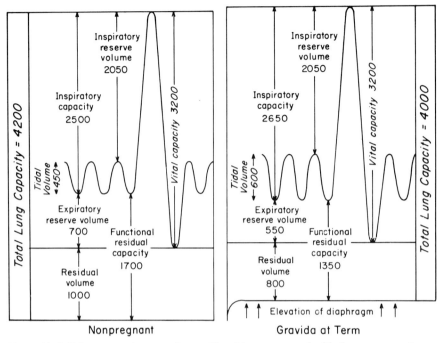

Figure 10–6. Pulmonary volumes and capacities at term compared with the nonpregnant state. (From Bonica JJ: Principles and Practice of Obstetric Analgesia and Anesthesia. Philadelphia: FA Davis, 1967; 24. With permission.)

laryngeal mucosa. This increases the likelihood of bleeding if the nasal route is used for the passage of tubes. Also, the narrowed upper airway may not be able to accommodate standard-size endotracheal tubes; a tube one size smaller than normal is recommended for the pregnant patient.

Renal Physiology in Normal Pregnancy

Renal plasma flow and glomerular filtration rate are 50% above normal by the end of the second trimester, resulting in lower values for blood urea nitrogen (8 mg/dl) and creatinine (0.46 mg/dl). However, during the third trimester, renal plasma flow and glomerular filtration rate tend to return toward nonpregnant levels, primarily as a result of aortic compression by the gravid uterus. Both mild glucosuria and moderate proteinuria (<300 mg/ day) are very common during pregnancy. Neither condition necessarily indicates underlying disease.

Gastrointestinal Physiology in Normal Pregnancy

Pregnancy is associated with a loss of competency of the gastroesophageal junction, leading to reports of "heartburn" and esophagitis in roughly half of all pregnant patients. This effect occurs early in pregnancy and is caused in part by increased levels of progesterone, a smooth muscle relaxant. Gastric acidity and volume are elevated in late pregnancy as a result of increased gastrin levels, probably arising from the placenta. Gastric emptying may be slightly delayed during late pregnancy owing to increased levels of progesterone, decreased levels of the hormone motilin, and mechanical displacement of the pylorus by the uterus. However, it is the pain of labor that has the greatest retardant effect on gastric emptying. All these factors combine to increase the likelihood and the severity of pulmonary aspiration of gastric contents, an event that continues to contribute to maternal morbidity and mortality in association with general anesthesia during pregnancy.

Nervous System Physiology in Normal Pregnancy

Anesthetic requirement or minimum alveolar concentration (MAC) is decreased approximately 40% during pregnancy. This is most likely due to increased maternal endorphins, since the decreased MAC is reversible with naloxone hydrochloride. A smaller amount of agent is also required for epidural and subarachnoid blockades in pregnancy. Although a number of factors have been implicated in this, including engorgement of the epidural veins and acid-base changes in the spinal fluid, the onset of the decrease in anesthetic requirement during early pregnancy adds credence to another explanation: Progesterone alters the nerve membrane to make it more easily penetrated by local anesthetic molecules.[9]

Hemostasis in Normal Pregnancy

The blood of pregnant patients becomes slightly hypercoagulable as gestation progresses, a useful adaptation to decrease blood loss at delivery. Factor I (fibrinogen) levels and factor VIII (antihemophilic factor) activity are increased 50–100%. Other coagulation factors increase slightly or not at all. Although the platelet count decreases 20%, no clinically significant change in bleeding occurs.

MATERNAL MONITORING IN LOW-RISK PREGNANCY

Antepartum Monitoring

Routine antepartum monitoring in low-risk pregnancies consists of periodic examinations with particular attention to blood pressure, weight, uterine size, hematocrit, blood glucose, urinalysis (particularly for protein), and cultures and blood serology for sexually transmitted diseases. Increasingly, ultrasonography is included in routine antepartum monitoring, although the

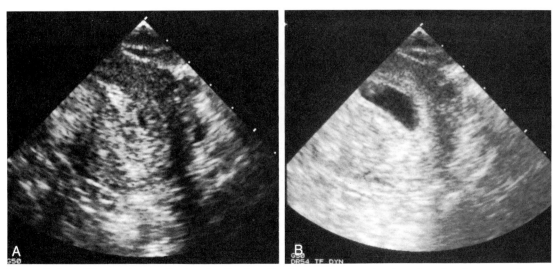

Figure 10–7. *A,* Ultrasound scan allowing visualization of an intrauterine gestational sac 3 weeks after conception. The sac is the small black spot in the center of the scan. The dark shadows on both sides of the sac outline the uterus. *B,* Twelve days later. The gestational sac is much larger, and a tiny fetus is visible. Real-time ultrasonography is able to record the beating of the fetal heart at this early stage.

maternal indications are rather limited. The image produced by ultrasound can identify a gestational sac as early as 3 weeks following conception, and it can help in the diagnosis of an ectopic pregnancy (Fig. 10–7). Placental problems such as placenta previa and abruptio can be diagnosed using ultrasound. If amniocentesis is necessary, ultrasound is required in order to locate fluid for aspiration and to avoid the placenta, the umbilical cord, and the fetus.

Blood pressure monitoring is important, since maternal hypertension in pregnancy is a major risk factor affecting fetal outcome. Unfortunately, this extremely important vital sign is subject to considerable error in both measurement and interpretation.[10] The diastolic pressure appears to be more critical in establishing a diagnosis of pregnancy-induced hypertension, yet this value has the greatest variability of measurement. Even with accurate measurement, blood pressure measurements often fail to correctly identify patients with preeclampsia, as hypertension tends to be a late manifestation of the disease.

Monitoring during Labor and Delivery

Maternal monitoring during labor and delivery in low-risk pregnancies is a controversial subject. Because the incidence of complications in such pregnancies is low, one can use absolutely no monitoring and demonstrate a high probability of a good outcome. In addition, opponents of maternal monitoring criticize the costs and the unnatural atmosphere created by electronic equipment connected to the mother. However, the working hypothesis of this chapter is that effective monitoring improves maternal and fetal outcomes. In addition, our experience is that effective monitoring is not inconsistent with an intimate birthing experience and that the attitude of the caregivers is much more important than the presence of electronic hardware.

Because low-risk pregnancies can abruptly attain high-risk status, and because it is usually impossible to identify those patients in whom this is likely to occur, the following guidelines apply to all healthy parturients. Fetal monitoring is discussed later.

The most important maternal monitor is continuous observation and frequent assessment by an experienced obstetric nurse. A patient complaint of chest pain or shortness of breath without evidence of impaired gas exchange must be recognized as suggestive of amniotic fluid embolism. Unusual abdominal or shoulder pain must be distinguished from normal labor pains, as the former may herald uterine rupture. Frequent visual inspection and occasional digital examination of the vaginal canal are necessary to detect prolapse of the umbilical cord.

The purpose of routine monitoring is to detect abnormal events or trends at a stage early enough to allow intervention; since many obstetric events can happen with great rapidity, frequent monitoring is essential. Blood pressure should be monitored at least every hour in all patients in labor. Low blood pressure due to vena caval obstruction is usually accompanied by clinical signs of light-headedness or nausea. Hypertension is usually asymptomatic. Heart rate and respiratory rate should be monitored along with blood pressure. Temperature is measured every 4 hours. Once maternal membranes are ruptured, the frequency of temperature measurement is increased to every 2 hours for detection of chorioamnionitis. An initial urine examination for protein, glucose, and cellular elements should be performed.

The frequency of uterine contractions can be monitored noninvasively by manual palpation of the abdomen or use of an external tocodynamometer. However, internal monitoring of the uterine cavity is necessary in order to accurately assess the quality of contractions.

Monitoring during Lumbar Epidural Analgesia

Monitoring during lumbar epidural analgesia is focused upon detection of the possible complications of the technique: hypotension, intravascular injection, and subarachnoid injection.

Maternal hypotension is infrequent in patients who are adequately prehydrated (at least 1000 ml of crystalloid), maintained in the lateral recumbent position, and given limited amounts of local anesthetic (8 ml of 0.25% bupivacaine hydrochloride). However, blood pressure should be monitored once every 5 minutes after initiation of lumbar epidural analgesia for 15 minutes, and then once every 15 minutes for the duration of the block. More important than the recorded blood pressure is the response of the patient. Hypotension is usually heralded by nausea, signs of cerebral hypoperfusion, and slowing of the heart rate (right atrial reflex).

Intravascular injection of large amounts of local anesthetic can result in loss of consciousness, seizures, arrhythmias, and cardiovascular collapse. For this reason, 0.75% bupivacaine hydrochloride is no longer considered safe as an epidural agent, although it is still appropriate for subarachnoid anesthesia. Incremental doses (2–3 ml) of 0.25% bupivacaine hydrochloride produce blood levels well below the seizure threshold if accidentally injected intravascularly during performance of an epidural block. An aspiration test should be performed before every injection of local anesthetic, including repeat doses administered through an indwelling catheter. It is possible for a catheter to migrate into an epidural vein at any time. Total failure of an apparently correctly placed epidural catheter is also suggestive of an intravascular position, as are patient complaints of tinnitus, perioral tingling, or mental confusion. The use of epinephrine in an epidural test dose in order to detect an intravascular injection has proponents as well as detractors.

Unsuspected subarachnoid injection of a volume of drug sufficient for epidural blockade can produce total spinal anesthesia, with loss of diaphragmatic function and protective airway reflexes in a patient who probably has a significant volume of acidic gastric fluid. This possibility can be greatly reduced by the incremental administration of small doses of local anesthetic and testing for evidence of subarachnoid block between each injection.

When epidural analgesia is administered by continuous infusion, the lack of need for frequent redosing should not eliminate frequent reassessment by the anesthesiologist. Development of significant lower extremity weakness or sensory loss above the T-8 level warrants slowing of the rate of infusion. Loss of previous analgesia despite an adequate rate of infusion requires aspirating the catheter for blood before administering a supplemental bolus injection, since the catheter may have migrated to an intravascular location. Rapid increases in the level of block may be due to subarachnoid catheter penetration. Infusion pumps must be frequently checked to make sure the correct infusion rate is set and that the correct volume of drug is being delivered. The safety of continuous infusion techniques is increased by the use of the lowest effective concentration of local anesthetic, often supplemented with small concentrations of epidural narcotics.

Monitoring during General Anesthesia

In the healthy parturient receiving general anesthesia for cesarean delivery, the special monitoring considerations include the likelihood of a "full stomach" in all patients, regardless of the timing of the last oral intake; the shorter time to hypoxia if gas exchange is interrupted; potential difficulties in intubation due to obesity, breast engorgement, and airway mucosal swelling; the decreased anesthetic requirement; and the possibility of amniotic fluid embolism. Because it is difficult to monitor gastric contents, gastric acid prophylaxis is recommended in all patients, and may include nonparticulate antacids, histamine$_2$-receptor blockers, and metoclopramide hydrochloride. Essential operating room monitoring includes electrocardiogram, blood pressure, and pulse oximetry. Because of the persistence of maternal deaths due to unsuspected esophageal intubation, capnography is useful for documenting intratracheal placement.

MATERNAL MONITORING IN HIGH-RISK PREGNANCIES

Preeclampsia

Perhaps no other disorder of pregnancy involves such extensive maternal physiologic derangement as that associated with preeclampsia. Most invasive hemodynamic monitoring in obstetric units occurs in patients with preeclampsia.

Definition of Preeclampsia

The hypertensive disorders of pregnancy have been classified by the American College of Obstetricians and Gynecologists as listed in Table 10–3.[11] Hypertension is defined as an increase in blood pressure of 30 mmHg systolic or 15 mmHg diastolic, or a blood pressure greater than 140/90 if the previous blood pressure is unknown. Hypertension occurring before the twentieth week of gestation is classified as chronic hypertension. Preeclampsia is defined as hypertension plus proteinuria or edema, or both, occurring after the twentieth week of gestation. Eclampsia refers to the new onset of seizures in the setting of preeclampsia in the absence of other central nervous system pathology. The degree of hypertension in preeclampsia does not necessarily correlate with the severity of the disease, and 20% of patients who become eclamptic do not have preeclampsia by this definition. On the other hand, some patients are extremely hypertensive, with blood pressure in the range of 250/150.

Preeclampsia is defined by nonspecific clinical signs. As a consequence, the validity of many scientific studies of preeclampsia is questioned. When preeclampsia is defined solely by clinical signs, some patients who do have the disease are excluded and others who do not have preeclampsia are included. For example, in one study 25% of patients with a diagnosis of preeclampsia were found to have evidence of unsuspected chronic renal disease when a renal biopsy was performed.[12] Also, it is possible to have preeclampsia with blood pressure in the normal range or to have preeclampsia without edema or proteinuria.

The following definition, although lacking in brevity, addresses both the

---

Table 10–3. CLASSIFICATION OF
HYPERTENSIVE DISORDERS OF
PREGNANCY

Chronic hypertension
Preeclampsia/eclampsia
Preeclampsia superimposed upon chronic hypertension
Transient hypertension
Unclassified

---

pathophysiologic and the clinical aspects of the disease. Although pre-eclampsia is classified as a hypertensive disorder of pregnancy, this definition makes no direct reference to elevated blood pressure.

Preeclampsia is a condition of reversible systemic arteriolar vasoconstriction initiated in the presence of trophoblastic tissue. Compared with normal pregnancy, preeclampsia is characterized by an imbalance of thromboxane A_2 and prostacyclin, an increased sensitivity to vasopressors, a contracted intravascular volume, and a potential for impaired perfusion of vital tissue beds, including the placenta. It is frequently associated with coagulation disorders. Generalized edema and proteinuria may be present, and the untreated patient is always at risk for convulsions.

Preeclampsia is further categorized into mild and severe forms. Criteria for the severe form include blood pressure >160 mmHg systolic or >110 mmHg diastolic while at bed rest, proteinuria >5 gm in 24 hours (3 + or 4 + on qualitative examination), oliguria (<500 ml urine in 24 hours), cerebral or visual disturbances, epigastric pain, and pulmonary edema or cyanosis. Rather than discrete categories, there is actually a continuum of disease. It is important to be aware of these quantitative signs of preeclampsia. For example, knowledge of urine output and urinary protein during the previous 24 hours is much more clinically useful than a "mild" or "severe" label. Epigastric pain can signal impending rupture of the liver and is an ominous finding irrespective of other signs and symptoms.

Cardiovascular Physiology in Preeclampsia

In preeclampsia, the expected increase in plasma volume is impaired, and the degree of impairment is related to the severity of the disease.[13] Two studies using different techniques found plasma volume increases of 10–15% in patients with preeclampsia compared with increases of 45–50% in normal pregnancies.[1,14] The normal increase in red cell mass is also impaired in preeclampsia, but it parallels the modest increases in plasma volume. The hematocrit level more closely approximates that of the nonpregnant patient.[1] Preeclamptic patients have the same increase in total body water as is seen in normal pregnancies.[15] However, since less of this volume is distributed to the intravascular space, it must be accounted for by abnormal increases in interstitial or intracellular water, or both. Much of this increased volume represents edema fluid that coexists with a state of contracted intravascular volume. The edema is generalized, as opposed to the dependent edema typically seen in normal pregnancy. This generalized edema is one of the main reasons for mismanagement of patients with preeclampsia. The usual treatment of edema is fluid restriction and diuretics, which is inappropriate treatment in preeclampsia. Although these patients are edematous, their intravascular volume is decreased.

Studies of maternal hemodynamics in severe preeclampsia are often obscured by the presence of confounding variables, such as the onset of labor or prior therapy with agents such as magnesium sulfate, intravenous fluids, or antihypertensive medications, all of which have significant effects on maternal hemodynamics. In a very important study, Groenendijk and

Table 10–4. HEMODYNAMIC DATA (MEAN [RANGE]) IN CONTROLS AND PATIENTS WITH SEVERE PREECLAMPSIA

	Preeclamptic Patients (*n* = 10)					Control Subjects (n = 4)
	Initial	*After Volume Expansion*	*p**	*After Vasodilatation*	*p†*	
Diastolic blood pressure (mmHg)	106 (100–120)	102 (90–120)	NS‡	85 (75–100)	<0.01	77 (70–90)
Mean arterial pressure (mmHg)	121 (113–136)	116 (103–136)	<0.02	102 (97–116)	<0.01	95 (93–106)
Heart rate (beats/minute)	100 (90–130)	81 (60–110)	<0.01	82 (70–100)	NS	84 (70–90)
PCWP (mmHg)	3.3 (1–5)	8 (7–10)	<0.01	8 (7–9)	NS	9 (6–12)
SVR (dynes-second/cm^{-5})	1943 (1480–2580)	1284 (1073–1600)	<0.01	947 (782–1028)	<0.01	886 (805–1021)
Cardiac index (L/minute/m^2)	2.75 (1.97–3.33)	3.77 (3.26–4.05)	<0.01	4.40 (3.94–5.00)	<0.01	4.53 (3.96–4.97)

Wilcoxon signed-ranked test (two-tailed):
  * As compared with initial values.
  † As compared with values after volume expansion.
  ‡ NS, Not significant.
  From Groenendijk R, Trimbos JB, Wallenburg HCS: Hemodynamic measurements in preeclampsia: Preliminary observations. Am J Obstet Gynecol 1984; 150:232–236. With permission.

coworkers performed hemodynamic measurements in women with severe preeclampsia prior to the initiation of therapy and the onset of labor.[16] These findings are summarized in Table 10–4. Cardiac index was decreased in preeclampsia patients compared with normal pregnant women. Mean blood pressure and heart rate were both increased approximately 25% compared with controls. SVR was markedly elevated at twice the normal value for pregnancy. PCWP was low in all preeclamptic patients.

Fluid and Vasodilator Therapy. Figure 10–8 graphically depicts the hemodynamic responses of individual patients in the Groenendijk study to sequential therapy of volume expansion and vasodilatation. A synthetic colloid administered to preeclamptic patients until the cardiac index approached 4 L/minute/m^2 with a maximum PCWP of 10 mmHg resulted in the following hemodynamic changes: blood pressure decreased slightly, heart rate decreased 20%, PCWP increased to 8 mmHg, and, most importantly, SVR decreased 34%. Thus, expansion of intravascular volume in preeclampsia, independent of any other therapy, primarily increases cardiac index and decreases SVR.

Vasodilator therapy with dihydralazine after volume expansion further decreased mean blood pressure and increased cardiac index, but it produced no increase in PCWP or heart rate (Fig. 10–8). The improvement in cardiac performance resulted from an additional decrease in SVR to a normal range for pregnancy. Data from such studies have confirmed the physiologic rationale for using volume and vasodilator therapy in the management of patients with preeclampsia. Without an understanding of the underlying pathophysiology of this disease and the response to fluid therapy, administration of several liters of fluid to a massively edematous patient would appear to violate usual standards of medical practice. However, volume expansion is

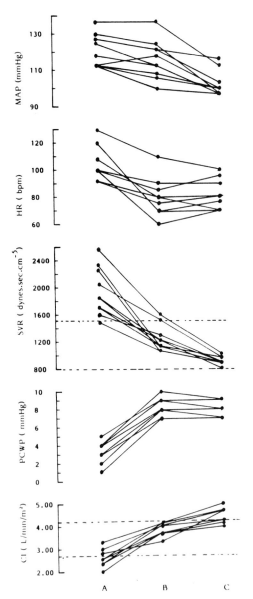

Figure 10–8. Hemodynamic responses in patients with severe preeclampsia (A) prior to treatment; (B) following volume expansion; (C) after vasodilation. (MAP = mean arterial pressure, HR = heart rate, SVR = systemic vascular resistance, PCWP = pulmonary capillary wedge pressure, CI = cardiac index.) (From Groenendijk R, Trimbos JB, Wallenburg, HCS: Hemodynamic measurements in preeclampsia: Preliminary observations. Am J Obstet Gynecol 1984; 150:234. With permission.)

essential prior to treatment of severe hypertension, since vasodilation in a hemoconcentrated, hypovolemic, hypertensive patient may result in cardiovascular collapse.[17]

In a subsequent study, Clark and colleagues confirmed the findings of Groenendijk and coworkers[16] and further characterized the range of hemodynamic abnormalities found in severe preeclampsia.[18] Studies were made in patients who were oliguric (<30 ml of urine/hour for 3 consecutive hours) in spite of maintenance fluid therapy of 100–125 ml/hour and a fluid bolus of 300–500 ml of crystalloid. One subset of patients (category I, Table 10–5) had an average cardiac index of 3.8 L/minute/m², a PCWP of 4 mmHg,

Table 10–5. HEMODYNAMIC DATA FROM NINE PREECLAMPTIC PATIENTS WITH PERSISTENT OLIGURIA

	Patient No.—Category I					Patient No.—Category II			Patient No.—Category III
	1	*2*	*3*	*4*	*5*	*6*	*7*	*8*	*9*
Following Unsuccessful Fluid Challenge									
Mean arterial pressure (mmHg)	120	110	101	118	107	117	129	130	140
PCWP (mmHg)	7	3	4	5	1	9	10	18	18
CVP (mmHg)	6	1	0	2	2	5	9	9	3
Cardiac index (L/minute/m^2)	3.5	4.2	3.5	4.1	4.0	4.8	5.1	6.4	2.6
SVR (dynes-second/cm^{-5})	1378	1245	1393	1497	1135	1093	1043	921	2790
Left ventricular stroke work index	54	90	54	66	59	88	94	89	33
Therapy	Fluid	Fluid	Fluid	Fluid	Fluid	Fluid/hydralazine	Fluid/hydralazine	Nitroglycerin	Hydralazine
Following Therapy and Resolution of Oliguria									
Mean arterial pressure (mmHg)	117	123	120	107	107	110	107	105	104
PCWP (mmHg)	11	7	11	9	11	9	15	2	8
CVP (mmHg)	11	5	4	—	—	8	10	—	—
Cardiac index (L/minute/m^2)	4.6	4.5	4.1	5.0	4.4	5.4	5.1	5.6	4.0
SVR (dynes-second/cm^{-5})	961	1237	1367	1138	1049	884	843	910	1867
Left ventricular stroke work index	66	111	65	59	50	65	60	65	51

From Clark SL, Greenspoon JS, Aldahl D, Phelan JP: Severe preeclampsia with persistent oliguria: Management of hemodynamic subsets. Am J Obstet Gynecol 1986; 154:490–494. With permission.

and an SVR of 1330 dynes-second/cm^{-5}. A diagnosis of hypovolemia was made and, following administration of an additional volume of crystalloid, oliguria resolved in these patients. After additional volume therapy, mean arterial pressure was 115 mmHg; cardiac index, 4.5 L/minute/m^2; PCWP, 10 mmHg; and SVR, 1150 dynes-second/cm^{-5}.[18]

These values are very consistent with those of Groenendijk and co-workers after fluid therapy but prior to the use of vasodilating agents. However, two other subsets of patients identified in the Clark study had persistent oliguria following a fluid challenge with crystalloid. Because one subset (category II) had normal or elevated PCWP and low SVR, it was postulated that selective renal artery vasoconstriction maintained the oliguric state in these patients. The administration of hydralazine hydrochloride and additional fluid was followed by resolution of the oliguria in the patients with normal PCWP. In one patient with a PCWP of 18 mmHg and a cardiac index of 6.4 L/minute/m^2, the diagnosis of volume overload was established, and the patient given an infusion of nitroglycerin to decrease both preload and afterload. Nitroglycerin decreased blood pressure and resolved the oliguria.

Nitroglycerin is usually an inappropriate vasodilator for patients with preeclampsia. It acts on the venous side of the circulatory bed to a greater degree than it acts on the arterial side. The vasoconstriction of preeclampsia is primarily arteriolar. Thus, one could predict that giving nitroglycerin would result in venous dilatation with pooling of blood and decreased return to the heart. Although this may be desirable in a patient who is volume overloaded, it is poorly tolerated by patients with intravascular volume depletion, such as in preeclampsia. Although such therapy may lower blood pressure, it does so primarily because of decreased cardiac output and not decreased SVR. This impairs uterine perfusion and may lead to fetal hypoxia.[19]

The third subset in the Clark study included only one patient but one who helps to illustrate an important aspect of preeclampsia. This oliguric patient had a mean arterial pressure of 140 mmHg, a cardiac index of only 2.6 L/minute/m², a PCWP of 18 mmHg, and an SVR of 2790 dynes-second/ cm[-5]. This patient demonstrated left ventricular dysfunction and was managed with fluid restriction and aggressive afterload reduction with hydralazine hydrochloride.

Colloid Osmotic Pressure. The decrease in colloid osmotic pressure (COP) seen in normal pregnancy is even more pronounced in preeclampsia.[20] This decrease results in a greater likelihood of pulmonary edema, should PCWP increase. Such increases are very common after endotracheal intubation and extubation, and the development of acute pulmonary edema is not uncommon at such times. The COP continues to decline in the immediate postpartum period, a time when there is an increase in the PCWP due to involution of the uterus. Overly zealous volume administration in this period can elevate the PCWP and result in pulmonary edema.[21]

Alteration in Vascular Reactivity. The arteriolar vasoconstriction that characterizes preeclampsia is associated with increased responsivity to vasopressors such as epinephrine, norepinephrine, and angiotensin II, whereas in normal pregnancy vasopressor responsivity decreases.[4] In Figure 10–9, the response of patients with pregnancy-induced hypertension to angiotensin II is compared with the normal response, which was presented in Figure 10–5. This differential sensitivity has been utilized to identify women with preeclampsia prior to the onset of clinical symptoms.[22] However, because of the complexity of infusing angiotensin II and uncertain safety in pregnant patients, this test is not yet widely used clinically. The significance of the increased vasopressor response for the anesthesiologist is that it applies to exogenous vasopressors as well and requires the careful titration of reduced dosages, if such agents are required.

In addition to altered pharmacologic reactivity, the uterine vessels are anatomically altered in preeclampsia. The blood supply to the placenta travels through the uterine muscle via an arterial network that includes the spiral arteries. In normal pregnancy, the trophoblast, which derives from the fertilized ovum and is thus of fetal origin, invades the wall of the spiral arteries and replaces the encircling vascular smooth muscle and the internal elastic lamina. The resultant large-lumen vessels lose the ability to vasoconstrict.

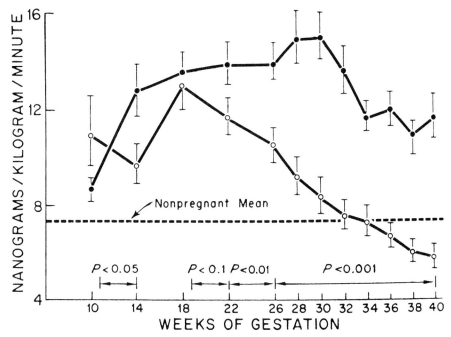

Figure 10–9. Increased angiotensin II sensitivity in patients with preeclampsia. Although normal pregnancy (*closed circles*) is associated with a decreased sensitivity to vasopressors such as angiotensin II, patients with preeclampsia have an increased sensitivity, such that small doses produce a marked pressor response. (From Gant NF, Daley GL, Chand S, et al: A study of angiotensin II pressor response throughout primigravid pregnancy. Reproduced from *The Journal of Clinical Investigation*, 1973; 52:2682–2689, by copyright permission of the American Society for Clinical Investigation.)

Thus, in normal pregnancy, the uterus becomes a very low resistance vascular bed with minimum ability to vasoconstrict and autoregulate blood flow in response to changes in maternal blood pressure. The fact that uterine flow is normally pressure-dependent is why so much attention is paid to preventing even modest hypotension during anesthesia for the pregnant patient.

However, in preeclampsia, the invasion of the spiral arteries by the trophoblast does not occur, and the vessels maintain their encircling smooth muscle and the ability to vasoconstrict. In preeclampsia, uterine perfusion is primarily a function of uterine vascular resistance. Blood pressure may be markedly elevated, but if resistance is increased to a greater extent, uterine flow decreases.

Therapy of Maternal Hypertension. A lack of understanding of these relationships between maternal blood pressure and uterine flow may lead to suboptimal management in patients with preeclampsia. The standard of practice on many obstetric services is that maternal hypertension is not treated until the diastolic pressure exceeds 110 mmHg; hypertension is maintained in order to "ensure adequate uterine perfusion."[23] However, in preeclampsia, hypertension does not maintain adequate uterine perfusion. Despite elevated blood pressure, uterine blood flow is reduced 50% and, in severe cases, reduced 70%;[24] the highest blood pressures are often associated with the lowest uterine blood flows. Decreasing maternal blood pressure by decreasing peripheral vascular resistance, using vasodilating agents such as hydralazine hydrochloride or epidural blockade, also dilates the uterine vessels such that placental flow is not impaired so long as maternal hypotension is avoided.[25]

Allowing the maternal blood pressure to remain elevated has consequences for the mother as well as the fetus. The upper limit of cerebral blood flow autoregulation occurs at a mean perfusion pressure of 150 mmHg; above this the blood-brain barrier begins to break down and cerebral injury results. Many patients with severe preeclampsia have mean pressures close to this limit and exceed it during painful labor. Also, untreated hypertension increases the workload on the left ventricle. It is not uncommon for preeclampsia patients to develop acute left-sided heart failure during the stress of labor or in association with endotracheal intubation and surgery. Sodium nitroprusside is the drug of choice for acute control of severe hypertension in preeclampsia and has no detectable adverse effects on the fetus.[26,27] Nitroprusside has seen limited use in obstetrics, in part because of misinterpretation of animal studies in which supraclinical doses were given to pregnant ewes in order to produce acidosis in fetuses.[28] Thus, antihypertensive therapy improves the margin of maternal safety and, as discussed later, may actually increase uterine and fetal blood flow.

Renal Physiology in Preeclampsia

Renal function in preeclampsia is affected adversely by numerous factors. Decreased cardiac output, discussed previously, decreases renal blood flow and glomerular filtration rate. There may also be selective renal artery vasoconstriction, further impairing renal perfusion.[18,29] There may also be direct injury to the glomeruli and renal tubules.

Renal tubular injury can be estimated by following uric acid levels, a substance handled by the tubule.[30] The injury to the glomerulus is reflected by the degree of proteinuria, defined as 0.1 gm/L of protein in a random sample or 0.3 gm/L in a 24-hour specimen. Severe preeclampsia is diagnosed in the presence of proteinuria of 5 gm or more in a 24-hour period. Fetal mortality is directly related to the degree of proteinuria and the uric acid levels, suggestive of a common etiology of injury to both the kidney and the placenta. However, the presence and severity of proteinuria do not correlate with the occurrence of seizures (eclampsia), suggesting a different mechanism for central nervous system injury.

Decreased urine output is a usual feature of preeclampsia, and it correlates with the severity of the disease. In most patients, volume and vasodilator therapy, guided by invasive cardiovascular monitoring when required, corrects the prerenal causes of oliguria. If this does not correct the problem, the diagnosis of acute renal failure must be considered. This diagnosis may be difficult to establish, since urinary diagnostic indexes, such as the fractional excretion of sodium and urinary sodium concentration, may not correlate with measurements of effective intravascular volume as determined by the PCWP.[29] Management of a preeclamptic patient in renal failure is very challenging and usually demands immediate delivery of the infant and, possibly, renal dialysis.

Central Nervous System in Preeclampsia

Generalized central nervous system irritability is associated with preeclampsia and may be documented by the presence of hyperreflexia or clonus on physical examination. Part of the therapy of the disease involves minimizing stimulation of the patient in order to decrease the risk of convulsions. Seizures may occur in patients with seemingly mild disease in terms of blood pressure, proteinuria, and edema. Although patients with preeclampsia are at risk for cerebral edema, edema is probably not the etiology of the convulsions. Autopsy findings usually show only petechial hemorrhages. It is possible that seizures are due to platelet microthrombi blocking tiny capillaries in the brain and increasing central nervous system irritability on an ischemic basis. The standard seizure prophylaxis in the United States is magnesium sulfate. Since magnesium also affects the neuromuscular junction, reduced dosages of both depolarizing and nondepolarizing neuromuscular-blocking drugs are indicated.

Should a seizure occur, it can be terminated with a small dose of barbiturate or benzodiazepine. Oxygen by mask should be given and cricoid pressure maintained to protect the airway. This is one instance in which succinylcholine chloride and an endotracheal tube may not be indicated. The extreme hypertensive response associated with tracheal intubation in an unanesthetized patient may pose a greater risk to the mother than aspiration does, and the seizure can usually be terminated rapidly using intravenous drugs. Although gastric acid neutralization therapy is not standard, it would seem prudent to administer some form of it to all patients with preeclampsia, since they are at risk for convulsions.

One large series of hypertensive pregnant patients was managed during labor with lumbar epidural analgesia and no anticonvulsant medications.[31] In 1106 patients, there were no convulsions in any patient treated with effective lumbar epidural analgesia. This is a considerably better result than that experienced with magnesium. In the study, two patients experienced seizures after catheter placement but before onset of analgesia. Four patients had seizures in the postpartum period, hours after the termination of the local anesthetic effect. Although the authors do not so speculate, it may be that this beneficial effect, if real, relates to epinephrine effects on platelet aggregation. Epinephrine is a well-known activator of platelet aggregation, a process that may contribute to small vessel occlusion and organ ischemia in preeclampsia. Lumbar epidural analgesia decreases epinephrine concentrations and may favorably affect platelet function.

Hemostasis in Preeclampsia

Preeclampsia is associated with a wide range of coagulation abnormalities, with the most extreme being disseminated intravascular coagulation. The HELLP syndrome of *h*emolysis, *l*iver enzyme abnormalities, and *l*ow *p*latelets is also well recognized. However, platelet dysfunction is the most frequent abnormality. Bone marrow analysis demonstrates increased platelet production in preeclampsia, but this may still be insufficient to keep up with increased platelet consumption. A falling platelet count is often an ominous sign in a patient with preeclampsia. There may also be a qualitative platelet defect, as patients may have prolonged bleeding times in spite of adequate numbers of platelets. Platelet activation, which results in aggregation and consumption, is favored by the imbalance between thromboxane and prostacyclin and by increased sympathetic nervous tone associated with elevated plasma catecholamines.

Plasma epinephrine levels are elevated during labor in both normal and preeclampsia patients. Epidural analgesia during labor decreases maternal epinephrine levels, which may have a favorable effect upon platelet aggregation.[32] Although it is unstudied and unproved, effective epidural analgesia prior to the onset of labor may decrease the likelihood of the development of severe platelet dysfunction.

Impaired platelet function increases the risk of an epidural or subarachnoid hematoma, as do other coagulation defects. There are insufficient data to even suggest the risk associated with epidural analgesia and anesthesia in preeclamptic patients with clotting abnormalities. One case report describes epidural bleeding (but no hematoma) in a patient with the HELLP syndrome and a bleeding time in excess of 15 minutes in association with an epidural catheter.[33] No treatment was required. It is also important to recognize that epidural hematomas may occur spontaneously in patients with impaired clotting mechanisms, so that the avoidance of an epidural needle does not prevent this complication. It is critical to recognize the symptoms of back pain in association with neurologic deficits in the legs and urogenital region, since prompt evacuation of an intraspinal hematoma is crucial in order to avoid permanent injury. Long-term neurologic sequelae are unlikely as long as high-risk patients are properly observed and evaluated.

There is no consensus on the minimum acceptable platelet count prior to performing regional anesthesia, in part because platelet function depends upon both quantity and quality. A bleeding time is a more meaningful test, since it is an *in vivo* test of platelet function. Severely thrombocytopenic patients may require platelet transfusions prior to surgery. If platelet infusion restores the bleeding time to normal, there is less risk of bleeding complications associated with epidural anesthesia. Prolonged bleeding times are frequently found in patients with otherwise normal coagulation profiles. Since bleeding times are not routinely obtained in most patients with preeclampsia, it is likely that thousands of patients with prolonged bleeding times have received regional anesthesia without reported complications. Thus, although there is an increased risk of epidural bleeding in patients with disorders of coagulation, the risk is very small and must be weighed against the risks associated with general anesthesia in patients with preeclampsia, which include pulmonary edema, heart failure, and cerebral hemorrhage as well as the ever-present risk of pulmonary aspiration of gastric contents.

The placenta in normal pregnancy produces roughly equal amounts of thromboxane A_2 and prostacyclin. In the setting of preeclampsia, placental prostacyclin production is decreased and thromboxane A_2 production increased, with a resulting thromboxane/prostacyclin ratio of 7:1.[34] This imbalance favors platelet aggregation, vasoconstriction, decreased uteroplacental blood flow, and increased uterine activity, factors detrimental to both

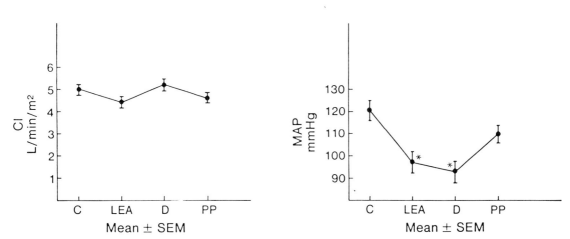

Figure 10–10. Cardiac index (*left*) and mean arterial pressure (*right*) in patients with severe preeclampsia at control (C), following lumbar epidural anesthesia (LEA), at delivery (D), and 2 hours postpartum (PP). * indicates statistical significance, $p \leq 0.05$. (SEM = standard error of the mean.) (Reprinted with permission from the International Anesthesia Research Society from Severe preeclampsia: Hemodynamic effects of lumbar epidural anesthesia, by Newsome LR, Bramwell RS, Curling PE, Anesthesia and Analgesia, 1986; 65:32.)

fetus and mother. However, the imbalance may be reversible with drugs affecting prostaglandin synthesis. Several small studies have suggested that low-dosage aspirin (60 mg/day) prevents or ameliorates the symptoms of pre-eclampsia in women identified to be at high risk, if therapy is begun early in the course of the disease. At this aspirin dosage, there is no clinically significant impairment of hemostatic mechanisms in either the mother or the fetus. In the near future, preeclampsia may become a treatable disease as monitoring is directed at earlier detection with routine screening for prostaglandin metabolites.

Cardiovascular Physiology during Epidural Analgesia and Anesthesia in Preeclamptic Patients. Epidural blockade has the potential for producing profound hypotension in patients with severe preeclampsia, as it does in any patient with a severe intravascular volume deficit. This concern has led to a blanket condemnation of epidural blockade by some,[35] whereas others have demonstrated that the risk of serious hypotension can be greatly reduced by intravascular volume repletion prior to performance of the block. This is true for both lumbar epidural analgesia for labor,[36] with a segmental block to T-8–10, and epidural anesthesia for cesarean section,[37–39] with a T-4–6 level.

Figures 10–10 and 10–11 illustrate the modest and beneficial decrease in maternal blood pressure following epidural blockade in adequately hydrated preeclampsia patients. As long as cardiac filling pressures are maintained, there is no significant decrease in cardiac output to impair uterine perfusion. On the contrary, lumbar epidural analgesia has the unique potential to actually increase uterine blood flow while decreasing maternal blood pressure. Most vasodilators affect both the maternal systemic and the uterine circulations fairly equally, so that the flow relationships remain constant.[25,40] Lumbar epidural analgesia selectively blocks the sympathetic innervation of the uterus without blocking sympathetic innervation of other

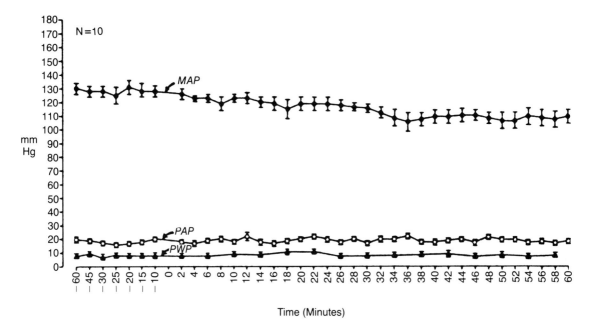

Figure 10–11. Hemodynamic response to lumbar epidural anesthesia for cesarean section in patients with severe preeclampsia. Injection of epidural anesthetic was at time zero. *Closed circles* represent mean arterial pressure (MAP); *open circles*, pulmonary artery pressure (PAP); *solid squares*, pulmonary wedge pressure (PWP). (From Hodgkinson R, Husain FJ, Hayashi RH: Systemic and pulmonary blood pressure during caesarean section in parturients with gestational hypertension. Can Anaesth Soc J 1980; 27:392. With permission.)

vascular beds, particularly the splanchnic bed. This preferentially reduces uterine vascular resistance relative to maternal SVR, thereby increasing the fraction of flow through the low-resistance bed. In one study of severe preeclamptics in labor, lumbar epidural analgesia resulted in a 77% increase in intervillous blood flow over controls, when maternal blood pressure was maintained at pre–lumbar epidural analgesia levels (Table 10–6).[36]

Cardiovascular Physiology during General Anesthesia in Preeclamptic Patients. General anesthesia is associated with potentially dangerous increases in maternal blood pressure and cardiac filling presssures. The most extreme elevations are related to tracheal intubation and extubation, an absolute requirement in anesthetized pregnant patients. Hodgkinson and coworkers documented a 45 mmHg increase in mean arterial pressure and a 20 mmHg increase in PCWP during both intubation and extubation of the trachea in patients with severe preeclampsia (Fig. 10–12).[38] Severe and abrupt pulmonary and systemic hypertension of this magnitude has been associated with acute heart failure, pulmonary edema, and cerebral hemorrhage in patients with preeclampsia.

Monitoring in Patients with Preeclampsia

The risk/benefit ratio of invasive cardiovascular monitoring in patients with preeclampsia, as well as with other cardiovascular disorders, must reflect the skill and experience of the physicians and nursing staff as well as

Table 10–6. EPIDURAL ANALGESIA IN SEVERE PREECLAMPSIA: INTERVILLOUS BLOOD FLOW, MATERNAL BLOOD PRESSURE, AND NEONATAL APGAR SCORES

Patient	Gestational Age (wk)	Birth Weight (gm)	Apgar Score		Blood Pressure (mmHg)		IVBF* (ml/minute/dl)		Percentage Change of IVBF
			1 Minute	5 Minute	Before Epidural	After Epidural	Before Epidural	After Epidural	
1	40	3600	9	9	150/100	145/90	197	471	+139
2	39	2200	8	9	160/110	160/100	72	68	−6
3	39	2980	9	9	170/105	160/90	292	352	+21
4	37	3000	8	8	140/100	130/80	55	170	+209
5	38	3180	9	9	150/100	145/110	121	227	+88
6	39	2600	9	9	140/70	150/80	273	358	+31
7	38	3050	8	10	180/110	170/110	430	697	+62
8	38	3080	9	9	140/90	150/100	128	282	+120
9	38	3140	8	9	170/130	200/140	196	257	+31
Mean ± SD	38.4 ± 0.9	2980 ± 390	8.6 ± 0.5	9.0 ± 0.5	155/100 ± 15/16	155/100 ± 20/19	196 ± 120	320 ± 183	+77 ± 69

* IVBF = intervillous blood flow.

From Jouppila P, Jouppila R, Hollmen A, Koivula A: Lumbar epidural analgesia to improve intervillous blood flow during labor in severe preeclampsia. Reprinted with permission from The American College of Obstetricians and Gynecologists. (Obstetrics and Gynecology, vol. no. 59, 1982, pp 158–161.)

369

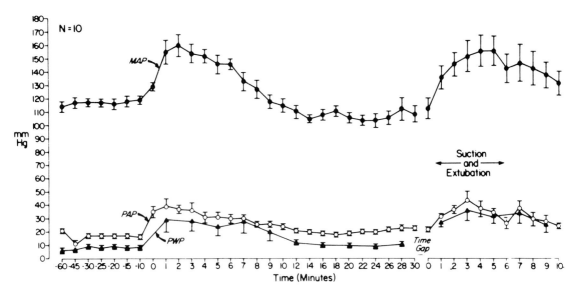

Figure 10–12. Hemodynamic responses in patients with severe preeclampsia undergoing cesarean section under general anesthesia. The first zero indicates induction; the second, suction and extubation. (MAP = mean arterial pressure, PAP = pulmonary artery pressure, PWP = pulmonary wedge pressure.) (From Hodgkinson R, Husain FJ, Hayashi RH: Systemic and pulmonary blood pressure during caesarean section in parturients with gestational hypertension. Can Anaesth Soc J 1980; 27:392. With permission.)

the severity of the patient's disease. Placement of intra-arterial and pulmonary artery catheters in a patient with preeclampsia is not warranted, regardless of her status, if the obstetric and anesthetic decision makers are either unable or unwilling to incorporate the information to be obtained into the medical and anesthetic management of the patient. Likewise, intra-arterial and pulmonary artery catheters should not be used without the continuous presence of personnel experienced in recognizing the significance of various arterial waveforms.

Central Venous Pressure. In patients with coagulation problems, introduction of central venous and pulmonary arterial catheters through the median basilic vein in the antecubital fossa or an external jugular vein is preferable to an internal jugular vein approach in order to minimize the risk of a neck hematoma in the event of carotid artery cannulation (see Chapter 5). Although the blood of preeclamptic patients is often hypocoagulable, as compared with the hypercoagulability of normal pregnancy, axillary vein thrombosis may occur with brachial venous catheters.

A central venous catheter is important in patients with moderate to severe preeclampsia in which there is reduced urine output. If the initial central venous pressure (CVP) is low (0–5 mmHg), it is appropriate to assume that the oliguric patient has persistent intravascular volume depletion and to continue with fluid and arteriolar vasodilator therapy. It is inappropriate to use volume therapy alone in the face of persistent oliguria, as demonstrated in the study of Clark and colleagues.[18] If fluid and vasodilator therapy are ineffective in establishing adequate urine output, a pulmonary artery catheter is warranted in order to guide further therapy.

Pulmonary Artery Pressure. Although most oliguric patients have low to normal PCWP, a minority have markedly increased wedge pressures in spite of low CVPs. These patients have left-sided heart dysfunction and need careful hemodynamic management. If the initial CVP in an oliguric patient is high (>15 mmHg), a diagnosis of left-sided heart failure must be considered, and a pulmonary artery catheter is necessary for further assessment and management. It must be stressed that the more severe the preeclampsia, the lower the degree of correlation between CVP and PCWP, and a low CVP does not preclude volume overload.[21]

Disparities between right-sided and left-sided heart filling pressures may occur in the absence of any underlying cardiac abnormality. For example, an increase in SVR may initiate increases in left ventricular and left atrial pressures and PCWP as higher filling volumes are utilized to maintain cardiac output by moving further out on the Starling curve. However, in preeclampsia, pulmonary vascular resistance is not normally increased despite sharply increased SVR. Thus, right-sided cardiac output remains equal to left-sided output without a change in cardiac filling pressures. Although CVP may not correlate with PCWP in patients with preeclampsia, CVP may be a better estimate of effective intravascular volume than PCWP, which may be more reflective of SVR.[17] Compared with CVP, PCWP provides a better estimate of the risk of pulmonary edema, particularly if the COP is known.[41]

A pulmonary artery catheter is recommended for management of preeclamptic patients with pulmonary edema. This allows more accurate determination of the cause of the pulmonary edema and the underlying hemodynamic state. Increased PCWP and cardiac output with decreased to normal SVR, particularly in the immediate postpartum period and with a history of aggressive fluid therapy, suggest volume overload. Increased PCWP and SVR with decreased cardiac output are consistent with acute left-sided heart failure. A low PCWP and a normal COP can be associated with pulmonary edema on the basis of altered capillary permeability.[20]

Volume loading prior to epidural or spinal anesthesia is guided by CVP in the absence of oliguria. However, if CVP fails to increase after administration of 1500 ml of crystalloid and the catheter position is confirmed, it is likely that there is poor correlation between the CVP and the PCWP. Further fluid management should be based upon clinical assessment or a pulmonary artery catheter.

Arterial Pressure. In severe preeclampsia, an in-dwelling arterial catheter is warranted for beat-to-beat assessment of maternal blood pressure during either regional or general anesthesia. Both tracheal intubation and extubation may cause extreme systemic and pulmonary hypertension (see Fig. 10–12); direct arterial monitoring is necessary in order to guide antihypertensive therapy with rapid-acting agents. During epidural or spinal anesthesia, direct arterial monitoring allows for earlier correction of possible hypotension. Such prompt therapy is mandated in the setting of a compromised fetus with minimal cardiovascular reserve, as is the usual case in severe preeclampsia.

Noninvasive Monitors. In the future, noninvasive cardiovascular monitoring will probably be increasingly used in patients with preeclampsia. This approach offers desirable benefits in terms of patient safety, particularly in patients with coagulation defects. In oliguric patients with preeclampsia, noninvasive monitoring of cardiac output and intrathoracic fluid volumes may be able to reliably differentiate the patient with intravascular hypovolemia from the patient with myocardial dysfunction. Current technologies for obtaining this information include Doppler ultrasound measurement of blood velocity combined with M-mode echocardiography[42,43] and electrical bioimpedance devices.[44]

Maternal Heart Disease

The normal hemodynamic changes associated with pregnancy may have severe adverse consequences for patients with cardiac disease, even those with previously asymptomatic lesions. Increases in blood volume (40–50%) and cardiac output (40–50% during pregnancy and 80% during labor and delivery) may precipitate pulmonary edema and heart failure in patients with mitral valve disease, whereas patients with aortic stenosis or right-to-left shunt are most imperiled by systemic hypotension. Thus, in managing patients with cardiac disease, it is essential that the exact nature of the heart lesion be known, since inappropriate intrapartum management can result in sudden cardiac decompensation in a patient who has tolerated pregnancy quite well. The underlying pathophysiology of various cardiac lesions, as well as their expected physiologic effects during pregnancy, labor, and delivery, and the consequences of anesthetic interventions are discussed later.

Indications for Invasive Cardiovascular Monitoring in Parturients with Heart Disease

Since most of the increase in cardiac output occurs before the twenty-fourth week of gestation, the parturient presenting with a viable fetus has already undergone a prolonged and quite strenuous cardiac stress test. The response of the mother to the stress of pregnancy can be ascertained by the obstetric anesthesiologist from a careful history and physical examination. In many cases, this information alone is sufficient to determine the need for invasive cardiovascular monitoring. Asymptomatic patients who have had an uneventful pregnancy without worsening of their cardiopulmonary status can be expected to tolerate the additional stress of labor and delivery *as long as obstetric and anesthetic management is appropriate for the specific cardiac lesion.* In such cases, invasive hemodynamic monitoring is usually not required. Some suggested exceptions to this rule include any parturient with a right-to-left shunt, primary pulmonary hypertension, severe coarctation of the aorta, or severe aortic stenosis.[45]

Use of data obtained from a pulmonary artery catheter requires an understanding of the limitations inherent in measurements made in patients with cardiac abnormalities. In many cases, trends provide more reliable information than any one absolute value, underscoring the importance of frequent observation and early recognition of ominous trends.

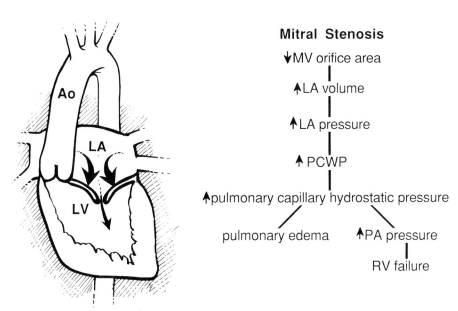

Mitral Stenosis

↓MV orifice area

↑LA volume

↑LA pressure

↑ PCWP

↑pulmonary capillary hydrostatic pressure

pulmonary edema   ↑PA pressure

RV failure

Figure 10–13. Mitral stenosis (diastole). Restricted flow through the narrowed mitral valve orifice results in elevated blood volumes in the cardiopulmonary circuit proximal to the mitral valve. (MV = mitral valve, LA = left atrium, PCWP = pulmonary capillary wedge pressure, PA = pulmonary artery, RV = right ventricle, LV = left ventricle, Ao = aorta.)

Mitral Stenosis

Pathophysiology. In mitral stenosis, there is an impediment to filling of the left ventricle due to narrowing of the mitral valve orifice (Fig. 10–13). The normal gradient of 3–5 mmHg across the valve is increased several fold, and gradients in excess of 25 mmHg are present in patients with severe mitral stenosis. The obstruction to left atrial outflow increases pressures in the left atrium, pulmonary veins, and pulmonary capillaries.

Pulmonary congestion accounts for the symptoms of dyspnea and orthopnea that occur as the disease progresses in severity. Chronic cardiac decompensation usually presents as right ventricular failure with hepatic congestion. Thus, the presence of right ventricular hypertrophy on electrocardiogram carries a significant risk of pregnancy-related cardiac failure. Acute volume overload in pregnant patients with mild to moderate stenosis is more likely to overstress the left ventricle.[46]

Atrial contraction contributes 33% of left ventricular filling in mitral stenosis, compared with 20% in normal hearts. Thus, sinus rhythm is important for maintaining cardiac output. The distention of the left atrium in mitral stenosis predisposes patients to atrial fibrillation, which can rapidly result in pulmonary edema and cardiac insufficiency for two reasons: the loss of atrial contraction, and decreased diastolic filling time if the heart rate increases during atrial fibrillation. Also, the sluggish flow of blood through the distended left atrium favors thrombus formation. The risk of systemic embolization is further enhanced by the presence of atrial fibrillation.

Patients with mitral stenosis may not tolerate the normal physiologic changes of pregnancy, particularly the increase in pulmonary blood volume.

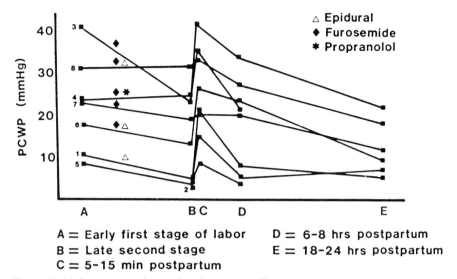

Figure 10-14. Intrapartum changes in pulmonary capillary wedge pressure (PCWP) in eight patients with mitral stenosis. Delivery is consistently associated with an abrupt increase in PCWP and the risk of pulmonary edema. (From Clark SL, Phelan JP, Greenspoon J, et al: Labor and delivery in the presence of mitral stenosis: Central hemodynamic observations. Am J Obstet Gynecol 1986; 67:157–168; as reproduced in Mangano DT: Anesthesia for the pregnant cardiac patient. *In* Shnider SM, Levinson G [eds]: Anesthesia for Obstetrics, 2nd Ed. Baltimore: Williams & Wilkins Co., 1987.)

Labor, delivery, and the immediate puerperium are considered the times of maximum risk. Tachycardia during painful uterine contractions is poorly tolerated. Each uterine contraction increases central blood volume by 15–25%, worsening any pulmonary congestion. The further distention of the left atrium by this increased blood volume increases the probability of atrial fibrillation. The greatest increase in central blood volume occurs immediately after delivery, as a result of uterine involution and relief of vena caval obstruction. Clark and colleagues documented a 10 mmHg (±6 mmHg) mean increase in PCWP after vaginal delivery in a series of patients with severe mitral stenosis (Fig. 10–14).[47] However, the range (0–18 mmHg) was wide, and the greatest increases occurred in patients beginning labor with the highest wedge pressures. Cunningham and coworkers reported four patients with mitral stenosis among a series of patients with unsuspected and asymptomatic cardiac disease who developed peripartum congestive heart failure.[48] All four patients with mitral stenosis became symptomatic *after* delivery (within 48 hours).

Monitoring. Parturients with mild mitral stenosis without episodes of pulmonary edema or atrial fibrillation do not require invasive monitoring during labor and delivery. However, the electrocardiogram should be monitored continually during this period, and equipment for direct current cardioversion must be available. Volume status must be carefully assessed in the postpartum period. All patients with mitral stenosis should be considered to be at risk for development of pulmonary edema, regardless of the severity of their lesion. Pulse oximetry is useful for early detection of worsening pulmonary congestion in such patients.

Symptomatic patients should be monitored with both a peripheral arterial and a pulmonary artery catheter. In Clark and colleagues' study, very poor correlation was found between CVP and PCWP, with differences of 10 mmHg or greater in 85% of patients studied.[47] Clark recommends maintaining the PCWP in the 14 mmHg range.[49] This value is based upon predicted increases in PCWP following delivery and the observation that clinically significant pulmonary edema does not usually occur with wedge pressures below 28–30 mmHg. Attaining a PCWP of 14 mmHg may require diuresis in some patients, but this must be done with extreme caution, as the PCWP does not accurately reflect left ventricular filling volumes in the presence of mitral stenosis.[50] Treating increased PCWP when in fact the left ventricular end-diastolic pressure is decreased may severely impair cardiac output. Many patients with mitral stenosis require elevated left atrial pressures for adequate ventricular filling. Therapeutic alterations in intravascular volume should be guided by additional information, such as blood pressure and cardiac output.

Anesthetic Considerations. Because of the severity of the consequences of atrial fibrillation, pregnant patients with mitral stenosis usually receive prophylactic digitalis. Drugs causing tachycardia, such as atropine, ketamine hydrochloride, and pancuronium bromide, should be avoided. If tachycardia does occur, it may be treated with verapamil or beta-blocking drugs such as propranolol or esmolol.

Epidural analgesia is beneficial for preventing increases in heart rate associated with painful contractions. Perineal analgesia blocks the urge to push, a beneficial effect since Valsalva maneuvers are detrimental. The venodilatation resulting from epidural anesthesia is likewise helpful in reducing central blood volume.[51] Hypotension should be treated with a pure alpha$_1$ agonist such as phenylephrine hydrochloride, since ephedrine produces tachycardia. The addition of epinephrine to solutions of local anesthetics for epidural injection may also increase the risk of tachycardia.

General anesthesia utilizing a standard rapid intubation sequence and a potent inhalational agent is acceptable only for patients with mild disease. This regimen may precipitate rapid cardiac decompensation as a result of tachycardia and increased pulmonary artery pressure and worsen pre-existing right ventricular dysfunction. Patients with severe stenosis and cardiac compromise requiring general anesthesia are more safely managed with topical anesthesia of the pharynx and trachea (such as regional blockade of the glossopharyngeal and superior laryngeal nerves),[52] a narcotic induction, and tracheal intubation. Although such an approach may be associated with a slightly increased risk of pulmonary aspiration of gastric contents, this risk can be decreased by proper antacid prophylaxis and maintenance of cricoid pressure until the airway is secure. Antagonism of narcotics in the infant may be required.

Pulse oximetry is particularly important if general endotracheal anesthesia is utilized, because of the potential for rapid worsening of pulmonary function. Pulse oximetry is also useful for evaluation of adequacy of oxygenation prior to extubation of the trachea postoperatively.

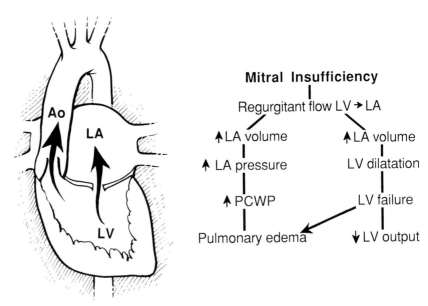

Figure 10–15. Mitral insufficiency (systole). Part of the left ventricular output is ejected in a retrograde manner back into the left atrium, resulting in increased blood volume in the pulmonary venous circuit. During diastole, this extra volume overloads the left ventricle, resulting in chamber enlargement. (LV = left ventricle, LA = left atrium, PCWP = pulmonary capillary wedge pressure, Ao = aorta.)

Mitral Regurgitation

Pathophysiology. Incompetence of the mitral valve permits regurgitant flow from the left ventricle into the left atrium (Fig. 10–15). The compliant atrial walls readily distend to accommodate the increased blood volume, and, until late in the course of the disease, there is no significant pressure increase in the pulmonary vascular bed. Forward flow through the aortic valve depends on the resistance across this valve compared with the resistance across the incompetent mitral valve. Factors that lower SVR tend to favor forward flow and improve cardiac output. For this reason, normal pregnancy is usually well tolerated by individuals with isolated mitral regurgitation. However, parturients with longstanding mitral regurgitation may have increased left atrial pressures and left ventricular dysfunction based on chronic volume overload. The elevated left atrial pressures are transmitted to the pulmonary circulation, predisposing the patient to pulmonary congestion. In such patients, labor can be quite hazardous, since the enhanced sympathetic nervous system activity increases SVR and worsens the regurgitant flow, and further pulmonary blood volume overload occurs with the autotransfusion associated with each uterine contraction. This combination of factors may precipitate acute left-sided heart failure and pulmonary edema.

Atrial fibrillation may occur in mitral regurgitation, but it has less adverse effect on cardiac output than that seen in patients with mitral stenosis. Tachycardia decreases regurgitant volume.

Monitoring. Monitoring concerns are similar to those for mitral stenosis.

Figure 10–16. Intrapartum hemodynamic changes in a parturient with mitral and aortic valvular disease. For pulmonary and systemic arterial pulse pressures, the upper border of the shaded area represents systolic pressure and the lower border represents diastolic pressure. Note that from time 22:20 to 23:20 central venous pressure (CVP) (*solid triangles*) was essentially unchanged, and pulmonary capillary wedge pressure (PCWP) (*open circles*) almost doubled, increasing from 19 torr to 37 torr. (Reprinted with permission from the International Anesthesia Research Society from Anesthetic management of a parturient with mitral and aortic valvular disease. by Lynch C, Rizor R, Anesthesia and Analgesia, 1982; 61:789.)

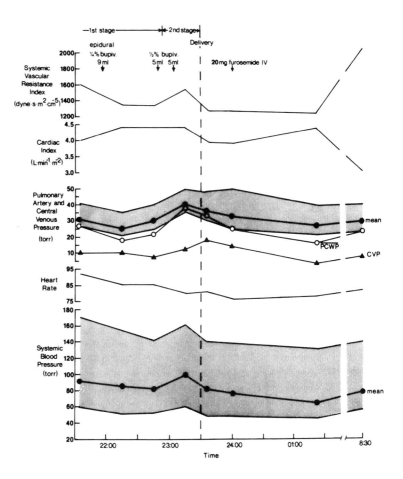

The amount of regurgitant flow parallels the intensity of the insufficiency murmur as well as the size of the V wave on the PCWP tracing. These findings may be a better guide to hemodynamic management than the PCWP is, since there may be little correlation between left atrial pressure and left atrial volume in a chronically dilated atrium. Such lack of correlation precludes any valid estimate of left ventricular end-diastolic volume. Also, as illustrated in Figure 10–16, there may be a wide disparity in preload between the right and the left sides of the heart; in one patient, an initial CVP of 10 mmHg was obtained at the time the PCWP was 27 mmHg.[53]

Anesthetic Considerations. Epidural anesthesia is beneficial in decreasing SVR. Since bradycardia can be harmful, it is appropriate to use epinephrine in local anesthetic solutions, taking care to slowly administer incremental doses in order to avoid hypertension should an accidental intravascular injection occur. Care must be taken as the epidural block rises above the T-7 level, producing splanchnic venodilatation and decreased blood pressure. Contrary to what one might expect, the response of the right side of the heart and the sinoatrial node to acute hypovolemia is bradycardia. Only in this manner can the right ventricle fill enough to maintain an adequate fiber length in order to permit contraction. If the hypovolemia persists, sympathetically mediated responses dominate, and tachycardia ensues. However, the sudden decrease in cardiac filling volume coupled with slowing of the heart rate severely decreases cardiac output. This can be minimized by pretreating with an anticholinergic drug to prevent bradycardia, judicious volume administration as the epidural anesthetic is being administered, maintaining the patient in the left lateral decubitus position until the block reaches T-7, and steeply elevating the patient's legs at the first sign of hypotension (nausea, slowing of heart rate). Small doses of ephedrine are also useful, providing both inotropic and chronotropic support without an excessive increase in afterload.

Figure 10–16 documents the beneficial effect of epidural analgesia in a parturient with mitral and aortic insufficiency who had experienced two episodes of cardiac decompensation during pregnancy. SVR index decreased and cardiac output increased with onset of the block. The deterioration in cardiac performance during the second stage of labor resulted from maternal propulsive efforts.

The same concerns for hypertension with tracheal intubation apply as were discussed for mitral stenosis. The capability for careful titration of a rapid-acting vasodilator such as sodium nitroprusside must be present. Potent agents may cause excessive myocardial depression in already compromised patients.

Mitral Valve Prolapse

Pathologic mitral valve prolapse is a connective tissue abnormality of the leaflets, annulus, and chordae tendineae of the mitral valve, and it must be distinguished from the normal superior displacement of the mitral valve leaflets. This latter condition is very common, occurring in 5–15% of healthy patients examined using two-dimensional echocardiography.[54] Diagnostic criteria for identifying patients with pathologic mitral valve prolapse are given in Table 10–7. One or more major criteria are necessary and sufficient to establish the diagnosis of pathologic mitral valve prolapse. Patients with one or more minor criteria do not warrant this diagnosis, but they still may have cardiac abnormalities, particularly in the presence of a holosystolic murmur.

Fortunately, mitral valve prolapse remains asymptomatic in most patients, and pregnancy, labor, and delivery are well tolerated.[55,56] Pregnancy may present complications for the small percentage of patients with significant mitral regurgitation.

Pathophysiology. In mitral valve prolapse, the chordae tendineae are elongated, allowing the mitral valve leaflets to prolapse into the left atrium when the ventricular volume decreases during systole (Fig. 10–17). This accounts for the mid- to late-systolic click and murmur of mitral regurgitation that are characteristic of mitral valve prolapse. The volume status of the left ventricle affects the degree of regurgitant flow and is a variable that is subject to some therapeutic manipulation. Conditions that augment left ventricular volume tend to decrease regurgitant flow and include hypervolemia, increased afterload, bradycardia, and decreased myocardial contractility. Regurgitant flow increases when left ventricular volume decreases (hypovo-

Table 10–7. CRITERIA RELATED TO THE
DIAGNOSIS OF MITRAL VALVE PROLAPSE

**Major criteria that establish the diagnosis of mitral valve
prolapse**
Auscultation
Mid to late systolic clicks and a late systolic murmur at
the cardiac apex
Mobile mid to late systolic clicks at the cardiac apex
Late systolic murmur at the cardiac apex in the young
patient
Auscultation plus Echocardiography
Apical holosystolic murmur of mitral regurgitation plus
echocardiographic criteria
Two-Dimensional/Doppler Echocardiography
Marked systolic displacement of mitral leaflets with coap-
tation point at or on the left atrial side of the annulus
Moderate systolic displacement of the leaflets with at least
moderate mitral regurgitation, chordal rupture, and an-
nular dilatation
Two-Dimensionally Targeted M-mode Echocardiography
Marked (≧3 mm) late systolc buckling posterior to the
C-D line (annular plane)

**Minor criteria that arouse suspicion but do not establish the
diagnosis of mitral valve prolapse**
History
Focal neurologic attacks or amaurosis fugax in the young
patient
First-degree relatives with major criteria
Recurrent supraventricular tachycardia (documented)
Auscultation
Soft, inconstant, or equivocal mid to late systolic sounds
at the cardiac apex
Other Physical Signs
Low body weight, asthenic habitus
Low blood pressure
Thoracic bony abnormalities
Two-Dimensional/Doppler/Color Flow Echocardiography
Moderate superior systolic displacement of mitral leaflets
with Doppler mitral regurgitation
Two-Dimensionally Targeted M-mode Echocardiography
Moderate (2 mm) late systolic buckling posterior to the
C-D line (annular plane)
Holosystolic displacement (3 mm) posterior to the C-D line
(annular plane)

From Perloff JK, Child JS: Clinical and epidemiologic
issues in mitral valve prolapse. Am Heart J 1987; 113:1324.
With permission.

lemia, sustained increases in intrathoracic pressure, venodilatation, and
tachycardia with resultant decreased filling time).

Monitoring. Invasive cardiovascular monitoring is rarely necessary in
patients with isolated mitral valve prolapse. Dysrhythmias are common,
particularly supraventricular tachyarrhythmias, and continuous electrocardiogram monitoring during labor allows prompt treatment of dysrhythmias.

Anesthetic Considerations. Preload should be maintained in patients with
mitral valve prolapse. Epidural anesthesia is appropriate as long as sym-

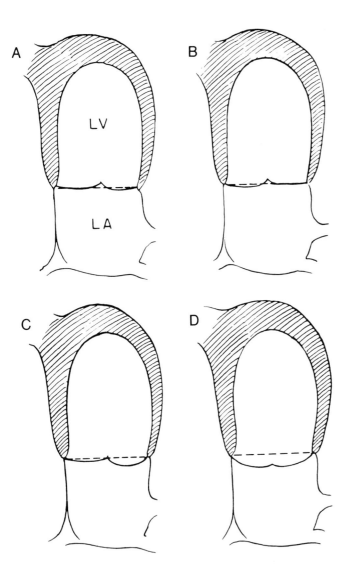

Figure 10–17. Mitral valve prolapse: Schematic echocardiographic views illustrating (*A*) mild displacement of the posterior leaflet superior to the annular plane (*dotted line*), (*B*) mild displacement of the anterior leaflet, (*C*) moderate displacement, (*D*) marked displacement. (From Perloff JK, Child JS, Edwards JE: New guidelines for the clinical diagnosis of mitral valve prolapse. Am J Cardiol 1986; 57:1127. With permission.)

pathetic blockade (decreased SVR) is induced slowly, and intravascular volume is carefully evaluated.[55] Ephedrine is not advisable for treating hypotension, because its inotropic and chronotropic properties are undesirable in the setting of mitral valve prolapse. Antibiotic prophylaxis against subacute bacterial endocarditis is recommended for all patients with pathologic mitral valve prolapse.[54] Antiarrhythmic medications should be continued, regardless of anesthetic technique. The hyperdynamic cardiac response to tracheal intubation can worsen the degree of prolapse, and control of tachycardia and hypertension is important for optimal management.

Aortic Stenosis

Pathophysiology. Aortic stenosis is rarely symptomatic during the childbearing years. However, in symptomatic patients, pregnancy causes severe

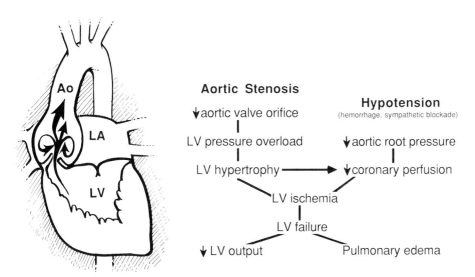

Figure 10–18. Aortic stenosis (systole). The narrow aortic valve orifice requires elevated left ventricular pressures to overcome the increased resistance to ejection. There is turbulent flow just distal to the valve, resulting in dilatation of the aortic root. (LV = left ventricle, LA = left atrium, Ao = aorta.)

hemodynamic derangements. As the aortic valve narrows from a normal cross-sectional area of 2.6–3.5 mm^2 to less than 1 mm^2, increasing left ventricular pressures are required to maintain cardiac output (Fig. 10–18). This leads to concentric hypertrophy of the left ventricle. The elevation in end-diastolic pressure combined with a thickened left ventricular wall impairs subendocardial blood flow, resulting in myocardial ischemia.

The outflow tract obstruction results in a relatively fixed stroke volume, so that increases in cardiac output are determined primarily by increases in heart rate. However, decreased diastolic compliance may be the major pathophysiologic abnormality in many patients with aortic stenosis, and tachycardia with resultant decreased ventricular filling times may actually worsen cardiac output.[57]

Monitoring. Invasive hemodynamic monitoring is required in patients with severe stenosis (gradient >50 mmHg), symptoms of congestive failure, angina, or a history of syncopal episodes.[45] However, because of decreased left ventricular compliance, left ventricular end-diastolic pressure may be elevated although actual chamber volume is low. Higher than normal PCWP may be necessary to maintain cardiac output, but such increases in pressure increase the likelihood of pulmonary edema. Electrocardiogram monitoring is recommended in order to detect evidence of myocardial ischemia.

Anesthetic Considerations. Pregnant patients with aortic stenosis may not tolerate large decreases in preload (filling volumes), afterload (peripheral vascular resistance), or heart rate. Thus, epidural anesthesia, which has the potential for causing all three of these undesirable responses, must be administered carefully, with attention given to adequate fluid pretreatment and prompt correction of hypotension. The treatment for this is administration

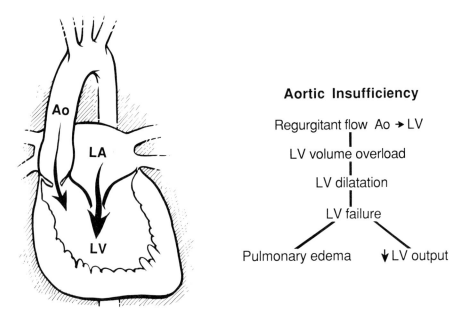

Aortic Insufficiency

Regurgitant flow Ao → LV
|
LV volume overload
|
LV dilatation
|
LV failure

Pulmonary edema   ↓ LV output

Figure 10–19. Aortic insufficiency (diastole). The incompetent aortic valve allows ejected blood to flow back into the left ventricle during systole, at the same time that the ventricle is being filled from the left atrium. This volume overload causes the left ventricle to enlarge and possibly fail. (Ao = aorta, LV = left ventricle, LA = left atrium.)

of an arteriolar vasoconstrictor such as phenylephrine to elevate aortic root pressures.

Light general anesthesia such as that typically used for cesarean section is usually tolerated quite well, since both blood pressure and heart rate are well maintained. The hemodynamic response to laryngoscopy and tracheal intubation can precipitate left ventricular dysfunction, and alfentanil (35 µg/kg) has been recommended for use in blocking this response.[58] However, this dose is associated with maternal hypotension and neonatal respiratory depression. Regional and topical anesthesia of the airway prior to induction, as described for patients with mitral stenosis, coupled with reduced dosages of intravenous induction agents, offer another option for minimizing excessive hemodynamic alterations. In patients with evidence of left ventricular failure, the use of potent inhalational agents should be avoided, owing to their propensity for myocardial depression.

Aortic Regurgitation

Pathophysiology. In aortic regurgitation, the incompetent valve allows blood in the aorta to flow back into the left ventricle (Fig. 10–19). This "runoff" lesion decreases diastolic pressure and widens pulse pressure. Volume overload of the left ventricle and, if chronic, dilatation of the left ventricle occur in aortic regurgitation. Thus, left ventricular end-diastolic pressure may remain normal despite an abnormally high left ventricular end-diastolic volume. With progressive distention, the left ventricle eventually fails and left ventricular end-diastolic pressure increases. Bradycardia allows more time for regurgitant flow during diastole and should be avoided. Increased SVR favors regurgitant flow and may precipitate congestive heart failure.

Pregnancy is well tolerated in patients with mild to moderate aortic insufficiency, since the pregnancy-induced decrease in SVR decreases the ratio of regurgitant volume to total stroke volume. However, in patients with myocardial dysfunction, increased blood volume worsens pulmonary congestion, and the increase in SVR associated with labor occurring in such a patient can lead to acute decompensation.

In severe aortic regurgitation, there are abnormalities of coronary flow, with phasic coronary flow being mainly during systole,[59] reversal of flow during part of diastole, and redistribution of coronary flow from the endocardium to the epicardium.[60] Systemic hypotension may precipitate myocardial ischemia and cardiac failure.[61]

Monitoring. Isolated aortic regurgitation is usually asymptomatic in patients of childbearing age. In patients with left ventricular dysfunction or evidence of a significantly dilated left ventricle based on echocardiographic examination, invasive hemodynamic monitoring is warranted in order to guide titration of vasodilator and inotropic therapy. The dilated ventricle accommodates a large end-diastolic volume without an increase in pressure, and thus PCWP fails to accurately assess ventricular volume. However, any increase in PCWP must be investigated and promptly treated, if necessary, since such a change may herald a rapid deterioration in cardiac function.

Anesthetic Considerations. The anesthetic considerations in aortic insufficiency are similar to those for mitral insufficiency: avoid increased SVR, bradycardia, or myocardial depression. Carefully administered epidural anesthesia is well tolerated for labor and delivery in patients with aortic regurgitation.

Intracardiac and Extracardiac Shunts

Left-to-Right Shunts

Pathophysiology. Atrial septal defect, ventricular septal defect, and patent ductus arteriosus differ in the location of the shunt site, yet they have in common an increase in pulmonary blood flow due to a left-to-right shunt. Small defects produce small shunts and minimum symptoms, whereas large defects, in which the pulmonary blood flow may be four to five times systemic flow, eventually overload the pulmonary circuit, leading to pulmonary hypertension and right ventricular failure. Increases in SVR normally worsen the shunt.

The increased blood volume associated with pregnancy adds to the already excessive pulmonary blood flow, but this effect is offset somewhat by the decrease in SVR occurring in normal pregnancy. Maternal and fetal outcomes are usually satisfactory.[62]

Monitoring. Invasive hemodynamic monitoring is not required in patients with small defects and no symptoms. However, patients with pulmonary hypertension and right ventricular dysfunction warrant pulmonary and peripheral arterial monitoring and, in the case of an atrial septal defect, right atrial pressure monitoring.

Anesthetic Considerations. Patients with shunts are always at risk for systemic embolization of any air introduced into a blood vessel, regardless of the normal direction of the shunt. For example, in patients with an atrial septal defect with a left-to-right shunt, air bubbles introduced into the right atrium may traverse the septal defect and gain access to the systemic circulation, notably the cerebral vessels and coronary arteries.

Epidural and spinal anesthesia result in peripheral vasodilatation and decreased SVR, conditions that generally benefit patients with left-to-right shunts. Extreme arterial hypotension, however, can cause shunt reversal and hypoxemia. Conversely, general anesthesia and the necessity for tracheal intubation carry the risk of sharp elevations in peripheral resistance and worsening of the left-to-right shunt.

Right-to-Left Shunts

Pathophysiology. In right-to-left shunts, deoxygenated blood bypasses the pulmonary capillary bed, resulting in systemic arterial desaturation and cyanosis. The shunt can occur at any level in the cardiopulmonary circuit— atrial, ventricular, aortopulmonary, or intrapulmonary. Right-to-left shunts also develop as a consequence of pulmonary hypertension in lesions normally resulting in left-to-right shunting. This reversal of shunt flow is known as Eisenmenger's syndrome. Cyanosis and reversed shunt flow carry a high risk for both maternal and fetal morbidity and mortality.[62]

In tetralogy of Fallot, the pulmonic stenosis can be either fixed or dynamic, the latter involving infundibular hypertrophy. In cases of fixed obstruction, increased right ventricular contractility is necessary to maintain adequate pulmonary blood flow. On the other hand, if there is dynamic infundibular obstruction, increases in right ventricular contractility tend to worsen the outflow obstruction, as does hypovolemia and tachycardia.

Pregnancy is deleterious for patients with right-to-left shunts and even more so in the presence of pulmonary hypertension. In a recent study, deterioration of cardiac status occurred in all pregnant patients with pulmonary artery pressures greater than 50 mmHg.[46] The thickened pulmonary vessels are minimally responsive to the factors producing peripheral vasodilatation in pregnancy, and pulmonary vascular resistance does not decrease. The imbalance between pulmonary vascular resistance and SVR worsens the right-to-left shunt. This can produce severe cyanosis, with detriment to both the mother and the fetus. In patients with tetralogy of Fallot and right ventricular infundibular hypertrophy, the sympathetic nervous system response to labor increases right ventricular contractility and pulmonary vascular resistance, conditions that worsen the degree of right-to-left shunt.

Monitoring. Pulse oximetry is one of the most useful monitors in patients with right-to-left shunts. These patients tend to be on the steep portion of the oxygen-hemoglobin dissociation curve, and thus they are very sensitive to any of the factors adversely affecting oxygen saturation (Sao_2): (1) decreased inspired fraction of oxygen, (2) increased right-to-left shunting, (3) increased oxygen consumption, (4) decreased cardiac output, and (5) decreased mixed venous oxygen tension.[63] Pulse oximetry correlates well with *in vitro* Sao_2 determined by co-oximetry in children with cyanotic congenital heart disease over an oxygen saturation range of 35–95%.[64] Measurement of CVP is helpful in patients with tetralogy of Fallot and infundibular hypertrophy, since it is important to maintain an adequate central volume.

Anesthetic Considerations. Epidural and spinal anesthesia carry the risk of decreased SVR with consequent worsening of right-to-left shunting. This can be managed with careful volume and appropriate vasopressor therapy. For example, ephedrine, with its beta$_1$ enhancement of cardiac contractility and inotropy, should not be used to correct venodilatation in patients with tetralogy of Fallot and infundibular hypertrophy. Rather, a pure alpha$_1$ agent is preferable.

Light general anesthesia for cesarean section tends to maintain peripheral resistance, a desirable goal in patients with a right-to-left shunt. Halothane is particularly efficacious in reducing right ventricular contractility in patients with tetralogy of Fallot and dynamic outflow tract obstruction, but it might prove deleterious in patients with tetralogy of Fallot and fixed pulmonary valvular obstruction. Factors increasing pulmonary vascular resistance, such as hypercapnia, hypoxia, and extremes of lung volume,[65] must be assiduously avoided in patients with right-to-left shunts. For example, prolonged coughing on an endotracheal tube empties the lung to residual volume and may lead to hypoxia and tachycardia, conditions adversely affecting pulmonary flow in patients with right-to-left shunts.

MONITORING OF PATIENTS RECEIVING EPIDURAL NARCOTICS

Epidural narcotics are used extensively for postoperative analgesia following cesarean section, and epidural and intrathecal opiates are being increasingly utilized in combination with local anesthetics for labor analgesia and anesthesia for cesarean section.[66] The advantages of spinal opiates include good pain relief without motor blockade, prolonged duration of action compared with other routes of administration, and negligible narcotic blood levels in the fetus. The disadvantages include pruritus, nausea, urinary retention, and the potential for respiratory depression. All these side effects are reversible with naloxone hydrochloride at dosages that do not reverse the analgesic effects.[67]

After the initial injection of an epidural opiate, there is some systemic absorption through the epidural vessels that is related to the lipophilicity of the particular opiate and is roughly equivalent to an intramuscular injection of the same dose of drug. There is also the potential for an unsuspected intravascular or intrathecal injection when administering epidural opiates. Thus, patients should be continuously observed following each injection for the possibility of immediate respiratory depression, in the same manner that patients should be monitored after parenteral narcotic administration.

However, it is the potential for delayed respiratory depression that has been the main factor limiting the widespread use of epidural narcotics.[68] This effect is thought to be caused by the interaction of the narcotic with respiratory centers in the central nervous system, whereas the analgesic effects are postulated to occur in the dorsal horn of the spinal cord. The narcotic reaches this area of the brain through the cerebrospinal fluid rather than through the systemic circulation, and the flow characteristics of spinal fluid are such that it takes several hours for usual doses of lumbar epidural morphine to reach the brain. Since pruritus and nausea are also centrally mediated, these side effects exhibit the same delay.[69] The peak time period for delayed respiratory depression is from 4 to 8 hours after epidural morphine administration, although Abboud and coworkers have demonstrated 30–50% depression of ventilatory response to CO_2 beginning 1.5 hours after administration of 5 mg of epidural morphine sulfate and lasting 24 hours.[70] Rawal, however, found that a naloxone hydrochloride infusion (5 μg/kg/hour) reversed the ventilatory depression produced by 10 mg of epidural morphine in healthy volunteers, a morphine dose twice that used clinically.[71]

Other narcotics that are more lipid-soluble than morphine sulfate is, such as fentanyl citrate and meperidine hydrochloride, appear to penetrate the lipid membranes of the spinal cord and epidural vessels more rapidly and more extensively than morphine sulfate does, and, consequently, less drug is available for rostral migration to the brain.[69] Use of the lipid-soluble agents reduces the likelihood of delayed respiratory depression, but it also reduces the duration of analgesia. For example, epidural fentanyl citrate (75 μg) has a duration of analgesic action of approximately 6 hours, whereas epidural morphine sulfate (5 mg) has a duration of 18–24 hours.

It is likely that postpartum patients receiving epidural narcotics are at less risk for delayed respiratory depression than other patients, owing to the respiratory stimulant effects of elevated progesterone levels that accompany pregnancy. Also, obstetric patients tend to be young and free of concurrent lung disease, factors also reducing the likelihood of delayed respiratory depression. For additional safety, a naloxone citrate infusion (0.05–0.1 mg/hour) in all patients receiving epidural morphine sulfate effectively eliminates the risk of delayed respiratory depression. In addition, this practice lessens the severity of nausea and pruritus. However, naloxone citrate infusion is not standard practice at many leading obstetric centers, and the financial costs are not insignificant.

An alternative approach to the problem of narcotic-induced respiratory depression is apnea monitoring. However, this approach has been largely abandoned in favor of naloxone citrate infusion.

FETAL MONITORING

Fetal Physiology

An understanding of fetal cardiovascular physiology is important in the evaluation of fetal heart rate patterns, one of the most fundamental aspects

Figure 10–20. The fetal circulation. *Dark arrows* indicate oxygenated blood; *stippled arrows*, deoxygenated blood. (P = placenta, UV = umbilical vein, IVC = inferior vena cava, DV = ductus venosus, RHV = right hepatic vein, LHV = left hepatic vein, PV = portal vein, PS = portal sinus, RA = right atrium, LA = left atrium, SVC = superior vena cava, RV = right ventricle, LV = left ventricle, MPT = main pulmonary trunk, DA = ductus arteriosus, AAo = ascending aorta, PA = pulmonary artery, DAo = descending aorta.) (From Heymann MA: Biophysical evaluation of fetal status. *In* Creasy R, Resnik R [eds]: Maternal-Fetal Medicine. Philadelphia: WB Saunders, 1984; 260.)

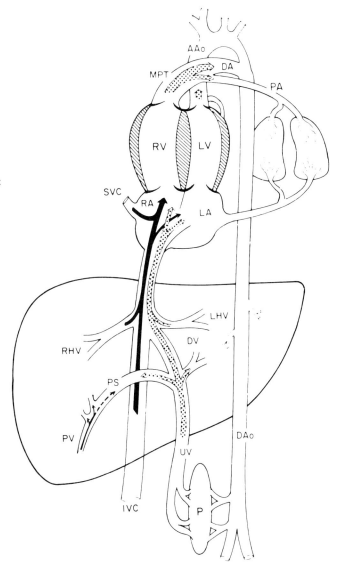

of fetal monitoring. Oxygenated blood from the placenta has a normal oxygen tension of about 30 mmHg. However, owing to the presence of fetal hemoglobin, this represents a saturation of 80%. The saturated blood is carried by the umbilical vein (Fig. 10–20). A portion goes to the liver, but the majority bypasses the liver by traversing the ductus venosus and empties into the inferior vena cava. Streaming occurs, so that much of the oxygenated blood from the placenta is directed across the foramen ovale into the left atrium and, subsequently, the left ventricle. This oxygenated blood is then preferentially supplied to the brain and myocardium. Desaturated blood from the head and upper body returns via the superior vena cava and is directed into the right ventricle, where it mixes with saturated blood from the placenta. Because of the high pulmonary vascular resistance, most of the right ventricular output crosses the ductus arteriosus and enters the descending aorta. A portion of this blood then goes to the placenta via the umbilical arteries to be reoxygenated. The normal oxygen tension of this desaturated umbilical artery blood is 20 mmHg, with a saturation of approximately 55%.

Fetal Hypoxic Response

The response of the fetus to hypoxia consists of a redistribution of blood flow to essential organs, decreased oxygen consumption, and anaerobic glycolysis. The favored organs are the brain, heart, placenta, and adrenal glands. With hypoxia, heart rate decreases owing to increased vagal stimulation, and overall oxygen consumption decreases. Fetal pH decreases owing to a metabolic acidosis resulting from lactic acid being produced in vascular beds when vasoconstriction (and thus decreased flow) occurs. Asphyxia with a marked decrease in placental flow impairs carbon dioxide exchange and contributes a respiratory component to the acidosis.

ANTENATAL FETAL MONITORING

Fetal well-being is assessed by a range of techniques that may be as simple as the mother's reporting of fetal movements or as complex as invasive entry into the amniotic cavity in order to sample tissue or view the fetus with a fetoscope. Equally important is the assessment of fetal maturity, which also has both simple and complex technologies associated with it. Fetal well-being and maturity are not the same thing. A fetus can be mature and not well or very immature and quite well as long as it continues an intrauterine existence. For practical purposes, most assessments of fetal well-being focus on the presence or absence of central nervous system asphyxia, whereas maturity refers primarily to lung maturity. These assessments are certainly appropriate, since lung disease due to prematurity and permanent neurologic impairment due to intrauterine asphyxia account for a disproportionate share of neonatal morbidity and mortality.

It is also significant that both intrauterine asphyxia and prematurity, when present, can be reliably diagnosed, and maternal-fetal management based on this information may decrease the likelihood of a bad outcome. In the case of prenatal diagnosis of congenital disorders, the opportunity to alter an adverse outcome is limited to a very small number of conditions.

Certain high-risk fetuses warrant assessment of well-being before the onset of labor. The most frequent pregnancies so monitored are those complicated by hypertension, diabetes, or a growth-retarded fetus. How early in pregnancy monitoring should be initiated depends upon how soon one is willing to intervene if a distressed fetus is detected. The beginning of the third trimester is usually the earliest time that this type of assessment is undertaken.

Ultrasound in Fetal Assessment

Ultrasound refers to sound waves whose frequency exceeds 20,000 Hz. Diagnostic ultrasound involves the application of electrical current to a crystal in order to produce vibrations, thus emitting ultrasonic waves that are reflected off target tissues and returned to the crystal to be converted back to electrical energy. The timing and the intensity of the returning echo allow the electrical signals to be displayed on a two-dimensional cathode ray tube, with time (distance) on one axis and intensity on the other. In modern obstetric ultrasonography, the electrical signal is converted to a spot on the oscilloscope, and the brightness of the spot varies with the intensity of the signal. This display is referred to as B-mode or brightness-mode. Real-time imaging displays the echoes so rapidly that it is possible to visualize target motion. Thus, real-time B-mode ultrasound imaging allows a dynamic view of the fetus, permitting both structural and functional evaluations.

Ultrasound can document an intrauterine pregnancy as early as 3 weeks after impregnation (see Fig. 10–7). It is also valuable for estimating gestational age and measuring such features as gestational sac volume at 4–8 weeks, crown-rump length at 6–12 weeks, and biparietal diameter at 12–26 weeks.[72] Accurate estimation of gestational age is important in determining fetal maturity and reducing the incidence of respiratory distress syndrome of prematurity following elective cesarean section. Fetal growth can be documented using ultrasound, and the finding of intrauterine growth retardation may, in cases in which the cause is uteroplacental insufficiency, demand an early delivery. Ultrasound imaging is used to determine fetal position, such as breech presentation.

Ultrasound permits detection of a wide range of congenital disorders, both structural and functional, with a high degree of precision.[73] In some cases, early detection permits beneficial therapy. Fetal supraventricular tachycardia can be treated with maternal propranolol, thus avoiding heart failure. A new area of fetal medicine emerged after the performance by Harrison and associates of bilateral ureterostomies in a 21-week fetus.[74] Since this time, numerous surgical procedures have been performed upon fetuses to correct lesions that, if left untreated, would cause further damage to the newborn.[75] An example is hydrocephalus due to aqueductal stenosis. Insertion of a ventriculoamniotic shunt *in utero* prevents the development of hydrocephalus in some fetuses. In other cases, ultrasound reveals lethal anomalies, such as anencephaly, and prevents unnecessary maternal surgery and morbidity.

Elevated maternal alpha-fetoprotein levels are suggestive of either neural tube or abdominal wall defects. Ultrasonography can confirm a suspected diagnosis (Fig. 10–21) and allow for appropriate delivery room management and prompt surgical intervention, if necessary.

Combination real-time and Doppler ultrasonography has recently permitted hemodynamic studies of the fetus in late pregnancy. This technology has been used to evaluate blood velocity waveforms in the pulsatile fetal and uteroplacental vessels and has identified fetal distress in hypertensive pregnancies.[76]

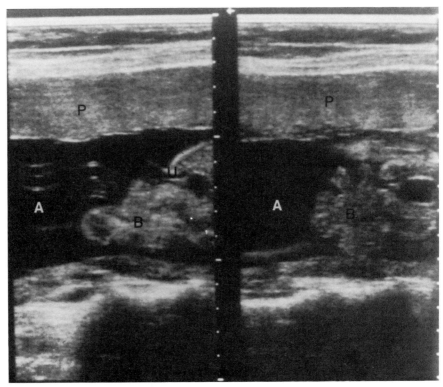

Figure 10–21. Ultrasonographic visualization of a fetus with gastroschisis, two views. The lesion is distinguished from omphalocele by the lack of an amniotic membrane, the cauliflower appearance of the extruded bowel (B), and the lateral location relative to the umbilicus (U). This distinction is significant, since omphalocele is associated with a high rate of associated anomalies, whereas gastroschisis tends to be an isolated lesion. (P = placenta, A = amniotic fluid.)

Amniocentesis

Amniocentesis performed early in the second trimester allows the antenatal determination of the cytogenetic constitution of the fetus, the diagnosis of inborn errors of metabolism, and the detection of neural tube and abdominal wall defects (identified by elevated alpha-fetoprotein levels in the amniotic fluid). In late pregnancy, amniocentesis is utilized to assess the severity of Rh-isoimmunization, predict fetal lung maturity, and decompress polyhydramnios.

Fetoscopy

Fetoscopy involves passing a viewing instrument into the amniotic cavity in order to observe the contents. It allows visualization of small defects, such as a cleft lip. Operative procedures such as liver and skin biopsies can be done using the fetoscope.

Xenon-133 Clearance Studies

Intervillous blood flow can be measured using xenon-133 clearance techniques. This technique has been used to validate the beneficial effect of lumbar epidural analgesia upon uteroplacental blood flow, particularly in the presence of maternal hypertension.[36]

Antepartum Fetal Heart Rate Monitoring

The nonstress test monitors fetal heart rate variability and accelerations with fetal movement over a 20-minute period. If the baseline variability is less than 6 beats/minute and heart rate acceleration is less than 15 beats/minute with fetal movement, the test is considered nonreactive. Heart rate values greater than this are classified as "reactive" and correlate highly with fetal well-being. A "nonreactive" test does not necessarily indicate a depressed fetus, but it does require further evaluation. This is most commonly done with an oxytocin challenge test in which the fetal heart rate pattern is evaluated in response to uterine contractions induced by oxytocin. The appearance of abnormal heart rate slowing (late decelerations) with contractions indicates a "positive" test. A nonreactive positive contraction stress test is indicative of a distressed fetus. It demands immediate intervention in order to either reverse the maternal condition causing the distress or deliver the fetus if the gestational age is greater than 30 weeks.[77]

Assessment of Fetal Maturity

Prematurity is still the most significant cause of perinatal morbidity and mortality. Fetal maturity in present perinatal practice is synonymous with pulmonary maturity. This is the rate-limiting step in the process that allows the fetus to become independent of the placenta. Until recently, the standard method for assessing lung maturity was the lecithin/sphingomyelin ratio. It compares the concentrations of two phospholipids, lecithin and sphingomyelin, in amniotic fluid obtained by amniocentesis. Before 34 weeks, both substances are present in approximately equal amounts. After 34 weeks, the amount of lecithin increases and the amount of sphingomyelin decreases (Fig. 10–22). A lecithin/sphingomyelin ratio of 2:1 is indicative of lung maturity, but a significant number of fetuses with mature studies still, if delivered at that point, develop respiratory distress syndrome of prematurity. This is thought to be due to a lack of phosphatidylglycerol, which appears to stabilize lecithin in surfactant. Phosphatidylglycerol measurements of 3% or greater in the amniotic fluid indicate functional lung maturity. Phosphatidylglycerol is not present in blood, vaginal secretions, or meconium, so these contaminants do not confuse the interpretation.

INTRAPARTUM FETAL MONITORING

Evaluation of fetal heart rate patterns remains the cornerstone of monitoring for the purpose of assessing fetal well-being during labor. Auscul-

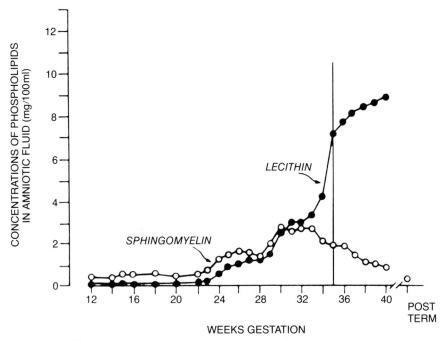

Figure 10–22. Changes in concentrations of lecithin and sphingomyelin in amniotic fluid over the course of normal pregnancy. (From Gluck L, Kulovich MV: Lecithin/sphingomyelin ratios in normal and abnormal pregnancy. Am J Obstet Gynecol 1973; 115:541. With permission.)

tation of the fetal heart rate using a stethoscope provides very limited information, other than identifying extremes of heart rate and dysrhythmias. Owing to the intermittent nature of this technique, significant pathology may be present but undetected. Maximum benefit from fetal heart rate monitoring occurs with continuous beat-to-beat monitoring for an extended period of time using electronic monitoring equipment.

Fetal Heart Rate Changes

Fetal heart rate changes consist of baseline changes and periodic changes. Baseline changes include beat-to-beat variability, tachycardia, and bradycardia. Periodic changes refer to deceleration patterns: early, late, and variable.

Baseline Fetal Heart Rate Changes

Beat-to-Beat Variability. The baseline fetal heart rate is normally 120–160 beats/minute. However, in the healthy fetus, there is a slight difference in the interval between successive heart beats. This is referred to as beat-to-beat variability or short-term variability. Beat-to-beat variability produces the irregular line seen on recordings of the fetal heart rate (Fig. 10–23). The

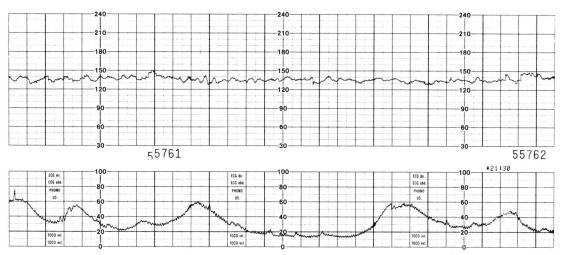

Figure 10–23. Normal fetal heart rate tracing (upper trace) showing good beat-to-beat variability, a baseline rate of 135 beats/minute, and no heart rate changes with uterine contractions (lower trace).

physiologic origin and significance of this variability are not known with certainty, but clinical evidence suggests that its presence confirms an intact pathway from cerebral cortex to midbrain to vagus nerve to the cardiac conduction system.[78] Sporadic input from various areas in the cerebral cortex is transmitted to the cardiac centers in the medulla oblongata. This results in continuously varying levels of vagal stimulation, and the heart rate reflects this uneven input. Cerebral asphyxia causes decreased heart rate variability (Fig. 10–24), possibly because of decreased cerebral input to the midbrain. Absent beat-to-beat variability is seen in anencephalic infants, in whom there is an absence of cerebral cortex. It may also be caused by drugs, such as narcotics and sedatives, that depress higher brain centers. Use of such agents

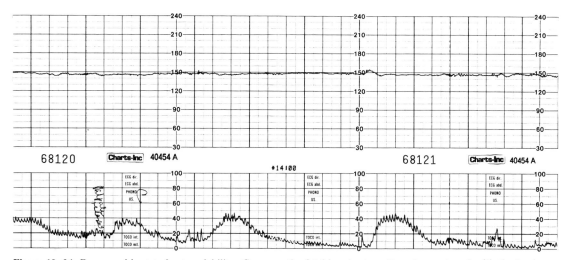

Figure 10–24. Decreased beat-to-beat variability. Compare the fetal heart rate pattern (upper trace) with the tracing in Figure 10–23.

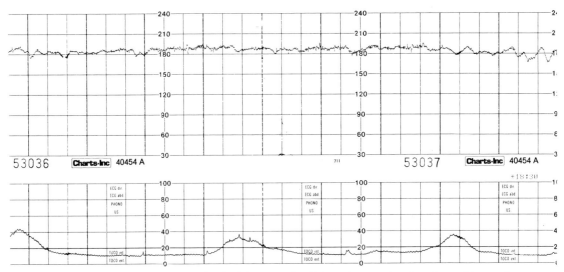

Figure 10–25. Fetal tachycardia. The baseline fetal heart rate is 190 beats/minute, but there is good beat-to-beat variability and there are no decelerations.

during labor thus removes an important indicator of fetal cardiopulmonary reserve. Anticholinergic drugs in high doses decrease variability. Defects in the fetal cardiac conduction system also cause loss of variability.

Fetal Tachycardia. Fetal tachycardia is defined as a heart rate greater than 160 beats/minute. If normal variability is present, tachycardia does not indicate asphyxia (Fig. 10–25). It may be seen in the recovery phase following a period of asphyxia and represents catecholamine activity. Other causes of tachycardia are maternal or fetal infection, especially chorioamnionitis, drugs such as beta$_2$ agonists or parasympathetic blockers, tachydysrhythmias, and thyrotoxicosis.

Fetal Bradycardia. Bradycardia is the initial response of a normal fetus to acute hypoxia. Moderate bradycardia is defined as a heart rate between 100 and 120 beats/minute. If good variability is present, it indicates that the fetus is able to tolerate mild hypoxic states by the compensatory mechanisms already discussed, namely, redistribution, decreased oxygen consumption, and anaerobic glycolysis. In some patients, moderate bradycardia is idiopathic and benign and does not represent hypoxia. A heart rate below 80 beats/minute eventually results in fetal decompensation. In the fetus, cardiac output is primarily determined by heart rate, and a decrease in heart rate signifies a decrease in cardiac output. Severe bradycardia thus results in inadequate cardiac output to support tissue oxygen demand. Fetuses lack the myocardial reserve present in older children and adults and cannot substantially increase cardiac contractility.

Moderate bradycardia may result from prolonged head compression and is vagally mediated. Other causes of bradycardia are less common. Complete heart block, a condition associated with a significant incidence of structural heart disease, may be present. Congenital heart block may also be seen in the offspring of mothers with systemic lupus erythematosus. Bradycardia can be caused by maternal medications, such as beta-blockers or local an-

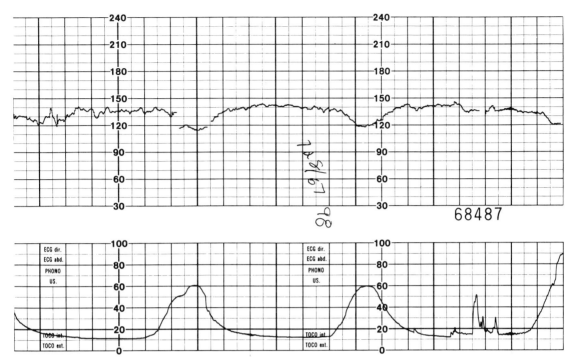

Figure 10–26. Early decelerations. The onset of the fetal heart rate slowing corresponds to the onset of the uterine contraction. Although early decelerations may resemble late decelerations, pictured in Figure 10–27, this pattern is not associated with fetal distress but is attributed to vagal discharge, possibly in response to fetal head compression. The infant was subsequently delivered by cesarean section for prolonged bradycardia. At delivery, the infant had a tight nuchal cord but Apgar scores of 9 and 9 at 1 and 5 minutes.

esthetics. Of particular note is the high incidence of fetal bradycardia following paracervical block.

Periodic Fetal Heart Rate Changes

Periodic changes are those patterns that occur in association with uterine contractions. There are three specific periodic patterns: early decelerations, late decelerations, and variable decelerations. It should be emphasized that heart rate changes with contractions are not normal. Thus, as is shown in Figure 10–23, a normal fetal heart rate pattern shows a baseline rate between 120 and 160 beats/minute with good beat-to-beat variability and no periodic changes, that is, no heart rate decelerations with contractions.

Early Decelerations. Early decelerations occur concomitantly with uterine contractions. They start at the same time, are smooth, and are a mirror image of the uterine contraction (Fig. 10–26). Early decelerations are mild (less than 20 beats/minute below baseline). The etiology is unknown, although the usual explanation is fetal head compression.

Late Decelerations. Late decelerations are also smooth and associated with contractions, but the onset and recovery are delayed 10–30 seconds. The onset usually coincides with the peak of the uterine contraction, and the fetal heart rate is slowest at the end of the contraction (Fig. 10–27). This

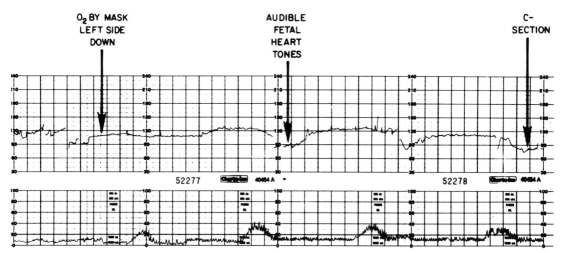

Figure 10–27. Late decelerations. The slowing of the fetal heart rate coincides with the peak of the uterine contraction. The absence of beat-to-beat variability during the first 3 minutes of the recording (each bold line indicates 1 minute) is indicative of a decompensated fetus. Slight improvement is achieved following repositioning of the mother and administration of oxygen. The persistence of late decelerations and a low baseline heart rate compared with the earlier rate of 145 beats/minute prompted an emergency cesarean section. The infant was severely depressed; Apgar scores were 1 (1 minute), 2 (5 minutes), and 6 (10 minutes).

pattern is indicative of uteroplacental insufficiency. Uterine blood flow decreases during the contraction, and fetal blood returning from the placenta is not adequately oxygenated. Chemoreceptors sense the low oxygen tension and trigger vagal discharge. As long as cerebral oxygenation is maintained, fetal heart rate variability should also remain normal, in spite of the late decelerations. However, if the deoxygenation is severe enough, it may affect not only the central nervous system but the myocardium as well. In this case, beat-to-beat variability is decreased or absent (Fig. 10–27). The latter pattern often occurs in the setting of an already impaired placental reserve, such as preeclampsia or intrauterine growth retardation. Again, the key to assessing the severity of the pattern is the degree of variability present. The combination of late decelerations with absent variability is an ominous pattern, since it indicates that each contraction stresses the fetus beyond its compensatory capacity.

The treatment of the maternal-fetal unit when late decelerations occur consists of efforts to optimize placental blood flow and oxygenation. Maternal position should be changed, particularly if the mother is lying supine, in order to eliminate the mechanical effects of the uterus on the aorta or vena cava. In Figure 10–27, note that the response to the fetal heart rate of 110 beats/minute but with absent variability was to administer oxygen, place the patient on her left side, and notify the obstetrician. If the mother is hypotensive after correct positioning, then volume and blood pressure support with ephedrine is indicated. In patients with significant mouth breathing, as is often taught in prepared childbirth courses, oxygen should be delivered to the mother by a sealed face mask rather than by nasal prongs. Uterine activity can be reduced by stopping oxytocin if it is being infused or by the use of tocolytic agents. These measures usually correct late decelerations

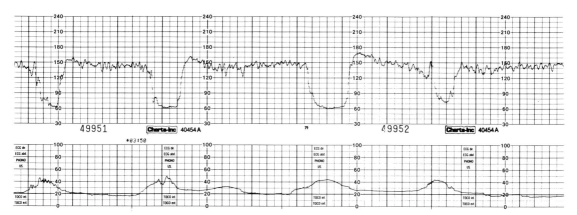

Figure 10-28. Variable decelerations. The deceleration tends to mirror the uterine contraction. Fetal heart rate often overshoots the baseline at the termination of the deceleration. Note the variable appearance of each deceleration tracing relative to the preceding tracing. This infant was delivered vaginally and had Apgar scores of 7 (1 minute) and 9 (5 minutes).

in which good beat-to-beat variability is still present. However, in a decompensated fetus, these measures are usually not effective, and immediate delivery is required.

Variable Decelerations. Variable decelerations differ in duration, depth, and shape from contraction to contraction. Onset and termination of the deceleration are usually very abrupt. There is no definite relationship to uterine contractions (Figs. 10-28 and 10-29). Severe variable decelerations are defined as those that decrease 60 beats/minute below baseline, decrease below 60 beats/minute, or last longer than 60 seconds. Variable decelerations are felt to represent vagal firing in response to cord compression or sustained head compression, as when the mother is pushing during the second stage of labor. Again, the presence or absence of baseline variability correlates with the oxygenation of central tissues and is indicative of the severity of

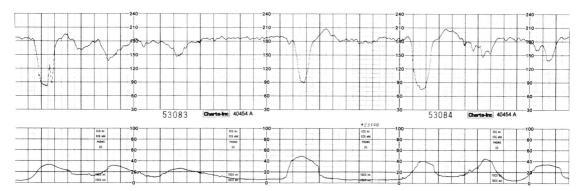

Figure 10-29. Variable decelerations. Compared with Figure 10-28, there is less beat-to-beat variability. Note also the lack of uniformity of the deceleration tracings. This heart rate tracing is from the same infant as in Figure 10-25 but 5 hours later. The baseline tachycardia is still present, but there is less variability and variable decelerations are persistent. The mother was an insulin-dependent diabetic. She was allowed to deliver vaginally. The infant weighed 3680 gm and had a 1-minute Apgar score of 3 and a 5-minute score of 8.

the stress producing the decelerations. The same techniques used to treat late decelerations are applicable—treatment of hypotension and maternal oxygenation.

Predictive Value of Fetal Heart Rate Patterns

A normal fetal heart rate pattern (rate 120–160 beats/minute with good beat-to-beat variability and no late or variable decelerations) during the last 30 minutes of labor is predictive of a vigorous infant at birth greater than 98% of the time, even in high-risk pregnancies, assuming that the delivery is atraumatic and the infant has no congenital malformation inconsistent with extrauterine life, such as tracheal atresia or aplastic lungs.[79] However, the converse is not true. Heart rate patterns of variable or late decelerations do not guarantee a depressed newborn. Earlier studies of late and variable decelerations showed very little correlation between these patterns and depressed newborns. One reason for this is that these studies failed to subdivide patient population based on heart rate variability.[80] Patients with decelerations with adequate variability often have a low 1-minute Apgar score but usually have a 5-minute Apgar of 8 or above. The presence of decelerations and decreased variability increases the risk for significant neonatal depression. Severe deceleration patterns plus the absence of variability are almost always associated with an asphyxiated fetus requiring active resuscitation.

The vast majority of fetuses with major congenital anomalies have normal fetal heart rate patterns. Exceptions are anencephaly and congenital heart disease with complete heart block.

Techniques of Fetal Heart Rate Monitoring

Meaningful fetal heart rate monitoring requires both the fetal heart rate pattern plus the pattern of uterine contractions in order to assess the relationship between the two. There are four methods for obtaining fetal heart rate. Intermittent stethoscopic auscultation remains the main form of surveillance during labor in low-risk pregnancies and continues to be used in many high-risk pregnancies despite the fact that there is no auscultatory pattern of early fetal distress. Auscultation is able to identify only the extreme condition. The patterns of variable and late decelerations were only described in 1967 with the advent of electronic monitoring techniques.[81] They were never recognized through the stethoscope by generations of skilled clinicians. The reason that stethoscopic surveillance is acceptable is that the true incidence of fetal distress is so low—about 2%. Thus, 98% of low-risk mothers monitored in this fashion, or any other manner, can be expected to deliver vigorous infants. Despite its widespread use, there are no scientific studies to validate the use of stethoscopic auscultation.[82]

Phonocardiography and Doppler ultrasound are both noninvasive and detect sounds produced by the fetal heart valves. Neither technique is adequate for assessing beat-to-beat variability, but both detect deceleration patterns.

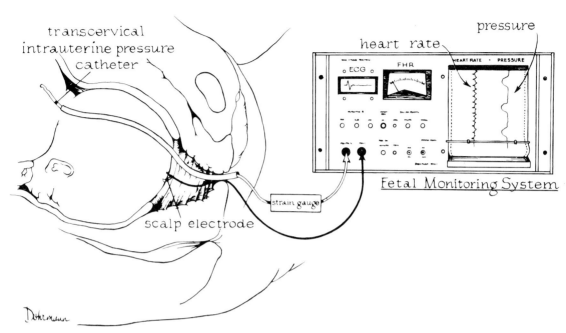

Figure 10–30. Fetal heart rate and intrauterine pressure are recorded from a fetal scalp electrode and a transcervical pressure catheter in the uterus. (From Parer JT: Biophysical evaluation of fetal status: Fetal heart rate. *In* Creasy R, Resnik R [eds]: Maternal-Fetal Medicine. Philadelphia: WB Saunders, 1984; 292.)

Electrocardiography can be either indirect from the maternal abdomen or direct from stainless steel spiral electrodes placed in the infant's scalp (Fig. 10–30). This latter technique is invasive and requires rupture of the maternal membranes. It carries the risk of fetal scalp infection, facial injury (particularly the eye), and bleeding. However, it is the best way to get dependable data on beat-to-beat variability for clinical decision making.

Uterine contractions may be monitored either externally or internally. External monitors document the frequency and duration of contractions but not the intensity. Internal monitors are able to quantify the intensity of contractions but require that the amniotic membranes be ruptured in order to place an intrauterine catheter (Fig. 10–30).

Fetal Scalp pH Sampling

When a fetal heart rate pattern is suggestive of fetal compromise, fetal scalp pH is often recommended in order to confirm the suspected acidosis. This requires that the amniotic membranes be ruptured. The normal range for fetal capillary blood pH is 7.25–7.35 (Fig. 10–31); below 7.2, the fetus is definitely acidotic. Between 7.2 and 7.25, a clinical interpretation is required. What is the maternal pH? What is the type of acidosis? A metabolic acidosis suggests that anaerobic glycolysis is present, possibly as a result of tissue asphyxia due to placental failure. Respiratory acidosis is more likely to reflect umbilical cord compression.[83] Was there any preceding maternal

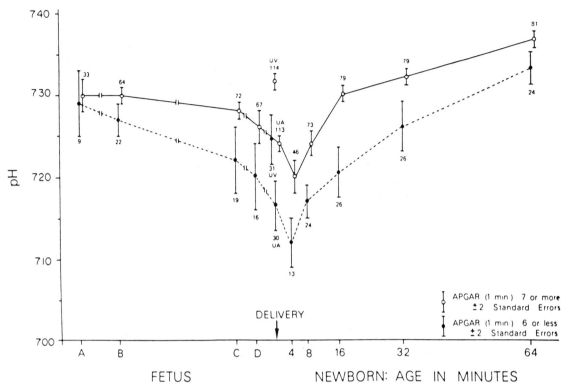

Figure 10–31. Mean fetal and newborn pH values. The *open circles* (upper trace) reflect newborns with 1-minute Apgar scores of 7 or above; the *solid circles*, those with scores below 7. Sample times were (A) early labor, (B) 5-cm cervical dilatation, (C) complete dilatation, (D) delivery. (From Modanlou H, Yeh SY, Hon EH: Fetal and neonatal biochemistry and Apgar scores. Am J Obstet Gynecol 1973; 117:942–951. With permission.)

event, such as a seizure or anesthetic-induced maternal hypotension, to account for the fetal acidosis? Also important is the timing of the fetal scalp sampling in relation to maternal contractions. The best information regarding the well-being of the fetus is obtained by sampling just before a contraction.

Mild to moderate decelerations with good variability have not been shown to correlate with fetal acidosis, whereas moderate and severe decelerations with decreased baseline variability are predictive of an acidotic fetus.[84] The presence of normal fetal heart rate variability predicts a vigorous fetus in close to 100% of cases. In contrast, a normal pH (above 7.25) predicts a vigorous fetus in 90% of cases, and a very low pH (below 7.15) predicts a depressed fetus with a reliability of only 80%. Thus, there is little point in performing fetal scalp sampling in a situation in which there is good fetal heart rate variability. Also, there is little benefit to be gained in scalp sampling when the fetal heart rate pattern is ominous and persistent. Fetal blood sampling should not be done when there is any known or suspected bleeding disorder such as hemophilia or von Willebrand's disease. Sampling in such cases has resulted in fetal death.

Some indications for sampling are (1) presence of moderate to severe decelerations with somewhat decreased fetal heart rate variability that do not respond to standard treatment, (2) need to monitor a fetus during labor when maternal drug therapy affecting fetal heart rate variability is required, and (3) absence of beat-to-beat variability without obvious cause on initial measurement of heart rate.

Influence of Monitoring on Rates of Cesarean Section

It is unclear whether monitoring has increased the rate of cesarean sections. The number has increased, but it reflects factors other than monitoring, such as changed management for genital herpes and breech presentation, as well as the decline of midforceps interventions. There are studies that support both views, but most indicate that monitoring is associated with higher rates of cesarean sections.[79,85] It is likely that part of this difference results from inadequate interpretation of the fetal heart rate patterns.

Monitoring and Fetal Outcome

There are as yet no randomized controlled trials establishing the benefits of fetal monitoring. Because of the small numbers of affected fetuses, it takes very large numbers to generate meaningful studies. Such numbers (>100,000 births) have been obtained from nonrandomized surveys, and the following information was generated. The intrapartum stillbirth rate decreased from 2.4 to 0.5 per 1000 with monitoring (p <0.0001), and the neonatal death rate decreased from 8.1 to 3.6 per 1000 with monitoring (p <0.0001).[79] The data are suggestive but not conclusive that routine fetal monitoring improves neonatal outcomes.

NEONATAL ASSESSMENT

With severance of the umbilical cord at delivery, the infant must rapidly make the transition from intrauterine dependency to extrauterine independence. Careful monitoring of the fetus during this period is essential if one is to intervene promptly in the event of failure of transition, the consequences of which are devastating and lifelong.

Apgar Score

The standard method for assessing the immediate well-being of a newborn is by the Apgar score. Although many think that this is a mnemonic for appearance, pulse, grimace, activity, and respiration, others know that it is actually named for Virginia Apgar, the anesthesiologist who first proposed the scoring system.[86] The Apgar scoring system assigns a score of 0, 1, or 2 in the categories listed (Table 10–8). For example, an absent heart rate results in a score of 0, any heart rate below 100 gets a score of 1, and

Table 10–8. APGAR NEONATAL SCORING SYSTEM*

	Score		
Sign	*0*	*1*	*2*
Heart rate	Absent	Under 100 beats/minute	Over 100 beats/minute
Respiratory effort	Absent	Slow, irregular	Good, crying
Color	Blue, pale	Acrocyanosis (pink body, blue extremities)	Completely pink
Reflex irritability (response to nasal catheter)	Absent	Grimace	Cough, sneeze
Muscle tone	Limp	Some flexion of extremities	Active motion

* Each sign is evaluated and scored from 0 to 2 at 1 and 5 minutes after birth. The sum of each individual score is the Apgar score for that time period.

a heart rate over 100 gets a score of 2. The Apgar score is assessed at 1 and 5 minutes and occasionally at 10 minutes. A 1-minute score of 0–2 is indicative of a severely depressed neonate who is in need of active resuscitation. A score of 3–7 is indicative of a moderately depressed infant who will probably respond to oxygen administration by mask, possibly with positive pressure ventilation. Infants with scores greater than 8 rarely need

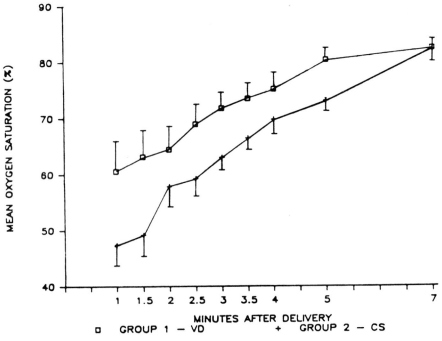

Figure 10–32. Oxygen saturation in the immediate newborn period. *Open squares* represent infants delivered vaginally (VD); *crosses* indicate cesarean delivery (CS). The lower saturation in infants delivered by cesarean section is accounted for by increased lung fluid in these infants. (From Harris AP, Sendak MJ, Donham RT: Changes in arterial oxygen saturation immediately after birth in the human neonate. J Pediatr 1986; 109:117–119. With permission.)

respiratory assistance. The Apgar score is not a good predictor of long-term neurologic outcome. For any individual infant, a very low score at 5 minutes is of little value in predicting either the likelihood of survival or the neurologic outcome.[87]

In addition to the Apgar scoring system, newborn assessment in the delivery room requires the same clinical observations used in other critical care settings. It is essential to recall the ABCs of basic life support: airway, breathing, circulation. Is the airway patent? Are there bilateral breath sounds? What is the quality of respiratory effort? Are there sternal retractions or nasal flaring? Is the abdomen distended? Is there adequate capillary refill?

Oxygen Saturation

Recently, pulse oximetry has been introduced into the delivery room as a monitor of newborn oxygen saturation (Sao_2).[88] This allows an immediate assessment of the infant's initial oxygen saturation, as well as documentation of the normal transition from the low saturation state found *in utero* to the much higher saturations associated with pulmonary gas exchange. Pulse oximetry has been shown to be unreliable at low saturations ($<60\%$) in sick neonates, and it should not replace direct arterial blood gas sampling in such infants.[89] However, it is a valuable trend monitor and an early indicator of the efficacy of various therapeutic interventions. When pulse oximetry is utilized in the delivery room, it is important to be aware that an oxygen saturation of 80% at 5 minutes is normal (Fig. 10–32) and does not warrant aggressive respiratory intervention in the absence of clinical signs of respiratory distress.

References

1. Blekta M, Hlavatý V, Trnková M, et al: Volume of whole blood and absolute amount of serum proteins in the early stages of late toxemia of pregnancy. Am J Obstet Gynecol 1970; 106:10–13.
2. Wilson M, Morganti AA, Zervoudakis I, et al: Blood pressure, the renin-aldosterone system and sex steroids throughout normal pregnancy. Am J Med 1980; 68:97–104.
3. Sachs BP, Brown DA, Driscoll SG, et al: Maternal mortality in Massachusetts. Trends and prevention. N Engl J Med 1987; 316:667–672.
4. Gant NF, Daley GL, Chand S, et al: A study of angiotensin II pressor response throughout primigravid pregnancy. J Clin Invest 1973; 52:2682–2689.
5. Davison JM: Renal haemodynamics and volume homeostasis in pregnancy. Scand J Clin Lab Invest [Suppl] 1984; 169:15–27.
6. Cotton DB, Gonik B, Spillman T, Dorman KF: Intrapartum to postpartum changes in colloid osmotic pressure. Am J Obstet Gynecol 1984; 149:174–177.
7. Huch A, Huch R, Schneider H, Rooth G: Continuous transcutaneous monitoring of fetal oxygen tension during labor. Br J Obstet Gynaecol (Suppl 1) 1977; 84:1–39.

8. Russell IF, Chambers WA: Closing volume in normal pregnancy. Br J Anaesth 1981; 53:1043–1046.

9. Datta S, Lambert DH, Gregus J, et al: Differential sensitivities of mammalian nerve fibers during pregnancy. Anesth Analg 1983; 62:1070–1072.

10. Redman CWG: Hypertension in pregnancy. *In* deSwiet M (ed): Medical Disorders of Pregnancy. London: Blackwell Scientific, 1984; 149–191.

11. Hughes EC (ed): Obstetric-Gynecologic Terminology. Philadelphia: FA Davis, 1972; 422–423.

12. McCartney CP: Pathological anatomy of acute hypertension of pregnancy. Circulation 1964; 30 (Suppl 2):37–42.

13. Goodlin RC, Quaife MA, Dirksen JW: The significance, diagnosis, and treatment of maternal hypovolemia as associated with fetal/maternal illness. Semin Perinatol 1981; 5:163–174.

14. Hayes PM, Cruikshank DP, Dunn LJ: Plasma volume determination in normal and preeclamptic pregnancies. Am J Obstet Gynecol 1985; 151:958–966.

15. Gallery EDM: Pregnancy-associated hypertension: Interrelationships of volume and blood pressure changes. Clin Exp Hypertens 1982; B1:39–47.

16. Groenendijk R, Trimbos JB, Wallenburg HCS: Hemodynamic measurements in preeclampsia: Preliminary observations. Am J Obstet Gynecol 1984; 150:232–236.

17. Wasserstrum N, Cotton DB: Hemodynamic monitoring in severe pregnancy-induced hypertension. Clin Perinatol 1986; 13:781–799.

18. Clark SL, Greenspoon JS, Aldahl D, Phelan JP: Severe preeclampsia with persistent oliguria: Management of hemodynamic subsets. Am J Obstet Gynecol 1986; 154:490–494.

19. Cotton DB, Longmire S, Jones MM, et al: Cardiovascular alterations in severe pregnancy-induced hypertension: Effects of intravenous nitroglycerin coupled with blood volume expansion. Am J Obstet Gynecol 1986; 154:1053–1059.

20. Benedetti TJ, Carlson RW: Studies of colloid osmotic pressure in pregnancy-induced hypertension. Am J Obstet Gynecol 1979; 135:308–311.

21. Benedetti TJ, Kates R, Williams V: Hemodynamic observations in severe preeclampsia complicated by pulmonary edema. Am J Obstet Gynecol 1980; 152:330–334.

22. Oney T, Kaulhausen H: The value of the angiotensin sensitivity test in the diagnosis of hypertensive disorders in pregnancy. Am J Obstet Gynecol 1982; 142:17–20.

23. Roberts JM: Pregnancy-related hypertension. *In* Creasy R, Resnik R (eds): Maternal-Fetal Medicine. Philadelphia: WB Saunders, 1984; 739.

24. Lunell NO, Lewander R, Mamoun I, et al: Uteroplacental blood flow in pregnancy induced hypertension. Scand J Clin Lab Invest [Suppl] 1984; 169:28–35.

25. Jouppila P, Kirkinen P, Koivula A, Ylikorkala O: Effects of dihydralazine infusion on the fetoplacental blood flow and maternal prostanoids. Obstet Gynecol 1985; 65:115–118.

26. Shoemaker CT, Meyers M: Sodium nitroprusside for control of severe hypertensive disease of pregnancy: A case report and discussion of potential toxicity. Am J Obstet Gynecol 1984; 149:171–173.

27. Stemple JE, O'Grady JP, Morton MJ, Johnson KA: Use of sodium nitroprusside in complications of gestational hypertension. Obstet Gynecol 1983; 60:533–538.

28. Naulty J, Cefalo RC, Lewis PE: Fetal toxicity of nitroprusside in the pregnant ewe. Am J Obstet Gynecol 1981; 139:708–711.

29. Lee W, Gonik B, Cotton DB: Urinary diagnostic indices in preeclampsia-associated oliguria: Correlation with invasive hemodynamic monitoring. Am J Obstet Gynecol 1987; 156:100–103.

30. Shuster E, Weppelmann B: Plasma urate measurements and fetal outcome in preeclampsia. Gynecol Obstet Invest 1981; 12:162–167.
31. Merrell DA, Koch MA: Epidural anesthesia as an anticonvulsant in the management of hypertensive and eclamptic patients in labor. S Afr Med J 1980; 58:875–877.
32. Abboud T, Artal R, Sarkis F, et al: Sympathoadrenal activity, maternal, fetal, and neonatal responses after epidural anesthesia in the preeclamptic patient. Am J Obstet Gynecol 1982; 144:915–918.
33. Sibai BH, Taslimi MM, El-Nazer A, et al: Maternal-perinatal outcome associated with the syndrome of hemolysis, elevated liver enzyme, and low platelets in severe preeclampsia-eclampsia. Am J Obstet Gynecol 1986; 155:501–509.
34. Walsh SW: Preeclampsia: An imbalance in placental prostacyclin and thromboxane production. Am J Obstet Gynecol 1985; 152:335–340.
35. Lindheimer MD, Katz AI: Hypertension in pregnancy. N Engl J Med 1985; 313:675–680.
36. Jouppila P, Jouppila R, Hollmen A, Koivula A: Lumbar epidural analgesia to improve intervillous blood flow during labor in severe preeclampsia. Obstet Gynecol 1982; 59:158–161.
37. Newsome LR, Bramwell RS, Curling PE: Severe preeclampsia: Hemodynamic effects of lumbar epidural anesthesia. Anesth Analg 1986; 65:31–36.
38. Hodgkinson R, Husain FJ, Hayashi RH: Systemic and pulmonary blood pressure during caesarean section in parturients with gestational hypertension. Can Anaesth Soc J 1980; 27:389–393.
39. Ramanathan J, Bottorff M, Jeter JN, et al: The pharmacokinetics and maternal and neonatal effects of epidural lidocaine in preeclampsia. Anesth Analg 1986; 65:120–126.
40. Jouppila P, Kirkinen P, Koivula A, Ylikorkala O: Labetalol does not alter the placental or fetal blood flow or maternal prostanoids in preeclampsia. Br J Obstet Gynaecol 1986; 93:543–547.
41. Cotton DB, Gonik B, Dorman K, Harrist R: Cardiovascular alterations in severe pregnancy-induced hypertension: Relationship of central venous pressure to pulmonary capillary wedge pressure. Am J Obstet Gynecol 1985; 151:762–764.
42. Robson SC, Dunlop W, Moore M, Hunter S: Combined Doppler and echocardiographic measurement of cardiac output: Theory and application in pregnancy. Br J Obstet Gynaecol 1987; 94:1014–1027.
43. Easterling TR, Watts DH, Schmucker BC, Benedetti TJ: Measurement of cardiac output during pregnancy: Validation of Doppler technique and clinical observations in preeclampsia. Obstet Gynecol 1987; 69:845–850.
44. Siekmann U, Heilmann L, Klosa W, et al: Simultaneous investigations of maternal cardiac output and fetal blood flow during hypervolemic hemodilution in preeclampsia—preliminary observations. J Perinat Med 1986; 14:59–69.
45. Mangano DT: Anesthesia for the pregnant cardiac patient. In Schnider SM, Levinson G (eds): Anesthesia for Obstetrics, 2nd Ed. Baltimore: Williams & Wilkins, 1987; 345–381.
46. Sugishita Y, Ito I, Kubo T: Pregnancy in cardiac patients: Possible influence of volume overload by pregnancy on pulmonary circulation. Jpn Circ J 1986; 50:376–383.
47. Clark SL, Phelan JP, Greenspoon J, et al: Labor and delivery in the presence of mitral stenosis: Central hemodynamic observations. Am J Obstet Gynecol 1985; 152:984–988.
48. Cunningham FG, Pritchard JA, Hankins GD, et al: Peripartum heart failure: Idiopathic cardiomyopathy or compounding cardiovascular events? Obstet Gynecol 1986; 67:157–168.

49. Clark SL: Labor and delivery in the patient with structural cardiac disease. Clin Perinatol 1986; 13:695–703.
50. Nadeau S, Noble WH: Misinterpretation of pressure measurements from the pulmonary artery catheter. Can Anaesth Soc J 1986; 33:352–363.
51. Hemmings GT, Whalley DG, O'Connor PJ: Invasive monitoring and anaesthetic management of a parturient with mitral stenosis. Can J Anaesth 1987; 34:182–185.
52. Woods AM, Longnecker DE: Endoscopy. In Marshall BE, Longnecker DE, Fairley HB (eds): Anesthesia for Thoracic Procedures. Boston: Blackwell Scientific, 1988; 338–341.
53. Lynch C, Rizor R: Anesthestic management of a parturient with mitral and aortic valvular disease. Anesth Analg 1982; 61:788–792.
54. Perloff JK, Child JS, Edwards JE: New guidelines for the clinical diagnosis of mitral valve prolapse. Am J Cardiol 1986; 57:1124–1129.
55. Alcantara LG, Marx GF: Cesarean section under epidural analgesia in a parturient with mitral valve prolapse. Anesth Analg 1987; 66:902–903.
56. Shapiro EP, Trimble EL, Robinson JC, et al: Safety of labor and delivery in women with mitral valve prolapse. Am J Cardiol 1985; 56:806–807.
57. Dineen E, Brent BN: Aortic valve stenosis: Comparison of patients with to those without chronic congestive heart failure. Am J Cardiol 1986; 57:419–422.
58. Redfern N, Bower S, Bullock RE, Hull CJ: Alfentanil for caesarean section complicated by severe aortic stenosis. Br J Anaesth 1987; 59:1309–1312.
59. Karp RB, Roe BB: Effects of aortic insufficiency of phasic flow patterns in the coronary artery. Ann Surg 1966; 164:959–966.
60. Buckberg GD, Kattus AA: Factors determining the distribution and adequacy of left ventricular myocardial blood flow. In Bloor CM, Olsson RA (eds): Current Topics in Coronary Research. New York: Plenum, 1975; 95.
61. Alderson JD: Cardiovascular collapse following epidural anaesthesia for caesarean section in a patient with aortic incompetence. Anaesthesia 1987; 42:643–645.
62. Shime J, Mocarski EJM, Hastings D, et al: Congenital heart disease in pregnancy: Short- and long-term implications. Am J Obstet Gynecol 1987; 156:313–322.
63. Laishley RS, Burrows FA, Lerman J, Roy WL: Effect of anesthetic induction regimens on oxygen saturation in cyanotic congenital heart disease. Anesthesiology 1986; 65:676–677.
64. Boxer RA, Gottesfeld I, Sharanjeet S, et al: Noninvasive pulse oximetry in children with cyanotic congenital heart disease. Crit Care Med 1987; 15:1062–1064.
65. Simmons DH, Linde LM, Miller JH, O'Reilly RJ: Relationship between lung volume and pulmonary vascular resistance. Circ Res 1961; 9:465–471.
66. Hughes SC: Intraspinal opiates in obstetrics. In Schnider SM, Levinson G (eds): Anesthesia for Obstetrics, 2nd Ed. Baltimore: Williams & Wilkins, 1987; 123–141.
67. Rawal N: Nonnociceptive effects of intraspinal opioids and their clinical applications. Int Anesthesiol Clin 1986; 24:75–91.
68. Gustafsson LL, Schildt B, Jacobsen K: Adverse effects of epidural and intrathecal opiates: Report of a nationwide survey in Sweden. Br J Anaesth 1982; 54:479–485.
69. Bromage PR, Camporesi EM, Durant PAC, Nielsen CH: Rostral spread of epidural morphine. Anesthesiology 1982; 56:431–436.
70. Abboud TK, Moore M, Zhu J, et al: Epidural butorphanol or morphine for the relief of post-cesarean section pain: Ventilatory responses to carbon dioxide. Anesth Analg 1987; 66:887–893.

71. Rawal N, Wattwil M: Respiratory depression after epidural morphine—an experimental and clinical study. Anesth Analg 1984; 63:8–14.
72. Manning FA: Ultrasound in fetal medicine. *In* Creasy R, Resnik R (eds): Maternal-Fetal Medicine. Philadelphia: WB Saunders, 1984; 210.
73. Campbell S, Pearce JM: The prenatal diagnosis of fetal structural anomalies by ultrasound. Clin Obstet Gynecol 1983; 10:475–505.
74. Harrison MR, Golbus MS, Filly RA, et al: Fetal hydronephrosis: Selection and surgical repair. J Pediatr Surg 1987; 22:556–558.
75. Touloukian RJ: What's new in pediatric surgery. Pediatrics 1988; 81:692–696.
76. Jouppila P, Kirkinen P: Blood velocity waveforms of the fetal aorta in normal and hypertensive pregnancies. Obstet Gynecol 1986; 67:856–860.
77. Freeman RK: Contraction stress testing for primary fetal surveillance in patients at high risk for uteroplacental insufficiency. Clin Perinatol 1982; 9:265–270.
78. Martin CB: Physiologic and clinical use of fetal heart rate variability. Clin Perinatol 1982; 9:339–351.
79. Parer JT: Biophysical evaluation of fetal status: Fetal heart rate. *In* Creasy R, Resnik R (eds): Maternal-Fetal Medicine. Philadelphia: WB Saunders, 1984; 285–319.
80. Paul EH, Suidan AK, Yeh SY, et al: Clinical fetal monitoring. VII. The evaluation and significance of intrapartum baseline FHR variability. Am J Obstet Gynecol 1975; 123:206–210.
81. Hon EH: Instrumentation of fetal heart rate and fetal electrocardiography. Obstet Gynecol 1967; 30:281–286.
82. Schifrin BS: The fetal monitoring polemic. Clin Perinatol 1982; 9:393–407.
83. Wible JL, Petrie RH, Koons A, Perez A: The clinical use of umbilical cord acid-base determinations in perinatal surveillance and management. Clin Perinatol 1982; 9:387–397.
84. Miller FC: Prediction of acid-base values from intrapartum fetal heart rate data and their correlation with scalp and fundic values. Clin Perinatol 1982; 9:353–361.
85. Haverkamp AD, Orleans M, Langendoerfer S, et al: A controlled trial of the differential effects of intrapartum fetal monitoring. Am J Obstet Gynecol 1979; 134:399–412.
86. Apgar V: A proposal for a new method of evaluation of the newborn infant. Anesth Analg 1943; 32:260–267.
87. Cohen SE: Evaluation of the neonate. *In* Schnider SM, Levinson G (eds): Anesthesia for Obstetrics, 2nd Ed. Baltimore: Williams & Wilkins, 1987; 489–507.
88. House JT, Schultetus RR, Gravenstein N: Continuous neonatal evaluation in the delivery room by pulse oximetry. J Clin Monit 1987; 3:96–100.
89. Fanconi S: Reliability of pulse oximetry in hypoxic infants. J Pediatr 1988; 112:424–427.

Computerized Monitoring

chapter eleven

Computerized Monitoring in Anesthesia

ALAN W. MURRAY, M.B., Ch.B., F.F.A.R.C.S.
■ GAVIN N. C. KENNY, B.Sc. (Hons.), M.D., F.F.A.R.C.S.

The computer, now a well-established tool in medicine, is used for a wide variety of functions ranging from simple clerical tasks, such as word processing, to complex clinical simulations for undergraduate and postgraduate teaching.[1] The ability to perform data acquisition; signal processing, storage, and analysis; and number manipulation is especially appropriate in anesthesia. Interpretive calculations can be performed in real time as the data are acquired, and derived information can be displayed almost instantaneously with its collection. Detection of detrimental changes in physiologic functions and production of appropriate warnings distinguish computerized monitoring from simple data capture. Modern sophisticated monitors frequently contain on-board microprocessors to perform calculations of this type. Microprocessor-based drug- and anesthesia-delivery systems permit collection of physiologic data and adjustment of drug administration based on hemodynamic parameters.[2] Computerized monitors also provide storage for many hours of data and thus produce graphic trend displays of information. Although humans are adept at pattern recognition (interpretation of electrocardiogram or electroencephalogram), their limitation of short-term memory reduces data management capability.

Development of computerized monitoring systems requires considerable skill in engineering and programming, owing to the necessity for performing data capture and analysis in real time and for producing a system that is simple for relatively untrained operators to use. Many different groups have described monitoring and records systems, and most have approached the problems involved in different ways.

TYPES OF COMPUTERS

Before computer applications in anesthesia are discussed, the basics of computing must be considered. Two distinct types of computers are used in monitoring anesthesia: analog and digital. Their structures and functions are completely different.

Analog Computers

These machines are based on a unit known as an operational amplifier. Operational amplifiers cannot handle alphanumeric data (letters and numbers) but can process fixed or variable waveforms almost instantaneously when these are presented as voltages. Connecting different circuits to an operational amplifier alters the characteristics of the system and allows data manipulations such as summation, subtraction, division, multiplication, integration, and differentiation. The output from the analog computer is a voltage proportional to that of the input, and display of the calculated result occurs virtually instantaneously with the input signal.[3]

The most frequent use of analog computers in anesthesia is to calculate cardiac output from a bolus injection of dye or cold dextrose solution (thermodilution) into the circulation with blood sampling downstream from the injection site. When the concentration of the indicator is measured and plotted against time, a curve is produced. Cardiac output can then be obtained by calculating the area under the curve. Manual calculation of this is tedious and time-consuming. Application of a computer to the problem results in almost instantaneous calculation of the result by integration of the curve in real time (see Chapter 7).

One major drawback of analog computers is the inability to use alphanumeric data. A second major disadvantage is the difficulty of changing the function of the computer. This can only be achieved by rewiring or changing the input circuit, which may require a high degree of technical skill. Analog computers have almost completely been replaced by digital computers, and most modern cardiac output computers now use digital techniques for collection of the temperature waveform and calculation of the final result.

Digital Computers

The components of a digital computer system—keyboard, central processor unit, memory circuits, visual display unit, and output devices—are collectively known as computer hardware. Software is the term applied to data and programs used by the machine that determine the functions performed by the computer. Programs are stored usually on some form of magnetic medium such as a floppy disk and must be loaded into the computer before use. Firmware is an arrangement in which programs are stored permanently on a reprogrammable integrated circuit and are therefore available for immediate use.

Method of Operation

Digital computers deal directly with numbers, and all information used is coded and stored in numeric form. The computer then applies a program to process the data. A program is a series of instructions that directs the computer precisely how to perform the required tasks. Thus, a finite time is required to perform a calculation or to process data. The program may consist of several thousand individual steps, each of which must be correct for the system to function appropriately. Correction or "debugging" and maintenance of programs can require considerable time, and errors may not appear until some unusual combination of circumstances arises.

Until a digital computer is provided with a program, it cannot perform any useful operation. With a change in the program, the computer can be used for a completely different task. This provides a unique degree of flexibility, so that the same machine can be used for a wide variety of different functions simply by changing the program it executes.

Binary System

The binary system is used to encode information. Thus, only two "states" are required to represent information. These states represent the digits 1 and 0. The digits can be represented as arbitrarily defined voltages, the open or closed positions of a switch, the presence or absence of an electrical impulse, or the change of north-south orientation of a magnetic field. Each individual 1 or 0 is known as a *bit* of information. A group of 8 bits is known as a *byte*. One byte can represent decimal numbers between 0 and 256. Values in this range are used to represent letters and control codes for activating special functions and output devices. Numbers are represented in scientific notation by a combination of two or more bytes that contain information related to the sign of the number and the exponent.

Forms of Digital Computers

Digital computers are produced in three main forms: main frame, minicomputers, and microcomputers. The principles of operation, however, remain similar. Classification of computers is based on the complexity and capacity of the system.

Mainframe Computers

Mainframe computers are the largest systems. They can support several dozen users simultaneously by sharing processor time among active terminals. Each terminal consists of a keyboard with which the operator enters information and controls the functions performed by the computer and a visual display unit, which displays the results on a screen. Switching between terminals occurs so rapidly that there is usually no noticeable delay during use of any one terminal. However, if many users each require considerable processor time or frequent disk access, the response time can increase to an unacceptable level.

The advantage of mainframe computing is that it allows sharing of data, and expensive output and peripheral devices such as printers and plotters can be used efficiently. These systems are thus centralized systems, and their use is controlled by professional computing staff. Combined with the high purchase and maintenance costs, this results in a highly expensive system. Attempts have been made to link all departments within a hospital to a centralized computer, but these have rarely been successful.[4]

Minicomputers

Minicomputers are also capable of serving several users simultaneously, and their architecture and operation are similar to those of the mainframe. Running costs of the minicomputer are also significant but much lower than the mainframe, and response time of the processor can be unacceptably long with these systems. However, when many users must have access to a large central store of information, minicomputers can provide the hardware requirements for a satisfactory system.

Microcomputers

Microcomputers were designed initially for single users. They are relatively simple devices with smaller memory capacity and slower processing speeds than either minicomputers or mainframe computers. However, microcomputers are sufficiently powerful to handle applications when few simultaneous demands are made on the system. Their simplicity allows nonexperts to write their own programs if necessary. Microelectronic developments have resulted in microcomputers whose performance approaches that of minicomputer systems at a fraction of the cost.

Networking of microcomputers allows communication between autonomous units over short distances (local area network), thus sharing information, output, and storage devices. In contrast to minicomputers and mainframe systems, if one microcomputer within a network fails, the remainder of the network continues to function normally.

Sections of Digital Computers

Functionally, the digital computer can be divided into four sections: the central processing unit, memory system, input, and output devices.

Central Processing Unit

The central processing unit (CPU) or microprocessor provides the arithmetic and decision-making capabilities of the computer. The CPU executes the programs and is also responsible for the correct transfer of information among the input, output, and memory devices.

The CPU and other integrated circuits are usually connected in such a way that data can be passed among them one byte at a time. The connection consists of many parallel tracks, one of which carries a timing signal that synchronizes the actions of the integrated circuits and others that carry the byte of data, one bit per track. Data are passed rapidly via this system, which is known as a data bus. More recent processors handle 16- and 32-bit data, which allows much more rapid computation than the original 8-bit data bus.

When the power supply is switched on at the start of a computing session, the CPU initiates a routine that checks the functions of the system and prepares the computer for use. This is known as *booting* the system.

The Memory Systems

Memory systems are required to hold the computer operating systems, the programs, and the data to be acted on by the programs. Memory within the computer is arranged on several types of specialized integrated circuits.

Random Access Memory (RAM) is a form of memory that allows retrieval or storage of data one byte at a time as required. Data are transferred to a specific area of RAM by an address bus (a parallel collection of wires of high or low voltage corresponding to binary number bits). Data movement from RAM is very rapid. Modern microcomputers now have memory capacities of up to 4 million bytes (4 megabytes). The disadvantage of RAM is that it requires a constant power supply in order to maintain its integrity. However, battery-backed RAM is available and can last for up to 10 years, depending on battery type.

Read Only Memory (ROM) is a type of memory device that contains the operating system and the start-up instructions of the computer. ROM memory is not usually available to the user for storing information, and its contents cannot be altered by the program. Its contents are unaffected by interruptions of the power supply.

More permanent storage is available using magnetic media to make a record of information that can be reloaded into the computer when required. Magnetic tape storage is possible, but since storage of data is sequential, retrieval is slow.

Disks coated with magnetic material are available for information storage. The data are stored on concentric tracks, and, when retrieval is required, any part of the disk can be accessed within one rotation of the disk. Floppy disks are relatively inexpensive and can store between 100,000 and 2 million characters per disk. Hard disks are more expensive, but they can hold up to 80 million characters and are capable of much faster data storage and retrieval. A character is a letter, digit, or other special symbol. Magnetic media can be reused many times but are sensitive to damage by magnetic fields generated by electrical equipment of all kinds.

Laser disk storage, called compact disk ROM (CD ROM), has storage capacity in excess of 4 billion characters per disk. At present, the system can only record information once, but it can be retrieved an unlimited number of times. This is known as Write Once Read Many Times or WORM technology.

Input Devices

Input devices can be divided into two groups: off-line and on-line. Off-line devices allow data entry after all the information has been collected, and on-line collection of data obtains the information directly from a source such as a blood pressure monitor. Off-line entry of data involves an operator transcribing from a print-out or graph; thus human error is possible. Selection of the most appropriate type of input device is essential in order to make the program simple and convenient to use.

Off-Line Devices

Keyboard. A keyboard is present on most computer systems and is therefore an inexpensive, readily available route for data entry. It requires no special software to support its use, although some skill is required to enter data accurately and at an acceptable speed. However, in a study comparing data entry by keyboard, light pen, and voice recognition in a group of nurses, it was found that keyboard data entry was quickest.[5] Data accuracy with the keyboard was good and comparable to the light pen. Voice recognition was three times slower than keyboard entry, owing to the high number of errors that occurred. In a separate study, medical students also expressed a preference for keyboard use when asked to compare keyboard and light pen control of teaching programs.[5] This acceptability may be the result of the increased use of computers in schools and homes and the greater familiarity with a standard keyboard, since 53% of the medical students had previous computer experience.[6]

Keypad. The keypad is similar to a keyboard but is restricted to fewer keys, which may be labeled with predefined functions or numbers according to the application involved. Each key may be labeled either permanently or with an overlay that can be changed for the entry of different types of data such as fluids, drugs, or anesthetic procedures. The keypad allows rapid selection of any desired item, but it is essentially less flexible than a standard keyboard. However, its simplicity of use allows those unfamiliar with a typewriter keyboard to operate the computer with minimum training.

Monitor Screen. Data selection from lists of "menus" *directly displayed on a monitor screen* is increasingly popular, especially with nontypists. Whereas a standard keyboard or keypad can be used to select from a list of possible items displayed on the screen by using only the numeral keys, three devices are available—a light pen, a mouse, or a touch screen—that allow the required item to be selected simply by touching the screen display directly.

Light Pen. A light pen can be interfaced with the computer. When specific blocks of light are touched on the screen, selection of the appropriate item from the screen menu is made.[7]

Mouse. A mouse is a small box with wheels that is now available on many microcomputers. It is moved across a work surface by the operator. As the mouse is moved, a ball on the under surface transmits the x and y coordinates to the computer via two optical sensors. Using this information, the computer's operating system moves a pointer (cursor) on the monitor screen in an equivalent direction and distance. When the pointer tip is over the required item, a button on the mouse is pressed and the selection is made.[8] Other similar input devices are track balls and joy sticks.

This is known as the *wimp* environment and refers to the combination of *w*indows (areas of the monitor screen that can show parts of a document that is much larger than the whole screen could display), *i*cons (pictures representing items such as disk drives), *m*ouse, and *p*ointer. This user interface enables very rapid and easy use of the program with minimum computer knowledge.

Touch Screen. The touch screen is the third method of selecting information. This system involves use of a special monitor screen that contains horizontal and vertical arrays of light sources and detectors. When the operator touches a specific item on the screen, the x and y coordinates are detected by interruption of the appropriate light beams and thus recognized by the computer's operating system.

These methods allow rapid and accurate selection from screen lists but are relatively restricted by the number of items that can be displayed on the screen at any one time. The touch screen is also relatively expensive. It is available on the Ohmeda Automated Anesthetic Record Keeper (AARK), described below.

Bit Pad. A bit pad allows entry of x-y coordinates into the computer by touching the pad with a stylus connected to the pad. The pad can then be covered with a printed sheet containing diagrams. Touching the appropriate part of the diagram enters information into the computer. A system has been described in which calculation of fluid balance was performed using the bit pad.[9]

Bar Codes. Bar codes are used increasingly to enter data into computer systems in areas such as supermarkets and have been employed to collect anesthetic information. The bar codes indicating the items available for selection may be printed on sheets of paper or attached directly to a syringe. Passing the bar code reader over the parallel bars of the code enters the selected item into the computer.

Voice Recognition. Voice recognition at present tends to be inaccurate, especially in areas with high background noise.[10] However, development of voice input is progressing rapidly, and one computerized anesthetic record system, which is described later, has this form of data entry available as an option. With anticipated future developments in hardware and software, this may eventually offer the easiest and most natural form of off-line data input.

On-Line Data Collection

During on-line data collection, the computer is connected directly to the data source. This means that data transfer is rapid, complete, and free

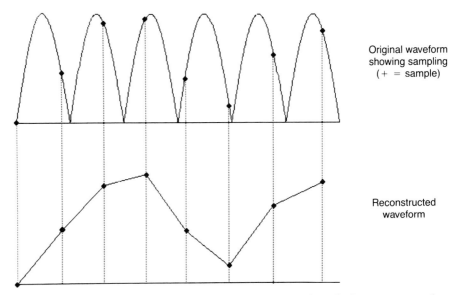

Figure 11–1. Sampling of the waveform at an incorrect rate (top) results in a reconstructed waveform (bottom) that differs markedly from the original waveform.

from human interference. Data may be made available on-line in an analog or digital form.

Analog Data Collection

Most signals from medical equipment are presented as varying *analog voltages,* e.g., an arterial pressure waveform. The signal must therefore be changed to a digital form that the computer can accept. This is achieved by an analog-to-digital converter (ADC) that produces binary output in proportion to the voltage received by the unit. The signal can be sampled at varying rates; sampling too slowly gives an inaccurate representation of the original signal (Fig. 11–1), whereas frequent sampling provides more accuracy (Fig. 11–2).

Complex waveforms can be analyzed to produce a set of simple sine waves of different frequencies and amplitudes (Fourier transformation). In order to produce an accurate representation of any waveform, sampling must occur at twice the rate of the highest frequency in the waveform (Nyquist theorem). A blood pressure wave, for example, requires a sampling rate of 50–100 samples/second, and electrocardiogram complex, about 200–1000 samples/second.

The ADC must be calibrated or scaled according to the amplitude of the waveform. Provision must be made for a negative phase on the wave, such as may occur when recording a central venous pressure wave. The maximum resolution of the waveform amplitude depends on the type of ADC used. An 8-bit ADC allows resolution of two to the power eight, or 256 steps, which is adequate for analysis of a blood pressure wave. For higher resolution, 16-bit converters are available and are capable of giving a resolution

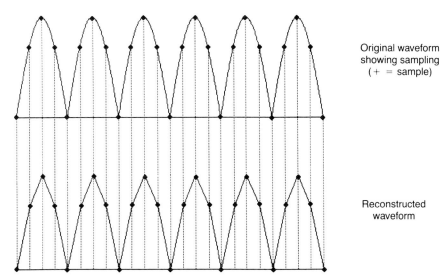

Original waveform showing sampling (+ = sample)

Reconstructed waveform

Figure 11–2. When the waveform is sampled at the correct rate, the reconstructed waveform closely resembles the original.

in excess of sixty-four thousand steps. An ADC may require special software that interrupts the computer's main program to look for data from the converter. Thus, on-line data collection using an ADC can range from relatively simple capture of a slowly changing voltage to complex programs needed to collect and analyze rapidly varying signals.

Digital Data Collection

An increasing number of modern patient monitors contain their own dedicated microprocessor. Preprocessed information can therefore be transferred to the computer. The computer processor load is reduced, and signal analysis programs are not required. Dedicated processors within monitoring equipment often have the ability to signal the computer when information is available for transfer.

RS 232. Special types of interfaces have been developed to transfer information between processors. The most common of these is known as the RS 232 interface. This consists of a multicore cable connector that allows transfer of data one bit at a time. The rate of data transfer, known as the baud rate, has to be preset and identical in both systems. Standard baud rates are 300, 1200, 4800, and 9600 bits/second. A baud rate of 300 signifies transfer of about 30 characters/second. The pattern of the bits to be transferred must also be identical, as data may be sent as 5, 6, 7, or 8 bits/ character. The system can also be configured to check whether data have been received correctly by the second system.

Medical Information Bus. A system known as the Medical Information Bus is under development to allow standardization of data transfer protocols, data structure, and connectors. Medical Information Bus greatly reduces the effort required to interconnect monitoring systems and subsequently extract information from these systems. Electrical safety is extremely important if devices are connected to patients, and all equipment must conform to international standards (IEC 601/1). These standards emphasize the problems of leakage current and electrical isolation when connecting computers to medical instrumentation. Isolated power supply, isolating transformers, and optical links have been used to provide isolation of patients from computer equipment.[11]

Advantages of On-Line Collection. The advantages of on-line data collection include rapid transfer of the information into the computer. Since this is totally independent of the operator, bias and interpretation of the data do not occur. Information can also be obtained from several different signal sources almost simultaneously, and derived data can be calculated and displayed rapidly. However, the computer system must be able to detect and reject artifacts in the signals, and it can be relatively difficult to produce programs that perform detailed pattern recognition.[12]

If the information is supplied to the computer in digital form that has been preprocessed by a patient monitor, it is more difficult to validate the data. When it is essential to ensure accurate data, such as during closed loop control of blood pressure, the raw analog signal may have to be acquired and analyzed directly by the host computer.

Output Devices

The output is the result of the computer's activities as presented to the user. Several devices provide useful output for a system.

Screen Displays

Temporary display of output can be achieved with a visual display unit (cathode-ray tube). The display is created in the same way as in a domestic television set, by the interaction of electron beams on phosphor dots on the screen, and may be either monochrome (two colors such as black/white, black/green, and so on) or multicolor. The quality of the display is improved by increasing the density of the phosphor dots. This is referred to as the *resolution* of the display, high resolution referring to higher quality display. Most microcomputers can produce graphic displays of data, and the quality of the display depends on the number of points that the computer can address on the screen. Each point is termed a pixel, and the number of pixels determines the smoothness of curved graphs. In a monochrome system, each pixel may be on or off, whereas with a color system, each pixel can be used to display the number of colors available from the computer.

Some portable computers use a display based on liquid crystal (LCD), similar to those found in digital watches. LCD consumes very little power, which is a major advantage in a battery-operated system. A significant disadvantage is that the angle from which the display is viewed can be critical. A small change in the viewing angle causes the display to become virtually invisible. Backlighting the display helps to overcome this problem.

Light-emitting diodes (LEDs) arranged in a large array can also be used for display purposes. A LED is a small semiconductor device that emits light when a current is passed through it. The advantage of this system is that it can be used in poor lighting conditions.

The type of screen display used in any computer application depends on whether graphics will be used, what degree of resolution is required from the graphic display, and whether a color display is necessary. Power consumption, robustness, and visibility in poor ambient light may also be factors.

Printers and Plotters

Permanent copies of the computer output can be made using printers or plotting devices. Printers of different types provide different qualities of output. The most inexpensive are dot matrix printers that, as the name suggests, produce output as a series of dots in a pattern corresponding to the desired character. Daisy wheel printers are similar to electronic typewriters and contain the raised patterns of letters and characters on a wheel that spins in front of the paper. The appropriate letter is selected by the printer, and an imprint is made on the paper by pushing that part of the wheel against an ink-impregnated ribbon and then onto the paper. The daisy wheel printer is limited to the characters contained on the wheel and thus cannot print satisfactory graphics. Impact printers may be excessively noisy for use in the operating environment. Alternatives to impact printers are thermal dot matrix printers, which make dot images on heat-sensitive paper, and ink jet printers, which eject a stream of ink to form each individual character.

Graphic plotters produce their output via a pen that is moved across the paper according to the computer's instructions. Plotters produce high-quality drawings and are capable of drawing on transparencies as well as on paper. However, the quality of characters produced by pen plotters is rarely totally satisfactory. Laser printers produce their output by marking the paper with a low-power laser and then passing it through a toner similar to that used in photocopying machines. The laser-based machine produces very high quality print and graphics but is much more expensive than other printers. Bubble jet printers, which are relatively quiet, produce good quality output, and are less expensive than laser printers, are a very recent development.

Information output can also be in digital form for transmission to another computer. The machines may be sufficiently close for the connections to be made directly, or a modem can be used. Modem is an abbreviation for *mod*ulator-*dem*odulator. This is a device that converts electrical binary pulses into sound tones. The sounds can be transmitted by telephone and permit communication among computers almost anywhere in the world.

PROGRAMMING AND LANGUAGES

Digital computers require specific instructions in order to perform any useful function. Conventional programs organize information into data with instructions that act on the data. The step-by-step process that assures that a given input goes through a series of simplified procedures in order to solve a complex problem and deliver the solution is called an algorithm. A number of algorithms are combined as a program. Programs are structured in many different ways according to the syntax of the programming language used.

Languages

Computer languages are structurally similar to human languages, but with two important differences. First, they tend to be considerably simpler, with perhaps no more than several hundred "words" in their vocabulary. Second, the syntax rules are precise and must be obeyed rigidly, whereas in human language they can sometimes be disregarded without loss of meaning. Programs are known as software and are stored in the computer's RAM along with data.

Many different programming languages have been developed for different applications. For example, FORTRAN, a contraction of *for*mula *tran*slation, was developed to handle scientific and technical calculations. COBOL (*com*mon *b*usiness *o*riented *l*anguage) was developed for business applications such as data base management and accounting. PASCAL is a highly structured multipurpose language, but it can be difficult for nonprogrammers to use. BASIC (*b*eginners *a*ll *s*ymbolic *i*nstruction *c*ode) is a simple language that is very similar to English, and it was developed to introduce people to computer programming. Modern versions of BASIC are approaching the structured approach of PASCAL but are retaining the ease of use of BASIC.

A new generation of higher-level languages including LISP (*list* processing) has been produced that is the basis of the developing field of artificial intelligence. Artificial intelligence attempts to create thought processes similar to those of a human within a computer. Traditional programming deals with information on two levels: the program (instructions) and the data, which are acted on by the program. Artificial intelligence programs have an additional level containing knowledge. This results in a program of much greater power and complexity that may be able to make judgments on a situation.

At present, artificial intelligence development is progressing in three main fields. Visual recognition, natural language recognition, and expert systems development are being researched. Of the three, only expert systems are developing at a significant rate. The aim of an expert system is to achieve a level of decision making and judgment similar to human skills in a specialized field. Problem-solving expert systems already exist in areas such as medical diagnosis and prescription. Development of an expert system involves high cost because of the considerable amount of programming time required, especially in acquiring and representing knowledge in the system. Requirements for rapid instruction execution and large memory capacity can still exceed the most advanced systems. Thus, widespread application of artificial intelligence may not occur for several years.[13]

INTERACTION WITH COMPUTERS

The ease of use of a computer without detailed knowledge of the operating principles of the system is referred to as the user friendliness of the system. This can be achieved by incorporating several features into the program controlling the computer. It is extremely important to prevent the user from entering inappropriate data by checking all information as it is put into the computer. Values that are outside the expected range can be indicated for confirmation or reentry, and the facility for easy correction of data must be allowed. Careful design of screen displays can assist medical and nursing staff to assimilate information quickly and accurately. The essential feature of any computer application is that it should either reduce the effort of performing a task or undertake a task that cannot be readily performed without a computer.

ANESTHETIC RECORDS

Accurate and detailed records form an integral part of the practice of anesthesia. The ever increasing complexity of modern anesthetic techniques and equipment may leave insufficient time to record and chart cardiorespiratory variables as frequently and accurately as required.[14,15]

Anesthetic records appeared as early as 1894. Details of the patient's physical condition and anesthetic drugs used were recorded for future reference. During the intervening years, the anesthetic record has become more complex. However, the basic principles have remained similar to the format described by Cushing.

Purposes

The anesthetic record can provide information in three broad categories: clinical care, historical data, and quality assurance.

Clinical Care

Data concerning the preoperative health of the patient and any specific risks that may be anticipated prior to administration of an anesthetic are noted. During administration of an anesthetic, records are made concurrently with patient management. Information such as administration of drugs is recorded, as are cardiorespiratory responses, loss and administration of fluids, and blood products. Any unexpected events such as an idiosyncratic reaction to a drug or an unexpected difficult intubation are usually carefully recorded. Analysis of the electrocardiogram for dysrhythmias or ischemia is frequently performed by computer and recorded automatically (see Chapters 1 and 2). Information about the respiratory system such as respiratory rate, gas composition, and flow is determined by computers and recorded directly. Accurate intraoperative information is also immediately available to assist staff involved in postoperative care.

Many clinical research projects require a large amount of data to be collected simultaneously. The use of a computer can greatly simplify this process as well as provide completely unbiased data recording. Data that are stored automatically on magnetic media are much simpler and less time-consuming to analyze.

Historical Data

Retrospective examination of anesthetic records is important for revealing potential hazards noted during previous anesthetics. Early repeat use of certain anesthetic agents can be avoided. However, manual records can be lost from the patient's chart, or the chart itself may be lost.

Administrative data must be extracted from which operating room utilization and staffing levels can be determined and billing of the patient or his or her insurance carrier can be performed. The degree of supervision of junior staff and the adequacy of their training require documentation in order to ensure that adequate experience has been gained in different techniques and types of operations.

Review of Quality of Care (Quality Assurance)

Clinical review of anesthetic records may be undertaken for estimation of quality of care and for educational purposes, especially when unusual problems are encountered. The use of different anesthetic techniques and drugs and the frequency of complications should be documented. However, review of manual records is so tedious to perform that it is very rarely undertaken on a large scale.

The use of an anesthetic record for medicolegal purposes requires accuracy, legibility, and completeness in recording details. In a court of law, the quality of a clinical record is taken as a reflection of the quality of the anesthetic given. Missing data and badly kept records allow conjecture by expert witnesses and reduce the chance that the anesthesiologist will be defended successfully. The basic premise is that if measurements were not recorded, they were not performed. Manually produced records can have major disadvantages in this respect, since, during a period of crisis, the anesthesiologist is more concerned with correcting the situation than in making notes. Computerization of the anesthetic record may therefore offer many advantages to the practicing anesthesiologist.

COMPUTERIZED ANESTHETIC RECORDS

During the conduct of an anesthetic administration, the anesthesiologist spends a great deal of time examining the monitors that display information concerning the patient, determining whether the data are within an acceptable range, and, if not, deciding whether the data are accurate. The data must then be recorded on the anesthetic chart. Most of this activity is mechanical and repetitive and requires little decision-making ability.

Automatic collection of information results in greater precision of information and fewer errors from transcription. An automatic system collects data from monitors accurately and rapidly. However, data collected directly on-line from a monitor can contain artifacts that do not accurately reflect the patient's true status. With modern monitors, artifact rejection is very efficient, and so the need to correct data is rarely a problem. However, provision should be made to correct or annotate any spurious result.

Automated data collection is much faster than that obtained with manual methods, and it continues when the clinician is fully occupied with other aspects of patient care. Both the American Society of Anesthesiologists and the Association of Anaesthetists of Great Britain and Ireland recommend the recording of anesthetic data every 5 minutes. Clearly, in many situations this would be very difficult, if not impossible, without a suitable automated anesthetic record system (Fig. 11–3).

The computer record is absolutely objective and records transient fluctuations in physiologic parameters with complete accuracy. A human operator may "smooth" fluctuations, such as a single low blood pressure reading, to produce a more acceptable record.[16] Such fluctuations are very common and would appear to have little significance, but demonstration by an automatic system may be considered to have medicolegal implications. Widespread use of automatic systems and regular demonstration of such events would reassure the legal profession of the benign nature of these transient changes. Many anesthesiologists express the fear that an automatic anesthetic record may require more explanation than a conventional manual record. However, most legal experts consider that the overall cost of anesthetic litigation would be reduced by the use of such systems.

Large quantities of data can be stored on magnetic media, resulting in a major reduction in space required for paper storage.[17] Once data have been stored in computers, recall and analysis of data are many times faster than manual searches and calculations. Design of the record system should be organized in such a way that useless data do not fill valuable storage capacity. Equally important, useful information should not be missed. The problem of what data to store and what to reject has not been completely resolved. Most departments usually begin by storing excessive information but realize within 6–12 months what is actually valuable and worth storing for the long term.

Desirable Features

For successful complete computerization of anesthetic records, several attributes must be considered, including accurate and complete data entry from monitors, easy manual data entry, real-time record generation, adaptability, easy interfacing with existing equipment in available work space, and use of standard anesthesia record forms.

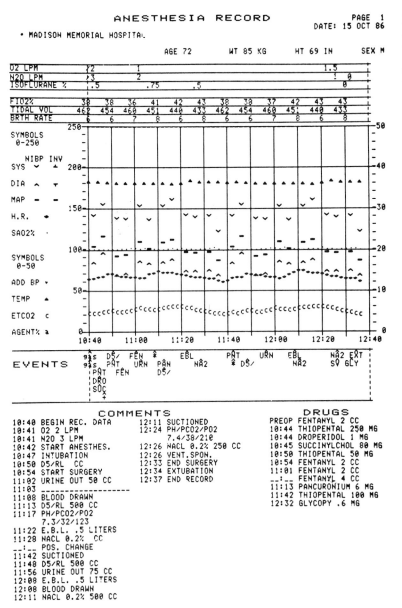

Figure 11–3. A computer-generated automated anesthesia record. The Ohmeda AARK (*A*utomated *A*nesthetic *R*ecord *K*eeper) generates not only a legible record but also a summary with total amounts of drugs and fluids administered. (Reprinted with permission of Ohmeda, A Division of The BOC Group Inc.)

Accurate and Complete Recording of Data

Direct transfer from patient monitors via ADC or RS 232 using suitable software achieves complete data recovery. The Medical Information Bus may assist in the future with standardization of interfacing to medical instrumentation.

The rate of data acquisition should be considered. Frequent sampling of physiologic variables generates a large data file. If the operation is prolonged and the patient is stable, much of this information is unnecessary.

Infrequent sampling, however, may miss transient events or sudden rapid deterioration of the patient's condition.

In practice, sampling at 5-minute intervals provides adequate information for a complete anesthetic record. Any changes within this time can obviously still be detected by the vigilant anesthesiologist. Data compression techniques assist and greatly reduce the volume of data stored, with only minimum loss of resolution of the data.

Manual Data Entry

Manual data entry should be simple and easy. Systems have been described using standard computer keyboards with single key selection of data from menus, touch screen entry, and voice recognition. The system should ideally require no more time to enter information than is required with a manual method.

Real-Time Recording

Data should be easily available for examination during anesthesia. Physiologic data are best represented graphically as trend plots; however, provision should also be made for entry of drug and fluid data and free text information.

Adaptability and Interfacing

The system must be easily adaptable for the individual user. Individual anesthesiologists should be able to preselect their individual requirements and recall these at the beginning of a working session. Standard monitors should be interfaced easily in order to provide data for the record system. As previously stated, most modern monitors have signal or data output as standard, and so connection to a computerized system is relatively straightforward. The system should function in the available work space. Modern operating rooms are often filled with sophisticated equipment, and space is limited. Computers used in the operating environment should therefore be as unobtrusive as possible. Some records systems are manufactured as an integral part of the anesthetic machine, obviating the need for the use of further floor space. Other systems have used portable or laptop computers for this task.

Finally, it should be possible to use existing record sheets to provide a hard copy of the computer-generated record. A graphic plotter is capable of accepting a standard $8\frac{1}{2}'' \times 11''$ anesthetic record and, with appropriate software, is capable of completing a record form.

Available Anesthetic Record Systems

Many automated records systems of varying degrees of sophistication are commercially available. Automatic data acquisition from patient monitors is common to all systems, but off-line data entry, data display, data storage, and record production vary according to the manufacturer's perception of what is desirable in a records system.

Three systems are considered that demonstrate the simplicity of the Datatrac system; the total integration of anesthetic machine, monitoring system, and records keeper in the Ohmeda AARK; and the highly sophisticated Diatek ARKIVE patient management system.

Datascope Datatrac

Datatrac is a semiautomated system. At the beginning of a record, the system prepares a record sheet by pulling it onto the front panel of the system. The left part of the record is covered by clear plastic, and physiologic data collected from patient monitors are recorded automatically. Manual data entry is achieved by writing on the right side of the paper record in an "event" box. Pressing a function key on the record keeper marks the event on the automated record.

The Datatrac is a relatively simple, yet flexible, system, and, compared with other fully automated systems, it is inexpensive to purchase. However, storage of data on magnetic media is not available on this system, and the record is limited to the final copy printed out at the end of the operation.

Ohmeda AARK

The Ohmeda AARK is an integrated anesthetic machine, monitoring system, and computerized record keeper. Standard Ohmeda pulse oximeter, oxygen analyzer, capnograph, ventilation, volatile agent, and blood pressure monitors can be included. Further analog and digital inputs are available to connect other monitoring units to the system. Off-line data entry is via a touch screen and menu system, which is preprogrammable by the user. The paper record is generated by a thermal dot matrix plotter that automatically updates when new data are made available. There was no data storage or other output facility available on the initial version of the system, making any attempted analysis difficult and tedious, since manual data extraction from the paper record had to be performed. Connection of monitors other than those specified by Ohmeda was unfortunately difficult or impossible to achieve owing to the system design.

However, a new version of this system, which offers serial output to a remote device such as a microcomputer of all data collected for the anesthetic record, is at the prototype stage. In addition, it incorporates a central hierarchic alarm display system, which is an important feature that will become universal on integrated anesthetic-monitoring systems in the future.

The advantages of the AARK result from the integrated design, which requires minimum excess wiring to connect the recorder to the monitors. Separate monitoring and recording system units are not present in order to reduce valuable floor space in the operating room.

Diatek ARKIVE

The ARKIVE is a free-standing system that allows patient monitors to be mounted on top of the record keeper. It accepts input automatically from up to 25 commonly used monitors simultaneously but allows manual correction of erroneous entries. Off-line data can be entered either by the standard touch screen and menu system or by an optional voice recognition system. The system also has the capacity for preconfiguration by individual users.

Data display is via a flat plasma screen that presents the anesthesiologist with second-to-second update on values from the connected monitors. Physiologic data can be displayed as trend graphs, the time scale of which can be altered during the procedure as required. Drug information is also displayed on the same scale as the physiologic data. The display can be pulled outward from the main body of the system and positioned according to the anesthesiologist's preference.

Data output from this system is to a Microsoft data operating system–compatible floppy disk that allows analysis on standard IBM microcomputers. Hard copy of the anesthetic record is provided by a dot matrix printer at the end of the procedure.

Other Systems

Whereas these systems represent the commercial state of the art, many others have been produced by anesthesiologists and bioengineers in their own hospitals. Because they have been produced in-house, they can be readily altered to fulfill local needs; new approaches can be tested and valuable experience gained as to the actual requirements of anesthesiologists working in the operating environment.

Three levels of computerization of anesthetic records have emerged. At the simplest level, features concerning the anesthetic such as duration, type of operation, monitoring used, and complications are entered onto a separate card or sheet. The sheets are then collected at a central point and the data entered into the computer database. The number of features can range from a few dozen to over a hundred. The frequency of occurrence of each item in the database can then be printed out at suitable intervals to form a record of work activity, operating room utilization, or junior staff experience. Problems with this type of record system are concerned with data collection and entry into the computer. It can be difficult to ensure total compliance of all members of staff, and it may be tedious to enter large volumes of relatively uninteresting information.

The next level includes portable computers situated on the anesthetic machine to collect the relevant data at the source. In addition to purely administrative information, more clinical details of drugs and fluids can be entered. The information can then be downloaded into the database of a larger system for analysis.

Finally, the goal of an anesthetic record system is to capture all patient information at the source. For this purpose, an automated computerized system of the AARK or ARKIVE type is necessary. These are quite expensive at present, but with recognition of the need for such systems and volume production, the cost will decrease.

INTENSIVE CARE MONITORING SYSTEMS

Anesthetists are involved increasingly in intensive care, and many forms of monitoring are common to both operating room and intensive care units. It is well recognized that diagnostic accuracy increases when more relevant data are presented.[18] In the management of critically ill patients, large amounts of data are produced over short periods of time in order to detect detrimental changes as quickly as possible. To recognize significant changes, it is important that the data are presented in an informative manner. Properly applied computer techniques greatly assist in the process of trend plotting (see Chapter 12).

Several workers have shown dramatic increases in the amount of time spent in direct patient care by nurses following implementation of automatic data collection by computer.[19,20] The computerized data collection system continues to function through critical situations when medical and nursing staff are fully occupied and otherwise unable to record data. In the operating room, the endless gathering, recording, and processing of data are relegated to the ever attentive, tireless computer, freeing the anesthesiologist to provide corrective action when required.

Many systems have been described that have had varying degrees of success. Most successful are systems based on modern microcomputers and microcomputer networks.[21,22] The requirements of such systems are (1) The output of the system must provide relevant, accurate, reliable, accessible, and familiar information at the patient's bedside. (2) The output must be appropriate to local requirements. (3) Retrieval of information must be simple for all users. (4) Data entry must be simple in order to improve accuracy and prevent reduction in time spent in patient care.

These systems work satisfactorily only if they are seen to benefit the patients and if there is no opposition to the system by staff.

FUTURE DEVELOPMENTS IN COMPUTERIZED MONITORING

All monitors have integral alarm systems for their variables. Alarm limits are set by the clinician to detect unexpected changes in variables, changes without reason, and instrument failure. During an anesthetic procedure, a minimum of five alarms may be in use, and in more complex cases, over ten system alarms can be present.

Integration of alarms by a computer would minimize (1) the time taken to identify which monitor is in the alarm state, (2) the time taken to manage the alarm state, and (3) confusion caused by several alarms sounding simultaneously. In the case of equipment alarms, the source of the problem can be rapidly identified and acted upon. The precise cause of deterioration in vital signs can be difficult to detect, and detrimental changes can develop slowly.

Intelligent alarm systems are at an early stage of development using expert systems. Software development using a cardiovascular and respiratory database with artificial intelligence techniques could identify detrimental trends and suggest appropriate courses of action before critical events occurred. Considerable effort is being made to develop such systems, and this may represent one of the major benefits in terms of patient safety that will accrue from the use of such technology.

Anesthetic machines are approaching a new stage of development in which more functions will be performed by closed loop feedback control based on microprocessor technology. They should offer improved control and safety checking of gas flow and composition and improved monitoring of vital functions (see Chapter 13). This approach has already been extended to the aircraft industry, which has many similarities to administration of anesthesia. Automation of the production of the clinical record will become a standard feature of these systems. This readily available, detailed information is necessary in order to plan and demonstrate the efficient use of the expensive human resources required to operate a department of anesthesia. The requirement for these data may be the driving force behind the acquisition of such systems.

References

1. Dickinson CJ: A Computer Model of Human Respiration. Lancaster: MTP, 1977.
2. Smith NT, Quinn ML, Flick J, et al: Automatic control in anesthesia: A comparison in performance between the anesthetist and the machine. Anesth Analg 1984; 63:715–722.
3. Blackburn JP: Computers and the anaesthetist. *In* Scurr C, Feldman S (eds): Scientific Foundations in Anaesthesia. London: William Heinemann, 1982; 600–609.
4. Zissos A, Strunin L: A micro-computerized anaesthetic record system. Can J Anaesth 1982; 29:168–173.
5. Murchie JC, Kenny GNC: Comparison of keyboard, light pen and voice recognition as methods of data input. Int J Clin Monit Comput, in press.
6. Prentice JW, Kenny GNC: Medical students' attitudes to computer assisted learning in anaesthesia. Med Educ 1986; 29:57–59.
7. Kenny GNC, Madsen S, Davis PD: Data entry by light pen. Int J Biomed Comput 1985; 17:27–30.
8. Colvin J, Kenny GNC: Automatic control of blood pressure after cardiac surgery. Anaesthesia 1989; 44:37–41.
9. Bailey JS, Wyatt R, Allwood JM: The nurse to computer interface. *In* Paul JP, Jordan MM, Ferguson-Pell MW, Andrews BJ (eds): Computing in Medicine. London: Macmillan, 1982; 289–293.
10. Sarnat AJ, Quinn ML, Smith NT: A preliminary evaluation of computerized speech recognition for anaesthesia. Anaesthesia 1981; 55 (Suppl):A128.
11. Kenny GNC, Davis PD: Computer techniques in critical care medicine. *In* Ledingham IMcA, Hanning CD (eds): Recent Advances in Critical Care Medicine. Edinburgh: Churchill Livingstone, 1983; 197–209.
12. Beneken JEW, Blow JA, Meijler AP: Computerized data acquisition and display in anaesthesia. *In* Parkash O (ed): Computing in Anaesthesia and Intensive Care. Boston: Martinus Nijhoff, 1984; 25–43.

13. Zissos A, Strunin L: Computers in anaesthesia. Can J Anaesth 1985; 32:374–384.

14. Prentice JW, Kenny GNC: Microcomputer-based anaesthetic record system. Br J Anaesth 1984; 56:1433–1437.

15. Lunn JN, Mushin WW: Mortality Associated with Anaesthesia. London: Nuffield Provincial Hospitals Trust, 1982.

16. Block FE. Automated record keeping. Medical Innovations Quarterly Review 1987; 1:1–3.

17. Hunter AR: Computing in anaesthesia and intensive care. Anaesthesia 1984; 39:487–490.

18. Jenkin MA, Cheezum L, Essick V, et al: Clinical patient management and the integrated health care system. Med Instrum 1968; 12:217–221.

19. Miller J, Preston TD, Dann PE, et al: Charting versus computer in a post-operative cardiothoracic intensive care unit. Nurs Times 1978; 74:1423–1425.

20. Sheppard LC: The computer in the care of the critically ill patient. Proc IEEE 1979; 67:1300–1306.

21. Phillips GD: Computer-based monitoring and data analysis in anaesthesia and intensive care. Anaesth Intensive Care 1982; 10:229–232.

22. Reid JA, Kenny GNC: Data collection in the intensive care unit. Journal of Microcomputer Applications 1984; 7:257–269.

chapter twelve

Patient Data Management Systems

JOHN W. HOYT, M.D. ■ HARRY COMERCHERO, M.Sc.

The intensive care unit (ICU) is a technologic environment for the monitoring and life support of critically ill patients. Monitoring implies the collection of information about the patient's condition. Life support implies the use of medications and equipment to assist or replace failing or failed body systems. The type or dose or degree of life support must be monitored, leading to more information. The critical care environment is a veritable sea of information or data that must be analyzed and then synthesized into a clinical picture. Appropriate therapeutic decisions and plans can be made only when relevant data have been considered.

SUBJECTIVE DATA

Critical care data can be divided into subjective and objective determinations. For example, the physical examination provides a large body of subjective information. The information is descriptive and only rarely is quantitative. The examination of the eyes might lead to the subjective statement that the pupils are round, of equal size, and reactive to light. Occa-

433

sionally one may find an attempt at quantifying a physical finding such as a grade 2/4 systolic murmur or 3 + pitting edema. These findings are placed in the patient's chart—first in the history and physical examination section and subsequently in the progress notes, when repeated examinations reveal changing information. Trending of this information is difficult, because it is not systematically filed in the usual patient chart, and it requires the laborious reading of many handwritten daily progress notes. There is much observer variation in recording physical findings, and the fact that most of the physical examination information is not quantified means that tables and graphs cannot be conveniently constructed.

OBJECTIVE DATA

Most of the information collected in the ICU can be classified as objective data. For example, the hourly measurement of vital signs such as heart rate, blood pressure, temperature, central venous pressure, and pulmonary artery pressure constitutes objective measurements of patient condition made at the bedside and recorded on the chart. This information is normally gathered automatically in today's busy ICU or operating room by calibrated bedside monitors using various sensors such as temperature probes or saline-filled catheters. The information is continuous but is only intermittently recorded on a paper record to become part of the patient's chart. In the automated ICU or anesthesia record, the quality of these signals is very important in order to have accurate patient information.[1]

Physiologic Measurements

Another type of objective data is physiologic measurements such as thermal dilution cardiac output, arterial blood gases, and pulmonary capillary wedge pressure. This information is not always available from the bedside monitor and requires the intervention of a nurse, technician, or physician. A volume of thermal indicator must be intermittently injected to obtain cardiac output (see Chapter 7). Blood must be withdrawn from the patient and taken to the laboratory for blood gas analysis (see Chapter 17). A balloon on the tip of the pulmonary artery catheter must be inflated to occlude blood flow in order to measure pulmonary capillary wedge pressure (see Chapter 5). These activities lead to numeric information that must be recorded on the patient's chart and can be trended for interpretation of patient status.

Information from continuously available vital signs can be combined with information from intermittent physiologic measurements to provide calculations of more objective data. Calculations for cardiac index, systemic vascular resistance, stroke work, and shunt are common cardiopulmonary evaluations in the contemporary ICU.[2] These calculations lead to a more accurate assessment of the patient (see Chapter 7).

Intake and Output

One of the most complex data units in the ICU is the patient's fluid input and output information. On the input side, there is an enormous array of solutions in the ICU. They start with the simple dextrose and water and go to the exceedingly complex three-in-one total parenteral nutrition solutions that have carbohydrate, amino acids, fat, vitamins, trace elements, insulin, H_2 receptor antagonist drugs, and electrolytes, all contained in a 3-L bag to be delivered over 24 hours. Not only is it important to record the volume of fluid administered but, particularly in the case of parenteral nutrition, the data on delivered carbohydrate and fat calories, grams of protein, milliequivalents of electrolytes, and the like must be recorded as well. There is, in addition, a wide variety of output fluids to record. Beyond simple urine output, there are a variety of tubes and drains carrying various kinds of fluids that must be recorded in character and amount.

Continuous Arteriovenous Hemofiltration

Recently, continuous arteriovenous hemofiltration has been added to the ICU armamentarium. A large arterial catheter and a large venous catheter are connected through a filter that removes an electrolyte filtrate (of about the composition of plasma without protein) from the blood. The patient's arterial blood pressure serves as the driving pressure for the system. Blood flows continuously through the filter, removing 300–500 ml/hour. If the clinician wants the patient to be in a 200-ml negative fluid balance, then intravenous fluid must be returned to the patient for the next hour in order to leave a negative 200 ml balance when all other intravenous fluids and drains have been calculated. Continuous arteriovenous hemofiltration is a major assistance in the fluid balance of overloaded patients with compromised renal function, but it is a record-keeping nightmare that creates stacks of information.

Medication Records

Another significant source of objective data recorded by the nursing staff comes from medications. There are two forms of medication delivery in the ICU, intermittent and continuous. Record keeping for intermittent medications is standardized throughout any hospital. Some medication is delivered at a fixed interval in a known amount by one of several routes. On the other hand, continuous medication delivery is more difficult to chart and tends to be more frequent in the ICU. The best example is the continuous administration of a drug like nitroprusside for decreasing blood pressure and systemic vascular resistance. This medication is given in micrograms/kilogram/minute with the dose titrated to maintain a prescribed blood pressure. Changes in dosage occur every few minutes in an unstable patient, and the charting of these frequent changes is essentially impossible. As a result, the nurse usually records a dosage of medication at the hourly time when a blood pressure is recorded, and other information about dosage is lost.

Laboratory Data

Laboratory data are collected more frequently on ICU patients than on any other hospitalized patient. Usually electrolytes, hematocrit, and arterial blood gases are measured one to three times daily, depending upon the patient's status. Other laboratory information, such as coagulation studies and chemical profiles, is gathered two to three times per week in order to trend laboratory data. Some laboratory values, such as blood sugar or serum potassium, can be measured every 2–4 hours for several days, until an abnormality is corrected. This frequency of sampling blood for laboratory information requires a tabular presentation for clinical interpretation.

Frequently, not all this laboratory information comes from the same area of the hospital. Typically, central chemistry runs blood in batches and reports patient data in the morning, whereas an ICU STAT laboratory takes care of the tests when results are needed quickly. This can lead to reporting problems if both laboratories do not use the same tabular forms.

Miscellaneous Data

Finally, objective data are collected from various life support settings. When arterial blood gases are reported, they must be interpreted in the context of ventilator tidal volume, rate, oxygen concentration, and positive end-expiratory pressure, if respiratory support is being used. Likewise, hemodynamic data must be interpreted in the light of the setting for the intra-aortic counterpulsation balloon, if such a device is being employed. One must be able to trend these life support settings in order to make clinical judgments about patient improvement or deterioration.

ASSESSMENT DATA

The physician progress notes represent another important source of data. House officers, primary physicians, and consultants write their opinions of the collected information. These opinions could be called assessment data. All the data mentioned previously represent isolated data points in the patient's chart that must be synthesized into a clinical picture set down in the progress notes. From the assessment information, therapeutic plans are developed and finally translated into physician orders. The nursing staff formulates orders using something such as a Kardex system to signal when to give medications, measure vital signs, and collect blood for laboratory tests. Thus, we have come full circle in the data collection system that represents medical charting.

THE PATIENT'S CHART

Components

The simultaneous evolution of the patient's chart and the ICU has not always been cooperative in nature. As a result, when one walks into an ICU to see a patient, there is no reliable standard for the location or presentation of information. Usually the bedside chart contains physician orders, progress notes, and some laboratory reports. Other laboratory reports, if they have come from an ICU laboratory, may not be in the chart at all. ICUs use a separate laboratory board for information that has been called back from the ICU laboratory, and this information is never transcribed onto either the bedside flow sheet or the patient's chart. The customary ICU system is to provide some sort of flow sheet that is generally used only in the critical care areas and not on regular hospital wards. This flow sheet may be as simple as two sides of one page containing vital signs or as complicated as a fold-out, four-sheet spread using both sides for eight different data areas.[3]

Device Check Sheets

Commonly, there exists a life support device check sheet. Hanging on each ventilator is a check sheet used by the respiratory therapist. Hourly checks of ventilator and alarm settings are recorded on this sheet and, on occasion, transcribed onto a blood gas sheet to make interpretation of arterial blood gases clinically meaningful. Likewise, there can be a check sheet for the intra-aortic balloon.

Nursing Notes

Nurses' notes, helpful observations about patient status and explanations for physiologic changes, can be anywhere. Some hospitals separate nursing notes from physician progress notes. Nursing notes can be on the bedside flow sheet or, in some hospitals, in sequence with the physician notes. In a poorly organized ICU, a physician may have to go to as many as five or six sources in order to assemble a clinical picture. This is time-consuming, inefficient, and, many times, misleading, if items are not carefully labeled with data and time. In the ICU, it is essential to be able to assemble time-specific information from many sources to explain sudden clinical events such as dysrhythmias or hypotension.

Lost Data

Many data are lost in the usual technology-oriented ICU. Once-an-hour sampling of vital signs, mixed venous oxygen saturation, or the dosage of a continuously infused drug can leave out an enormous amount of valuable clinical information. The use of trending strip-chart recorders or computers to sample vital sign data every 15–30 seconds can markedly improve the quality of the collected data. Ease of data review and assessment is essential for ICU technology.[4] Other data are lost because of the absence of a systemized charting technique. Many times, textual information is lost because of illegible handwriting on the part of the physician or nurse.

Comprehensive Flow Sheet

Every 24 hours, the critical ICU patient accumulates over 1000 objective data points on a comprehensive flow sheet. There are many more subjective data points from nurse and physician observations written in the progress notes. The more organized the system and the more efficient the format of presentation, the better the bedside nurse and physician can make accurate decisions and effective therapeutic plans. This organized system and efficient format is a database management system, or, in clinical terms, it has been known as a patient data management system (PDMS).[5,6]

In most busy ICUs, the chart is not the center of information. Instead, the 24-hour critical care flow sheet represents the most up-to-date information. Most ICUs keep the present day's and the previous day's flow sheets at the bedside of the critically ill patient. Older flow sheets become part of the chart. The most current information is not in the chart but rather at the bedside on the flow sheet.

There is one reason that the critical care flow sheet is so valuable in the ICU—integration of information. Relatively speaking, information on the floor patient comes back slowly, and the clinical picture evolves over days. Not so in the ICU. Here changes occur minute to minute, and there must be minute-to-minute integration of information in order to facilitate decision making.

Computerized hospitals that are using hospital information systems continue to use the chart both for computer print-outs of information such as laboratory data and for hand-entered data such as progress notes. There are plans for bedside terminals and the use of a paperless record, but for most hospitals that step is far off.[7] Many large hospitals have yet to install hospital information systems to facilitate the handling of laboratory, pharmacy, and central supply information.

Juxtaposition of Data

Another way of looking at integration of information is the concept of juxtaposition, which is defined as either side by side, or close together. The critical care flow sheet must provide juxtaposition of important and related information in a proper time sequence. One of the best and oldest examples of the need for juxtaposition is the reporting of arterial blood gases. The arterial blood gas report gives pH, Pa_{CO_2}, Pa_{O_2}, and Sa_{O_2} as direct measurements, with some other calculations such as base excess or bicarbonate. These numbers are meaningless unless juxtaposed with the respiratory support setting. It is impossible to interpret a pH, Pa_{CO_2}, Pa_{O_2}, or Sa_{O_2} if the mode of ventilation, respiratory rate, FI_{O_2}, positive end-expiratory pressure, tidal volume, and minute volume are unknown. The critical care flow sheet provides the place for the proper time sequence juxtaposition of ventilator settings with arterial blood gases.

The critical care flow sheet is a place for the integration of information through the juxtaposition of data. In that sense, it becomes a hand-done, paper PDMS. Each hospital is likely to design its own critical care flow sheet, which is commonly divided into systems. For example, there may be cardiovascular, respiratory, neurologic, renal and fluid, and laboratory sections.

In many busy ICUs, the cardiovascular section is the largest. It contains routine vital signs such as blood pressure, heart rate, respiration, and temperature. For sicker patients, there are spaces for pulmonary artery pressures, central venous pressure, and cardiac output. One also juxtaposes calculations from the hemodynamic profile, such as cardiac index, systemic vascular resistance index, pulmonary vascular resistance index, stroke volume index, left ventricular stroke work index, and oxygen transport. In order to interpret all this basic and advanced information, the bedside nurse and the physician must understand what life support techniques were in place when these measurements and calculations were made. As a result, there must be a side-by-side space for recording the infusion of cardiac drugs and the settings on the intra-aortic balloon. Finally, it is helpful to have an adjacent area for text comments, where the nurse can enter other information to assist in understanding and interpreting the cardiovascular data.

Likewise, the neurologic section needs juxtaposition of data from the neurologic examination side by side with other measurements and calculations such as intracranial pressure and cerebral perfusion pressure. Again, there should be space for comments.

The need for juxtaposition of respiratory information has already been discussed. This section is a place to record both arterial and mixed venous blood gases plus calculations such as shunt, arterial oxygen content, mixed venous oxygen content, arterial-venous content difference, CO_2 production, and the ratio of dead space to tidal volume. This information should be side by side with ventilator and oxygen therapy settings. Safety checks on the ventilator can be recorded on the same sheet, in the respiratory section. From a liability standpoint, this is quite helpful should a hypoxic episode occur, because there is documentation of quality control of the equipment.

As mentioned previously, one of the most difficult sections is the renal-fluid balance section. This section crosses over many systems such as gastrointestinal, hematologic, and renal. Here there is juxtaposition in urine output, nasogastric drainage, chest tube losses, and so on, in order to look at fluid balance. Daily weight must be recorded with this fluid balance in order to aid in interpreting any positive or negative balances. Laboratory tests, such as analyzing nasogastric drainage for blood and pH, are done on some of these fluids and recorded in this section.

Finally, most critical care flow sheets have a laboratory section to record some information from central chemistry as well as all information from the ICU laboratory. Most ICU laboratories perform hematocrits and sodium, potassium, glucose, and ionized calcium studies. This information needs to be juxtaposed with central laboratory information and nursing comments (see Chapter 18). For example, if the ICU laboratory reports a serum potassium level of 3.0 mEq/L, this information should be next to the nurses' note that 20 mEq of potassium chloride was given intravenously in 100 ml of fluid over 1 hour.

The patient's chart must be added to the critical care flow sheet in order to complete the patient picture. Some laboratory results such as cultures may not be kept on the flow sheet, because the results come back several days after being sent to the laboratory. The chart then serves as a better source of documentation of a patient's bacteriologic evaluation. The critical care flow sheet is also not a good source of documentation of routine medications. Continuous infusions of medications are on the flow sheets, but intermittent medications may be better kept on the patient's chart. Investigative reports that come from the pharmacy on pharmacokinetic dosing of aminoglycosides are normally kept on the chart. These reports are developed over several days as peak and trough levels of antibiotics are measured; the critical care flow sheet is designed for hourly information and changes, not daily information. Of course, narrative information from physician and nurse progress notes remains on the patient's chart. The nurse makes brief documentation notes associated with an episode of patient care on the flow sheet, but the initial patient evaluation and final shift summary are in a chart progress note.

Clearly, then, the critical care flow sheet and patient chart represent a PDMS, but of an unintegrated fashion. Attempts to automate and computerize this record into one paperless record have been associated with many frustrations and defeats. For the most part, only large medical centers with significant engineering and computer staffs have successfully automated this system, and, even then, there are residual questions about how much one has gained over a well-organized critical care flow sheet.[8]

COMPUTERIZATION

There is little doubt that computers have made a major impact on critical care medicine. They are everywhere in the ICU but commonly transparent to the user. There is computer power in bedside monitors, venous infusion pumps,[9] cardiac output devices, and so on. However, there are few fully integrated computers providing juxtaposed information for better ICU decision making.

History

The manufacturers of bedside monitoring equipment were among the first to attempt to "computerize" the ICU. This started in the early 1970s when systems evolved for the trending of vital signs such as heart rate, temperature, blood pressure, pulmonary artery pressure, and respiratory rate. This was information that could be easily collected from the bedside

Table 12–1. TRADITIONAL PDMS
FOCUS

Extension of monitoring systems
Automating the flow sheet (vital signs)
Clinical calculations
Centralized minicomputer architecture

monitor, using various patient sensors. Initially, this information was collected frequently, every 5–10 seconds, and trended for hours or days, depending on the memory of the computer. Trends could be analyzed on a central station cathode-ray tube, which usually had hard-copy capability. In this setting, the computer acted as an electronic strip-chart recorder. Some meager attempts were made on this system to note clinical events such as starting drugs, but there were severe limitations on the type and amount of information that could be entered. Few hospitals incorporated this information into the final medical record, and, as a result, its value, other than for teaching or research, was questionable (Table 12–1).

During the evolution of vital sign trend plotting, computerized cardiac arrhythmia systems also developed. These systems looked at the bedside electrocardiogram and analyzed the QRS complexes for premature ventricular contractions or more serious rhythms such as ventricular tachycardia or fibrillation in coronary care units. The number of premature ventricular contractions occurring per hour and a permanent record of other serious cardiac events were available from these systems. Again, there was little ability to juxtapose other information such as treatment for arrhythmias.

After the evolution of thermodilution pulmonary artery catheters, calculation of hemodynamic profiles from cardiac output measurements became popular. First, programmable calculators were used. As personal computers came into use, they replaced the calculator. Many of the newer bedside cardiac output computers were also equipped with computer packages for doing hemodynamic calculations. This information was then transcribed by the bedside nurse onto the critical care flow sheet.

Computerized laboratory, pharmacy, and hospital information systems evolved in the late 1970s and helped to automate the management of an overwhelming amount of data[10] in the ICU. Unfortunately, all these various computerized instruments and systems are not integrated except by the effort of the bedside nurse, who is now the central processing unit of this partially computerized, but mostly manual, PDMS centered on the critical care flow sheet.

"Advice" Systems

One of the brightest potentials for ICU computer application is the evolution of "advice" systems.[11] The hospital information systems discussed so far are "communicative" systems that are capable of storing, retrieving, and formatting information. An "advice" system uses collected information in order to help physicians make better decisions and provide better patient care.[12] For example, an ICU "advice" system might know that a patient is on digoxin by integration of information from the "communicative" system. When a serum potassium level of 2.8 mEq/L is reported, the "advice" system would warn the physician that this patient is at particular risk from hypokalemia because of concomitant use of digoxin. Many other "advice" systems are possible with a full integration of all ICU data by a single computerized PDMS.

PATIENT DATA MANAGEMENT

There have been several attempts to combine aspects of ICU patient data into a single, ccordinated PDMS. Only the one developed by Hewlett-Packard enjoyed much commercial success.

Hewlett-Packard PDMS

This PDMS used a central mainframe computer with transfer of analog information from the bedside monitor to the central system. An analog-to-digital converter at the computer converted the bedside waveform information to digital information to be stored in the mainframe system. Information could be recalled from the bedside, using a computer pad and bedside cathode-ray tube. Other information not automatically collected was entered with keyboard and cathode-ray tube by hand at the bedside.

Retrieval of data was done on a menu basis, partially because of the limitations of the keyboard system. The various bedside terminals were in a time-sharing relationship on the mainframe computer, frequently leading to significant delays if many users tried to interact with the system at one time. Reports were generated by printers on the mainframe computer. These reports could be requested or printed out on schedule, depending on the needs of the ICU. There was a need for a back-up mainframe system nearly identical to the primary system in order to prevent loss of data and function should the main computer fail.

One of the greatest drawbacks of the system was the difficulty in interacting with other hospital computer systems such as those in laboratory and pharmacy departments. As a result, there was need for expensive, time-consuming hand entry of laboratory information. Despite that, a number of hospitals successfully implemented this system and modified it to their own needs, allowing an early look at the benefits of a partially integrated ICU computer system (Table 12–2). The knowledge gained from this most important effort is now being incorporated into a full integration of ICU patient data by using fast and independent bedside computerized work stations.

NEED FOR AUTOMATION

The economics of the health care delivery system in the United States have changed significantly in recent years. Hospitals are finding themselves

Table 12–2. PDMS PROBLEMS

Degraded performance under peak load
Poor response time
Primitive user interface (menu-driven)
Lack of development/research tools
Not very tailorable/configurable
High cost to upgrade
Reliability
Interfaceability

under increasing pressure to contain costs and still maintain a high level of patient care. With the institution of the medical program of prospective payment based on diagnosis-related groups, hospitals are under pressure to minimize patient care costs. Hospitals are also feeling the pressure of increased competition, not only from other hospitals but also from other health care delivery systems, such as outpatient clinics and surgicenters. Third-party payors are demanding that hospitals control their escalating costs in order to manage insurance costs (Fig. 12–1).

Such pressures are having a profound effect upon hospitals. Nationwide, bed occupancy has fallen in institutions of all sizes. Patient acuity is rising, and the length of stay of the acutely ill patient is becoming shorter. This is occurring while institutions have reduced staff in order to minimize direct labor costs. The highest-acuity patients are found in the ICU.

As bleak as this picture appears, it has renewed attention to the role that automation can play in the hospital. Computer systems increase productivity, achieving greater results with fewer staff. The capture and accounting of billable treatments and supplies can be improved. By handling the more mundane clerical tasks automatically, automation contributes greatly to increased morale, which, in turn, profoundly affects staff retention and recruitment. By providing timely, accurate, and comprehensive

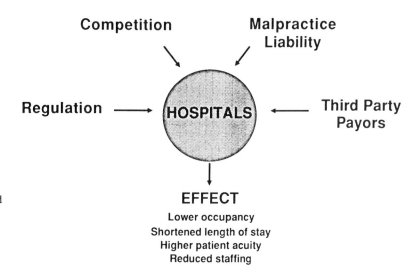

Figure 12–1. Government regulations, insurance companies, competition from other health care systems, and medical liability—all have forced hospitals to provide more sophisticated intensive care at lower costs, with fewer people, and in a short time, leading to increased automation.

organization of clinical information, computers help the medical staff deliver higher-quality patient care.

Because the ICU is a complex and costly clinical setting, automation of information management in the ICU provides significant benefits. On average, ICU beds represent approximately 8% of all hospital beds, but they often incur three or four times the cost of a general ward bed.[13,14] The nurse-to-patient ratio is 1:1 or 1:2. The ICU generates a large amount of communication with ancillary departments, such as the laboratory, pharmacy, and radiology. Consequently, in the ICU, nurses face the greatest clerical and documentation load.

INFORMATION FLOW

Clearly, computers can have a dramatic impact on the many aspects of ICU operation. It is useful to examine the different categories of information flow in the ICU. Managing information in the ICU can be segmented into three categories: charting, planning, and communications.

Charting is the documentation of patient information on the flow sheet and patient chart. Such information may be derived from bedside instrumentation, clinical observations, and interventions performed.

Planning consists of the tasks necessary to derive a treatment plan for the patient. This includes the writing of physician orders, the maintenance of the Kardex, the development of care plans, the preparation of nursing task lists, and the like. Staff scheduling and therapeutic intervention scoring are also parts of the planning process in the ICU.[15,16]

Communications is the dissemination of requests for services to and reports of results from other departments within the hospital. A patient requires certain medications from the pharmacy. Tests are performed by the laboratory. The patient must be sent to radiology for an x-ray or computed tomography scan. Efficient protocols must be established to assure that such requests are received accurately and in a timely fashion by the ancillary departments and that results are reported back to the unit as needed.

Previous generations of PDMSs focused primarily on the charting aspects of managing patient information in the ICU. As outgrowths of monitoring systems, their primary purpose was to capture data from instruments and present those data in more useful forms. However, simply automating the collection and organization of flow sheet data did not really solve the information management problem in the ICU.

The information management problem in the ICU is much broader (Fig. 12–2). A very complex "paper trail" exists in the critical care unit. The writing of physician orders initiates multiple transcription steps. This clerical task typically falls upon the ward clerk or the nurse. A simple medication order requires transcription onto the Kardex as well as the flow sheet, a request for medication initiated to the pharmacy, an entry into a task list, and so on. Communication with ancillary departments is required. Clearly, errors can occur as this information is repeatedly transcribed from form to

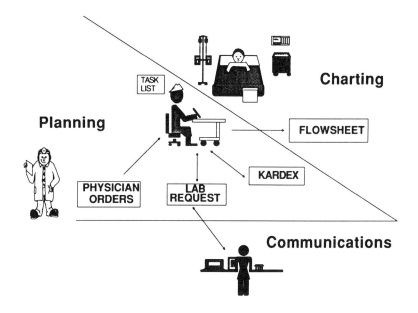

Figure 12–2. The triad of information management problems in intensive care units—charting, communications, and planning.

form. Transcription can take a tremendous amount of time, time that a nurse could spend more productively caring for patients. Nurses typically spend as much as 30–40% of their time performing clerical and communication tasks.[17] With the proliferation of new technologies at the patient's bedside, the amount of information to be captured and processed has certainly increased in recent decades.[18]

NEW AUTOMATED SYSTEMS

The next generation of automated systems for critical care will not only focus on the capture of data but also provide facilities for managing a wide variety of patient information. For that reason, such systems are typically denoted as Clinical Information Management Systems (CIMSs). They are being designed with the power and flexibility to meet the complex needs of the critical care environment. The CIMSs incorporate very advanced hardware and software architectures. The breadth of clinical functionality has been greatly extended to encompass all aspects of information collection and documentation found in the ICU, not just the flow sheet.

Whereas yesterday's PDMS was built around a centralized minicomputer, the current generation of CIMS typically uses a distributed architecture, supporting multiple bedside-oriented work stations (Fig. 12–3). Each work station is a high-performance, high-resolution terminal connected via a local area network. A typical work station might include a powerful processor such as the Motorola 68030 and contain several megabytes of memory and 60–100 megabytes of local Winchester disk storage. Displays can be as large as 19 inches and offer 1024 × 780 bit mapped graphics resolution. The

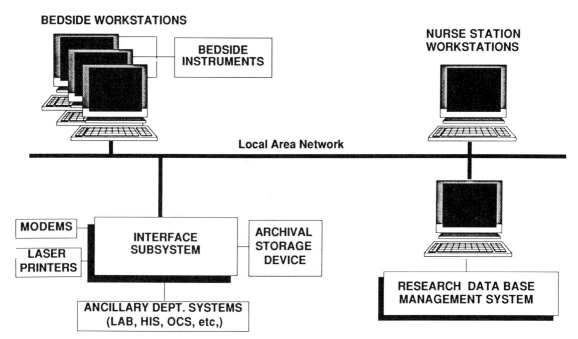

Figure 12–3. The architecture of a clinical information management system (CIMS). (Reprinted with permission from EMTEK Health Care Systems, Inc. © 1989.)

local area network might be an Ethernet, token bus, or token ring network, operating at 5–10 megabaud bandwidth.

In order to achieve the ultimate goal of the "paperless ICU," work stations are placed where one previously found the flow sheet—at the patient's bedside. Additional work stations can be located in areas where entry or review of patient information is required, such as at the central nurses' station or nursing lounge. Work stations may be configured in self-contained, mobile carts, which can be positioned within the patient's room for maximum convenience.

The systems are designed to interface with a variety of bedside instrumentation. Today, most manufacturers of patient monitors, infusion pumps, ventilators, and other monitoring devices provide computer-compatible interfaces to allow host computers to easily acquire measured values as well as status and alarm indicators. These values can be automatically retrieved by the CIMS and documented directly into the appropriate portions of the patient flow sheet.

An interface subsystem typically handles all necessary bidirectional communications to ancillary department systems. Results derived by a laboratory computer are transmitted automatically to the clinical system, and the results are placed directly into the appropriate lab form for review. Interfaces to hospital information systems facilitate the transfer of admission discharge transfer information and the exchange of information relative to orders and billing. In addition, the interface subsystem provides the necessary support for laser printers and modems. Although an automated system might alleviate the need for ongoing management of paper forms in the ICU, the patient charts are still printed once per shift or once per day for inclusion in the medical record. High-resolution, quiet laser printers facilitate printing/outputting this information in a format similar to the current paper chart. In addition, modem support allows the system vendor to provide remote diagnostic services as well as updates to the system on-line. More significantly, clinical staff with access to personal computers in their home or office could, provided the proper security precautions were taken, access the system for information from a remote location. Most recent lab results or current vital signs information can be easily retrieved for presentation on an IBM PC or Apple MacIntosh computer.

Once information is captured in the system through routine clinical use, it can also be made available for research purposes. Using rational database management software, researchers can perform retrospective studies on various patient populations for both clinical and administrative purposes. By replicating the storage of information on large disk drives at a research data management node, studies can be performed concurrent with the clinical use of the system for the clinical users.

A major benefit of a fully distributed architecture for a CIMS is that it puts the maximum power of the computer at each user location. The system can support any number of users entering or reviewing patient information without noticeable degradation. With the appropriate design and distribution of the software, one can expect subsecond response time for all displays. In addition, data can be shadowed such that patient data are stored on more than one physical device, assuring a high degree of reliability. Unlike architectures based on centralization of processor capability, a distributed system is not vulnerable to a single point of failure, resulting in a system that becomes unusable.

A CIMS for the ICU should automate the entire manual charting process, beginning with the on-line entry of physician orders (Fig. 12–4). Entry of orders makes sense only if the system is extremely fast and makes the order entry process even more efficient than its paper counterpart. Major advances in software technology and user interface design, as typified by the pioneering efforts reflected in the MacIntosh interface, have indeed revolutionized how users communicate with computers.[19] Pop-up windows and pull-down menus facilitate very rapid presentation of data and selection of choices. Not only can a physician very rapidly specify a medication order, for example, but while this is being done, a pop-up window can present for selection a subset of the hospital's pharmacy formulary tailored to the specific requirements of the particular ICU. Using a pointing device such as a mouse or track ball, a physician can rapidly specify all elements of a medication order, aided by supporting lists presented in a fraction of a second. As a result, the order can be more complete, more legible, and automatically transcribed to other appropriate forms, without any nurse or ward clerk interventions.

Once an order is signed and acknowledged, the content of the order is automatically transcribed to the Kardex. In addition, in the case of a medication or intravenous order, an entry is automatically created in the appropriate portion of the flow sheet. Column labels are created and data fields reserved to allow subsequent charting of intervention.

The flow sheet becomes a highly automated document (Fig. 12–5). A

PATIENT DATA MANAGEMENT SYSTEMS

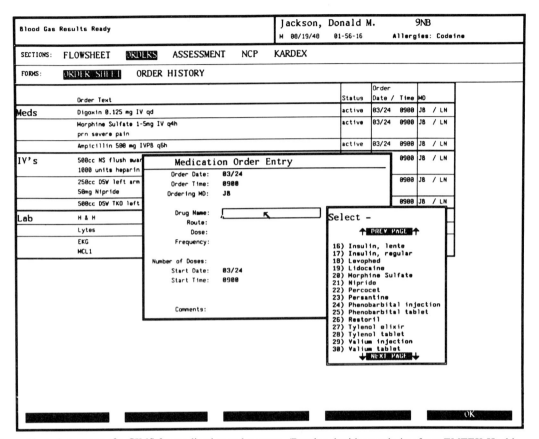

Figure 12–4. A segment of a CIMS for medication order entry. (Reprinted with permission from EMTEK Health Care Systems, Inc. © 1989.)

nurse, ready to chart vital signs, instructs the system to acquire data, alarm, and status information from all bedside instrumentation. The nurse need not transcribe data from digital displays of instruments into the system. The data are automatically displayed in the appropriate column of the flow sheet and simply require validation and signature. Nursing notes can be written directly into the computer, using word processing capabilities. Clinical reference materials such as medication information (typical dosages, precautions, contraindications) are rapidly retrieved and presented within a pop-up window in the appropriate context.

Nursing task lists can be developed to provide a chronologic listing of all interventions and actions assigned to a nurse or a given nursing shift for each patient (Fig. 12–6). Entries into the task list originate from physician and nursing orders, unit protocols, or interventions specified as part of developing a nursing care plan. As tests are completed, the nurse simply and accurately documents each intervention directly into the appropriate forms without leaving the task list, using pop-up entry windows. The task list can be used to evolve therapeutic intervention scores in order to track patient acuity and staffing requirements.

In addition, a CIMS should facilitate patient admission into and dis-

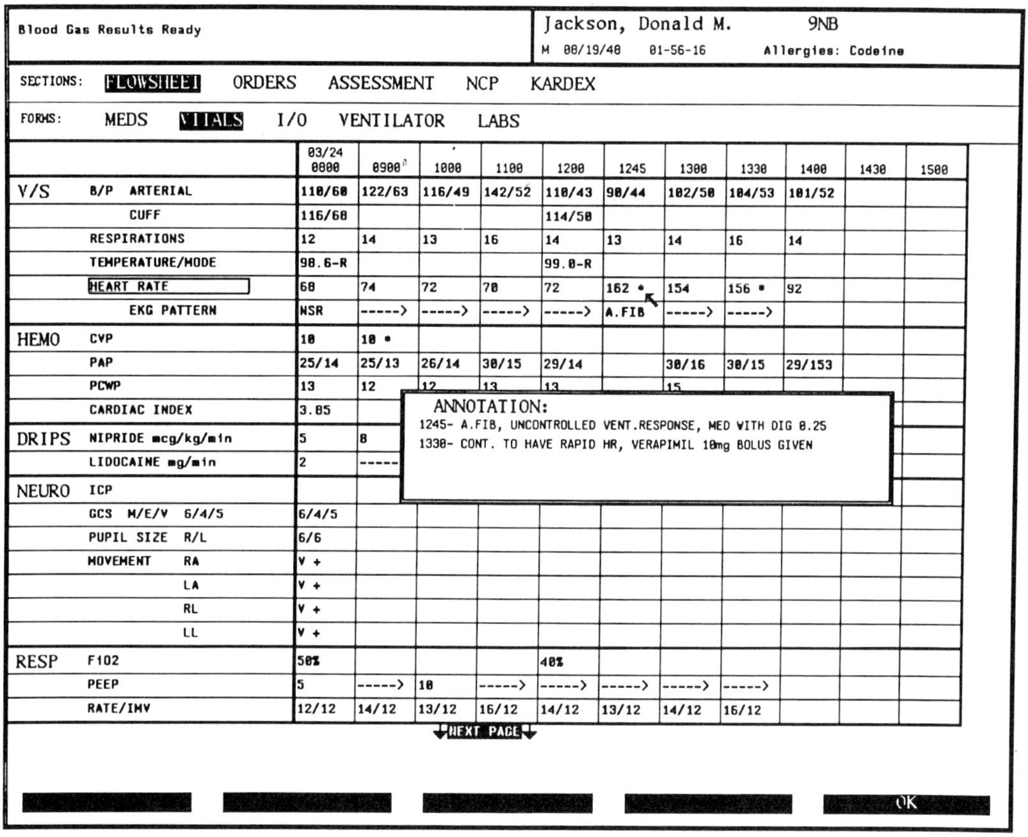

		03/24 0800	0900	1000	1100	1200	1245	1300	1330	1400	1430	1500
V/S	B/P ARTERIAL	110/60	122/63	116/49	142/52	110/43	90/44	102/50	104/53	101/52		
	CUFF	116/60				114/50						
	RESPIRATIONS	12	14	13	16	14	13	14	16	14		
	TEMPERATURE/MODE	98.6-R				99.0-R						
	HEART RATE	68	74	72	70	72	162 *	154	156 *	92		
	EKG PATTERN	NSR	----->	----->	----->	----->	A.FIB	----->	----->			
HEMO	CVP	10	10 *									
	PAP	25/14	25/13	26/14	30/15	29/14		30/16	30/15	29/153		
	PCWP	13	12	12	13	13		15				
	CARDIAC INDEX	3.85										
DRIPS	NIPRIDE mcg/kg/min	5	8									
	LIDOCAINE mg/min	2	-----									
NEURO	ICP											
	GCS M/E/V 6/4/5	6/4/5										
	PUPIL SIZE R/L	6/6										
	MOVEMENT RA	V +										
	LA	V +										
	RL	V +										
	LL	V +										
RESP	FIO2	50%				40%						
	PEEP	5	----->	10	----->	----->	----->	----->	----->			
	RATE/IMV	12/12	14/12	13/12	16/12	14/12	13/12	14/12	16/12			

Figure 12–5. An automated flow sheet in a CIMS. (Reprinted with permission from EMTEK Health Care Systems, Inc. © 1989.)

charge/transfer from the ICU, documentation of physician and nurse progress notes, and summary reports of patient assessments. The system should be flexible enough to accommodate whatever degree of user security the institution desires. Similar systems can also be used in operating rooms.

References

1. Divers RT: The quality of physiologic data for automated and alarm systems. *In* Gravenstein JS, Newbower RS, Ream AK, Smith NT (eds): The Automated Anesthesia Record and Alarm Systems. Stoneham, MA: Butterworths, 1987; 55–61.
2. Shabot MM: Software for computers and calculators in critical care medicine. Software in Healthcare 1985; Feb/Mar:26–39.
3. Augenstein JS: Computerization. *In* Shoemaker WC, Abraham E (eds): Diagnostic Methods in Critical Care. New York: Marcel Dekker, 1987; 87–110.
4. Hassett JJ: Technology's front line: The intensive care unit. *In* Reiser SJ, Anbar M (eds): The Machine at the Bedside. New York: Cambridge, 1984; 95–104.
5. Sawson JA: Computerized database management in critical care medicine: The

PATIENT DATA MANAGEMENT SYSTEMS

```
Blood Gas Results Ready                    Jackson, Donald M.        9NB
                                           M 08/19/48   01-56-16  Allergies: Codeine

SECTIONS:  FLOWSHEET   ORDERS   ASSESSMENT   NCP   KARDEX

FORMS:   TASK LIST   DIAGNOSTIC STUDIES   MEDICATIONS   GENERAL CARE   PERTINENT INFORMATION
```

DATE	TIME	ORDER NUMBER	ORDER TEXT
03/24	0800	207	Check Nipride infusion site
	0800	204	Neuro vital signs
	0800	202	Bag & suction using sterile technique
	0800	201	Assess lung sounds
	0900	103	Bed grounded and wheels locked
	0900	207	Check Nipride infusion site
	0900	208	Complete bed bath & skin care
	0900	516	Valium tablet 5 mg Oral qd prn restlessness
	1000	207	Check Nipride infusion site
	1000	212	Foley cath care per protocol
	1000	210	ET tube position change
	1200	508	Ampicillin 500 mg IVPB q6h
	1600	422	Morphine Sulfate 1-5mg IV q4h

START STOP	MEDICATION DOSE ROUTE	FREQUENCY	SCHED TIME	ACTUAL TIME	DOSE	ROUTE / SITE	COMMENTS	INITIAL
03/24 0900 04/02 0900	Valium tablet 5 mg Oral prn restlessness	qd	0900	0900	5 mg	Oral		

	P175	EO	Demonstrates a decrease in anxiety level
	P175	EO	Demonstrates a modification in behavior pattern Is less demanding of staff's time
	521	P175	Explain all procedures to patient

```
                          ↓ NEXT PAGE ↓
```

```
HOLD DOSE                                                      OK
```

Figure 12–6. The nursing task list in a CIMS, detailing orders, nursing protocols, and acute interventions. (Reprinted with permission of EMTEK Health Care Systems, Inc.)

problem of data retrieval. *In* Fein IA, Strosberg MA (eds): Managing the Critical Care Unit. Rockville, MD: Aspen, 1987; 198–227.

6. Dean JM, Booth FVM: Data collection and analysis: Controlling your id. *In* Dean JM, Booth FVM (eds): Microcomputers in Critical Care: A Practical Approach. Baltimore: Williams & Wilkins, 1985; 268–317.

7. Pesce J: Bedside terminals: Medtake. MD Comput 1988; 5:16–28.

8. Gardner RM: Computerized management of intensive care patients. MD Comput 1986; 3:36–51.

9. Alvis JM, Reves JG, Govier AV: Computer-assisted continuous infusions of fentanyl during cardiac anesthesia: Comparison with a manual method. Anesthesiology 1985; 65:41–49.

10. Bleich HL, Beckley RF, Horowitz GL: Clinical computing in a teaching hospital. N Engl J Med 1985; 312:756–764.

11. Rennels GD, Shortliffe EH: Advanced computing for medicine. Sci Am 1987; 257:154–161.

12. Schwartz WB, Patil RS, Szolovits P: Artificial intelligence in medicine: Where do we stand? N Engl J Med 1987; 316:685–687.

13. Hospital Statistics. Chicago: American Hospital Association, 1986; 196–203.

14. Russel LB: Technology in Hospitals: Medical Advances and Their Diffusion. Washington, DC: The Brookings Institution, 1979; 46–49.

15. Cullen DJ, Civetta JM, Briggs BA, et al: Therapeutic intervention scoring sys-

tem: A method for quantitative comparison of patient care. Crit Care Med 1974; 2:57–60.

16. Knaus WA, Draper EA, Wagner DP, et al: Apache II: A severity of disease classification system. Crit Care Med 1985; 13:818–829.

17. Richard RH: Evaluation of a hospital computer system. *In* Collen MF (ed): Hospital Computer Systems. New York: John Wiley & Sons, 1974; 379.

18. Brimm JE: Computers in critical care. Crit Care Nurs Q 1987; 9:53–63.

19. Philosophy. *In* Human interface guidelines: The Apple desktop interface. Reading, MA: Addison-Wesley, 1987; 1–18.

Monitoring the Anesthesia Machine

chapter thirteen

Monitoring the Anesthesia Machine

■ WILLIAM T. ROSS, Jr., M.D.

THE CONTINUOUS FLOW ANESTHESIA MACHINE

Continuous flow anesthesia machines available for use in the modern practice of anesthesia have resulted from prolonged development. The evolution of these devices can be traced through published reports of innovative technology spanning more than 100 years. More complete and specific information about anesthesia machines is reviewed in the several excellent texts,[1, 2] manufacturers' publications,[3-5] and extensive literature describing anesthesia equipment.

More important, descriptions of failures of anesthesia machines or of unexpected results from their operation have prompted many of the modifications influencing development of the anesthesia machines currently available for clinical use. To understand the circumstances in which equipment departs from its expected function, one needs to think in terms of the manner in which anesthesia equipment can fail. The operation of equipment after failure of a portion of the assembled apparatus is referred to as a failure mode. Understanding likely failure modes significantly enhances the anesthesiologist's appreciation of his or her equipment.

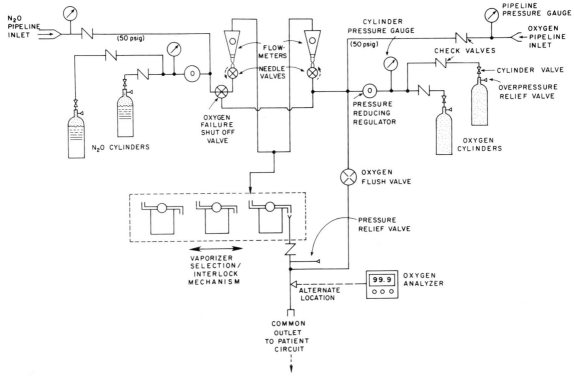

Figure 13–1. A "generic" continuous flow anesthesia machine. This diagram does not represent a specific machine but illustrates design features of various widely used machines.

Gas Supply

The continuous flow anesthesia machine (Fig. 13–1) is a device that allows accurate combination of several gases (or vapors) in order to provide the gas mixtures used in the clinical conduct of anesthesia. These machines, designed originally to be mobile, freestanding devices, were equipped with oxygen and nitrous oxide cylinders containing a few hundred liters of these gases at high pressure. Most modern hospitals in the United States now distribute gases through built-in piping systems. Today's anesthesia machines retain compressed gas cylinders to be used as reserve gas sources if pipeline gas supplies are lost.

Oxygen, nitrous oxide, and air may be delivered to anesthetizing locations via medical gas piping systems at pressures of 50–55 psi, or they may be supplied in high-pressure cylinders. When they are full, high-pressure cylinders contain oxygen or air as compressed gas at pressures approaching 2500 psi. The amount of oxygen or air contained in a cylinder is proportional to the pressure in the cylinder. Thus, the amount of oxygen in a compressed gas cylinder may be accurately estimated by measuring the pressure within the cylinder.

Nitrous oxide is supplied as a liquid with a vapor pressure of approximately 750 psi at room temperature. The amount of liquid nitrous oxide (or any fluid for that matter) contained in a cylinder can be accurately estimated from the weight of nitrous oxide (weight of cylinder plus nitrous oxide less the tare weight of the cylinder) contained within the cylinder. In practice, it is more convenient to measure the pressure within cylinders, and the tare weight of cylinders is typically unknown. During periods when nitrous oxide is used from cylinders, the vaporization of liquid nitrous oxide to gas results in sufficient cooling of the cylinder and its contents to significantly reduce the vapor pressure of the liquid remaining within the cylinder. For this reason, the pressure measured in cylinders of nitrous oxide that have been subjected to significant cooling is found to be as much as several hundred pounds below the expected 750 psi, even though the cylinders still contain liquid nitrous oxide.[6] Consequently, the amount of nitrous oxide available for use from cylinders is usually not accurately known.

Pressure and Flow Controls

The 50–55-psi pressure available in the supply pipeline may be used as the intermediate or "working" pressure within the plumbing of the anesthesia machine proximal to flowmeter control valves or on/off controls such as the oxygen flush valve. The flows set by flow control valves are monitored by observing the associated flowmeters. The flow control valves used in anesthesia machines to regulate gas flow perform as variable resistors and can provide constant gas flow at their outlets only if presented with constant inlet pressure. This relationship dictates a requirement to accurately reduce the high pressure available in high-pressure cylinders to a nearly constant working pressure. This is accomplished by pressure-reducing regulators that maintain a constant outlet pressure of slightly less than 50 psi while a variable but greater pressure is presented to the inlet. Likewise, variations in the pressure of gas in the piping system result in proportional variations in the flow of that gas through a flow control valve. A 10% variation in supply pressure produces a similar variation in the gas flow exiting the flow control valve, in the absence of compensating adjustments of the flow control valve.

Most anesthesia machines in production today are constructed so that the intermediate pressure section of the machine incorporates additional stage(s) of regulation to a pressure lower than the pipeline supply pressure of 50–55 psi. This is done in order to achieve superior regulation of the pressure being presented to the valves controlling gas flow to the flowmeters[4] as well as to permit the operation of master-slave controllers[3, 7] that serve to adjust oxygen flow, so that mixtures of oxygen and nitrous oxide containing less than 25–30% oxygen cannot be delivered.

Vaporizers

Agent-specific vaporizers are used to accurately add measured concentrations of volatile anesthetics to the gas stream. These devices must be used only with the anesthetic agent for which they were designed. Anesthesia machines having more than a single vaporizer should have an interlock/exclusion mechanism in order to prevent more than one vaporizer from being used at a time. The interlock mechanism also serves to isolate vaporizers not selected for use from the gas stream by disconnecting both inlets and outlets of unselected vaporizers from the gas stream. This prevents vapor from an upstream vaporizer being carried downstream and mixing with liquid anesthetic in the downstream vaporizer. Isolation of unselected vaporizers from the gas stream serves to prevent the addition of small amounts of volatile anesthetics to the gas stream as a result of continuing evaporation of these agents within the unselected vaporizers themselves in those machines in which the outlet of the vaporizer remains connected to the gas stream while the vaporizer is turned off.[8]

Oxygen Flush Circuit

The oxygen flush circuit permits the flushing of the gas machine with a high flow of oxygen. It should be noted that the operation of the flush valve simply admits a high flow of oxygen to the outlet of the machine; it neither turns off vaporizers nor provides anesthetic-containing gas mixtures during operation of the flush mechanism. Certain older machines had flush valves that were linked to include other functions, such as deselecting vaporizers. Often a check valve is installed in the anesthesia machine between the outlet of vaporizers and the junction of the oxygen flush line with the fresh gas stream (i.e., near the fresh gas outlet of the machine). This serves to prevent retrograde flow of appreciable volumes of gas back into the machine when positive pressure is applied to the machine outlet, as with positive pressure ventilation. This feature serves particularly to isolate vaporizers from the "pumping effect" of pressure fluctuations on the constancy of vaporizer output.[9]

Fresh Gas Outlet

Access to the gas stream emanating from the anesthesia machine is provided at the fresh gas port. This connector provides a standardized connecting point from which gas can be delivered to the patient breathing circuit.

RATIONALE FOR MONITORING THE ANESTHESIA MACHINE

In a broad sense, anesthesia machines fail to perform the functions for which they were designed when they provide incorrect concentrations or proportions of the various gases or deliver an incorrect amount of gas. This may lead to disastrous consequences if the resulting gas mixture is devoid of oxygen. Other serious failures can occur with less dire consequences; for example, the omission of the anesthetic agent from the gas mixture can result in failure to achieve an anesthetic state. Because gas flowing from the anesthesia machine is relied upon to fill reservoir bags in anesthetic circuits and ventilators, leaks that permit the loss of gas can result in the failure of ventilation in situations in which the volume of gas delivered is insufficient to adequately fill the reservoir or ventilator bag. Monitoring provides early, timely recognition of problems, which is essential for the prompt correction necessary to minimize the likelihood of an adverse outcome.

There is little debate that assurance of adequate delivery of oxygen to the patient breathing circuit is a crucial function of anesthesia machine monitoring. The assumption that operator vigilance can prevent the occasional accidental delivery of hypoxic or anoxic breathing mixtures has proved inaccurate.[10,11] The appreciation of this has resulted in extensive efforts to design machines that virtually do not permit the delivery of hypoxic gas mixtures. Efforts to achieve this have followed several paths. One approach has been to design machines that are not capable of delivering mixtures of oxygen that approach 0% oxygen. Another design approach has been to construct flow control valves so that the flow of oxygen cannot be reduced to less than some minimum value. In this way, anoxic mixtures are prevented, although hypoxic mixtures may be accepted at some nitrous oxide flowmeter settings.

More elaborate schemes have been devised to either monitor[3] or control[3,4] the concentration of oxygen being supplied to the patient breathing circuit as well as to analyze and report the concentration of oxygen within the patient breathing circuit.[12] North American Drager has offered pneumatic devices called oxygen ratio monitors (ORMs) that trigger an alarm when oxygen mixtures containing less than 30% ± 5% oxygen are selected. More recently, Drager has offered the oxygen ratio monitor/controllers (ORM/c) that control the concentration of oxygen actually delivered by the anesthesia machine (on Narkomed 2A, 2B, 3). The ORM/c[3] device includes oxygen and nitrous oxide flowmeters equipped with pneumatic resistors, each having a pressure sensing port. The pressure developed at the port is proportional to the flow through its associated flowmeter. The pressure developed at each flow resistor is applied to separate aneroid diaphragms that are mechanically coupled by a common shaft. A third diaphragm, also connected to the common shaft, actuates a valve regulating the amount of nitrous oxide supplied to the nitrous oxide flowmeter in such a way that the flow of nitrous oxide is reduced when the percentage of oxygen selected y the operation of the needle valves is sensed to be less than approximately 30%. On machines equipped with gases in addition to oxygen and nitrous oxide, the function of the ORM/c is altered when the selector switch indicates "All Gases." The Ohmeda Modulus anesthesia machine incorporates a mechanical linkage (Link 25—Proportional Limiting Control System) between the oxygen and the nitrous oxide flow control needle valves to provide a similiar function.

Another approach to the detection of low oxygen tension in the fresh gas mixture involves analysis of the gas stream for oxygen tension. This is commonly accomplished by an oxygen analyzer placed in the inspiratory limb of the patient breathing circuit or, alternatively, in the fresh gas line proximal to the breathing circuit (see Chapter 8).

MONITORING THE ANESTHESIA MACHINE

Monitoring the anesthesia machine for the conduct of anesthesia includes tasks occurring before using the device for patient care, during the conduct of the anesthetic procedure, and after completion of the procedure.

Preanesthetic Check-out

Preanesthetic check-out of the anesthesia apparatus is a prerequisite for the reliable conduct of safe anesthesia. The first step the anesthesiologist should take when planning to conduct an anesthetic procedure is to make sure she or he understands the general capabilities of the anesthesia machine proposed for use. The minimum information includes whether the machine has monitors that can be turned off independently from the gas flows available on the machine, and whether the machine is capable of producing hypoxic mixtures under any circumstances despite monitoring devices.

Although a number of anesthesia machine check-out procedures have been recommended, the most recent to appear and receive wide dissemination is published by the United States Food and Drug Administration (FDA) (Fig. 13–2)[13] and promoted by the American Society of Anesthesiologists.[14] When they are combined with effective preventive or progressive maintenance programs, the practices suggested by these procedures should reduce the incidence of critical machine failures to low rates.

The FDA check-out consists of the elements shown in Table 13–1. Most of these are directed toward the detection of potential leaks in the anesthesia apparatus and recognition of the loss of supply gases, especially the unforeseen loss of oxygen.

Visual Inspection

The initial survey of the machine should be visual—a "walk around" inspection. The operator should assure her- or himself that the apparatus has had a thorough preventive maintenance inspection within the interval established by the institution for such periodic inspection. This information should be available on an inspection sticker affixed to the machine in an obvious location. Other items to be checked during the visual inspection are the settings of controls and the absence of broken or otherwise obviously damaged machine components. Flowmeters should be observed for damage and the presence of bobbins, floats, or balls resting in the *bottom* of each flowmeter. Any sign of obvious damage to the machine should alert the operator to the possibility of a breach of the integrity of the device. For example, a damaged thermoplastic (Plexiglas) flowmeter shield should cause the operator to carefully seek evidence of damage to the flowmeters themselves (in addition to inspection in order to detect obvious gross damage, the check-out should include testing for leaks) and to search for the cause of the damage in order to prevent recurrence.

This checkout, or a reasonable equivalent, should be conducted before administering anesthesia. This is a guideline which users are encouraged to modify to accommodate differences in equipment design and variations in local clinical practice. Such local modifications should have appropriate peer review. Users should refer to the operators manual for special procedures or precautions.

*1. **Inspect anesthesia machine for:**
   machine identification number
   valid inspection sticker
   undamaged flowmeters, vaporizers, gauges, supply hoses
   complete, undamaged breathing system with adequate CO_2 absorbent
   correct mounting of cylinders in yokes
   presence of cylinder wrench

*2. **Inspect and turn on:**
   electrical equipment requiring warm-up. (ECG/pressure monitor, oxygen monitor, etc.)

*3. **Connect waste gas scavenging system:**
   adjust vacuum as required

*4. **Check that:**
   flow-control valves are off
   vaporizers are off
   vaporizers are filled (not overfilled)
   filler caps are sealed tightly
   CO_2 absorber by-pass (if any) is off

*5. **Check oxygen (O_2) cylinder supplies:**
   a. Disconnect pipeline supply (if connected) and return cylinder and pipeline pressure gauges to zero with O_2 flush valve.
   b. Open O_2 cylinder; check pressure; close cylinder and observe gauge for evidence of high pressure leak.
   c. With the O_2 flush valve, flush to empty piping.
   d. Repeat as in b. and c. above for second O_2 cylinder, if present.
   e. Replace any cylinder less than about 600 psig. At least one should be nearly full.
   f. Open less full cylinder.

*6. **Turn on master switch (if present)**

*7. **Check nitrous oxide (N_2O) and other gas cylinder supplies:**
   Use same procedure as described in 5a. & b. above, but open and *CLOSE* flow-control valve to empty piping.
   Note: N_2O pressure below 745 psig. indicates that the cylinder is less than ¼ full.

*8. **Test flowmeters:**
   a. Check that float is at bottom of tube with flow-control valves closed (or at min. O_2 flow if so equipped).
   b. Adjust flow of all gases through their full range and check for erratic movements of floats.

*9. **Test ratio protection/warning system (if present):**
   Attempt to create hypoxic O_2/N_2O mixture, and verify correct change in gas flows and/or alarm.

*10. **Test O_2 pressure failure system:**
   a. Set O_2 and other gas flows to mid-range.
   b. Close O_2 cylinder and flush to release O_2 pressure.
   c. Verify that all flows fall to zero. Open O_2 cylinder.
   d. Close all other cylinders and bleed piping pressures.
   e. Close O_2 cylinder and bleed piping pressure.
   f. CLOSE FLOW-CONTROL VALVES.

*11. **Test central pipeline gas supplies:**
   a. Inspect supply hoses (should not be cracked or worn).
   b. Connect supply hoses, verifying correct color coding.
   c. Adjust all flows to at least mid-range.
   d. Verify that supply pressures hold (45–55 psig.).
   e. Shut off flow-control valves.

*12. **Add any accessory equipment to the breathing system:**
   Add PEEP valve, humidifier, etc., if they might be used (if necessary remove after step 18 until needed).

13. **Calibrate O_2 monitor:**
   * a. Calibrate O_2 monitor to read 21% in room air.
   * b. Test low alarm.
   c. Occlude breathing system at patient end; fill and empty system several times with 100% O_2.
   d. Check that monitor reading is nearly 100%.

14. **Sniff inspiratory gas:**
   There should be no odor.

*15. **Check unidirectional valves:**
   a. Inhale and exhale through a surgical mask into the breathing system (each limb individually, if possible).
   b. Verify unidirectional flow in each limb.
   c. Reconnect tubing firmly.

††16. **Test for leaks in machine and breathing system:**
   a. Close APL (pop-off) valve and occlude system at patient end.
   b. Fill system via O_2 flush until bag just full, but negligible pressure in system. Set O_2 flow to 5 L/min.
   c. Slowly decrease O_2 flow until pressure *no longer rises* above about 20 cm H_2O. This approximates total leak rate, which should be no greater than a few hundred ml/min. (less for closed circuit techniques).
   CAUTION: Check valves in some machines make it imperative to measure flow in step c. above when pressure *just stops rising.*
   d. Squeeze bag to pressure of about 50 cm H_2O and verify that system is tight.

17. **Exhaust valve and scavenger system:**
   a. Open APL valve and observe release of pressure.
   b. Occlude breathing system at patient end and verify that negligible positive or negative pressure appears with either zero or 5 L/min. flow and exhaust relief valve (if present) opens with flush flow.

18. **Test ventilator:**
   a. If switching valve is present, test function in both bag and ventilator mode.
   b. Close APL valve if necessary and occlude system at patient end.
   c. Test for leaks and pressure relief by appropriate cycling (exact procedure will vary with type of ventilator).
   d. Attach reservoir bag at mask fitting, fill system and cycle ventilator. Assure filling/emptying of bag.

19. **Check for appropriate level of patient suction.**

20. **Check, connect, and calibrate other electronic monitors.**

21. **Check final position of all controls.**

22. **Turn on and set other appropriate alarms** for equipment to be used.
   (Perform next two steps as soon as is practical)

23. **Set O_2 monitor alarm limits.**

24. **Set airway pressure and/or volume monitor alarm limits (if adjustable).**

If an anesthetist uses the same machine in successive cases, the steps marked with an asterisk (*) need not be repeated or may be abbreviated after the initial checkout.

†† A vaporizer leak can only be detected if the vaporizer is turned on during this test. Even then, a relatively small but clinically significant leak may still be obscured.

FDA - August, 1986

Figure 13–2. Anesthesia machine check-out procedures published by the United States Food and Drug Administration.

Even if such damage is superficial, it should be reported so the general condition of the machine may be maintained by the assigned repair personnel.

Signal wires, power cords, and gas and vacuum tubing should be inspected for cracks or other damage. If there is any question concerning damage to these items, they should be replaced promptly. Transparent insulation and covers have been advocated as a means to facilitate inspection of electrical wires or connectors. This is particularly likely to identify im-

---

Table 13–1. ANESTHESIA MACHINE CHECK-OUT SUMMARY*

1. General inspection and turn on (items 1, 2, 11)
2. Connection, inspection, test, and adjustment of scavenging system (items 3, 17)
3. Confirmation of initial settings and function of adjustable controls (items 3, 4, 8, 19, 20)
4. Confirmation of the presence of gas in high-pressure cylinders (items 5–7)
5. Tests of oxygen monitor, ratio monitoring device, and ability of the fail-safe system to respond to loss of oxygen supply pressure (items 9, 10, 13)
6. Identification and confirmation of pressure for each gas in medical gas piping systems (item 11)
7. Test to confirm the absence of gases other than oxygen when only oxygen has been admitted to the patient breathing circuit (item 14)
8. Tests to confirm integrity and function of circle-absorbing breathing system, including interface with scavenging system (items 15–17)
9. Check position of controls and alarm settings on monitors (items 21–24)
10. Tests to confirm integrity and function of accessory apparatus (items 12, 18–20)

---

* Item numbers refer to FDA recommendations.

pending or actual breakage of conductors adjacent to points at which considerable mechanical flexing occurs. Transparent insulation of wiring allows the very fine metal dust produced as the result of repeated flexion to be identified as a gray discoloration adjacent to the conductor. Using this inspection aid, the experienced anesthetist can identify areas of high wear in signal wires before the conductor actually fails and produces erratic or unobtainable signals.

If the carbon dioxide (CO_2) absorbent contains an indicator, inspection of the canister can tell the operator whether the absorbent has been expended. Because different indicators may be used in different formulations of absorbing compounds, the operator must be aware of the expected color changes with the product in use.[15] Most CO_2-absorbing circle systems are equipped with two canisters in series with the gas flow in the circle. Net flow through the canisters is from top to bottom in machines of recent manufacture. When the color change indicating consumption of the absorbent extends into the downstream canister of the absorber, the absorbent should be changed in the upstream canister and that canister (with fresh absorbent) placed in the downstream (lower) position in the gas stream.

Scavenging System

The waste gas scavenging system should be examined during the early part of the machine check-out. The interface between the patient breathing circuit and the conduit to the removal route should be inspected for integrity and lack of occlusion. A common cause of partial obstruction in the scavenging system is the collection of water in dependent loops of the scavenger connecting tubing. If a closed scavenging system with a reservoir bag is used, it is necessary to ascertain that the suction venting the scavenger is adjusted to provide proper flow, so that the reservoir bag on the scavenging system is emptied only at the highest flows that the operator expects to use. Usually this is in the neighborhood of 10 L/minute. With the Y connection to which the patient will be connected occluded and the adjustable pressure-

463

limiting valve open, a 10 L/minute flow can be admitted to the breathing circuit while the scavenging suction is turned off. This should result in an increase in pressure within the breathing circuit of less than 5 cmH$_2$O, and it provides a functional test of the positive pressure relief valve in the scavenging system. Similarly, with zero fresh gas flow into the patient breathing circuit, the scavenger suction on, the patient connection occluded, and the adjustable pressure-limiting valve open, there should be less than 2 cmH$_2$O negative pressure detected in the patient breathing circuit with proper functioning of the negative pressure relief valve in the scavenging system.

Other scavenging systems, such as passive systems that carry waste gases to the return vent of the nonrecirculating air conditioning system, may not be equipped with pressure-relief valves. These systems rely on patent large-bore (typically 19–22 mm) tubing as a conduit. Occlusion of this tubing or the direct application of suction to it must be avoided in order to prevent excessive positive or negative pressure from being applied to the patient breathing circuit.[16]

Flowmeters

The floats should be observed to move smoothly within the bore of the flowmeter, and they should return smoothly to the base of the tube when the flow control valve is closed. Floats are designed to rotate during use. Failure to do so results in sticking or interference between the float and the tube wall and causes erroneous readings. A rough approximation of flowmeter accuracy may be conducted by setting a flow of several liters per minute and determining the time required to fill a breathing bag of known volume.

Adjustable Controls

Initially, the machine can be expected to be found with the pipeline gases connected and all flowmeters and vaporizers turned off. However, the operator must determine that adjustable controls on the machine are set to appropriate positions before proceeding with the initial check-out of the machine. A consistent confirmation of the setting of all adjustable controls assures that they have not been left in some unexpected configuration.

Cylinders

Cylinders mounted on the machine should be examined in their yokes for proper mounting and the presence of only one seat washer. Next, determine the amount of gas available in the cylinders mounted on the machine. If the high-pressure (cylinder) gauges indicate no pressure in the high-pressure portion of the machine, then this part of the machine is depressurized. Turning on a cylinder indicates the pressure available in that cylinder. On machines with multiple gas cylinders attached to high-pressure manifolds, an important condition routinely occurs that prevents the ready determination of gas pressure available in individual cylinders (see Fig. 13–1).

With the machine connected to the pipeline gas supply, approximately 50–55 psi is applied to the plumbing within the machine proximal to the valves controlling the flow of gas through the various flowmeters. In the typical machine, the high-pressure-reducing regulators have been set to deliver gas from the high-pressure cylinders at a pressure slightly lower than the pipeline pressure. This is done in order to keep the outlet of the reducing regulator closed so long as the design pressure (i.e., 50–55 psi) is maintained within the internal plumbing of the intermediate-pressure section of the machine by the pipeline gases. Thus, one can be assured that, even if the cylinder valves remain open, cylinder gas supplies are not depleted so long as there is adequate pipeline pressure. Since the high-pressure yokes are equipped with check valves (to allow cylinders to be changed without losing high-pressure cylinder gas while remaining cylinder[s] remain open in order to provide an uninterrupted supply of gas and to prevent transfilling of high-pressure cylinders containing gas at unequal pressures), the high-pressure gas is trapped between the yoke check valve and the reducing regulator. The high pressure sensed by the cylinder gauges can be relieved only by removing the machine from the pipeline gas supply and allowing flow to occur from the regulator while the cylinder valves remain off. Thus, the FDA protocol recommends disconnection of the machine from the pipeline supply. Additionally, this permits confirmation of proper operation of the "fail-safe" mechanism.

The FDA recommended check-out procedure, which calls for at least daily disconnection/reconnection of the anesthesia machine from the pipeline gas supply, gives rise to the following potential hazard. The diameter-indexed safety system connectors, widely used as fittings among machines, connecting hoses, and the pipeline supply, are constructed of brass, a soft metal, and they show appreciable wear after repeated cycles of connection/disconnection. Furthermore, crossthreading of the fittings with attendant damage to the connectors and the potential for development of gas leaks are more likely with frequent use.

In recent years, numerous recommendations have been made to minimize gas leaks, particularly to prevent nitrous oxide contamination of the operating room atmosphere.[17] As a result, connections are made with diameter-indexed safety system connectors tightened lightly, but more than finger tight, with a wrench. Quick connections are not standardized for use in medical gas piping systems and are prone to leakage or damage while disconnected. Suggestions of other ways to disconnect gas machines from the pipeline source of gases abound but may not be practically useful. Indeed, it seems that recommendation to disconnect the machine from its pipeline source of gas in order to permit measurement of pressure in the high-pressure cylinders and testing of the fail-safe mechanism often results in this portion of the machine check-out being overlooked. In addition, the wear of connectors caused by daily disconnection suggests that additional kinds of failure related to wear and damage to the connectors will appear more frequently. Individual cutoff valves for the medical gases, accessible at the front of the machine and incorporated in the design of the machine, may need to be considered.

Pipeline Pressures. The presence of adequate pipeline pressure should be confirmed by the indication of 50–55 psi pressure on the pipeline pressure gauges of the machine. The fail-safe mechanism[3, 4] is designed to automatically halt the delivery of nitrous oxide to the breathing circuit in the event of failure of the oxygen supply pressure within the intermediate-pressure section of the machine. Note that this system responds to oxygen supply *pressure rather than to the flow* of oxygen. With older machines, it is possible to continuously administer hypoxic gas mixtures by adjusting oxygen to low (or even to zero) flow, although the machine is equipped with a fail-safe mechanism. To check the operation of the fail-safe device, oxygen and nitrous oxide are turned on and the source of oxygen pressure is removed. The flow of nitrous oxide should decline in proportion to the fall in oxygen pressure or be interrupted as the oxygen pressure falls below approximately 25 psi. The abruptness of cessation of nitrous oxide flow varies with the particular implementation of the fail-safe function and may even vary among individual machines of the same model. After these checks, the sources of medical gases should be reconnected and the high-pressure cylinder valves turned off.

Gas Analysis

The initial check of the oxygen analyzer should follow the manufacturer's instructions and, after a suitable warm-up interval, confirm that it reads, or can be adjusted to read, near 21% when the sensor is positioned in ambient air, well away from sources of gases that may change the ambient oxygen concentration. The sensor should be repositioned to its place on the anesthesia machine, the circuit flushed with a high flow of 100% oxygen, and the monitor observed to read 100% ± 10%. If the analyzer calibration control is adjusted at 100%, it should be checked again to confirm its reading of 21% ± 2% in room air.

In order to confirm that oxygen is the only gas present in the fresh gas connected to the patient breathing circuit, the breathing circuit should be flushed with 100% oxygen, after which a flow of 3–5 L/minute of oxygen is delivered to the circuit. A reading of 100% should be noted on the oxygen analyzer, and no odor (suggesting that a vaporizer is leaking or has been left on) should be detected by a sniff of the gas exiting the distal end of the inspiratory limb of the circuit. A few breaths from the patient breathing circuit demonstrate proper operation of the unidirectional valves. If the machine is connected to gas analysis equipment, such as a mass or Raman spectrometer or an infrared analyzer, the composition of the gas being delivered from the metering portion of the machine to the patient breathing circuit may be determined with the capability of the equipment available. These devices and their limitations are discussed in detail in Chapter 14.

Checking for Leaks

Several maneuvers are useful for determining that the machine *and* the patient breathing circuit are free from significant leaks. For the purposes of this description, only the circle absorption system is considered. If other circuits are to be used, procedures to assess their suitability for use can be determined by studying the information supplied by the equipment manufacturer. The adjustable pressure-limiting valve should be closed, and the patient connecting port at the Y connector of the circle occluded. Then the circle reservoir bag should be filled until the pressure gauge indicates 30 cmH$_2$O, at which time the flow of oxygen should be reduced to the point at which the pressure within the circle no longer rises. The oxygen flow, which indicates the total leak rate downstream from the flowmeter valve, should be minimum. This test measures the total of all leaks in the gas machine *and* the breathing circuit. The American National Standards Institute Z79.8–1979 standard[18] for anesthesia machines specifies a leak of less than 30 ml/minute from the gas machine, exclusive of the patient breathing circuit.

Several qualifications concerning leak testing should be addressed. When machines having a minimum flow of oxygen (typically in the range of 200–500 ml/minute) are tested for leaks, it is not possible to measure leaks that are less than the minimum flow available from the machine. As a practical matter, leaks of a few hundred milliliters per minute may be accepted, so long as low flow or closed circuit techniques are not used, and sufficient total flow is available to assure adequate ventilation of the patient. Any machine with leaks of greater than 2 L/minute should be removed from service for repair. The reader must understand that leaks within accessory equipment that may be turned off by the operator (e.g., vaporizers) are not tested for unless that accessory is selected for use and is functionally connected to the anesthesia machine during the leak test.

Pressurization of the machine can result in appreciable volumes of gas being compressed into vessels such as vaporizers that have significant internal volumes. Therefore, depressurization at the completion of the leak testing should be accomplished fairly slowly in order to prevent the sudden occurrence of transient unequal pressures within the interior of the anesthesia machine. Test pressures within the anesthesia machine should be limited to less than 50 cmH$_2$O.

Unidirectional Valves. An additional element of pressure testing for leaks that one needs to appreciate concerns the effect of unidirectional valves on the interpretation of the meaning of certain test results. Consider the situation in which a test pressure gauge is positioned near the distal end of a segment of tubing to be pressure tested for leaks (Fig. 13–3). A source of intermittent gas flow at the proximal end of the tube causes the pressure in the tube to rise. As the gas flow is reduced, the rate of pressure increase measured by the gauge slows and becomes zero when the inlet gas flow exactly equals the loss of any gas through leaks. In the situation in which there is no leak, the measured pressure remains constant even when the inlet gas flow is zero.

Now consider the situation that results when a unidirectional valve ("check valve") is placed in the tubing between the leak and the site of pressure measurement. If the pressure is brought up to the desired test pressure and gas flow is not monitored, pressurized gas is trapped and pressure is maintained in the segment of tubing downstream from the check valve, even after the source of gas has been removed and the pressure is lost from the leaking portion of the apparatus upstream from the check valve. Thus,

Figure 13–3. The effect of a check valve on test procedures to determine leaks within a segment of tubing. (See text for discussion.)

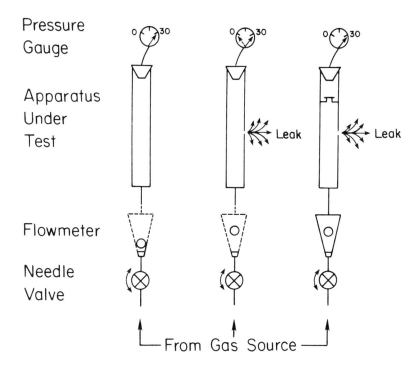

Pressure Gauge

Apparatus Under Test

Flowmeter

Needle Valve

From Gas Source

simply measuring pressure downstream from the check valve after flow into the proximal portion of the apparatus under test has ceased fails to suggest a leak. When the pressure is brought up to the test pressure *and* the flow of gas into the segment of the machine to be tested is monitored simultaneously, the presence of check valves does not obscure upstream leaks.

Check valves are used extensively in anesthesia machines to prevent reverse flow of gas in various portions of the machine. In particular, they are likely to be positioned (1) in the common gas line near the fresh gas outlet to the patient breathing circuit, just proximal to the point at which the oxygen flush line joins the gas stream;[19] (2) at the outlet of vaporizers to minimize the pumping effect of mechanical ventilation on vaporizer output; (3) between the pipeline connections and the junction with the outlet of the pressure-reducing regulators associated with the high-pressure yokes; and (4) between the high-pressure hanger yokes and the high-pressure manifold to prevent transfilling of high-pressure cylinders and to permit the removal of one high-pressure cylinder while others remain on. The operation of check valves is typically not tested in the daily check-out of the anesthesia machines but should be routinely tested by maintenance personnel during periodic maintenance.

INTRAOPERATIVE MONITORING OF ANESTHESIA MACHINES

Monitoring during the conduct of anesthesia requires careful attention to the status of the patient on a continuing basis. The following discussion addresses only those tasks that directly monitor the anesthesia machine. Patient, *per se,* monitoring is addressed in Chapters 1, 2, 4–10, and 15–22.

Intraoperative monitoring can be thought of as systematic verification of pressures within various portions of the machine, proper gas flows, and proper gas proportions, including vaporized volatile anesthetics. The operator should establish a pattern for scanning the different sources of data and should expect to check more frequently those that vary substantially over short intervals or that are judged to be particularly critical. As conditions change during the conduct of the anesthetic procedure, the order of the scan and the priority assigned to various monitoring tasks may need to be adjusted. For example, the initial portion of anesthetic administration demands frequent appraisal of the concentration of anesthetic agents while the uptake of the anesthetic agent proceeds toward equilibrium, as influenced by physiologic parameters (e.g., cardiovascular responses, pattern of ventilation, and absence of patient movement in response to surgical stimulation) and by measurement of the changing concentration of volatile agents in exhaled gas (e.g., mass spectroscopy and infrared analysis).

During a later phase of anesthetic maintenance, with the patient more nearly in equilibrium with the anesthetic agent, the anesthetic concentration might be monitored less frequently and attention (i.e., priority) might be directed toward lower-priority tasks such as ensuring that an adequate amount of liquid anesthetic is present in the vaporizer. Such examples illustrate a major difficulty of describing monitoring tasks during anesthetic administration. Various circumstances may dramatically affect the identification and description of criteria that one might use to set priorities for establishing those parameters to be tracked most closely as well as to set tolerances. Tolerances are the extremes of variation of individual variables that would be accepted before triggering action leading to adjustment of the variable being monitored (e.g., volatile anesthetic concentration) or adjustments of related variables (e.g., the administration of fluids).

Monitoring a number of parameters can lead to the continuing presentation of a large amount of data, requiring the anesthetist to sort out the important information. Experienced clinicians are able to perform these tasks fairly well, but the presentation of increasingly large volumes of information threatens to overload them. One sees this demonstrated when alarms sound on pieces of operating room equipment not related to the conduct of the anesthetic, and the anesthesiologist responds by searching the anesthesia machine for the source of the alarm. Manufacturers of anesthesia machines are responding to this problem by developing schemes for prioritizing the alarms that may be presented and having the alarms appear in a common location with instructions that help direct the operator's attention to the proper portion of the anesthetic apparatus.

Although a number of reports indicate that critical incidents that jeopardize patients arise from different sources, a common theme is that the causes relate most often to human error rather than to machine failure *per se* (see the Introduction of this book).[2, 10, 11] Understanding this, anesthesiologists should confirm their prior actions and continuously scan the machine for information concerning its status. The anesthesiologist who is idle for very long during the conduct of anesthesia is, at least, falling behind in

---

Table 13–2. VARIABLES REQUIRING MONITORING DURING
ANESTHESIA

---

1. Pipeline pressures of all gases connected to the anesthesia machine
2. Pressures within the high-pressure section of the anesthesia machine, when the cylinder supply of gas is in use
3. Flowmeter indication for each gas
4. Pressures within the patient breathing circuit
5. Concentration of oxygen within the patient breathing circuit
6. Concentration of anesthetic agents and other gases within the patient breathing circuit
7. Flow of gas within the patient breathing circuit
8. Pressures and flows associated with operation of the waste gas scavenging system

---

the gathering of information and runs the risk of frankly missing important changes in the status of the anesthetic procedure being conducted.

Table 13–2 provides an outline of those parameters that should be evaluated periodically during the conduct of clinical anesthesia in order to achieve ongoing monitoring of the anesthesia machine.

Pipeline Pressure Monitoring

Pipeline pressures should be monitored periodically, and the pressures should be confirmed to remain at 50 ± 5 psi. Major fluctuations may result from high resistance in the supply lines (e.g., multiple check valves in the pipeline system) producing a large pressure drop when higher flows are called for, such as when an oxygen-powered ventilator cycles or when the oxygen flush is activated. In installations in which such pressure drops are particularly large, the fail-safe system may be activated, resulting in intermittent changes in nitrous oxide flow. This situation indicates inadequate capacity of the pipeline system and should be corrected. It may interfere with the proper operation of oxygen-powered equipment, particularly anesthesia ventilators, and does not permit the high flow of oxygen necessary to provide adequate oxygen flush of the patient breathing circuit. In rare instances, low pipeline pressures are indicative of substantial leaks within the pipeline system.

Close monitoring of pressure within the high-pressure portion of the anesthesia machine (i.e., within gas cylinders) during the use of the cylinder gas supplies allows the operator to estimate the amount of gas remaining in the machine. This information, together with knowledge of the flow rate being employed, can be used to calculate the expected duration of the remaining gas supply. When this is done carefully and early in the procedure, additional cylinders can be delivered in a timely fashion or the anesthetic technique can be modified to conserve the available supply. Such estimates can be limited in several ways. The operator must recognize that the quantity of nitrous oxide remaining within the cylinders cannot be accurately estimated (see the previous discussion in this chapter). If oxygen-powered equipment is used (e.g., ventilators) or the oxygen flush valve is operated, then high and unmeasured oxygen expenditure does occur.

MONITORING THE ANESTHESIA MACHINE

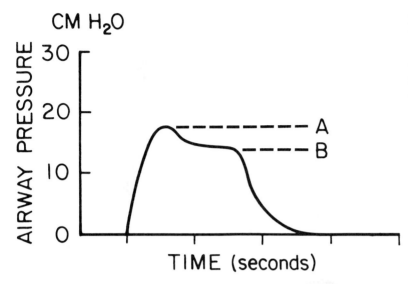

Figure 13–4. Typical airway pressure waveform during positive pressure ventilation when the initial flow delivered to the patient results in nonlaminar flow producing a pressure (A) greater than the plateau pressure (B) obtained when the inspiratory flow has decreased.

Breathing Circuit Pressure Monitoring

Monitoring pressures within the patient breathing circuit may confirm proper pressures, identify improper machine function, or indicate certain physiologic or physical problems with the patient or the tube used to provide access to the patient's airway. Although it has not been usual to have graphic display of airway pressures, the general shape of airway pressure waveforms during positive pressure ventilation can be determined from observation of the pressure displayed on the aneroid manometer in the patient breathing circuit (Fig. 13–4). With the onset of inspiration, the airway pressure increases at a rate determined by the rate of compression of the ventilator bellows and the characteristics of the flow of gas into the airways of the patient. Peak pressure may be easily obtained (Fig. 13–4A). When there is no further delivery of gas from the ventilator bellows or breathing bag, the pressure decreases to a value determined by the patient's pulmonary compliance and the volume of gas delivered to the patient (Fig. 13–4B). The peak pressure achieved is attributed to nonlaminar flow, primarily in larger airways during positive pressure ventilation. With the onset of exhalation, the airway pressure should rapidly decrease to less than 4 cmH$_2$O as the tidal volume is exhaled.

During spontaneous respiration, the pressure indicated by the breathing circuit pressure gauge should be low and not exceed 3–4 cmH$_2$O. Higher pressures during exhalation are most likely the result of the adjustable pressure-limiting valve being partially or completely closed. The extent of sustained elevated pressure within the breathing circuit can be great enough to cause barotrauma. If increased pressure remains during the expiratory phase of respiration and the adjustable pressure-limiting valve is known to be open, it is likely that there is obstruction of the outlet of this valve, the waste gas scavenger, or the scavenger conducting tubing. In scavenger installations equipped with a positive pressure relief valve, one may be able to hear that valve functioning during exhalation when there is occlusion of the scavenger tubing or inadequate flow provided by the scavenger suction.

Positive Pressure

The fact that positive pressure has been developed within the patient's airway does not assure that adequate ventilation has been achieved. The adequacy of ventilation can be accurately assessed by measuring the exhaled tidal or minute ventilation. This is usually accomplished by placing a spirometer in the patient breathing circuit. Until recently, mechanical spirometers in the breathing circuit were commonly employed (see Chapter 9). Recently, electromechanical spirometers have been introduced and are finding widespread acceptance.

The location of pressure- or flow-measuring apparatus within the patient breathing circuit bears an important relation to the information these devices can provide the anesthesiologist. The spirometric measuring devices are usually positioned in the expiratory limb of the circle absorbing system. In this position, they measure the sum of the volume of gas exhaled by the patient plus the volume of fresh gas flowing through the spirometer during the interval when the measurement is taken. Of interest is the fact that equipment manufacturers have recently begun to make the graphic display of airway pressure and flow waveforms available on some anesthesia machines. Pressure-measuring devices are typically located downstream from the exhalation unidirectional valve, between it and the inspiratory unidirectional valve. Conditions that elevate pressure within the patient's airway and the adjacent segment of the breathing circuit, as a positive end-expiratory pressure valve would, are not indicated on the pressure gauge in this location. This is because the positive end-expiratory pressure valve, in combination with a competent inspiratory unidirectional valve, serves to isolate the included segment of the breathing circuit from the pressure gauge that is functionally attached to the portion of the circle contiguous with the adjustable pressure-limiting valve or ventilator pop-off valve.

Negative Pressure

Negative pressures within the patient breathing circuit are abnormal and should be investigated and corrected promptly. Some causes are low total gas flow in combination with too-rapid descent of hanging bellows in certain anesthesia ventilators or application of too great a suction to the gas scavenging system. This latter effect may result in the removal of such large volumes of gas from the patient breathing circuit that the patient cannot be ventilated properly. Ventilators utilizing hanging (ascending during inspiration) bellows may create sufficient negative airway pressure that patients with airways having poor elastic support may suffer airway closure and interference with gas exchange. This can be managed by admitting a fresh gas flow to the breathing circuit that exceeds the maximum rate of filling of the bellows during its descent.

Breathing Circuit Gas Monitoring

Oxygen

The concentration of oxygen in the gas mixture being provided to the patient must be known. Adjustment of flowmeter settings can be made in a manner that minimizes the likelihood of accidental creation of hypoxic gas mixtures. It is suggested that anesthesiologists develop the habit of increasing the flow of oxygen first when increasing total flow and of decreasing the flow of nitrous oxide first when decreasing total flow. Information concerning the oxygen concentration is available directly from an oxygen analyzer (or other analytic instrument) or indirectly by calculation from knowledge of the flows of individual gases being employed.

Flow

The flow of each of the various gases used in the gas mixture being supplied to the anesthetized patient is usually monitored by the anesthesiologist observing the indications of flowmeters for each gas. This continues to be the primary monitor of gas flow. However, the incorporation of automated monitoring devices for gas flow is becoming increasingly widespread. In anesthesia machines that can deliver mixtures of oxygen and nitrous oxide containing less than 21% oxygen, several approaches have been used to enhance the safety of such machines. Some models of anesthesia machines have been equipped with oxygen ratio monitors. These devices often provide the first indication that an incorrect proportion of oxygen and nitrous oxide has been selected. They are pneumatic devices constructed to trigger an alarm when the concentration of oxygen in oxygen–nitrous oxide mixtures is less than 30%. It is important for the user of an anesthesia machine to recognize that such devices that purport to monitor flow or oxygen ratio in this fashion rely on the critical assumption that oxygen is being supplied to the apparatus. If the incorrect gas is supplied,[4, 7, 12] these devices, which rely on a pressure drop across a resistance to indicate flow, continue to report flow but, of course, do not indicate the gas being supplied.

For this reason, it is particularly critical that *analytic* instruments be included on anesthesia machines to measure oxygen concentration. Knowledge of the concentration of oxygen is so fundamental to the conduct of safe anesthesia that the use of analyzers specifically for oxygen seems destined to continue, even though other techniques (e.g., mass spectrometry) can serve to *identify* oxygen as well as to report its concentration in the gas mixture. Oxygen analyzers are cheap, reliable, specific, and accurate. Every anesthesia machine should be so equipped.

Carbon dioxide, nitrogen, and anesthetic gases are found in the patient breathing circuit, and the application of analytic techniques to monitor their concentration should be encouraged (see Chapter 14). Analysis of the concentration of gases other than oxygen can provide direct information about the progress of the patient toward equilibration with the anesthetic agents in use. This knowledge may be helpful in assessing the adequacy of ventilation or the state of the patient's cardiac function as well as being valuable for promoting a clear understanding of the manner in which uptake and distribution of anesthetic agents proceed. Measurement of end-tidal nitrogen can assist in understanding the extent to which a patient has been denitrogenated. Intraoperative increases in exhaled nitrogen provide evidence of air embolism. Measurement of carbon dioxide in exhaled gas provides clear evidence of the state of ventilation of the patient, as long as the production of carbon dioxide remains constant (see Chapter 9).[20, 21]

Because the sampling site has substantial effects on the concentration of different gases in different portions of the anesthetic circuit, it is important to know and understand expected concentrations in the patient breathing circuit, particularly as influenced by uptake, ventilation, and fresh gas flow. The details of instrumentation for the analysis and measurement of gases in the breathing circuit are discussed in Chapters 9 and 14.

Flow and pressure information may be converted to electrical signals that, in turn, can be put into monitoring devices. In anesthesia machines of recent manufacture, the monitoring of machine parameters is given a very high priority and is being developed to a high degree. Respiratory signals depicting pressure and flow within the breathing circuit may be displayed in real time on cathode-ray tube monitors. The signal produced by the concentration of CO_2 in exhaled gas may be used to provide important information concerning the adequacy of ventilation, including information that can lead to the rapid diagnosis of an incorrectly placed endotracheal tube (see Fig. 9–10). It is clear that it is becoming increasingly difficult to describe at exactly what point monitoring of the machine ceases and physiologic monitoring of the patient begins. Indeed, one of the issues now being confronted by those designing monitoring systems for larger surgical suites concerns resolution of questions related to monitoring priorities and display hierarchies for the integration of both physiologic monitoring of the patient and monitoring of parameters derived largely from the operation of anesthesia machines. Much of the problem relates to the need to present large amounts of monitoring information without overloading personnel.

Recently, Gaba and colleagues[11] presented a useful framework for developing a conceptual understanding of the manner in which anesthetic accidents evolve. They described the important elements leading to anesthetic mishaps in terms of the complexity of the interactions among "equipment, the anesthesiologist and the patient" and the tightness of the coupling between the various elements of a complex system. They further described a view in which simple incidents might interact and propagate within a complex system to develop into critical incidents or, when combined with a "substantive negative outcome," produce events that are generally recognized as accidents. Suggested strategies for recovery from such situations involve recognition and verification of a developing incident and the extent of the threat it represents, followed by the institution of life-sustaining functions and the initial application of diagnostic and corrective action, followed by specific diagnoses and treatment and adequate follow-up to assure continued correction throughout recovery.

INNOVATIVE APPROACHES TO ANESTHESIA MACHINE DESIGN

More than a decade ago, Cooper and coworkers[22] reported the development of a demonstration anesthesia system that incorporated new applications of electronic control of mechanical and pneumatic functions. They used electronically controlled digital valves to adjust the flow of gases and an electronically controlled injector for regulation of the amount of volatile anesthetic added to the gas mixture. For a variety of reasons, some of which were identified in their report, as well as high costs related to product liability, development, and proof of concept costs by potential manufacturers, the concepts used in the design of this apparatus have not been incorporated into the design of even the newest anesthesia machines. This is not to suggest that the refinement of anesthesia machines has ceased.

Most readers can appreciate that, with respect to the sophistication of monitoring machine functions, anesthesia machine development is proceeding rapidly. Today, anesthesia machines are being produced by only two domestic manufacturers, Ohmeda and Drager. A tendency toward the integrated monitoring of machine functions is strongly apparent. Integrated monitoring refers to designs such that, whether the monitoring functions are electrically or pneumatically based, turning on the machine master switch initiates monitoring of machine function, and one cannot use the machine without the monitoring apparatus in use—human ingenuity notwithstanding! For example, Drager has a back-up battery powering the machine monitoring functions on its Narcomed machines. In the event the machine is not connected to the 120 V alternating-current electrical service and battery power is used to power the monitoring functions, an advisory warning is provided to inform the operator of the limited power available from the battery.

Another clear direction in the development of anesthesia machines is the implementation of hardware such that it is not possible to administer gas mixtures containing less than 25–30% oxygen. Both manufacturers now provide machines that increase oxygen flow if an attempt is made to increase the flow of nitrous oxide to a degree that the percentage of oxygen in the resulting gas mixture would be less than approximately 30%.

Considerable attention is now being devoted to the manner in which the monitored information is displayed. Alarms are assigned priorities, so the anesthesiologist can rapidly assess and plan her or his response to monitor-generated messages. Schreiber and Schreiber described[5] a scheme in which all possible alarm conditions are prioritized into a three-level classification:

Warning: Requires immediate operator response
Caution: Requires prompt operator response
Advisory: Requires operator awareness that a condition exists

They have provided a detailed description of the display of such prioritized alarms in the form of audible, visual, and printed or cathode-ray tube–displayed messages that includes the suppression of lower-priority audible alarms until the higher-priority alarm conditions have been corrected. This style of alarm display has recently become available on Drager anesthesia machines.

It may soon be the norm to have monitored variables that fall outside of predetermined limits displayed in a central location on the anesthesia machine. Suggested courses of action might also be presented. The integration of the information resulting from monitoring anesthesia machine function with information resulting from physiologic monitoring of the patient will undoubtedly receive much attention. Whether these two lines of information will merge or not remains to be seen.

STANDARDS AND GUIDELINES

The continued evolution of anesthesia machines is confirmed by the ongoing development of new standards to describe their construction. The role of standards and guidelines in shaping the way anesthesia machines and related devices are used should be understood by those who use and who are involved in the acquisition of these devices. This discussion is not exhaustive but describes the principal standards now available.

Organizations

A number of organizations have written standards concerning various aspects related to the construction and use of anesthesia machines and of apparatus that supports the conduct of anesthetic practice. The standards characteristically represent the combined efforts of several groups (e.g., manufacturers, users, distributors, and regulators) concerned with the particular issues addressed by the given standard but do not, by themselves, have the force of law. They may, in some instances, be given the force of law by reference to state or local codes or laws. For example, the National Fire Protection Association's documents are often cited by building codes. Therefore, compliance becomes mandatory before a building can meet the requirements of the building code. In a general manner, whether mandated by law or not, compliance with published standards by practitioners and institutions assures the adherence to good practice as agreed upon by those intimately familiar with the field. In most instances, standards undergo periodic review and revision. Most institutions must plan for compliance with revisions of standards from time to time. This can be accomplished most easily if they stay abreast of trends in the field and develop practical plans for compliance with evolving standards. The responsibility for decision making in institutional policy, risk management, and purchasing resides with informed anesthesia clinicians, administrators, risk managers, and biomedical engineers.

Compressed Gas Association

The Compressed Gas Association is a voluntary organization of the manufacturers of compressed gases and products related to the use of compressed gases. This group has published standards describing the color coding of compressed gas cylinders, safety connecting systems (diameter-indexed safety system, thread-indexed safety system) to prevent the accidental cross-connection of gas cylinders and piping systems, the construction of cylinders for service as high-pressure gas storage, and the pin-indexed safety system to prevent the connection of improper gas cylinders to yokes intended for specific gases. Some of the Compressed Gas Association's standards provide examples of very specific methodologies to be used—for example, the descriptions of safety systems for interconnection of gas vessels and piping systems outline the fittings in such detail that different manufacturers are able to produce connectors that are compatible and interchangeable.

National Fire Protection Association

The National Fire Protection Association has prepared standards that are widely applicable to building design and construction, including, but not limited to, health care facilities. In the course of their work, this association has written standards dealing with electrical safety, the handling of medical gases, and medical gas piping systems that are the most widely recognized standards applied to health care facilities. Although these standards do not relate directly to anesthesia machines, understanding the underlying principles is of vital importance to those who provide anesthesia care.

American National Standards Institute

The American National Standards Institute assembles knowledgeable committees to define and publish standards in order to permit the interchange of information and ideas among groups having interests in a wide variety of technical disciplines. The work of the institute that relates to anesthesia equipment and machines was conducted by the ANSI Z79 Committee. The work of the Z79 Committee was transferred to the F-29 Committee of the American Society for Testing and Materials in 1983.

Other Organizations

Two additional organizations that have published standards that pertain to devices often used in conjunction with anesthesia machines or components are the Underwriters Laboratories and the Association for the Advancement of Medical Instrumentation.

A number of organizations have appeared over the last few years that promote the safety of medical devices and the dissemination of information concerning problems with or failure of various medical devices, including anesthesia machines. The Anesthesia Patient Safety Foundation is gaining prominence as an organization assuming responsibility for overseeing safety

Table 13–3. ORGANIZATIONS THAT HAVE
DEVELOPED STANDARDS APPLICABLE TO
ANESTHESIA MACHINES AND
EQUIPMENT

Compressed Gas Association
1235 Jefferson Davis Highway
Arlington, VA 22202
(703) 979–0900

National Fire Protection Association
Batterymarch Park
Quincy, MA 02269
(617) 770–3000

American National Standards Institute
1430 Broadway
New York, NY 10018
(212) 354–3300

American Society for Testing and Materials
1916 Race Street
Philadelphia, PA 19103
(215) 299–5400

Underwriters Laboratories, Inc.
333 Pfingsten Road
Northbrook, IL
(312) 272–8800

Association for Advancement of Medical Instrumentation
1901 North Fort Myer Drive
Suite 602
Arlington, VA 22209
(703) 525–4890

**Organizations Reporting Equipment Problems and
Promoting Safe Anesthesia Practices**
Anesthesia Patient Safety Foundation
515 Busse Highway
Park Ridge, IL 60068
(213) 825–5586

Emergency Care Research Institute
(Publisher of *Health Devices Alerts*)
5200 Butler Pike
Plymouth Meeting, PA 19462
(215) 825–6000

issues related to anesthesia, including those issues that pertain directly to anesthesia machines.

Table 13–3 lists the addresses and phone numbers of organizations that write standards applicable to the use of anesthesia machines. Most publish a directory of available publications and provide information concerning their areas of expertise.

References

1. Dorsch JA, Dorsch SE: Understanding Anesthesia Equipment: Construction, Care and Complications, 2nd Ed. Baltimore: Williams & Wilkins, 1984.

2. Petty C: The Anesthesia Machine. New York: Churchill Livingstone, 1987.

3. Schreiber P: Safety Guidelines for Anesthesia Systems. Telford, PA: North American Drager, 1984.

4. Bowie E, Huffman LM: The Anesthesia Machine: Essentials for Understanding. Madison, WI: Ohmeda/BOC Healthcare Group, 1985.

5. Schreiber P, Schreiber J: Anesthesia System Risk Analysis and Risk Reduction. Telford, PA: North American Drager, 1987.

6. Jones PL: Some observations on nitrous oxide cylinders during emptying. Br J Anaesth 1974; 46:534–538.

7. Epstein RM, Rackow H, Lee ASJ, Papper EM: Prevention of accidental breathing of anoxic gas mixtures during anesthesia. Anesthesiology 1962; 23:1–4.

8. Cook TL, Eger EI, Behl RS: Is your vaporizer off? Anesth Analg 1977; 56:793–800.

9. Keet JE, Valentine GW, Riccio JS: An arrangement to prevent pressure effect on the Vernitrol vaporizer. Anesthesiology 1963; 24:734–737.

10. Cooper J, Newbower R, Long C, McPeek B: Preventable anesthesia mishaps: A study of human factors. Anesthesiology 1978; 49:339–406.

11. Gaba DM, Maxwell M, DeAnda A: Anesthetic mishaps: Breaking the chain of accident evolution. Anesthesiology 1987; 66:670–676.

12. Mazze RI: Therapeutic misadventures with oxygen delivery systems: The need for continuous in-line oxygen monitors. Anesth Analg 1972; 51:787–791.

13. Anesthesia apparatus checkout draft recommendations. Federal Register Notices. March 28, 1986; 51:10673–10674.

14. Anesthesia apparatus checkout recommendations. American Society of Anesthesiologists Newsletter. October 1986; 50:5–6.

15. Anonymous: How to monitor Sodasorb exhaustion. Sodalines. Lexington, MA: Dewey and Almy Division of WR Grace, June 1987.

16. Hamilton RC, Byrne J: Another cause of gas scavenging line obstruction. Anesthesiology 1979; 51:365–366.

17. Whitcher C, Piziali RL: Monitoring occupational exposure to inhalational anesthetics. Anesth Analg 1977; 56:778–785.

18. American National Standard Z79.8–1979: Minimum performance and safety requirements for components and systems of continuous-flow anesthesia machines for human use. New York: American National Standards Institute, 1979.

19. Comm G, Rendell-Baker L: Back pressure check valves a hazard. (Letter.) Anesthesiology 1982; 56:327–328.

20. Weil MH, Bisera J, Trevino RP, Rackow EC: Cardiac output and end-tidal carbon dioxide. Crit Care Med 1985; 13:907–909.

21. Spargo PM: The use of end-tidal pCO_2 monitoring to detect pulmonary embolism during Swan-Ganz catheter removal. Anesthesiology 1985; 63:A293.

22. Cooper JB, Newbower RS, Moore JW, Trautman ED: A new anesthesia delivery system. Anesthesiology 1978; 49:310–318.

chapter fourteen

Monitoring Anesthetic Gases

KEITH D. KNOPES, M.D.
■ BERNICE R. HECKER, M.D.

With the revolution in technology, the role of the anesthesiologist now includes monitoring not only physiologic or pharmacologic variables but inspired and expired anesthetic and other respiratory gases as well. The routine monitoring of inspired and expired oxygen and carbon dioxide is standard in many operating rooms. This technology is also widely used in the intensive care unit (ICU).

The application of mass spectrometry to the field of monitoring anesthetic gases allows real-time measurement of multiple inspired and expired gases, including the anesthetic vapors. The cost of such instruments has necessitated the use of time-sharing. Time-sharing permits simultaneous monitoring of multiple operating rooms. Additional methods of measurement include infrared and Raman scattering spectrophotometry. The cost of these instruments permits their placement in individual operating rooms without the problems encountered with time-sharing.

In addition to monitoring patients during anesthesia, this technology is useful in assessing the occupational exposure to anesthetic gases in the operating room. The information obtained is helpful in analyzing the risk of exposure, in detecting leaks, and in determining the source of exposure.

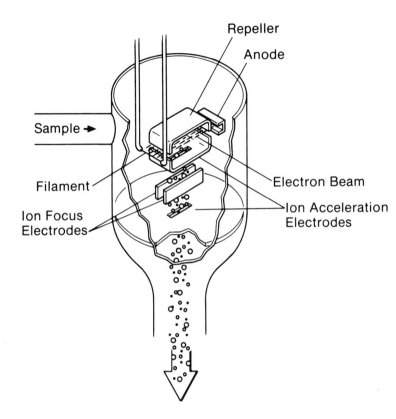

Repeller

Anode

Sample ➡

Filament

Ion Focus
Electrodes

Electron Beam

Ion Acceleration
Electrodes

Figure 14–1. The ion source is a stream of electrons generated by an incandescent filament that interacts with the sample to form ions of the parent molecule. (From McLafferty FW: Interpretation of Mass Spectrometry. Reading, MA: WA Benjamin, 1973; 6. With permission.)

MASS SPECTROMETRY: THEORY

Molecular Ion Generation

The basic purpose of the mass spectrometer is to provide measurable products of the ionization process. This results in a product that, when measured, is indicative of the content of the sample being measured. This process of ionization begins with the ion source (Fig. 14–1). A stream of bombarding electrons is generated by an incandescent filament. These electrons interact with a stream of vaporized sample molecules (sampled from the breathing circuit) to form ions of the parent molecules. These molecular ions may then go on to fragment, yielding the fragmentation mass spectrum.

Ion Separation

Once the ions are formed, they must be separated for counting based upon their mass-to-charge (M/C) ratios. Common techniques of separation are magnetic deflection, time-of-flight, quadrupole lens, radio frequency, cyclotron resonance, and cycloidal focusing. The most widely applied methods of separation of the molecular ions in clinical use are the quadrupole lens and magnetic sector techniques.[1]

Quadrupole Lens

The quadrupole lens makes use of a changing magnetic field induced between two electrodes charged with a combined direct and alternating current signal.[2] The stream of molecular ions is then directed through the magnetic field, which accomplishes the ion separation based upon the unique M/C ratio of each. A single detector collects and detects the ions. The results are synchronously reported, allowing the computation of the relative contribution of each ion to the mass spectrum.

Magnetic Sector

A different approach is used in a magnetic sector mass spectrometer. This method directs the stream of molecular ions through a magnetic field where the ions are deflected based upon their M/C ratio. After the separation, the individual ion paths end at a series of detectors that report the raw data for analysis based upon the relative amounts of each ion in the mass spectrum. An alternative design makes use of a varying magnetic field that changes the degree of ion deflection. This brings a different M/C ratio into focus on a detector slit that focuses the selected ion stream on the detector (Fig. 14–2).

Detector

Once the ions generated by the bombarding electrons in the ion source have been separated by these strategies, they are detected by collection plates. As the positive molecular ions contact the collector, a current of electrons is generated proportional to the number of molecular ions. The resulting current is amplified and presented for analysis. Research instruments can make use of electron multiplier circuits that make possible the detection of a single ion arriving at the collector. Instruments used in clinical monitoring are not required to be so sensitive, thus making the cost of an instrument more reasonable.

Spectral Interpretation

Once the ions in the mass spectrum have been generated, separated, and detected, the instrument must provide easily interpretable results. The molecular ion, M^+, is that ion produced with the highest M/C ratio in the mass spectrum. However, the detection of the molecular ion alone is insufficient to differentiate among the various gases encountered in the clinical setting, since some have the same mass number. Also, the ions generated during the fragmentation of various gases and vapors (especially halogenated

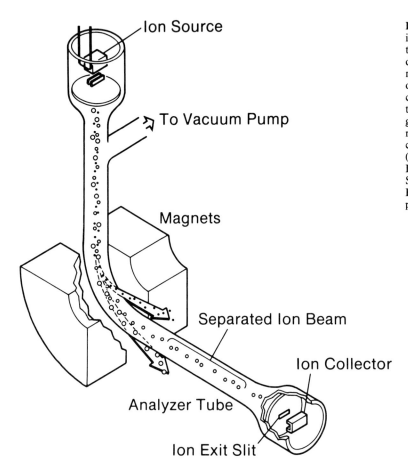

Ion Source

To Vacuum Pump

Magnets

Separated Ion Beam

Ion Collector

Analyzer Tube

Ion Exit Slit

Figure 14–2. The path of the ions is through a varying magnetic field that changes the degree of ion deflection so that ions of different mass-to-charge ratios are focused on the detector slit of the collection plates. As ions contact the collector, a current is generated in proportion to the number of molecular ions. The current is amplified and analyzed. (From McLafferty FW: Interpretation of Mass Spectrometry. Reading, MA: WA Benjamin, 1973; 7. With permission.)

hydrocarbons) cause generation of species that overlap the characteristic peaks of other components of the gas sample. Therefore, sophisticated computer programming for analysis of the mass spectrum is necessary in order to provide usable clinical data.

MASS SPECTROMETER SAMPLING

The mass spectrometer was adapted for measurement of respiratory gases in 1952.[3] It was not until the 1960s that routine commercial use of this technology became available. A key feature in the adaptation of mass spectrometry to the clinical arena is the development of multipatient applications.[4] The measurement of anesthetic gases during anesthesia required multiple samplings with a small time increment between measurements. The central placement of one instrument connected to multiple sampling sites by long capillary tubing makes this possible.[5] The small diameter of the capillary tubing allows multiple breath samples to be "stored" in the tubing with very little diffusion or mixing. The mass spectrometer may then sample

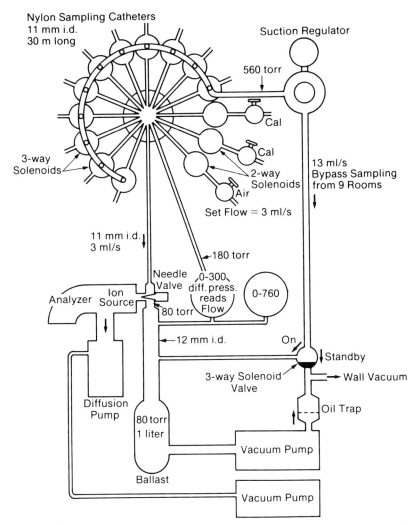

Figure 14–3. Time-shared mass spectrometer system allowing sampling from 10 rooms by way of the three-way solenoids. (From Ozanne GM, Young WG, Mazzei WJ, Severinghaus JW: Multipatient anesthetic mass spectometry: Rapid analysis of data stored in long catheters. Anesthesiology 1981; 55:62–70. With permission.)

each tube in turn. During the sampling interval, the instrument may quickly sample several breaths from the capillary tube and provide an analog display of the concentration-time profile with digital reports of the inspired and expired end-tidal values.

The application of multiline capillary sampling systems made the clinical use of mass spectrometry economical, easy to use, and reliable. The high cost of mass spectrometry makes individual patient monitoring impractical. A schematic of multipatient adaptation is in Figure 14–3. The use of long, small-diameter catheters and a bank of solenoid sampling valves allows systematic, time-shared sampling from multiple locations. A vacuum pump pulls the sample past the inlet. The introduction of plastic catheters for sampling presents the possibility of error introduced by the absorption of gases by the catheter. This error is considered so small as to be clinically insignificant. The use of disposable sampling apparatus eliminates the risk of infectious contamination. Sampling sites include the Y-piece of the circle system, a side port of the Rovenstine angle attached to the mask or endotracheal tube, or other portions of the anesthetic circuit.

INDICATIONS AND USES

Improved engineering designs have made mass spectrometry cost-effective through the use of time-shared sampling. With the advent of new applications of Raman scattering for gas analysis, it is possible to purchase single devices for single-patient monitoring at a reasonable cost. The availability of these respiratory gas monitors allows routine use in clinical, teaching, and research areas.

Clinical Indications

Routine use of mass spectrometry and Raman spectroscopy in clinical anesthesia permits continuous monitoring of all gases of interest to the practicing anesthesiologist. In addition to reporting values for the volatile anesthetic agents, these instruments simultaneously measure oxygen, carbon dioxide, nitrogen, and nitrous oxide. This technology provides a greater amount of information than does the use of polarographic devices for monitoring oxygen and infrared spectroscopy for detecting carbon dioxide. The use of oxygen and carbon dioxide analyzers, however, provides an additional layer of safety when used with mass spectrometry or Raman spectral analysis.

On-line measurement of respiratory and anesthetic gases is important to both clinical care and patient safety. The continuous measurement feature points out the difference between inspired and expired gas mixtures. An astute clinician makes use of these differences to draw conclusions that have direct consequences on patient care. Table 14–1 reviews some examples of critical events the detection of which often prevents anesthetic misadventures.

Construction of gas delivery systems for operating rooms is a complicated engineering project. A multitude of errors may occur during installation that include, but are not limited to, using improper fittings, mislabeling, crossing pipelines, and contamination by other gases, water, and foreign matter.[6] Deaths have occurred owing to errors in installation of gas delivery systems.[7] The gas source for delivery systems may be remote from the operating rooms in order to facilitate easy delivery of the gas supply. Therefore, a hospital remodeling project may introduce dangerous modifications to the gas delivery system that are unknown to the anesthesiologist. These critical incidents have been recognized by analysis of the inspired gas mix-

Table 14–1. CRITICAL
EVENTS DETECTED BY
MASS SPECTROMETER

Errors in gas delivery system
Anesthesia machine malfunction
Vaporizer malfunction
Errors in vaporizer contents
Anesthesia circuit leaks
Endotracheal cuff leaks
Poor mask fit
Hypoventilation
Airway obstruction
Air embolism

ture, before harm could come to the patient.[6] Obviously, a system that measures all the gases presented to the breathing circuit provides more information and perhaps improved safety for the patient than does an instrument measuring any single gas.

Clinical Uses

Measurement of Oxygen

The introduction of continuous monitoring of oxygen by mass spectrometry is redundant, as most anesthesia machines have polarographic monitors of the inspiratory oxygen concentration delivered to the anesthesia circuit (see Chapter 8). However, the additional inspired and expired values obtained by mass spectrometry confirm the adequate delivery of oxygen to the patient.

Measurement of Carbon Dioxide

The simultaneous monitoring of carbon dioxide allows continuous evaluation of ventilation (see Chapter 9). The mass spectrometer uses the detection of the CO_2 waveform to trigger various alarm states. The most important alarm is the "no breath" or apnea state. The rapid detection of CO_2 is used routinely to confirm tracheal intubation. During maintenance of anesthesia, the detection of CO_2 confirms the integrity of the circuit. If disconnection occurs, the "no breath" alarm sounds as the mass spectrometer fails to detect an expiratory waveform. The quantification of the analog waveform into digital information gives the anesthesiologist further information on the adequacy of ventilation.

Astute clinicians use end-tidal CO_2 measurements for important clinical observations. A recent example is the detection of higher than anticipated CO_2 measurements in a child undergoing repair of total anomalous pulmonary venous return.[8] While the patient was on cardiopulmonary bypass, the end-tidal CO_2 remained mildly elevated over expected levels of less than 0.5%. This suggested the presence of a systemic-to-pulmonary shunt to the clinicians caring for this child. Exploration of the great vessels revealed a patent ductus arteriosus. Ligation decreased the CO_2 to less than 0.2%. Careful observation and continuous gas analysis directly benefit patients.

Mass spectrometry measurement of CO_2 identifies problems with the anesthetic circuit.[9] Increased inspiratory CO_2 suggests inefficiency of the CO_2 absorber in a circle system. An alternative explanation is malfunction of the unidirectional valve on the inspiratory limb of the circuit. Therefore, increased inspired CO_2 requires direct inspection of the circle system of the anesthesia machine.

Measurement of Nitrogen

The continuous on-line measurement of nitrogen yields much useful information for the anesthesiologist. The standard of care for induction of patients with a full stomach is a rapid-sequence induction following denitrogenation of the patient. This may be accomplished by several minutes of quiet breathing of 100% oxygen via a tight-fitting mask.[10] Alternatively, four deep breaths of 100% oxygen may be used.[11] Mass spectrometry monitors nitrogen washout. When the end-tidal nitrogen is less than 5% of the exhaled gases, it is safe to proceed with the induction of general anesthesia.

Mass spectrometry is a very effective monitor of the integrity of anesthesia delivery systems. Nitrogen is washed out of the lungs in a matter of minutes. Although it may take hours for all the nitrogen to be washed out of body tissues, the end-tidal concentration is usually about 1–3% during the first few hours as the nitrogen diffuses out of the tissues and finds its way to the lungs for excretion and detection by the mass spectrometer. Therefore, a sudden rise in nitrogen percentage in the exhaled gas mixture is diagnostic of the introduction of air from outside the anesthesia gas delivery system. Sources of this air could be leaks in the circuit or endotracheal cuff or a venous air embolism.[12–14] In the case of venous air embolism, the increased end-tidal nitrogen precedes changes in precordial Doppler sounds. Mass spectrometry has been used to detect disconnection of the fresh gas "down-inflow."[15] This disconnection occurred in an anesthesia circuit with a descending bellows type of ventilator. The combination of this ventilator with a small-diameter fresh gas inflow prevented detection of the disconnection by the low-pressure alarm. The only indication was the rapid increase in nitrogen detected by the mass spectrometer. The additional information obtained by mass spectrometric analysis of all anesthetic gases simultaneously greatly benefits the anesthesiologist in the detection and diagnosis of critical incidents.

Measurement of Anesthetic Vapors

Vaporizers. The mass spectrometer is useful in the calibration and monitoring of vaporizer function. Uncalibrated vaporizers require knowledge of the vapor pressure, temperature, and gas flows to correctly calculate the concentration of anesthetic vapor delivered to the patient. Although multiple nomograms and pocket aids have been developed, the possibility of error is introduced, and the inadvertent overdose of anesthetic vapor is a real problem. The use of continuous computerized mass spectrometry significantly adds to patient safety by correctly reporting the delivered concentration of vapor.

Temperature-compensated and flow-calibrated vaporizers have been developed that allow the clinician to "dial-in" a desired percentage of vapor delivered. However, these are not without the possibility of malfunction. These complex devices require regular scheduled maintenance and calibration. Continuous mass spectrometry indicates when the vaporizer needs calibration. A routine check of vaporizer function is easily accomplished by connecting the sampling tube of the mass spectrometer to the fresh gas flow outlet at the anesthesia machine by means of a T-piece and directly sampling the vaporizer output.

The mass spectrometer also detects leaks in the vaporizer system. Many newer modes of anesthesia machines are equipped with more than one vaporizer in series. The possibility of leaking is detected by the mass spectrometer displaying a signal for an "unknown" vapor. This display occurs when the instrument simultaneously detects two vapors. The computer analysis display also reports "unknown" vapor conditions when a vaporizer has been contaminated by the addition of the wrong agent.[16] For example, if enflurane has been added to a vaporizer containing halothane, both agents are presented to the sampling port simultaneously. As in the situation for a leaking vaporizer, the mass spectrometer reports the detection of an "unknown" vapor.

Closed Circuit Anesthesia. The use of low-flow or closed circuit anesthesia has seen episodic popularity. The benefits include better respiratory gas humidification, clinically significant decrease in heat loss, and cost-effective anesthetic administration as less anesthetic vapors and gases are used. However, most anesthesiologists routinely use an open circuit with higher fresh gas flows primarily because of the fear of delivering a hypoxic inspiratory gas mixture. If the addition of oxygen to the circle system is less than that consumed by the patient, the rebreathed gases become hypoxic. This may occur quite rapidly if nitrous oxide is included in the gas mixture. It is obvious that continuous monitoring of the anesthetic gases alerts the anesthesiologist to the need to add more oxygen to the circuit.

Gas Analysis in ICU

The routine clinical use of mass spectrometry has extended from the operating room to the ICU.[17-20] Routine ICU use includes monitoring CO_2 to confirm tracheal placement of endotracheal tubes and regulating ventilation parameters to control hypo- and hyperventilation. Information from the mass spectrum has been used in calculating alveolar-arterial oxygen tension difference, minute volume, dead space, ventilation/perfusion ratio, and O_2 consumption (see Chapter 17). Derived variables have been used as extubation criteria. Routine ICU use is dependent upon the time-sharing of a mass spectrometer to be cost-effective. It seems unlikely that this costly instrument and installation will be a common feature in most ICU settings, as the information most necessary in patient care can be obtained in more cost-effective ways.

Teaching

Many teaching institutions have installed mass spectrometers to aid in the teaching of medical students and residents. The analog and trending displays are very useful in many demonstrations of normal and altered physiology during anesthesia. The concept of nitrogen washout is displayed on the user interface using the trend line for nitrogen. Alterations in ventilation and gas mixtures can be used to demonstrate simple principles used clinically to care for patients. The introduction of different anesthetic circuits, gas flows, and ventilation results in very different patterns of respiratory gas exchange. Attention to the change in anesthetic gas concentration with time improves student understanding of gas exchange.

The concept of uptake and distribution is a most difficult one for many students of anesthesiology. These complex pharmacokinetic principles are difficult to understand from texts or lectures. Mass spectrometer data are used by the clinical teacher to demonstrate these concepts to the student by examination of the gas concentration-time curves. A further extension of this teaching is the pharmacodynamic results of vaporizer, gas flow, and gas mixture manipulations. Alveolar concentrations can be adjusted to a specific fraction of minimum alveolar concentration. During closed circuit anesthesia, the calculation of metabolic oxygen requirements and their changes with depth of anesthesia give students insight into the physiologic changes caused by various anesthetic agents.

Research

In addition to the uses discussed previously, the mass spectrometer has a well-established place in clinical and basic research, but its full potential is yet to be discovered. It is very useful in establishing the steady state in studies involving the depth of anesthesia in humans and animals. Instruments have been adapted for measuring halothane metabolites[21] and examining tissue uptake of nitrous oxide.[22] This powerful technology will continue to widen our knowledge base about the pharmacokinetic, pharmacodynamic, and metabolic consequences of anesthetic vapors and gases.

SYSTEM MAINTENANCE

The time-shared mass spectrometer is a complex mechanical and electronic instrument that requires daily maintenance and calibration. The improvement in computer technology and its application to the user interface have made the daily care of these instruments much easier. However, meticulous care must be taken. The commercially available devices monitor themselves electronically to ensure that the values reported are within realistic parameters or an alert condition results. Daily logs of maintenance procedures and calibration are essential to aid in trouble-shooting should a major system failure occur.

Calibration and Standardization

A daily manual calibration is recommended for most commercial instruments. This involves establishing zero references of the electronics and calibrating sensitivities. If electrical steady state is confirmed by the absence of baseline drift, then gas calibration is performed. Gas calibration is accomplished by the use of standard gas mixtures (including oxygen, nitrous oxide, air, carbon dioxide, and a volatile agent) supplied in cylinders. The instrument samples a known gas mixture at regular intervals during operation and adjusts its own calibration.

Reliability and Sources of Error

Reliability

Clinical mass spectrometry has resulted in a surprisingly reliable instrument, given its great complexity. The system maintains close calibration without significant technician intervention for many days. However, service is still frequent and requires a qualified technical support person to maintain the instrument on a daily basis. In addition to daily calibration, gas cylinders need regular replacement, vacuum pumps require checking and changing of oil, and the user interface stations may get damaged in daily use. The most common problems involve the sampling systems, which may become blocked owing to tubing kinks or foreign matter. Mechanical damage to other parts of the sampling or measuring portions of the instrument also occurs. The spectrometer collecting plates and filaments require regular replacement over months or years.

Sources of Error

Commercial mass spectrometers have many ways of handling sampling sources of error. One problem is the overlap in the patterns of inspiratory and expiratory gases. A spectrum overlap eraser circuit is often used to help with this problem. However, these alterations in data analysis may themselves introduce error.[23]

A significant error in measurement occurs with the introduction of unmeasured ions into the sample stream. Commercially designed clinical mass spectrometers include collection plates and ion counters for the respiratory and anesthetic gases. Very low or high molecular weight species with limited fragmentation spectra are not detected by such instruments. An example of such a gas is helium.[24] Its low molecular weight prevents it from being measured. Therefore, any contribution that helium makes to the gas sample measured is not included in the calculated gas totals or percentages. Only dry gas totals are determined. Water vapor is ignored. If 50% helium were to be used in the inspired mixture, the mass spectrometer would report the totals and percentages of the remaining gas as twice their true values. This misinformation could lead the anesthesiologist to treat the incorrect information in ways injurious to the patient. For example, the end-tidal CO_2 would be reported as twice its true value. This might lead the anesthesiologist to hyperventilate the patient, with resultant metabolic alkalosis. As the use of helium (primarily for laser surgeries) and other gases is introduced into clinical practice, mass spectrometers require modification to remove these sources of error.

The sampling system, consisting of long distances of plastic tubing, may be a source of error.[2,25] The longer the tubing system, the greater is the error due to diffusion. Water vapor condenses on the walls of the tubing. This thin film of water absorbs small amounts of nitrous oxide, CO_2 and the volatile anesthetic agents, slowing their transit to the instrument. These sample tubing–induced errors are small and of no clinical significance. However, research data is influenced by even small sources of error. Thus, dedicated single-station instruments yield superior research data.

Condensate, blood, or secretions occasionally block the sampling tubing. A filter placed at the inlet of the sampling line minimizes obstruction from secretions, soda lime, or other particulate matter.

Errors in data interpretation are also common in the use of the mass spectrometer. Many anesthesiologists assume that the end-tidal concentration is always an accurate reflection of the arterial partial pressure. However, there are several conditions under which this is not the case.[26] Any barrier to anesthetic gas transfer in the lung is reflected in a higher end-tidal pressure than an arterial partial pressure. Ventilation-perfusion abnormalities represent such a situation. Increased ventilation-perfusion mismatch results in less uptake into the blood. When there are large differences between inspired and end-tidal values, the error is magnified. It is important to note that ventilation-perfusion abnormalities are exaggerated by anesthesia, thus further adding to the error.

Cost/Benefit

There is no doubt that the initial capital investment ($70,000–$100,000 range) is significant for a mass spectrometer installation. The cost per anesthetizing location decreases with the increasing number of locations serviced. However, as the number of sampling locations is increased, so are the service and maintenance costs. The requirement of a trained technician to perform daily service and trouble-shooting is an ongoing expense, as are parts and calibration gases. Improvements in design are moderating the cost and improving ease of use.

The addition of mass spectrometry introduces a certain redundance to existing monitoring equipment. Most anesthesia machines are equipped with inspiratory oxygen monitors, and many hospitals have invested in capnography for each operating room. Redundancy, however, improves safety. This has been proved over and over again in the aerospace field. The comparisons between operating an aircraft and performing an anesthetic have been made for many years. Redundancy in monitoring may be a safety feature common to both.

Sound clinical critical incident reporting and research have yet to be applied to the use of mass spectrometry in the operating room. Therefore, the dollar cost benefit is only speculation at this point. There can be little doubt, however, that prevention of harm secondary to a critical incident is worth a significant number of dollars, given the litigious nature of our society today. The benefits of improved anesthetic management with the use of continuous mass spectrometry are difficult to quantify. There are no data to support decreased recovery time, monetary savings from decreased anesthetic use, or better patient outcome during routine anesthesia uncomplicated by critical events. However, these data would also be difficult to obtain. Therefore, the case for the routine use of mass spectrometry must be made based upon the prevention of critical events related to anesthesia.

OTHER METHODS OF MONITORING ANESTHETIC GASES

Alternative methods, such as ultraviolet analysis and silicone rubber absorption method for detecting and quantifying anesthetic gases, have been used for decades. Oxygen analyzers are standard equipment on many anesthesia machines. A commonly used detector is designed around a polarographic method (see Chapter 8). Infrared spectrophotometry is used in most single-station capnographs for the monitoring of CO_2 (see Chapter 9).

As interest intensified for less expensive, smaller, more reliable, and easier to use instrumentation, new technologies were developed for operating room monitoring of anesthetic gases. Two such applications are Raman scattering spectroscopy[27] and piezoelectric quartz crystal[28] analysis of gases.

Raman Scattering Spectroscopy

Most of the commercial development of monitors of anesthetic gases followed long use of similar detection principles in the chemistry laboratory. This is certainly true for Raman scattering spectroscopy.

Raman scattering results when laser beam–generated photons strike gas molecules. The resultant collision yields light with characteristic frequency shifts. This shifted frequency is measured as Raman scattering. The scattered light is measured as separate peaks in the spectra, resulting in easy determination of the concentration of each of the respiratory gases and anesthetics of clinical interest.

There are some advantages to implementation of this type of analysis.

The cost of the instrument allows individual instruments at each location, providing continuous on-line data. The gases are unaltered by analysis and can be returned to the anesthesia circuit without harm to the patient. The technology has the theoretic possibility of very rapid response times.

The commercial success of Raman spectroscopy will depend upon improvements in engineering design. The instruments currently under development have higher signal-to-noise ratios than those of mass spectrometers. Their reliability compared with mass spectrometry has been established.[27] The laser source is an essential and costly element in the system. Therefore, the lifetime of the laser is important in the consideration of maintenance costs.

Piezoelectric Detectors

Piezoelectric quartz crystals have been recognized as an alternative detector of halogenated anesthetic gases.[28] The natural resonant frequency of a quartz crystal coated by a lipophilic layer changes in proportion to the partial pressure of a halogenated anesthetic gas. The instrument supplies the electric field to the piezoelectric quartz crystal and measures the changes in the resonant frequency. Data are reported as volumes-percent of anesthetic vapor. This method cannot distinguish among the different inhaled anesthetic vapors and must be calibrated for each agent individually by means of a dial on the instrument face.[28] Nitrous oxide and water vapor introduce error into the measurement, particularly for isoflurane.[29] If the nitrous oxide and water vapor are held constant, an electronic offset can be used to remove the error caused by them. However, the significance of the introduced error may influence clinical data for low concentrations of the anesthetic vapors, since heated, humidified gases increase the measured concentration.[29]

Piezoelectric quartz crystal instruments can be made available at each anesthetizing location at a very low cost. Cost and the ease of use of the instrument make piezoelectric quartz crystal monitors practical for limited installations. The Engstrom multigas monitor for anesthesia is an example of this technology.

OCCUPATIONAL EXPOSURE TO ANESTHETIC GASES

Analysis of Risk

Anesthesiologists have been aware of the effects of exposure to inhaled anesthetic gases for many decades. In the early portion of this century, when open-drop ether was still in use, operating room personnel experienced headache, nausea, and an inability to concentrate. The innovation of improved operating room ventilation greatly reduced these reactions. However, it was

Table 14–2. POTENTIAL* HEALTH
HAZARDS RESULTING FROM
OCCUPATIONAL ANESTHETIC
EXPOSURE

Increased spontaneous abortion rate[33, 34]
Increased rate of congenital malformations
  (teratogenicity)[35]
Increased risk of hepatic disease[39, 40]
Increased risk of renal disease[40]
Impairment of motor and cognitive skills[36, 37]
Increased incidence of cancer[30]
Headache, nausea[44]
Enzyme induction[41–43]

* Although some experimental and epidemiologic evidence strongly suggests a health hazard
from chronic anesthetic exposure, other causes
have not been completely excluded.

not until the last 20 years that there was greater awareness of the long-term
effects of trace anesthetics.

A higher incidence of malignancies in anesthesiologists than in the general population was one of the initial clues to this problem.[30] Up to this time,
trace anesthetics were thought to be inert and quickly eliminated, thus causing no harm. However, discoveries documenting the biotransformation of
these agents forced a review of this mistaken concept and strengthened
interest in improving scavenging techniques.[31] In 1974, *Anesthesiology* published a landmark study by Cohen and coworkers, who reported that working
in the operating room resulted in a significant risk to health.[32] This and
subsequent studies point to the role of chronic exposure to trace anesthetic
agents as a major health hazard, increasing the risk of spontaneous abortion,[33, 34] congenital anomalies in offspring,[35] cognitive defects,[36, 37] cancer,[30] and renal or hepatic disease.[38–40] Stimulation of drug-metabolizing
enzymes also occurs after anesthetic exposure.[41–43] Headache and nausea
are also reported after chronic environmental exposure.[44] However, more
recent studies fail to confirm some of these risks (Table 14–2).[45]

Routine use of scavenging systems minimizes such exposure. Industry-
wide standard practice now requires routine checks for sources of exposure,
detection of leaks, and implementation of techniques to minimize exposure.

Sources of Exposure

Anesthetic gases are supplied from the wall outlet and from the anesthesia machine itself with the vaporization of volatile anesthetics. Spilling
volatile anesthetics during vaporizer filling markedly increases environmental contamination. The trace contamination from the high-pressure sources
and anesthesia machine flowmeters is not adequately scavenged. The removal of this source of contamination requires detection of the leak and

A

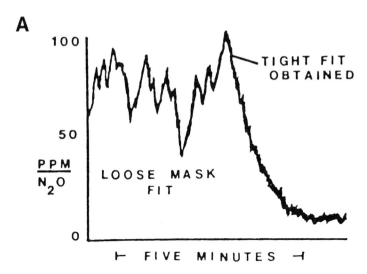

Figure 14–4. *A*, The effect of a poorly fitting mask on environmental concentrations of nitrous oxide (N_2O, parts per million). With proper mask application, the nitrous oxide concentration rapidly decreases. *B*, The benefits of endotracheal intubation on the maintenance of low environmental concentrations of N_2O. (From Lecky JH [ed]: Waste anesthetic gases in operating room air: A suggested program to reduce personnel exposure. Park Ridge, IL: American Society of Anesthesiologists Ad Hoc Committee on Effects of Trace Anesthetic Agents on Health of Operating Room Personnel; 9–10. Reprinted with permission from the American Society of Anesthesiologists, ASA 515 Busse Highway, Park Ridge, Illinois 60068.)

B

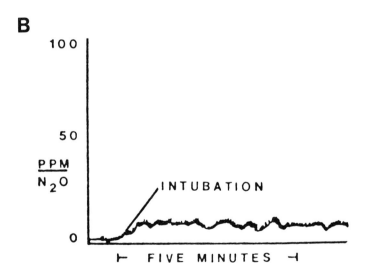

proper machine maintenance to prevent the occurrence of leaks. A program of regular simple testing detects these leaks, allowing their correction (see Chapter 13).[46]

The patient–anesthesia machine interface may be a significant source of operating room pollution. General anesthesia administered with a poorly fitting mask exposes every member of the operating team to large amounts of anesthetic gases. It is the duty of the anesthesiologist to use meticulous technique and provide a leak-proof mask fit (Fig. 14–4*A*). A good case may be made for the use of endotracheal intubation to protect operating room personnel from gas leaks due to poorly performed "mask" anesthesia (Fig. 14–4*B*). If the patient is intubated, care must be taken to ensure against cuff leaks. If positive pressure ventilation is used, a small cuff leak may allow significant amounts of gas to leak into the operating room environment.

Anesthetic gas flows should be discontinued prior to intubation or patient suctioning.

A significant advance in improving air quality in the operating room was the introduction of the routine use of well-designed scavengers. Scavenging systems consist of a gas capturing assembly, a disposal assembly, and an interface to allow positive and negative pressure relief. However, the scavenger itself may not work properly if neglected in the routine evaluation of the anesthesia machine (see Chapter 13). Most modern scavenging systems have multiple connections that may be sources for leaks. A reservoir bag made of rubber is often built into the system in order to protect the patient from the vacuum source. These reservoirs are often not replaced and are degraded by the very agents they are made to scavenge. Excess circuit gases must be disposed of properly, using a nonrecirculating air conditioning system, an independent vacuum system, an adsorber, or a passive through-wall system.

The anesthesia machine is only one source of operating room pollution. The use of volatile anesthetics during extracorporeal circulation has given rise to a new source of anesthetic gases. The extracorporeal circuit must be scavenged to prevent leakage of significant halogenated vapors into the operating room.[47-49] In orthopedic surgery, the plastic cements that are mixed in the operating room just before use are known to cause headaches and nausea among operating room personnel. These vapors are best handled by mixing the cement under a vacuum hood.

Detection of Leaks

The first step in detecting leaks is to establish that the operating room environment is polluted by anesthetic gases. Several methods have become accepted for monitoring exposure to anesthetic gases.[50-52]

In the average operating room, nitrous oxide leaking at about 3 L/minute results in a concentration of 160 ppm without scavenging.[50] An infrared analyzer for nitrous oxide can be used to detect the amount of operating room pollution by nitrous oxide.[51] An advantage to this technique is its ability to give real-time on-line data. This ability to report instantly the presence of leaks can also be used to pinpoint their sources. Samples obtained over a longer period of time give a better idea about the average concentration of the polluting agent.

Methods of Environmental Monitoring

Control concentrations of nitrous oxide should be measured at least every quarter year from the operating room after it has been out of use for 2 hours. Additional samples are also taken at various times during operating room use. Methods used for such sampling include continuous infrared (see Chapter 9),[51] time-weighted averaging, and "grab" samples.

Time-Weighted Average

The evacuated canister method of sampling is an example of time-weighted average sampling.[52] An evacuated canister fitted with a flow-controlled inlet valve continually samples the operating room air for later analysis. The canister is quite small and easily attached to a belt to sample air close to the carrier. The canister is "opened" in the laboratory where a mass spectrometer determines the average amounts and species of the operating room gases collected.

"Grab" Sampling

A leak-free inert container or syringe is used to obtain instantaneous samples of operating room air. When such samples are obtained intraoperatively, they evaluate the effectiveness of anesthetic techniques, equipment leakage, scavenger efficiency, and operating room ventilation. Grab samples can be analyzed by either infrared or chromatographic methods.

Acceptable Limits

The National Institute for Occupational Safety and Health proposes that acceptable environmental levels in operating rooms are time-weighted averages less than 25 ppm for nitrous oxide and 0.5 ppm for halogenated agents used with nitrous oxide.[53] When halogenated agents are used alone, the acceptable limit is 2 ppm.[53] When increased levels are detected, attention should be directed to modify anesthetic practice, check the anesthesia machine and gas hoses for leaks, and verify effective operation of the scavenging and ventilation systems.

References

1. McLafferty FW: Interpretation of Mass Spectrometry. Reading, MA: WA Benjamin, 1973.
2. Salamonsen RF, Tulloh AM, Boyd T: Adaptation of the quadrupole mass spectrometer to multipatient anaesthesia gas monitoring. Anaesth Intensive Care 1986; 14:163–173.
3. Comroe JH: The functions of the lung. *In* Harvey Lecture, vol 48. New York: Academic, 1952; 110–144.
4. Ozanne GM, Young WG, Mazzei WJ, Severinghaus JW: Multipatient anesthetic mass spectrometry: Rapid analysis of data stored in long catheters. Anesthesiology 1981; 55:62–70.
5. Severinghaus JW, Ozanne GM: Multi–operating room monitoring with one mass spectrometer. Acta Anaesthesiol Scand [Suppl] 1978; 70;186–187.
6. Krenis LJ, Berkowitz DA: Errors in installation of a new gas delivery system found after certification. Anesthesiology 1985; 62:677–678.
7. Feeley TW, McClelland KJ, Malhotra IV: The hazards of bulk oxygen delivery systems. Lancet 1975; 1:1416–1418.
8. Means LJ, Beckman DJ, Brown JW, King H: Detection of systemic to pulmonary

shunt by end-tidal carbon dioxide concentration. Anesth Analg 1987; 66:1055–1056.

9. Lichtiger M: Recent advances in clinical monitoring: Mass spectrometry. Curr Rev Clin Anesth 1985; 5:114–120.

10. Heller ML, Watson TR: The role of preliminary oxygenation prior to induction with high nitrous oxide mixtures. Anesthesiology 1962; 23:219–230.

11. Gold MI, Duarte I, Muravchick S: Arterial oxygenation in conscious patients after 5 minutes and after 30 seconds of oxygen breathing. Anesth Analg 1981; 60:313–315.

12. Lanier W: Intraoperative air entrainment with Ohio^R Modulus^{TM} anesthesia machine. Anesthesiology 1986; 64:266–268.

13. Matjasko J, Petrozza P, Mackenzie CF: Sensitivity of end-tidal nitrogen in venous air embolism detection in dogs. Anesthesiology 1985; 65:418–423.

14. Matjasko J, Gunzelman J, Delaney J, Mackenzie CF: Sources of nitrogen in the anesthesia circuit. Anesthesiology 1986; 65:229.

15. Ghanooni S, Wilks DH, Finestone SC: A case report of an unusual disconnection. Anesth Analg 1983; 62:696–697.

16. Munshi C, Dhamee S, Bardeen-Henschel A, Dhruva S: Recognition of mixed anesthetic agents by mass-spectrometer during anesthesia. J Clin Monit 1986; 2:121–134.

17. Roberts MJ, Boustred ML, Hinds CJ: A multipatient mass spectrometer based system for the measurement of metabolic gas exchange in artificially ventilated intensive care patients. Intensive Care Med 1983; 9:339–343.

18. Rikes JB, Haberman B: Expiratory gas monitoring by mass spectrometry in a respiratory intensive care unit. Crit Care Med 1976; 4:223–229.

19. Prakash O, Meij S: Use of mass spectrometry and infrared CO_2 analyzer for bedside measurement of cardiopulmonary function during anesthesia and intensive care. Crit Care Med 1977; 5:180–184.

20. Yakulis R, Snyder JV, Powner D, et al: Mass spectrometry monitoring of respiratory variables in an intensive care unit. Respir Care 1978; 23:671–679.

21. Sharp JH, Trudell JR, Cohen EN: Volatile metabolites and decomposition products of halothane in man. Anesthesiology 1979; 50:2–8.

22. Crocker D, Koka BV, Filler RM, et al: Tissue uptake and excretion of nitrous oxide in pediatric anesthesia. Anesth Analg 1974; 53:779–785.

23. Beatty PCW: Potential inaccuracies in mass spectrometry with spectrum overlap erasure units used during anaesthesia. Clin Phys Physio Meas 1984; 5:93–104.

24. Williams EL, Benson DM: Helium-induced errors in clinical mass spectrometry. Anesth Analg 1988; 67:83–85.

25. Davies NJH, Denison DM: The uses of long sampling probes in respiratory mass spectrometry. Respir Physiol 1979; 37:335–346.

26. Eger EI, Bahlman SH: Is the end-tidal anesthetic partial pressure an accurate measure of the arterial anesthetic partial pressure? Anesthesiology 1971; 35:301–303.

27. Westenskow DR, Smith KW, Coleman DL, et al: Clinical evaluation of a Raman scattering multiple gas analyzer. Anesthesiology 1989; 70:350–355.

28. Hayes JK, Westenskow DR, Jordan WS: Monitoring anesthetic vapor concentrations using a piezoelectric detector: Evaluation of the Engstrom EMMA. Anesthesiology 1983; 59:435–439.

29. Linstromberg JW, Muir JJ: Cross-sensitivity in water vapor in the Engstrom EMMA. Anesth Analg 1984; 63:75–78.

30. Bruce DL, Eide KA, Linde HW, Eckenhoff JE: Causes of death among anesthesiologists: A 20 year survey. Anesthesiology 1968; 29:565–569.

31. Cascorbi HF, Blake DA, Helrich M: Differences in the biotransformation of halothane in man. Anesthesiology 1970; 32:119–123.

32. Cohen EN, Brown BW, Bruce DL, et al: Occupational disease among operating room personnel: A national study. Anesthesiology 1974; 41:321–340.
33. Mazze RI, Fujinaga M, Rice SA, et al: Reproductive and teratogenic effects of nitrous oxide, halothane, isoflurane, and enflurane in Sprague-Dawley rats. Anesthesiology 1986; 64:339–344.
34. Cohen EN, Bellville JW, Brown BW: Anesthesia, pregnancy, and miscarriage. Anesthesiology 1971; 35:343–347.
35. Askrog V, Harvald B: Teratogen effect of inhalation anesthetics. Nord Med 1970; 83:498–500.
36. Bruce DL, Bach MJ, Arbit J: Trace anesthetic effects on perceptual cognitive and motor skills. Anesthesiology 1974; 40:453–458.
37. Bruce DL, Bach MJ: Psychological studies of human performance as affected by traces of enflurane and nitrous oxide. Anesthesiology 1975; 42:194–196.
38. Spence AA, Cohen EN, Brown BW, et al: Occupational hazards for operating room–based physicians. JAMA 1977; 238:955–959.
39. Burting JE, Hennekens CH, Mayrent SL, et al: Health experiences of operating room personnel. Anesthesiology 1985; 62:325–330.
40. Cohen EN, Brown BW, Bruce DL, et al: A survey of anesthetic health hazards among dentists. J Am Dent Assoc 1975; 90:2191–2196.
41. Brown BR, Sagalyn AM: Hepatic microsomal enzyme induction by inhalation anesthetics: Mechanism in the rat. Anesthesiology 1974; 40:152–161.
42. Linde HW, Berman ML: Nonspecific stimulation of dry-metabolizing enzyme by inhalation anesthetic drugs. Anesth Analg 1971; 50:656–667.
43. Ross WT, Cordell RR: Proliferation of smooth endoplasmic reticulum and induction of microsomal drug metabolizing enzymes after ether or halothane. Anesthesiology 1978; 48:325–331.
44. Whitcher CE, Cohen EN, Trudell JR: Chronic exposure to anesthetic gases in the operating room. Anesthesiology 1971; 35:348–353.
45. Ericson HA, Källén AJB: Hospitalization for miscarriage and delivery outcome among Swedish nurses working in operating rooms 1973–1978. Anesth Analg 1985; 64:981–988.
46. Lecky JH: The mechanical aspects of anesthetic pollution control. Anesth Analg 1977; 56:769–774.
47. Annis JP: Scavenging system for the Harvey blood oxygenator. Anesthesiology 1976; 45:359–360.
48. Miller JD: A device for the removal of waste anesthetic gases from the extracorporeal oxygenator. Anesthesiology 1976; 44:181–184.
49. Muravchick S: Scavenging enflurane from extracorporeal pump oxygenators. Anesthesiology 1977; 468–470.
50. Whitcher C, Piziali RL: Monitoring occupational exposure to inhalation anesthetics. Anesth Analg 1977; 56:778–785.
51. Isley AH, Crea J, Cousins MJ: Evaluation of infrared analysis used for monitoring waste anaesthetic gas levels in operating theatres. Anaesth Intensive Care 1980; 8:436–440.
52. Gray WM, Burnside GW: The evacuated canister method of personal sampling. Anaesthesia 1985; 40:288–294.
53. National Institute for Occupational Safety and Health: Criteria for a recommended standard . . . occupational exposure to waste anesthetic gases and vapors. DHEW (NIOSH) Publ No 77–140, 1977.

Miscellaneous Monitors

chapter fifteen

Stethoscopy, Thermometry, and Miscellaneous Monitors

■ CAROL L. LAKE, M.D.

STETHOSCOPY

Pathologic noises emanating from the body were noted in the seventeenth and eighteenth centuries. Initial efforts to hear these noises were by direct application of the physician's ear to the patient's chest or abdomen. Laënnec, faced with the inability to auscultate the heart of an obese patient, recalled the observation that a hollow tube amplified sounds. He placed one end of a rolled tube of paper against the patient's chest and the other in his ear, creating the first stethoscope.[1] Other landmarks in the development of stethoscopy are described in Chang's historical study[1] and the Introduction of this book.

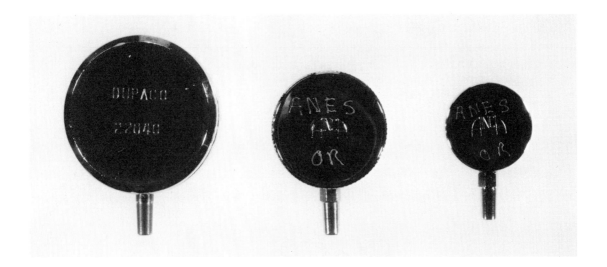

Indications

A precordial or esophageal stethoscope should be used in all anesthetic procedures, no matter how brief. Stethoscopy provides a nonelectric, uncomplicated method to qualitatively assess heart and lung function.

Types

Precordial

Weighted stethoscopes are available in three sizes, small, medium, and large, for application with double-sided tape disks to the precordium or sternal notch (Fig. 15–1). Various types of tubing, ranging from standard intravenous to small-bore rubber, connect the stethoscope to monaural or standard binaural earpieces. Information commonly obtained from precordial stethoscopes includes the presence and quality of heart and lung sounds. However, no data on the frequency response or effects of different types and lengths of tubing on the transmission of sounds exist.[2]

Esophageal

An esophageal stethoscope is an inexpensive, simple monitor of heart and lung sounds, introduced into anesthesia practice more than 3 decades ago (Fig. 15–2A).[3] It consists of a catheter fitted with openings in the distal 2–3 cm, which are covered by a rubber cuff. Esophageal stethoscopes do not require electricity or complicated technologic interpretation. Examples of clinical situations detectable with esophageal stethoscopy include dysrhythmias, ventilator disconnection or malfunction, wheezing, and quality

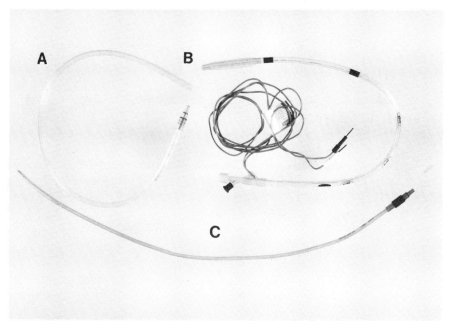

Figure 15–2. Esophageal stethoscopes of various types. *A* is an adult stethoscope. Stethoscope *B* is modified with two electrodes for monitoring the electrocardiogram. Stethoscope *C* has an integral thermistor for monitoring esophageal temperature.

of heart tones including murmurs.[4] More sophisticated versions of the esophageal stethoscope incorporate thermistors (Fig. 15–2C) and electrocardiogram (ECG) electrodes (Fig. 15–2B).[5] The advantages of monitoring the ECG from the esophagus are discussed in Chapter 2.[6] In addition to the risks of esophageal damage from passage of the probe, the possibility of esophageal burns from leakage currents is present when the stethoscope is connected to electrically powered ECG and temperature modules.[7]

Amplified

Small lightweight sterilizable microphones for attachment to precordial or esophageal stethoscopes amplify the heart and breath sounds through direct, hard-wired, or telemetric devices. Output can be monitored through headphones or an FM radio. They are battery-operated (Fig. 15–3).

Doppler

Doppler probes of 2.4 MHz transmit and reflect ultrasound from the heart in both fetuses and adults. The optimal location for cardiac monitoring is the third or fourth intercostal space to the right of the sternum. However, placement should be altered to the point at which sound transmission is best, particularly in response to rapid injection of fluid through a central venous catheter. Precordial Dopplers are not usually used for routine cardiac monitoring but rather are used for detection of venous air embolism. Unlike the

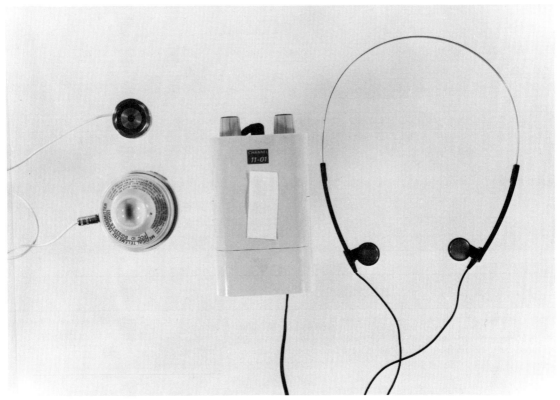

Figure 15–3. Amplified precordial stethoscope for telemetric monitoring of heart and breath sounds. Modifications allowing amplification and transmission of sounds from an esophageal stethoscope are also available.

normal swooshing cardiac sounds, air embolism causes a characteristic high-pitched scratching noise.[8] An unfortunate disadvantage of Doppler technology is interference by electrocautery.

Complications of Stethoscopy

Loss of an esophageal stethoscope into the stomach coincident to placement of a nasogastric tube and a second esophageal stethoscope has been reported.[9] Stethoscopes may fracture, with retention of fragments in the gastrointestinal tract. Misidentification of the esophagus containing a stethoscope for the trachea or for the internal jugular vein containing a ventriculojugular shunt catheter has been reported in children.[10] Misplacement of stethoscopes into the trachea instead of the esophagus causes significant gas leakage around the endotracheal tube cuff that may preclude adequate ventilation.[11] Loss of the cuff of the esophageal stethoscope can occur, especially with repeated use. Inadvertent fixation of the stethoscope during surgical repairs around the nasopharynx or esophagus can be avoided by using a precordial device or by verifying mobility of the stethoscope during surgical procedures in the area. Esophageal stethoscopes are flammable in both oxygen and nitrous oxide, if a source of ignition is nearby.[12] The oxidant O_2 index of flammability for the Portex esophageal stethoscope is 0.218, indicating flammability within the range of clinical use.[12]

THERMOMETRY

Physiology of Thermoregulation

Heat Gain

Body heat is primarily produced by metabolism in the liver and skeletal muscles. Basal heat production ranges from 65 to 85 kcal/hour. Heat is produced by voluntary muscle activity (exercise), involuntary muscle activity (shivering), and nonshivering thermogenesis (NST). During moderate work or exercise, heat production increases to 300 kcal/hour. With maximum work, heat production increases to 600 kcal/hour or more. Heat generated from muscular contraction is transferred to blood flowing through the muscle bed. The temperature of the body core as well as of blood exiting from the liver or lower extremities increases during exercise.

In infants, the major mechanism for heat production is NST, an oxygen-consuming, heat-producing mechanism stimulated by the sympathetic nervous system. NST results from byproducts of glucose metabolism, fatty acid metabolism, and gluconeogenesis. In infants, fatty acids are liberated from triglycerides owing to lipase release (stimulated by norepinephrine) in brown fat and are oxidized in muscle, white fat, brain, and liver or re-esterified or oxidized in brown fat. Brown fat, composing 2–6% of body weight, is located between the scapulae, around kidneys, adrenals, vertebrae, neck blood vessels, and mediastinum, and in the axillae. It causes the infant's neck and interscapular skin to be warmer than other body parts during exposure to cold. Microscopically, brown fat contains numerous mitochondria, densely packed with cristae and respiratory chain components.[13] NST is more energy-efficient than shivering thermogenesis, which is, nevertheless, fully developed in infants. It is unaffected by neuromuscular blockade[14] but is blocked by sympathectomy, ganglionic blockade, and beta-adrenergic blockade.

Heat Loss

Physiologic Mechanisms of Heat Loss

Convection, conduction, and radiation from the skin surface and lungs normally dissipate the heat produced by the body and protect it from thermal damage. The thermoregulatory center is located in the anterior and posterior hypothalamus; the anterior, temperature-sensitive area known as the Aronsohn-Sachs center; and the posterior, temperature-insensitive area known as the Krehl-Isenschmidt center.[15] Local blood temperature changes in the hypothalamus result as heated blood from muscle flows into the area. The

---

Table 15–1. PHYSIOLOGIC CONSEQUENCES
OF TEMPERATURE ALTERATIONS

Increased Temperature
Increased respiratory work
Increased cardiac work
Increased oxygen demand
Hypovolemia
Acidosis (respiratory and metabolic)

Decreased Temperature
Patient discomfort
Increased oxygen demand (shivering)
Decreased drug disposition
Decreased myocardial contractility and compliance
Cardiac dysrhythmias, conduction disturbances, and decreased rate
Peripheral vasoconstriction
Decreased cerebral blood flow and CMR_{O_2}
Central nervous system depression, delirium, and coma
Decreased oxygen availability (oxyhemoglobin dissociation curve shifted to left)
Sympathetic stimulation
Hyperglycemia
Thrombocytopenia

---

posterior hypothalamus receives sensory input of temperature changes, and the anterior hypothalamus adjusts the mechanisms controlling heat loss and production. The hypothalamic temperature change induces systemic changes (dilatation of skin vessels and secretion of sweat) to offset the alteration in central temperature, the Benzinger reflex.[16] Cold impulses arriving in the posterior hypothalamus initiate heat production by shivering. However, in the presence of normal or increased body temperature, the anterior hypothalamus overrides the posterior center, preventing heat production. Because hypothalamic temperature is integral to thermal equilibrium, this temperature should probably be regarded as the "core temperature."

Alterations in the core temperature away from its set point initiate changes in heat production or heat loss. In order to maintain a balance between heat production and heat loss, the autonomic nervous system varies the blood supply to the body surface, causing shivering or sweating.[17] If the environmental temperature is cool, a thermal gradient between the body surface and the environment allows rapid dissipation. If environmental temperature is increased to body surface temperature or greater, heat is lost only by vaporization of sweat. Maximum rates of sweat vaporization are limited by atmospheric humidity, air movement, and rate of sweating. At conditions of increased humidity, heat loss through sweat vaporization is limited, and body temperature increases. Practically, the amount of heat loss through sweating is about 650 kcal/hour.[18]

In addition to sweating, cardiovascular changes occur when humans are exposed to hot environments (Table 15–1). These changes include increased cardiac output, tachycardia, decreased hepatic and splanchnic blood flow, decreased systemic vascular resistance, and reduced effective arterial volume. In adequately conditioned and heat-acclimatized humans, maximum cardiac output increases, peak heart rate decreases, stroke volume increases, and sweat composition and volume change to limit volume and sodium loss. However, these compensatory mechanisms are overwhelmed by prolonged exposure to high environmental temperatures. Sweating ceases, cardiac output and stroke volume decrease, and cutaneous blood flow is reduced while core temperature increases. The end result is heat stroke, which is characterized by rectal temperature greater than 41.1°C, delirium, and coma.[18] Even physically conditioned and heat-acclimatized individuals may suffer heat stroke during extreme exertion.

Nonphysiologic Mechanisms of Heat Loss

Infants have considerable difficulty maintaining their core temperature in the face of changing ambient temperatures. They have a small body mass acting as a heat generator but a large surface area for heat loss (ratio of surface to mass = 3:1). Heat loss is increased in infants because of their lack of subcutaneous tissue, large surface-to-volume ratio, and decreased motor tone.

Thermoregulation increases oxygen consumption in infants in proportion to the ambient–to–skin surface temperature gradient.[19] Minimum ambient temperature for thermoregulation is 22°C in an infant compared with 0°C in an adult. Thus, their thermoregulatory range is significantly limited compared with that of the adult. Minimum oxygen consumption in infants occurs at environmental temperatures of 32–34°C, the neutral thermal state, in which there is less than a 2-degree gradient between environmental and abdominal skin temperatures.[20] Since operating room personnel have been shown to be most comfortable with relative humidities under 50%, temperatures of 18°C, and air changes 25 times per hour or more,[21] the usual recommendations are to maintain operating room temperature at 27°C for premature infants, 26°C for infants to 6 months of age, and 25°C for infants from 6 to 24 months of age.[22]

In humans, heat loss occurs in two phases: transfer of heat from body core to skin surface (internal temperature gradient), and heat dissipation (external temperature gradient). Heat loss is determined by the skin and environmental temperatures, the thermal transfer coefficient, and surface area. Tissue thickness, body size, and blood flow determine thermal transfer coefficients. Heat transfer from the core to the surface of the body creates an internal temperature gradient. Vasoconstriction decreases cutaneous blood flow and increases tissue insulation, attempting to increase the internal temperature gradient and reduce conductive and convective heat loss.

Heat loss across the external temperature gradient is affected by evaporation, convection, conduction, and radiation. Evaporative heat losses through the skin and respiratory systems depend upon minute ventilation, air flow velocity, and relative humidity (specifically the difference between vapor pressures in the environment and on the skin surface). The transfer of heat to the air currents (convection) is influenced by air velocity, specific heat of the flowing gas, surface area, and ambient temperature. Because of high air turnover rates in operating rooms, convection causes about 25% of body heat loss.[22,23] Trapping a layer of air between the skin and the environment reduces heat loss by convection.

Heat loss by conduction depends upon a temperature gradient between contacting surfaces and is affected by surface area and the thermal conductivity of the surface. Wetting increases conduction by 25–30-fold.[22] The transfer of heat between two objects in the form of electromagnetic energy is radiant heat loss. It is independent of environmental temperature but is dependent upon the radiating surface area and proportional to the temperature difference between skin and surrounding environment.[14,23] Radiation is the largest source of heat loss (65%) for the human body.[22]

Anesthesia. Although heat loss often occurs during anesthesia and anesthetic drugs may interfere with central and peripheral thermoregulation,[24] studies of the effects of anesthesia on heat loss disagree. Recent evidence suggests that thermoregulation is maintained during nitrous oxide–fentanyl and halothane anesthesia, although it does not occur until core temperature is about 2.5°C lower than normal.[25,26]

Core temperature usually decreases during the early minutes of anesthesia because of uncovering of the patient, wet and cold preparation solutions, and losses to the anesthetic administration system. Alterations in temperature at various measuring sites are shown in Figure 15–4. Holdcroft and Hall demonstrated no differences in heat loss in patients anesthetized with halothane, nitrous oxide and fentanyl, or nitrous oxide.[27] Engleman and Lockhart described greater temperature decreases during halothane than during ketamine anesthesia.[28] Patients receiving epidural anesthesia have greater initial heat loss than patients undergoing general anesthesia because of vasodilatation, decreased metabolic heat production, and abolition of shivering below the blocked spinal segments.[29] Peripheral thermal receptors, particularly the warm-sensitive receptors, are blocked by regional anesthesia.[23] Patients receiving regional anesthesia rewarm less readily in the postoperative period because of continued vasodilatation and muscle flaccidity.[30]

Other patients at increased risk for intraoperative hypothermia include the elderly[30] and those with major burns, paraplegia, quadriplegia, cachexia, and trauma. During anesthesia, temperature decreases about 1.1°C/hour at age 80 years versus only 0.3°C/hour at age 20.[31] Burned patients are unable to limit passage of water vapor through the skin, and their peripheral thermoregulatory mechanisms are impaired. Cachectic patients may have lost both muscle mass, responsible for heat production, and insulating fat. Paraplegia and quadriplegia disrupt the thermosensory pathways as well as the motor pathways responsible for shivering, thus impairing both autonomic and behavioral thermoregulation. Exposure of large surfaces of the abdominal or thoracic cavity increases intraoperative heat loss (Table 15–2).[32–34]

Indications for Temperature Measurement

The measurement of body temperature by some route is a standard of care during all anesthetic procedures, no matter how brief. The risk of both malignant hyperthermia and accidental hypothermia necessitates continuous

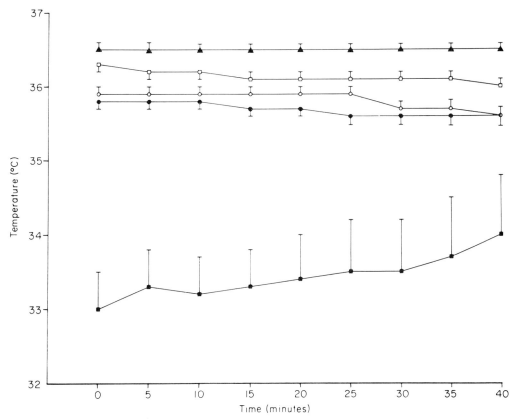

Figure 15–4. During the prebypass period, skin temperature (*solid squares*) is lower than internal body temperature as measured in the esophagus (*solid circles*), nasopharynx (*open circles*), rectum (*open squares*), and bladder (*solid triangles*). (From Bone ME, Feneck RO: Bladder temperature as an estimate of body temperature during cardiopulmonary bypass. Anaesthesia 1988; 43:181–185. With permission.)

observation of temperature. However, one specific indication for temperature monitoring is induced hypothermia, by either surface or perfusion (extracorporeal circulation) cooling and rewarming.

Methods

Body temperature was first measured by Hunter in 1776, using a mercury-in-glass thermometer under the tongue. Glass thermometers are still used in many clinical settings but are usually impractical in perioperative semiconscious patients.

Thermistors, Thermocouples

A thermistor or thermally sensitive resistor includes semiconductive elements (heavy-metal oxides such as manganese, iron, zinc, cobalt, nickel) in which electrical resistance varies with temperature. Electrodes are attached to a bead of the metal oxide, which is sealed into a small measuring

Table 15–2. CAUSES OF INTRAOPERATIVE
TEMPERATURE ALTERATIONS

Increased Temperature
Malignant hyperthermia, thyrotoxicosis, pheochromocy-
toma
Infections
Chemical reactions (hardening of plaster casts, methyl
methacrylate cement)
Excessive environmental warming (heating lamps, heated
humidifiers, blankets, heavy surgical drapes)

Decreased Temperature
Exposure to cold operating room environment
Intravenous, intraperitoneal, intrathoracic administration
of cold fluids
Skin preparation with cold solutions
Vasodilation secondary to spinal, epidural, or other re-
gional anesthesia
Hypothyroidism (myxedema)
Inability to compensate for heat loss in trauma or burn
patients
Deliberate hypothermia (surface or extracorporeal cool-
ing)

tip. Large changes in resistance correspond to changes in temperature, allowing a rapid response time. Thermistors are usually accurate to ± 5 degrees over a range from -80 to $+150°C$, although typically narrower ranges
improve linearity.[35]

In a thermocouple, voltage is produced by the electromotive force between two dissimilar metals (usually copper and constantan, a mixture of
copper and nickel), which depends upon the temperature difference between
two junctions maintained at different temperatures, a standard "cold" junction and the probe end of the thermocouple. One of the junctions is maintained as the "reference" junction, and the other becomes the "measuring"
junction, located within the probe. The current generated is proportional to
the temperature difference between the two junctions.[35] Thermocouples
have several advantages, including small size and reproducibility. Two problems with thermocouples involving the reference junction are the Seebeck
effect of electromotive force in the thermocouple and the Peltier effect,
which occurs when a current passed around the thermocouple circuit creates
cold at one junction and heat at the other.

Liquid-Crystal Devices

Stick-on liquid-crystal temperature detectors monitor skin temperatures
over ranges of 92–104°F and 34–40°C (Fig. 15–5A, B). Skin temperature on
the forehead is usually close to oral temperature, but it demonstrates considerable individual variation. Although temperatures measured with liquid-
crystal thermometry correlate well with forehead skin temperature, their
correlation with temperatures monitored at other sites is poor (r = 0.54
when compared with esophageal or tympanic probes).[36] Vaughan and col-

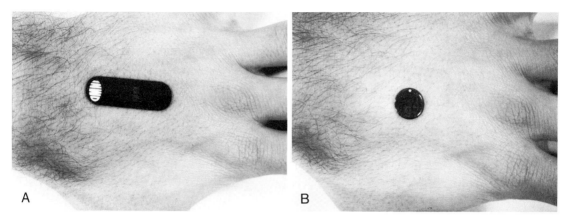

Figure 15–5. *A*, *B*, Two types of liquid-crystal thermometers measuring skin temperature on the hand. For perioperative monitoring, these devices are usually placed on the patient's forehead.

leagues reported that compared with tympanic membrane thermometry, liquid-crystal strips failed to accurately track temperature trends in postanesthetic patients.[37] Their data suggest that temperature in the body shell is an unreliable indicator of core temperature.[37]

Despite their inaccuracy, the convenience of liquid-crystal thermometers makes them useful for continuous temperature monitoring in operating rooms and postanesthesia recovery units and during sympathetic blockade during peripheral nerve blocks. For perioperative use, the sensors are applied to the forehead, whereas during sympathetic blocks, they are applied to the involved extremity. Advantages include safety (completely noninvasive) and low cost. Disadvantages include difficulties with adhesion secondary to skin secretions, susceptibility to external thermal influences such as radiant heat lamps or air currents, patient allergic reactions to adhesive backing, and inaccuracy and imprecision.[36–38]

Infrared Thermometry

A new method of clinical thermometry is an infrared tympanic probe that determines temperature by measuring the infrared radiation given off by an object. It consists of an otoscopelike probe covered by a disposable speculum, which is introduced into the external auditory canal like an otoscope. The sensor in the probe gathers emitted infrared radiation for about 1 second and then transfers that information to an analog-to-digital converter and microprocessor. A liquid crystal displays the resultant temperature on a base module. Accuracy of this technology has been documented with *in vitro* water baths as well as *in vivo*. Clinical trials demonstrate a correlation coefficient of the infrared tympanic probe with pulmonary artery thermistor of 0.98.[39] Advantages of this technology include the speed of determination, reduced potential for cross-contamination, and the absence of need for direct contact and temperature equilibrium of the device with the measuring surface.

Sites

Sites used for measurement of body temperature include the nasopharynx, skin, esophagus, rectum, and tympanic membrane. The choice of sites depends upon the purpose of the measurements. Usually, it is either specific organ temperature or core (total body) temperature that is needed. Temperatures measured in the tympanic membrane or nasopharynx estimate brain temperature. Esophageal temperature approximates myocardial temperature. Cork and coworkers report the greatest precision (correlation between tympanic membrane and other site temperatures) and accuracy (defined by difference from the tympanic membrane temperature) of temperature measurements in the urinary bladder, nasopharynx, and esophagus.[40] Axilla, great toe, and forehead temperatures are less accurate than those measured at other sites.[40]

Tympanic Membrane

The efficacy and convenience of tympanic thermometry were documented in the 1960s. Measurement of tympanic membrane temperature as an index of brain temperature is particularly prudent, since thermal homeostasis depends upon anterior hypothalamic temperature.[41] At the tympanic membrane, the thermoelectric sensor is in the vicinity of the internal carotid artery, the major cerebral blood supply.[42] The tympanic membrane and surrounding structures are supplied by branches of the external carotid artery, including the internal maxillary and posterior auricular arteries. Tympanic temperatures parallel temperatures measured from an ideally placed esophageal thermistor, except that tympanic temperatures are lower by about 0.2 degree.[42] The tympanic membrane temperature is probably the optimum site during profound hypothermia and circulatory arrest.[43]

An otoscopic examination to document patency of the tympanic membrane should precede tympanic or external auditory canal thermometry. The presence of cerumen may render measurements inaccurate.

Nasopharyngeal

Nasopharyngeal temperatures provide an estimate of brain temperature, particularly when the measuring device is carefully positioned behind the soft palate. Wedging of a thermistor in the roof of the nose provides satisfactory approximation of core temperature, the wedged nasal temperature. However, air leakage around an endotracheal tube cuff affects nasopharyngeal probe accuracy.[44] Another disadvantage is the possibility of epistaxis or adenoidal bleeding in children.

Esophageal

Esophageal temperatures are affected by ventilation (particularly when placed at the middle or upper esophagus),[44] thoracotomy, or rapid infusion of cold fluids and blood, which cools the heart and great vessels. Variations of as much as 1–6°C have been reported, depending upon the location of the tip of the probe within the esophagus,[42, 44, 45] varying with intubation, extubation, and intrathoracic manipulation. Kaufman noted that the coolest portion of the esophagus was the point at which both heart and breath sounds were best heard, and the warmest point was 12–16 cm past the position of best sounds.[45] As opposed to that measured in the lower esophagus, temperature at the tracheal bifurcation is about 1°C lower and in the region of the atrium about 0.5°C lower.[46] The ideal location for the thermistor is about 45 cm from the nostril, so that its tip is between the heart and the descending thoracic aorta and below the pulmonary veins.[47] However, this suggestion assumes that the distance between the teeth and the heart is similar in all individuals. Accurate positioning of the probe in relation to the heart is achieved by auscultation through esophageal stethoscopes combined with temperature thermistors (see Fig. 15–2C). In the lower esophagus, Whitby and Dunkin noted that temperatures approximated cerebral temperatures in the absence of rapid infusions of cold fluids or an open thorax.[44]

Contraindications to esophageal temperature measurements are bronchoscopy, esophagoscopy, laryngoscopy, certain facial or oral surgical procedures, and esophageal pathology (varices) or Zenker's diverticulum. However, Ritter and coworkers inserted esophageal stethoscopes in patients with varices undergoing hepatic transplantation without any incidents of bleeding.[48] Normal esophageal temperatures are from 36.9 to 37.7°C.[35]

Bladder

Urinary catheters with thermistor tips have been available for more than a decade, providing a safe, continuous, and convenient method for temperature measurement.[49] Both urine volume and bladder temperature are simultaneously measured. Bladder temperature is usually 0.2°C higher than rectal temperature, 0.7°C higher than esophageal temperature, and 3.5°C higher than skin temperature (thumb).[50] During extracorporeal cooling and rewarming, temperature in the urinary bladder changes more rapidly than does rectal temperature.[51] Lilly and associates noted excellent correlation between urinary bladder and esophageal, rectal, and pulmonary artery temperatures, with the strongest correlation with pulmonary artery temperatures during extracorporeal rewarming.[49] Nevertheless, the advantages of bladder temperature monitoring may be outweighed by the risks of bladder catheterization, if a urinary catheter is not otherwise indicated.

Rectum

The rectum is distant from the central nervous system and the heart and, therefore, has little thermal significance. Several sources of inaccuracy of rectal temperatures are the presence of heat-producing bacteria in the rectum, insulation by feces, or cold blood returning from the legs.[52] Temperatures measured in the rectum often differ substantially from those measured in other areas. For this reason, rectal temperatures should be considered erroneous if they differ from other points. However, rectal tem-

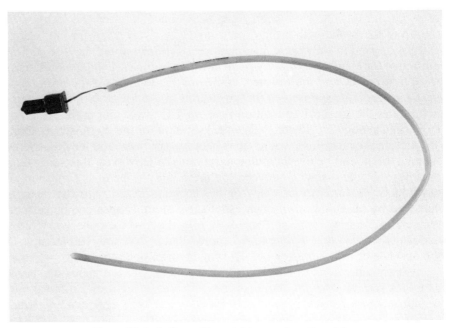

Figure 15–6. A disposable rectal temperature thermistor.

peratures may be useful indicators of the temperature of poorly perfused tissues (Fig. 15–6).[35] Rectal thermometry is often contraindicated during surgical procedures in the lower pelvis. The risk of rectal perforation should always be considered during placement of probes, particularly in infants and children. Normal rectal temperatures are 36.9–37.7°C.[35]

Other Sites

During cardiopulmonary bypass, temperatures of the venous blood returning to the extracorporeal circuit and arterial blood leaving the circuit are routinely measured. Muscle temperatures can be measured with a 25-gauge needle thermistor. Because a special probe is required, muscle temperatures are infrequently measured. However, muscle temperatures are quite responsive to blood flow. During extracorporeal cooling and rewarming, muscle remains warmer during hypothermia and cooler after rewarming.

Temperature can be measured in the pulmonary artery through the thermistor used for thermodilution cardiac output determinations. However, temperatures from this site are affected by ventilation, use of topical iced saline in the pericardium, and cold cardioplegia solutions. In the absence of topical hypothermia and cardioplegia, pulmonary artery temperatures are indicative of core temperatures. After discontinuation of cardiopulmonary bypass, pulmonary artery temperatures tend to be the lowest compared with nasopharyngeal, rectal, and other sites.[53]

During and after cardiac surgery, temperature in the great toe has been advocated as an indicator of peripheral perfusion, because its temperature depends on cutaneous blood flow. It also correlates well with cardiac output.[54] However, this temperature is not indicative of skin temperature.[55]

The axilla has been used as a site to monitor skin temperature. However, measurement is affected by pressure on the probe and sweat production and usually ranges from 35.3 to 36.7°C.[35]

Complications of Thermometry

Tympanic membrane temperature probes have a reported complication rate of less than 3%, with the primary complication being bleeding from the external auditory canal.[56] Other complications from the tympanic site include tympanic membrane perforation.[57] As described earlier, burns are possible with electrically operated equipment if leakage currents are present.[7]

Alterations in Temperature in the Perioperative Period

Induced Hypothermia

Hypothermia has been used in both neurosurgery and cardiac surgery to decrease the metabolic rate and allow complex intracranial and intracardiac repairs. However, it is infrequently used in neuroanesthesia at present, because of the prolonged time required for surface cooling and rewarming or the requisite anticoagulation if extracorporeal techniques are used. In cardiac surgery, some degree of hypothermia is used in most centers during cardiopulmonary bypass in both adult and pediatric patients. Profound hypothermia to esophageal temperatures of 10–12°C is used in children with congenital lesions or occasionally in adults with lesions of the aortic arch. Hypothermia with circulatory arrest provides ideal surgical conditions, decreases the duration of cardiopulmonary bypass, and prevents myocardial rewarming from washout of cardioplegia solutions by noncoronary collateral circulation.

Pathophysiologic responses to cold include intense stimulation of thermoregulatory mechanisms such as sympathetic stimulation and shivering. Responses in specific organ systems are discussed later, as they are similar in both induced and inadvertent hypothermia.

Anesthesia blunts both the sympathetic and the shivering responses to hypothermia.[58] During surgery, hypothermia is induced by either surface or core cooling. Core cooling with an extracorporeal circuit causes significant differences in the temperature measured at various sites (Fig. 15–7). The rate of decrease in temperature is greatest in the esophagus and least in the rectum.[50] During perfusion cooling, bladder temperature was similar to rectal temperature but differed significantly from nasopharyngeal, esophageal, and skin temperatures.[50] During hypothermia, renal oxygen consumption decreases more rapidly than does oxygen consumption in other organs, decreasing renal blood flow. Bladder temperatures represent an area intermediate between high and low blood flow. Rectal temperature changes

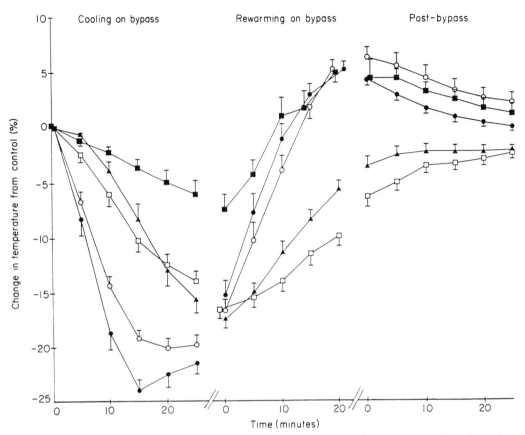

Figure 15–7. Changes in temperature as a percentage of control temperature during extracorporeal cooling and rewarming. Cooling and rewarming occurred most rapidly in the esophagus (*solid circles*). Rewarming also occurred more rapidly in the nasopharynx (*open circles*) than it did in the bladder (*solid triangles*), the rectum (*open squares*), or the skin (*solid squares*). Bladder temperature decreased more slowly during cooling and increased more slowly during rewarming than did esophageal temperature. Bladder temperatures remained below nasopharyngeal, esophageal, and skin temperatures after bypass. (From Bone ME, Feneck RO: Bladder temperature as an estimate of body temperature during cardiopulmonary bypass. Anaesthesia 1988; 43:181–185. With permission.)

slowly with cooling and rewarming, because the rectum is an area of reduced blood flow.[50]

During perfusion rewarming, esophageal and nasopharyngeal temperatures demonstrated the greatest rate of rise, with increases in bladder and rectal temperatures occurring more slowly (Fig. 15–7).[50] Lilly and associates noted that urinary bladder temperature consistently increased faster than rectal temperature and correlated well with pulmonary artery temperature during extracorporeal rewarming.[49] Changes in esophageal and nasopharyngeal temperatures reflect blood flow from the extracorporeal circuit to the vital organs. Temperatures measured from these sites tend to overshoot the control values during rewarming.[50]

After perfusion hypothermia and rewarming, core temperature often decreases following cessation of extracorporeal circulation. Ramsay and co-workers noted that the urinary bladder temperature at termination of bypass most closely indicated the amount of afterdrop (the difference between the nasopharyngeal temperature at the termination of bypass and the lowest nasopharyngeal temperature reached after bypass).[53] Afterdrop was minimized by a bladder temperature greater than 36.2°C. The subsequent period of rewarming occurring 2–4 hours after admission to the intensive care unit is accompanied by marked increases in oxygen consumption, carbon dioxide production, and shivering.[58, 59] Patients who do not exhibit shivering have lower oxygen consumption during this period.[58]

Accidental Hypothermia

Hypothermia is defined as a reduction of core temperature to less than 35–36°C. In hospital settings, hypothermia commonly occurs in neonates exposed to cold environmental conditions such as operating rooms or in adults transfused with unwarmed blood and fluids.[32, 60] About 60% of adult patients have hypothermia on arrival in postanesthetic care units.[30] Other causes include alcoholism and homelessness. Hypothermia also occurs in aged humans in cold climates and patients with hypothyroidism, adrenal insufficiency, diabetes, uremia, epilepsy, cirrhosis, and spinal cord lesions. Elderly patients are more prone to hypothermia in the perioperative period than are younger individuals.[30]

The human body loses heat by radiation, conduction, convection, evaporation, and through the respiratory tract. Decreases in environmental temperature are first sensed by cutaneous cold-sensitive thermoreceptors. Warm-sensitive receptors in the anterior hypothalamus are stimulated by temperatures greater than 44°C, whereas cold-sensitive receptors are inactive until the environmental temperature falls below 24°C.[23]

Neonates are particularly prone to hypothermia because of their large ratio of body surface area to heat-producing mass, decreased capacity to increase metabolic rate, limited energy stores, lack of insulating fat, and decreased shivering response. Elderly persons are likely to become hypothermic because of immobility, impaired sensation, decreased shivering response, loss of muscle mass, reduced vasoconstrictor response to cold, and inability to maintain a steep core–to–surface temperature gradient.

Effects of Hypothermia on Organ Systems

Total body metabolism decreases about 7–8% per degree Celsius as temperature decreases. Thus, metabolic rate is about 50% of normal at 28°C. Despite the decrease in metabolic rate, aerobic metabolism continues at low temperatures, provided adequate oxygen is delivered (see Table 15–1).

Heart and Circulation. In response to sympathetic activation during cooling, heart rate, stroke volume, and peripheral vascular tone increase and shivering occurs. Shivering, the involuntary rhythmic contraction of muscle, is mediated through hypothalamic pathways. It ceases at temperatures below 27°C. During shivering, oxygen consumption and calorigenesis are increased,[58] but convective and radiant heat losses are also increased by the increased muscular activity.[32] Ralley and coworkers noted significant reductions in mixed venous oxygen tension, even when cardiac output increased in shivering patients after cardiac surgery.[58] This finding indicates an imbalance between whole body oxygen supply and demand, mandating that shivering patients always receive supplemental oxygen.

Sinus bradycardia develops as temperature decreases below 33°C because of the effects of temperature on the spontaneity of the sinus node. Myocardial conduction abnormalities increase as the temperature decreases below 30 degrees (increased P-R interval, atrioventricular block, widening of the QRS complex). As temperature decreases below 30°C, elevation of the J point or a secondary wave following the S wave appears.[61] This wave is the J or Osborne wave. Both atrial and ventricular dysrhythmias increase and ventricular fibrillation often occurs around 28°C. The heart becomes more sensitive to electrolyte alterations such as hyperkalemia. With profound hypothermia, asystole ensues. Resuscitation from cardiac arrest due to hypothermia is difficult.

Compliance and myocardial contractility decrease below 28°C, although contractility initially increases as temperature decreases. Oxygen consumption per beat remains the same or actually increases, so that the decrease in myocardial oxygen consumption results from decreased rate.[62] Myocardial adenosine triphosphate stores and myocardial pH are maintained during induced hypothermia. However, autoregulation in the coronary vasculature is impaired by hypothermia, so that coronary perfusion is more dependent upon diastolic pressure.[62, 63]

As hypothermia develops, fluid shifts from the vascular space, increasing the hematocrit. Despite the shift of blood to the central compartment, cardiac output decreases beginning at 32°C. By 30°C, cardiac output is reduced by 30–40%.[23] Hypovolemia and increased blood viscosity may further reduce cardiac output. Systemic vascular resistance increases with hyperviscosity. Microcirculatory flow is reduced.

Central Nervous System. The effects of hypothermia on the central nervous system include depression of membrane conduction and neurochemical processes. As hypothermia progresses, alterations in electroencephalogram (EEG) occur. The EEG remains normal to a temperature of 35°C. Between 30 and 35°C, the predominant rhythm slows. At a temperature of 32°C, responses to stimuli are slowed, ataxia is present, and there is slight clumsiness. The amplitude of the EEG decreases below 32°C. Below 32°C, delirium followed by stupor and coma occurs. Pupillary dilatation is seen below 30°C. Slower EEG rhythms predominate between 24 and 29 degrees. Periods of isoelectricity of ever-lengthening duration develop below temperatures of 22°C.[64] Anesthetic requirements decrease so that minimum alveolar concentration decreases about 7% per degree Celsius.[65]

However, aerobic brain metabolism continues at low temperatures, although the cerebral metabolic rate for oxygen ($CMRo_2$) slows concomitantly with temperature reduction. Cerebral blood flow also decreases with hypothermia (about 7% per degree Celsius),[32] owing to decreased cardiac output, increased cerebrovascular resistance, and greater viscosity. At electrocerebral silence, there is no further reduction in $CMRo_2$. The preservative effects of hypothermia on the brain are greater than those predicted by decreased $CMRo_2$ alone.[66] The "no reflow" phenomenon after ischemia is prevented by hypothermia.

Respiratory Effects. Respiratory rate initially increases as hypothermia ensues. Between 30 and 34°C, the respiratory response to carbon dioxide decreases (CO_2 response curve shifts to right). Because carbon dioxide production decreases with hypothermia, respiratory alkalosis is often present. Dead space may increase owing to bronchodilatation as temperature decreases, if spontaneous respiration continues.

Hypoxic pulmonary vasoconstriction is reduced during hypothermia.[67] Ventilatory response to hypoxia may also be reduced, although it has been incompletely studied.[68] However, respiratory drive does not cease until 24°C.[32] Resistance in the pulmonary circulation increases with hypothermia. There is little change in lung compliance. Hypothermic patients should be fully rewarmed prior to extubation, because of these effects on the respiratory system.

The oxyhemoglobin dissociation curve shifts to the left, diminishing release of oxygen at the tissue level. The affinity of oxygen for hemoglobin increases about 6% per degree Celsius. The question of assessment of acid-base disturbances during hypothermia is controversial. Both correction and noncorrection of blood gases in hypothermic states are practiced (see Chapter 17). The consensus is that blood gases should not be corrected for body temperature. Instead, the samples should be analyzed at 37°C and interpreted as though they came from a normothermic patient.

Hepatic and Renal Effects. Renal blood flow and oxygen consumption are reduced by hypothermia. Glomerular filtration rate decreases progressively during cooling. Because both renal blood flow and glomerular filtration rate decrease, filtration fraction is unchanged. Because tubular function requires active enzymatic processes, tubular function decreases, reducing the concentrating effects of the renal tubules. Antidiuretic hormone release is suppressed because cold-induced vasoconstriction is interpreted by the kidney as volume overload, resulting in diuresis of urine produced by glomerular filtration. Hemoconcentration also results from capillary sequestration of fluid.

Hepatic enzymatic and excretory processes are reduced with hypothermia. Blood flow to the liver is reduced, but blood shifts from the periphery to the splanchnic circulation. Drug metabolism is reduced. The liver is also a site for sequestration of platelets during hypothermia. Coagulopathy during hypothermia results from thrombocytopenia, decreased activity of clotting cascade, and a slight decrease in platelet function.

Endocrine Effects. Because peripheral utilization of glucose and release of insulin decrease during hypothermia, blood glucose increases.[69] Parenteral insulin has little effect, but the hyperglycemia reverts to normal or nearly normal with rewarming. The stress response described previously causes release of adrenal cortical and medullary hormones (epinephrine and norepinephrine).[70, 71] In response to cold, the hypothalamus releases thyrotropin-releasing hormone, stimulating secretion of thyroxine and triiodothyronine to increase metabolic rate.

Profound hypothermia is compatible with life for brief periods of time because of the decreased metabolic rate and oxygen demand. However, prolonged hypothermia is not tolerated and usually causes death, because of cardiac electrical conduction disturbances. Rewarming in therapeutic applications of hypothermia is usually with extracorporeal circulation, at a gradient of no more than 10°C. In accidental hypothermia, surface methods are usually employed, coupled with supportive treatment of associated cardiac, respiratory, and coagulation problems.

Methods to Prevent or Minimize Perioperative Hypothermia

Postoperative hypothermia delays drug clearance, enhances peripheral vasoconstriction, and causes shivering. Shivering may occur because the patient is actually cold or because there is a discrepancy between the actual core temperature (normal) and the thermostat set point (elevated) that activates heat generation.[72] For these reasons, prevention and treatment are mandatory. Modalities to treat the mild-to-moderate hypothermia seen in the perioperative period include covering the patient, increasing the environmental temperature, using warmed respiratory gases and intravenous fluids, and using pharmacologic agents such as meperidine hydrochloride, chlorpromazine, droperidol, and nondepolarizing neuromuscular blockers to reduce shivering. Perioperative hypothermia is allayed by applying thermal blankets to the patient, wrapping the patient's limbs with polyester plastic film (Mylar), aluminum foil, or thermally occlusive materials, and placing the patient under radiant heating lamps.

Environmental Warming. Warmer operating rooms (greater than 21°C) minimize decreases in temperature in adults as compared with unwarmed rooms.[73-75] The "critical ambient temperature" appears to be 21°C or 70°F for stability of patient temperature between 36 and 37.5°C.[4,75] Room temperatures of 24–26°C are necessary in order to prevent any heat loss.[22] However, for a naked adult patient to maintain temperature without significant energy use requires ambient temperatures of 27–33°C.[22] The room temperatures must also be modified for patients having large surface area–to–body mass ratios, receiving large volumes of unwarmed intravenous fluids, or undergoing body cavity surgery and for those in a deeply anesthetized state.[74] However, Roizen and colleagues noted no difference in temperature in the postanesthetic period between patients undergoing surgical preparation and draping in a cold room and those in a warm operating room.[76] Temperatures at the beginning of surgery were lower in patients in the cold room.[76]

Since radiation and convection account for as much as 80% of heat loss perioperatively, covering the patient as much as possible is beneficial. Covering the scalp prevents the 50% radiation of heat from the head.[77] If 60% of the patient's body surface area is covered with reflective materials, body heat is conserved.[78] However, Radford and Thurlow were unable to prevent intraoperative hypothermia with reflective blankets.[79]

Murphy and coworkers demonstrated that radiant heat lamps stopped postanesthetic shivering (in animals) even without rewarming the core temperature.[80] Sharkey and colleagues showed that radiant heat lamps, but not warm blankets, terminated postanesthetic shivering within 10 minutes of application.[81] Other methods of radiant heat include frequently changed warm blankets or an active-warming blanket. Operations in infants can be performed in specially modified radiant warmers to minimize heat loss.

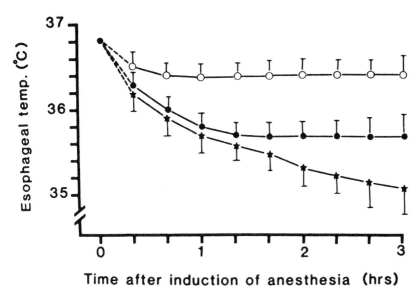

Figure 15–8. Combination of warming mattress and heated humidifier during abdominal aortic surgery (*open circles*) maintains esophageal temperature better than does humidifier alone (*closed circles*) or no active warming (*stars*). (From Tølløfsrud SG, Gundersen Y, Andersen R: Peroperative hypothermia. Acta Anaesthesiol Scand 1984; 28:511–515. © 1984 Munksgaard International Publishers Ltd., Copenhagen, Denmark. With permission.)

Thermal Mattresses. Thermal mattresses, which circulate thermostatically controlled water, minimize heat loss by increasing the conduction of heat from the environment to the patient. A layer of cotton sheet is placed over the mattress to prevent direct pressure of the fluid cells on poorly perfused skin. The level of the reservoir fluid should be noted before activating the unit. During operation, the temperature of the circulating fluid must be noted in order to prevent excessive temperatures and patient burns.

Although thermal mattresses are efficacious in infants,[82] they fail to maintain body temperature in adults.[73, 75, 83] This finding probably results from the lack of a highly perfused surface area in contact with the blanket.[83] Combination of a thermal mattress (38–40°C) and a heated humidifier preserved body heat better than did either method alone (Fig. 15–8).[84]

Vasodilators. Cardiac surgical patients are often hypothermic after surgery because their core temperatures are incompletely restored after cardiopulmonary bypass. Noback and Tinker demonstrated that administration of sodium nitroprusside during extracorporeal rewarming speeded rewarming and prevented postbypass cooling.[84]

Fluid and Blood Warming. Warming of room temperature intravenous fluids (1000 ml) to body temperature requires about 15 cal. In the anesthetized patient who is unable to increase caloric production, body temperature decreases.[22, 85] Body temperature decreases about 0.5°C after administration of 1 L of 4°C blood over 15 minutes.[22, 32] The efficacy of various blood warmers to deliver blood at temperatures above 32°C at rates of 150 ml/minute was reviewed by Russell.[60]

Humidifiers. Heated humidifiers are the best way to prevent and treat heat loss in the perioperative period.[83, 86–88] They save the patients from warming and humidifying cold, dry gases from the anesthetic circuit and maintain temperature compared with unwarmed patients.[83, 89] Preheating of the humidifier prior to use increases its effectiveness.[23] Airway temperature should always be measured and maintained at 38°C or less when humidifiers are used, in order to prevent airway burns or tracheobronchial edema.[22, 88]

Passive heat and moisture exchangers (artificial noses) fail to provide similar benefits.[90] They do limit the intraoperative temperature decrease by about 1°C.[91]

A recent study in outpatients noted that warmed, humidified gases during anesthesia resulted in warmer patients arriving in the postanesthetic unit; these patients also had shorter postoperative stays.[92] Ralley and colleagues noted the inability of heated, humidified gases to prevent decreases in temperature after discontinuation of hypothermic cardiopulmonary bypass.[93] However, humidified gases minimize damage to the cilia of the respiratory mucosal cells.

Other Methods. One method to limit perioperative hypothermia is the use of a GK-esophageal thermal tube, a specially designed 45-cm double-lumen tube with a thin, rigid inner tube surrounded by a 3-cm thin-walled outer tube through which thermostatically controlled warm water (41.7°C) is circulated at 3 L/minute.[94] In patients having major abdominal surgery, temperature was significantly higher when heat was transferred through the tube to the central core. However, the device has the disadvantages of thermal esophageal injury and gastric distention with water if tube leakage occurs.

Malignant Hyperthermia

The lethal upper limit of body temperature is 42–43°C. Crocker and colleagues noted that patients anesthetized with halothane who received succinylcholine chloride had higher temperatures during the first 30–45 minutes of anesthesia than those noted in patients not receiving halothane.[95] This finding suggests that malignant hyperthermia triggered by halothane and succinylcholine chloride represents an exaggeration of a normal response, as none of the patients studied developed malignant hyperthermia (see Table 15–2).[95]

Etiology

Malignant hyperthermia is often defined as a defect resulting in increased muscle metabolism that causes an increase in temperature of more than 1–2°C/hour. In susceptible patients, hyperthermia is triggered by various anesthetic agents, but it can also occur in nonanesthetic settings. Because a detailed discussion of this syndrome is beyond the scope of this chapter, the reader is referred to the review by Gronert.[96] Malignant hyperthermia is inherited as an autosomal dominant disorder with reduced penetrance and variable expressivity, but sporadic cases also occur.[96] An increased incidence has been noted in idiopathic scoliosis, muscular dystrophy, strabismus, ptosis, and certain congenital muscular disorders with myopathy. Susceptibility is determined by family history, by the presence of increased creatine kinase, and definitively by the response of muscle obtained by biopsy to caffeine (contracture). Frequency is variable, ranging from 1 in 14,000 to 1 in 190,000 anesthetic procedures.[97, 98]

The precise cellular location of the defect is unclear, with excessive release of calcium ion or defects in calcium uptake as likely mechanisms. Abnormally increased calcium ion in the cellular cytoplasm explains the heat production, muscle rigor, and glycogenolysis associated with the syndrome.[96]

Symptoms

Symptoms of malignant hyperthermia include spasm of the masseter muscles with difficulty opening the mouth for intubation, general muscular rigidity, tachycardia with dysrhythmias, increased carbon dioxide production, tachypnea, peripheral cyanosis, and hyperthermia. Myocardial oxygen consumption increases, but cardiovascular stability is present in many malignant hyperthermia episodes. However, the occurrence of sudden death in malignant hyperthermia–susceptible families raises questions about myocardial involvement.[96] Laboratory studies reveal severe metabolic acidosis with pH less than 7.0, hypercapnia, decreased mixed venous Po_2, and hyperkalemia. Adequate arterial oxygenation is usually present. As the syndrome proceeds, hyperphosphatemia, hemoconcentration, and hyperglycemia may occur.[99, 100] In later stages, acute renal failure results from acute tubular necrosis caused by excessive myoglobin release from muscle, disseminated intravascular coagulation, and central nervous system dysfunction resulting from brain temperatures exceeding 43°C.

Therapy

Therapy consists of general supportive treatment including hyperventilation with oxygen, administration of intravenous fluids, discontinuation of triggering agents, control of metabolic acidosis with bicarbonate, control of hyperkalemia with dextrose-insulin infusions, and control of dysrhythmias with procainamide hydrochloride or other agents. Attempts to cool the patient with external methods, gastric or peritoneal lavage, lavage of an open body cavity, or administration of iced intravenous fluids should be performed. Monitoring during the episode should include intra-arterial and central venous catheters, urinary bladder catheter, ECG, and if possible, a muscle temperature probe. Otherwise, temperature can be measured in the esophagus or other common sites. The definitive therapy is dantrolene sodium, given in initial doses of 2–2.5 mg/kg body weight, with additional increments every 5–10 minutes if no reduction of temperature, acidosis, tachycardia, or muscle rigidity occurs, to a total dose of 10 mg/kg. Therapy with dantrolene sodium should commence even while supportive measures are being applied, because it must be given while adequate muscle perfusion is present. Dantrolene sodium alters calcium release but does not affect its uptake. It causes muscle weakness and hepatic dysfunction.

Anesthetic agents that trigger malignant hyperthermia include succinylcholine chloride, halothane, enflurane, and isoflurane. Nitrous oxide was suggested as a triggering agent by Ellis and coworkers, but this has not been substantiated.[101] The choices for anesthesia in malignant hyperthermia–susceptible patients include local anesthetics of the ester type given in regional techniques, such as epidural or subarachnoid block, or thiopental sodium–nitrous oxide with narcotic and nondepolarizing neuromuscular-blocking drugs. An anesthesia machine with clean tubing, new soda lime, and empty vaporizers, whose fresh gas flow is analyzed by mass spectroscopy for absence of volatile anesthetics, is satisfactory for administration of anesthesia to a malignant hyperthermia–susceptible patient. Pretreatment with oral dantrolene sodium to a dosage of 4–7 mg/kg body weight during the 24 hours prior to surgery effectively prevents malignant hyperthermia.[102]

Other Causes of Intraoperative Hyperthermia

Endogenous pyrogens such as endotoxins and various microbial agents and hypersensitivity reactions to heterologous proteins such as bovine albumin elicit fever in some humans. Atropine blocks the cholinergic innervation of the sweat glands, preventing sweating, which may cause hyperthermia. Thyrotoxicosis and pheochromocytoma may cause hyperthermia. These conditions respond to treatment of the primary inciting causes. Specific antipyretic therapy is necessary only in children with very high temperatures.

OTHER MONITORS

Lower Esophageal Sphincter Pressure

The lower one third of the esophagus contains smooth muscle that is innervated by the vagus nerve. In the awake patient, it spontaneously and frequently contracts. A fluid-filled balloon esophageal catheter similar to a no. 24-F esophageal stethoscope can be used to measure esophageal contractions, and an air-inflatable balloon permits intermittent esophageal stimulation. The catheter is inserted to a distance of 35 cm from the teeth.

Two forms of esophageal activity are recorded: nonpropulsive tertiary and provoked secondary activity. Spontaneous contractions in the esophagus occur at the rate of four or more per minute, lasting 5 seconds with an amplitude of 10–100 mmHg (Fig. 15–9).[103] Contractions provoked by inflation of a pneumatic balloon to a diameter of 15 mm usually occur within 10 seconds of beginning balloon inflation. During anesthesia, esophageal contractility decreases, with the frequency of spontaneous and the amplitude of provoked activity correlating with minimum alveolar anesthetic concentration and clinical depth of anesthesia (Fig. 15–10).[104,105] With very deep anesthesia, both spontaneous and provoked contractions are absent. Changes in contractility occur before changes in EEG. These observations

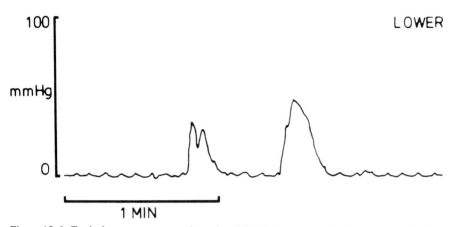

Figure 15–9. Typical spontaneous esophageal activity during anesthesia. (From Evans JM, Davies WL, Wise CC: Lower oesophageal contractility: A new monitor of anaesthesia. Lancet 1984; 1:1151–1154. With permission.)

form the basis for the use of lower esophageal tone to indicate anesthetic depth. Observation of esophageal motility reduces anesthetic dosage to that specifically required for the individual patient.

Although glycopyrrolate and metoclopramide hydrochloride do not interfere with detection of esophageal motility, atropine and scopolamine decrease motility. Absence of spontaneous esophageal contractility in the presence of provoked activity indicates brain death.[106]

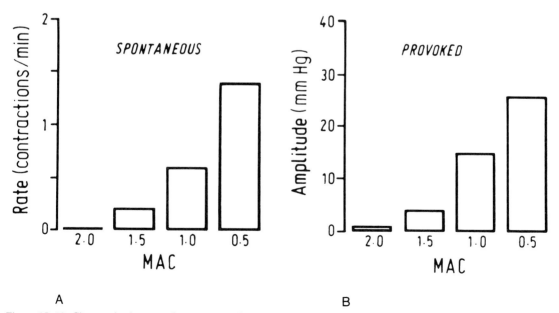

Figure 15–10. Changes in the rate of spontaneous lower esophageal contractions (*A*) correlate with the minimal alveolar concentration (MAC) of an anesthetic. The relation between the amplitude of esophageal contractions (*B*) provoked by balloon inflations and MAC demonstrates good correlation. (From Evans JM, Davies JM, Wise CC: Lower oesophageal contractility: A new monitor of anaesthesia. Lancet 1984; 1:1151–1154. With permission.)

The use of this device is contraindicated in primary or secondary esophageal diseases. The effects of such conditions as hiatal hernia or esophageal motility disorders on spontaneous and evoked contractions are unknown.

References

1. Chang L: Development and use of the stethoscope in diagnosing cardiac disease. Am J Cardiol 1987; 60:1378–1382.
2. Webster TA: Now that we have pulse oximeters and capnographs, we don't need precordial and esophageal stethoscopes. J Clin Monit 1987; 3:191–192.
3. Smith C: An endo-esophageal stethoscope. Anesthesiology 1954; 15:566.
4. Petty C: We do need precordial and esophageal stethoscopes. J Clin Monit 1987; 3:192–193.
5. Baker AB, McLeod C: Oesophageal multipurpose monitoring probe. Anaesthesia 1983; 38:892–897.
6. Kates RA, Zaidan JR, Kaplan JA: Esophageal lead for intraoperative electrocardiographic monitoring. Anesth Analg 1982; 61:781–785.
7. Parker EO: Electrosurgical burn at the site of an esophageal temperature probe. Anesthesiology 1984; 61:93–95.
8. Maroon JC, Albin MS: Air embolism diagnosed by Doppler ultrasound. Anesth Analg 1974; 53:399–402.
9. Kugler J, Stirt JA, Finholt D, Sussman MD: The one that got away: Misplaced esophageal stethoscope. Anesthesiology 1985; 62:643–645.
10. Schwartz AJ, Downes JJ: Hazards of a simple monitoring device, the esophageal stethoscope. Anesthesiology 1977; 47:64–65.
11. Goto H, Hackman LT, Arakawa K: Tracheal insertion of an esophageal stethoscope. Anesth Analg 1977; 56:584–585.
12. Simpson JI, Wolf GL: Flammability of esophageal stethoscopes, nasogastric tubes, feeding tubes, and nasopharyngeal airways in oxygen- and nitrous oxide–enriched atmospheres. Anesth Analg 1988; 67:1093–1095.
13. Himms-Hagen J: Cellular thermiogenesis. Annu Rev Physiol 1976; 38:315–351.
14. Davis PJ: Thermoregulation of the newborn. *In* Cook DR, Marcy JH (eds): Neonatal Anesthesia. Pasadena, CA: Appleton Davies, 1988; 63–70.
15. Hall GM: Body temperature and anesthesia. Br J Anaesth 1978; 50:39–44.
16. Benzinger TH: On physical heat regulation and the sense of temperature in man. Proc Natl Acad Sci 1959; 45:645–659.
17. Atkins E, Bodel P: Fever. N Engl J Med 1972; 286:27–34.
18. Knochel JP: Environmental heat illness. Arch Intern Med 1974; 133:841–864.
19. Adamson K Jr, Gandy G, James L: The influence of thermal factors upon oxygen consumption of the newborn infant. J Pediatr 1965; 66:495–508.
20. Heiser MS, Downes JJ: Temperature regulation in the pediatric patient. Semin Anesth 1984; 3:37–42.
21. Wyon DP, Lidwell OM, Williams REO: Thermal confort during surgical operations. J Hyg (Camb) 1968; 66:229–248.
22. Lilly RB: Inadvertent hypothermia. Refresher Courses in Anesthesiology 1986; 15:93–107.
23. Morley-Forster PK: Unintentional hypothermia in the operating room. Can Anaesth Soc J 1986; 33:516–527.
24. Hitt BA, Mazze RI, Cook TL, et al: Thermoregulatory defect in rats during anesthesia. Anesth Analg 1977; 56:9–15.

25. Sessler DI, Olofsson CI, Rubinstein EH, Beebe JJ: The thermoregulatory threshold in humans during halothane anesthesia. Anesthesiology 1988; 68:836–842.
26. Sessler DI, Olofsson CI, Rubinstein EH: The thermoregulatory threshold in humans during nitrous oxide–fentanyl anesthesia. Anesthesiology 1988; 69:357–364.
27. Holdcroft A, Hall GM: Heat loss during anesthesia. Br J Anaesth 1978; 50:157–164.
28. Engleman DR, Lockhart CH: Comparisons between temperature effects of ketamine and halothane anesthesia in children. Anesth Analg 1972; 51:98–101.
29. Stjernstrom H, Hennberg S, Tabow F, Wiklung L: Oxygen consumption and heat balance during TURP. Anesthesiology 1984; 61:A258.
30. Vaughan MS, Vaughan RW, Cork RC: Postoperative hypothermia in adults: Relationship of age, anesthesia, and shivering to rewarming. Anesth Analg (Cleve) 1981; 60:746–751.
31. Fox RH, Woodward PM, Exton-Smith AN, et al: Body temperatures in the elderly: A national study of physiological, social and environmental conditions. Br Med J 1973; 1:200–206.
32. Roe CF: Temperature regulation in anaesthesia. *In* Hardy JD, et al (eds): Physiological and Behavioral Temperature Regulation. Springfield: Charles C Thomas, 1970; 727–740.
33. Newman BJ: Control of accidental hypothermia: Occurrence and prevention of accidental hypothermia during vascular surgery. Anaesthesia 1971; 26:177–187.
34. Dyde LA, Lunn HF: Heat loss during thoracotomy. Thorax 1970; 25:355–358.
35. Holdcroft A: Body Temperature Control in Anaesthesia, Surgery, and Intensive Care. London: Balliere Tindall, 1980.
36. Lacoumenta S, Hall GM: Liquid crystal thermometry during anaesthesia. Anaesthesia 1984; 39:54–56.
37. Vaughan MS, Cork RC, Vaughan RW: Inaccuracy of liquid crystal thermometry to identify core temperature trends in postoperative adults. Anesth Analg 1982; 61:284–287.
38. Lees DE, Schuette W, Bull J, et al: An evaluation of liquid-crystal thermometry as a screening device for intraoperative hyperthermia. Anesth Analg 1978; 57:669–674.
39. Shinozaki T, Deane R, Perkins FM: Infrared tympanic thermometer: Evaluation of a new clinical thermometer. Crit Care Med 1988; 16:148–150.
40. Cork RC, Vaughan RW, Humphrey LS: Precision and accuracy of intraoperative temperature monitoring. Anesth Analg 1983; 62:211–214.
41. Benzinger TH: Clinical temperature: New physiological basis. JAMA 1969; 209:1200–1206.
42. Benzinger M: Tympanic thermometry in surgery and anesthesia. JAMA 1969; 209:1207–1211.
43. Hickey PR, Andersen NP: Deep hypothermia circulatory arrest: A review of pathophysiology and clinical experience as a basis for anesthetic management. J Cardiothorac Anesth 1987; 1:137–155.
44. Whitby JD, Dunkin LJ: Cerebral, oesophageal, and nasopharyngeal temperatures. Br J Anaesth 1971; 43:673–67.
45. Kaufman RD: Relationship between esophageal temperature gradient and heart and lung sounds heard by esophageal stethoscope. Anesth Analg 187; 66:1046–1048.
46. Severinghaus JW: Temperature gradients during hypothermia. Ann NY Acad Sci 1962; 80:515–521.

47. Piironen P: Effects of exposures to extremely hot environments on temperatures of the tympanic membrane, the oesophagus, and the rectum of men. Technical Documentary Report No AMRL-TDR-63-85. Wright-Patterson Air Force Base, OH: 6570th Aerospace Medical Research Laboratory, 1963.

48. Ritter DM, Rettke SR, Hughes RW, et al: Placement of nasogastric tubes and esophageal stethoscopes in patients with documented esophageal varices. Anesth Analg 1988; 67:280–282.

49. Lilly JK, Boland JP, Zekan S: Urinary bladder temperature monitoring: A new index of body core temperature. Crit Care Med 1980; 8:742–744.

50. Bone ME, Feneck RO: Bladder temperature as an estimate of body temperature during cardiopulmonary bypass. Anaesthesia 1988; 43:181–185.

51. Moorthy SS, Winn BA, Jallard MS, et al: Monitoring urinary bladder temperature. Heart Lung 1985; 14:90–93.

52. Stupfel M, Severinghaus JW: Internal body temperature gradients during anesthesia and hypothermia and effect of vagotomy. J Appl Physiol 1956; 9:380–386.

53. Ramsay JG, Ralley FE, Whalley DG, et al: Site of temperature monitoring and prediction of afterdrop after open heart surgery. Can Anaesth Soc J 1985; 32:607–612.

54. Joly HR, Weil MH: Temperature of the great toe as an indicator of the severity of shock. Circulation 1969; 39:131–138.

55. Matthews HR, Meade JB, Evans CC: Peripheral vasoconstriction after open-heart surgery. Thorax 1974; 29:343–348.

56. Webb GE: Comparison of esophageal and tympanic temperature monitoring during cardiopulmonary bypass. Anesth Analg 1973; 52:729–733.

57. Wallace CT, Marks WE, Adkins WY, Mahafey JE: Perforation of the tympanic membrane, a complication of tympanic thermometry during anesthesia. Anesthesiology 1974; 41:290–291.

58. Ralley FE, Wynands JE, Ramsay JG, et al: The effects of shivering on oxygen consumption and carbon dioxide production in patients rewarming from hypothermic cardiopulmonary bypass. Can J Anaesth 1988; 35:332–337.

59. Sladen RN: Temperature and ventilation after hypothermic cardiopulmonary bypass. Anesth Analg 1985; 64:816–820.

60. Russell WJ: A review of blood warmers for massive transfusion. Anaesth Intensive Care 1974; 2:109–130.

61. Okada M, Fumiaki N, Yoshino H, et al: The J wave in accidental hypothermia. J Electrocardiol 1983; 16:23–28.

62. Buckberg GD, Brazier JR, Nelson RL, et al: Studies of the effects of hypothermia on regional myocardial blood flow and metabolism during cardiopulmonary bypass. The adequately perfused beating, fibrillating and arrested heart. J Thorac Cardiovasc Surg 1977; 73:87–94.

63. McConnell DH, Brazier JR, Cooper N, et al: Studies of the effects of hypothermia on regional myocardial blood flow and metabolism during cardiopulmonary bypass. J Thorac Cardiovasc Surg 1977; 73:95–101.

64. Hicks RG, Poole JL: EEG changes with hypothermia and cardiopulmonary bypass in children. J Thorac Cardiovasc Surg 1979; 78:823–830.

65. Vitez T, White PF, Eger EI: Effect of hypothermia on halothane MAC and isoflurane MAC in the rat. Anesthesiology 1974; 41:80–81.

66. Hickey PR, Wessel DL: Anesthesia for treatment of congenital heart disease. *In* Kaplan JA (ed): Cardiac Anesthesia, 2nd Ed. Orlando: Grune & Stratton, 1987; 635–723.

67. Benumof JL, Wahrenbrock EA: Dependency of hypoxic pulmonary vasoconstriction on temperature. J Appl Physiol 1977; 42:56–58.

68. Regan MJ, Eger EI: Ventilatory responses to hypercapnia and hypoxia at normothermia and moderate hypothermia during constant-depth halothane anesthesia. Anesthesiology 1966; 27:624–633.

69. Benzing G, Frances PD, Kaplan S, et al: Glucose and insulin changes in infants and children undergoing hypothermic open heart surgery. Am J Cardiol 1983; 52:133–136.

70. Wood M, Shand DG, Wood AJJ: The sympathetic response to profound hypothermia and circulatory arrest in infants. Can Anaesth Soc J 1980; 27:125–131.

71. Turley K, Roizen M, Vlahakes GJ, et al: Catecholamine response to deep hypothermia and total circulatory arrest in the infant lamb. Circulation 1980; 62 (Suppl):175–179.

72. Flacke JW, Flacke WE: Inadvertent hypothermia: Frequent, insidious, and often serious. Semin Anesth 1983; 2:183–196.

73. Lewis DG, Mackenzie A: Cooling during major vascular surgery. Br J Anaesth 1972; 44:859–864.

74. Morris RH: Influence of ambient temperature on patient temperature during intra-abdominal surgery. Ann Surg 1971; 173:230–233.

75. Morris RH, Wilkey BR: The effect of ambient temperature on patients monitored during surgery, not involving body cavities. Anesthesiology 1970; 32:102–107.

76. Roizen MF, Sohn YJ, L'Hommedieu CS, et al: Operating room temperature prior to surgical draping: Effect on patient temperature in recovery room. Anesth Analg 1980; 59:852–855.

77. Hampston WR: Hypothermia in winter and high altitude sports. Conn Med 1981; 45:633–636.

78. Bourke D, Wurm H, Rosenberg M, Russell S: Intraoperative heat conservation using a reflective blanket. Anesthesiology 1984; 60:151–154.

79. Radford P, Thurlow AC: Metallised plastic sheeting in the prevention of hypothermia during neurosurgery. Br J Anaesth 1979; 51:237–239.

80. Murphy MT, Lipton JM, Loughran MB, Gieseke AH: Postanesthetic shivering in primates: Inhibition by peripheral heating and by taurine. Anesthesiology 1985; 63:161–165.

81. Sharkey A, Lipton JM, Murphy MT, Giesecke AH: Inhibition of postanesthetic shivering with radiant heat. Anesthesiology 1987; 66:249–252.

82. Goudsouzian NG, Morris RH, Ryan JF: The effects of warming blanket on maintenance of body temperature in anesthetized infants and children. Anesthesiology 1973; 39:351–353.

83. Tølløfsrud SG, Gundersen Y, Andersen R: Peroperative hypothermia. Acta Anaesthesiol Scand 1984; 28:511–515.

84. Noback CR, Tinker JH: Hypothermia after cardiopulmonary bypass: Amelioration by nitroprusside-induced vasodilation during rewarming. Anesthesiology 1980; 53:277–280.

85. Boyan CP, Howland WS: Blood temperature: A critical factor in massive transfusion. Anesthesiology 1961; 22:559–563.

86. Stone DR, Downs JB, Paul WL, Perkins HM: Adult body temperature and heated humidification of anesthetic gases during general anesthesia. Anesth Analg 1981; 60:736–741.

87. Pflug AE, Aasheim GM, Foster C, Marten RW: Prevention of postanesthesia shivering. Can Anaesth Soc J 1978; 25:43–49.

88. Tausk HC, Miller R, Roberts RB: Maintenance of body temperature by heated humidification. Anesth Analg 1976; 55:719–723.

89. Shanks CA: Humidification and loss of body heat during anaesthesia. II. Effects in surgical patients. Br J Anaesth 1974; 46:863–865.

90. Goldberg ME, Jan R, Gregg CE, et al: The heat and moisture exchanger does not preserve body temperature or reduce recovery time in outpatients undergoing surgery and anesthesia. Anesthesiology 1988; 68:122–123.

91. Haslam KR, Nielsen CH: Do passive heart and moisture exhangers keep the patient warm? Anesthesiology 1986; 64:379–381.

92. Conahan TJ, Williams GD, Apfelbaum JL, Lecky JH: Airway heating reduces recovery time (cost) in outpatients. Anesthesiology 1987; 67:128–130.

93. Ralley FE, Ramsay JG, Wynands JE, et al: Effect of heated humidified gases on temperature drop after cardiopulmonary bypass. Anesth Analg 1984; 63:1106–1110.

94. Kristensen G, Guldager H, Gravesen H: Prevention of perioperative hypothermia in abdominal surgery. Acta Anaesthesiol Scand 1986; 30:314–316.

95. Crocker BD, Okumura F, McCuaig DI, Denborough MA: Temperature monitoring during general anaesthesia. Br J Anaesth 1980; 50:1223–1228.

96. Gronert GA: Malignant hyperthermia. Anesthesiology 1980; 53:395–423.

97. Britt BA, Kalow W: Malignant hyperthermia. A statistical review. Can Anaesth Soc J 1970; 17:293–315.

98. Wilson ME, Ellis FR: Predicting malignant hyperpyrexia. Br J Anaesth 1979; 51:66P.

99. Britt BA, Kwong FHF, Endrenyi L: The clinical and laboratory features of malignant hyperthermia management: A review. *In* Henschel EO (ed): Malignant Hyperthermia: Current Concepts. New York: Appleton-Century-Crofts, 1977; 9.

100. Britt BA: Recent advances in malignant hyperthermia. Anesth Analg 1972; 51:841–850.

101. Ellis FR, Clarke IMC, Appleyard TN, Dinsdale RCW: Malignant hyperthermia induced with nitrous oxide and treated with dexamethasone. Br Med J 1974; 4:270–271.

102. Gronert GA, Milde JH, Theye RA: Dantrolene in porcine malignant hyperthermia. Anesthesiology 1976; 44:488–495.

103. Evans JM, Davies WL, Wise CC: Lower oesophageal contractility: A new monitor of anaesthesia. Lancet 1984; 1:1151–1154.

104. Evans JM, Bithell JF, Vlachonikolis IG: Relationship between lower oesophageal contractility, clinical signs and halothane concentration during general anaesthesia and surgery in man. Br J Anaesth 1987; 59:1346–1355.

105. Maccioli GA, Calkins JM, Greff R, Kuni D: The lower esophageal contractility index: A measure of anesthetic depth. J Clin Monit 1987; 3:302–303.

106. Sinclair ME, Suter PM: Lower oesophageal contractility as an indicator of brain death in paralyzed and mechanically ventilated patients with head injury. Br Med J 1987; 1:935–936.

chapter sixteen

Intraoperative Evaluation of Hemostasis

■ ROGER A. MOORE, M.D.

During every invasive surgical procedure, the hemostatic control mechanisms of the body are stimulated. For most operations, the intricate balances among the vascular, the coagulation factor, and the platelet control mechanisms are sufficient to ensure adequate intraoperative hemostasis; however, inherited conditions or acquired derangements in one or more of the hemostatic control mechanisms can lead to intraoperative situations requiring the intervention of the anesthesiologist. A primary problem in these situations is the need for rapid and accurate diagnosis of the problem, so that direct and specific therapeutic intervention can be initiated. The "shotgun approach" to blood component therapy (concomitant administration of plasma, platelets, and erythrocytes) is no longer acceptable. In addition to the older tests such as platelet count, prothrombin time, and partial thromboplastin time, a variety of recently developed medical devices are used in the intraoperative management of hemostasis.

The initial step in the evaluation of hemostasis is the measurement of blood loss. Blood in operative suction containers, if it is not contaminated with irrigating solutions, is directly measured. The amount of blood on sponges, surgical drapes, surgeons' gowns, and the operating room floor is more difficult to determine. Usually, an estimate by visual inspection is made. In the case of sponges, the cumbersome measurement of hemoglobin concentration in the effluent of washed sponges can be performed. An estimate based on the difference between the wet and dry weights of sponges (assuming 1 ml of blood weighs 1 gm) is more commonly used.

The first medical devices brought into the operating room for the evaluation of hemostasis were in answer to the need for monitoring anticoagulation during the extracorporeal circulatory techniques of open heart surgery. Complete inhibition of the coagulation system with heparin is an absolute requirement during extracorporeal circulation. More recently, the development of transplant surgical techniques has been a major impetus for having other medical instrumentation to allow more accurate diagnosis and management of the severe coagulation derangements that occur. At present, there is no "perfect" medical device or test for the intraoperative evaluation of coagulation. Each device or test has certain advantages and limitations. In order to adequately understand these devices, one should have a thorough understanding of the basic principles governing hemostatic control mechanisms.

MECHANISMS OF HEMOSTASIS

Vascular Integrity

The first line of defense in hemostasis is maintenance of vascular integrity. However, the elderly patient, the debilitated patient, or the patient receiving certain pharmacologic agents (e.g., steroids) may have compromised vascular defenses, increasing bleeding tendency. The patient with compromised vascular defenses may be brought to the anesthesiologist's attention preoperatively by the presence of a prolonged bleeding time (elevation of the bleeding time might also be due to platelet dysfunction).

Once a blood vessel is incised, unless hemostatic control mechanisms intervene, the intravascular fluids pour from the vessel. The driving force for the blood loss is the difference between the pressure inside the vessel and the pressure outside. Vascular mechanisms that come into play for the control of bleeding can be divided into immediate effects and delayed effects.[1]

Immediate Effect

An immediate effect is constriction of the vessel wall at the site of injury, thereby reducing blood flow to the severed vessel. The primary mechanism for inducing this vascular constriction is release of a cyclo-oxygenase product of arachidonic acid metabolism called thromboxane A_2 (Fig. 16–1). Thromboxane A_2 is released from granules within activated platelets and serves as both a potent vasoconstrictor and an inducer for platelet aggregation.

Figure 16–1. The metabolism of arachidonic acid by the cyclo-oxygenase pathway leads to the production of thromboxane A_2 in platelets and prostacyclin in vascular endothelial cells. These two products of arachidonic acid metabolism have opposite effects on vascular wall reactivity and platelet activity. The cyclo-oxygenase metabolism of arachidonic acid can be inhibited with aspirin.

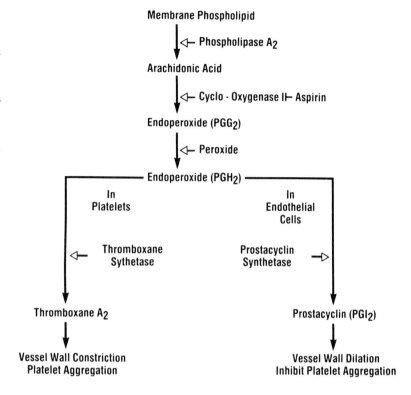

Delayed Effects

A delayed vascular mechanism for limiting blood loss is the increased extravascular tissue pressure resulting from the extravasation of blood into the surrounding tissues as well as the leakage of edema fluid into these tissues. The increase in extravascular tissue pressure from the extravasated blood and edema fluid balances the intravascular pressure, thereby nullifying the primary determinant promoting bleeding. The increased extravascular tissue pressure serves the same physiologic function as pressure bandages applied directly to a bleeding site or the use of positive end-expiratory pressure for intrathoracic bleeding.[2]

If a large vessel is severed, preventing normal hemostatic mechanisms from controlling the bleeding, the continued blood loss eventually leads to contraction of the intravascular volume and a resultant decrease in blood pressure. The decrease in blood pressure in combination with a reflex redistribution of blood flow away from the periphery and to the vital organs by the central nervous system serves as an extremely effective end-stage hemostatic control mechanism. The value of these mechanisms for the limitation of blood loss is well known in anesthesia, a field in which techniques using anesthetic agents[3] or other pharmacologic hypotensive agents[4] to produce deliberate hypotension have been effective in reducing intraoperative blood loss.

Coagulation Factors

One of the first events leading to hemostasis is formation of a hemostatic plug through activation of the coagulation cascade. The coagulation cascade allows a small stimulus for coagulation to be amplified by a series of sequential enzymatic steps leading to the formation of a fibrin clot at the bleeding site. This enzymatic amplification of coagulation stimuli can occur through two pathways: the intrinsic pathway and the extrinsic pathway (Fig. 16–2). The end result of activation of either pathway is the conversion of fibrinogen to fibrin, but each pathway is initiated by different stimuli. Upon contact with foreign surfaces, including such diverse substances as collagen, glass, and denuded vascular endothelium, the intrinsic pathway is activated with conversion of inactive factor XII to active factor XIIa. This is followed by sequential activation of factor XI and factor IX, with factor IX combining with factor VIII, calcium, and platelet factor 3. This latter conglomerate leads to the conversion of inactive factor X to its activated form (Xa), which is the first step in the final common pathway.

As an alternate method for activation of the final common pathway, the extrinsic coagulation pathway can be induced through the activation of factor VII by contact with tissue phospholipid. Tissue phospholipid is commonly released by damaged tissue as well as during platelet activation. The end result of activation of the extrinsic pathway is the same as activation of the intrinsic pathway, stimulation of the final common pathway and formation of a fibrin clot. In this discussion, the activities of the intrinsic and extrinsic pathways are rigidly separated, but in reality, crossovers between these pathways can occur, with activated factor VIII producing direct activation of intrinsic pathway factors.[1]

The final common pathway consists of conversion by activated factor X (Xa) of prothrombin (II) to thrombin (IIa), which induces the conversion of fibrinogen (I) to fibrin (Ia). The initial fibrin clot that results from activation of the final common pathway is helpful in providing hemostasis, but this clot is relatively unstable and friable. Through the action of factor XIIIa, increased cross-linkage between the fibrin strands is stimulated, thereby converting the unstable clot into a solid, insoluble plug providing better hemostatic control.

Although the coagulation cascade's ability to amplify a small stimulus for clot formation through a series of enzymatic steps is a major advantage, its complexity can be a primary weakness. Interruption of any of the enzymatic steps, through congenital abnormalities, pharmacologic interventions, or acquired conditions, results in abnormal clot formation. For the most part, a relative deficiency in the serum level of a coagulation factor does not play a major role in reducing hemostasis, since normal clot formation only requires between 10% and 50% of the normal amount of each factor.[5, 6] A decrease of a coagulation factor below the required level, how-

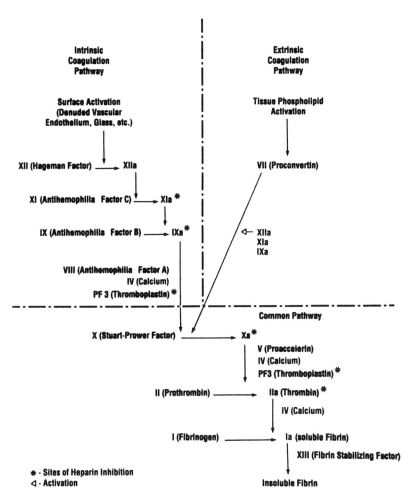

Figure 16–2. The coagulation cascade allows a small stimulus for clot formation to be amplified, resulting in the formation of a fibrin clot. The coagulation cascade is made up of three pathways—the intrinsic pathway, the extrinsic pathway, and the final common pathway. Heparin's effect is exerted primarily on the activated serum proteases (XIa, IXa, Xa, IIa) and thromboplastin (platelet factor 3).

ever, can compromise overall clot formation, even though a direct cause-effect relationship between the level of coagulation factor and the adequacy of clot formation does not always exist. For example, in classic factor VIII–deficient hemophilia, the bleeding tendency is *usually* inversely related to the serum level of factor VIII.[6] Some patients with extremely low factor VIII levels undergo surgery without hemostatic difficulty, whereas others with seemingly adequate factor VIII levels develop major hemostatic problems. Despite the growing knowledge of the coagulation system, whether or not an individual patient with an individual factor deficiency will have intraoperative bleeding problems is not easily predicted. Fortunately, one factor not found to directly affect most coagulation-promoting or -inhibiting systems is the commonly used anesthetic agents.[7]

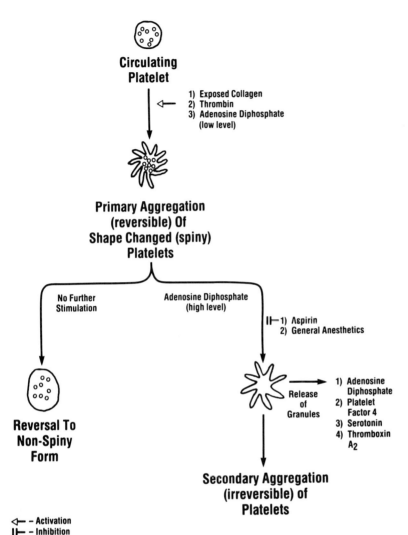

Figure 16–3. Smooth-surfaced circulating platelets can be stimulated to undergo a shape change to a spiny form by exposure to collagen, thrombin, and low levels of adenosine diphosphate. Spiny platelets can undergo primary aggregation, which is completely reversible in the absence of further stimulation. However, in the presence of continued adenosine diphosphate stimulation, platelet granule release occurs, leading to irreversible secondary aggregation.

Platelets

As important to the hemostatic process as the coagulation cascade is platelet activation. Normally, platelets circulate through the blood vessels in an inactive smooth-surfaced form. When an inactive platelet comes into contact with a damaged blood vessel, the platelet immediately changes from its smooth-surfaced form to a spiny-surfaced form (Fig. 16–3). This change to the spiny-surfaced form increases the platelet's adhesiveness and leads to primary aggregation.[8] The cause of the platelet's shape change is thought to be the release of adenosine diphosphate from the injured vessel's wall.

The primary aggregation induced by adenosine diphosphate is potentially reversible; if no further stimulation for platelet activation occurs, the primary platelet aggregate dissipates, with reversion of the platelets to their inactive smooth-surfaced form. However, if the stimulus for aggregation persists and reaches a threshold level, a release reaction occurs and the platelets discharge cytoplasmic granules containing a variety of substances, including adenosine diphosphate, serotonin, platelet factor 4, and catechols. The increased level of platelet activation leads to irreversible or secondary aggregation.

The secondary platelet aggregate acts as a base for the formation of a hemostatic plug, and during secondary aggregation, platelets release platelet factor 3. Platelet factor 3 is a cofactor with IXa, VIII, and ionized calcium to form a complex that activates the final common pathway in the coagulation cascade.[8] Platelet factor 3 may also initiate the extrinsic coagulation pathway. Therefore, platelets not only are involved in producing the initial hemostatic plug but also act as major modifiers and modulators of the coagulation cascade.[9] In addition, during secondary aggregation, thromboxane A_2 is released from the platelets, leading to constriction of the vessel wall and further stimulation of platelet aggregation. Although the role of thromboxane A_2 in maintenance of hemostasis is obviously advantageous in peripheral vessels, its release in coronary vessels may play a central role in initiating unstable angina episodes[8] as well as coronary thrombosis.[10] Thromboxane A_2 synthesis inhibitors, such as low-dose acetylsalicylic acid, are suggested prophylactic measures for prevention of myocardial infarctions[11, 12] in patients with coronary artery disease.

Functional platelets counts of greater than $100,000/\mu l$ are necessary in order to have normal template bleeding times.[13] Below functional platelet counts of $50,000-75,000/\mu l$, intraoperative hemostasis may be inadequate. The major point is that *functional platelets* are the primary determinant of platelet adequacy, and absolute platelet counts are not adequate indicators of circulating platelet function. Platelets are usually counted using phase-contrast microscopy. A variety of clinical conditions adversely affect platelet function, including such diverse conditions as von Willebrand's disease and uremia, as well as a number of commonly used pharmacologic agents. Conversely, hyperactive platelet function can be found in a variety of clinical situations, including idiopathic thrombocytopenic purpura and postchemotherapeutic bone marrow recovery. Qualitative tests of platelet function, not quantitative tests of platelet number, should be used to make clinical decisions regarding the need for platelet infusions. The Ivy bleeding time (whole blood) has been used to indicate both platelet and vascular competency, but the results of this test do not correlate consistently with the potential for increased intraoperative bleeding.[14, 15] One reason for the inconsistency with the Ivy bleeding time is that the technique for performing the test must be followed rigorously and exactly.

During performance of a bleeding time, venous pressure is maintained at 40 mmHg using a sphygmomanometer cuff. Standard incisions of 9 mm length and 1 mm depth are made on the volar surface of the forearm. Every 30 seconds, the bleeding edges are blotted with filter paper until bleeding ceases. The normal bleeding time is 4.5 ± 1.5 minutes. The Ivy bleeding time is relatively insensitive as an indicator of hemostasis. Bleeding times return to normal in 2 days after aspirin ingestion, whereas more sensitive platelet function tests are adversely affected for 6 days or more.[15]

The question of adequate platelet function is even more confusing. Unlike coagulation factors, platelet function can be adversely affected by a number of preoperative medications.[8, 16] The choice of anesthetic agent may also have a major effect on intraoperative platelet function. Although all investigators do not agree,[17] the general consensus from both *in vitro* and *in vivo* studies is that all of the commonly used inhalation anesthetic agents cause a dose-dependent inhibition of platelet function.[18–21]

MECHANISMS OF ANTICOAGULATION

The body's mechanisms for providing hemostasis are intricately related through positive and negative feedback systems. The mechanisms for formation and lysis of thrombus, for aggregation and inactivation of platelets, for activation and inhibition of plasminogen, and for dilation and constriction of vessels are all in delicate balance.

Protein C System

Equally as important to hemostasis as the clot-promoting systems are the activities of the balancing systems of clot inhibition and lysis. The role of the protein C system in inhibition of clot formation has been elucidated only relatively recently (Fig. 16–4). Protein C is a naturally occurring vitamin K–dependent anticoagulant that contains the protein residue gamma-carboxyglutamic acid, as do the other vitamin K–dependent factors (II, VII, IX, X).[22] The inactive, zymogen form of protein C is converted to its active, enzymatic form (Ca) through enzymatic cleavage by thrombin. The activated protein C then functions as a potent anticoagulant through inactivation of coagulation factors V and VIII. Thrombin is normally only a mild activator of protein C, but when thrombin combines with a capillary endothelial receptor (thrombomodulin), protein C conversion to an active state increases some 20,000-fold.[23] In addition, the combination of thrombin with thrombomodulin removes thrombin from the circulation, thereby reducing the amount of fibrinogen converted to fibrin. Protein C also has an effect on the fibrinolytic pathway. Activated protein C neutralizes tissue plasminogen inhibitors with the direct result of increased fibrinolysis.

The activity of the protein C system is made even more complex by the presence of an additional vitamin K–dependent plasma protein called protein S.[22] The purpose of protein S is the modulation of protein C's conversion to its active form. Therefore, a genetic or an acquired deficiency of either protein C or protein S could lead to a hyperthrombotic state.[22] Derangements in the protein C system during extracorporeal circulation have been linked to increased bleeding tendencies in patients following open heart surgery.[24] Infusions of activated protein C have been suggested as a possible alternative

Figure 16–4. The protein C system is actively involved in promoting fibrinolysis and anticoagulation. In the presence of calcium chloride, thrombin, and an endothelial cell wall molecule (thrombomodulin), protein C is rapidly converted to its enzymatically active form, C_a. Protein C_a neutralizes tissue plasminogen inhibitors, thereby promoting fibrinolysis. In addition, with the help of protein S, protein C_a inactivates factors V and VIII, leading to an increased anticoagulant state.

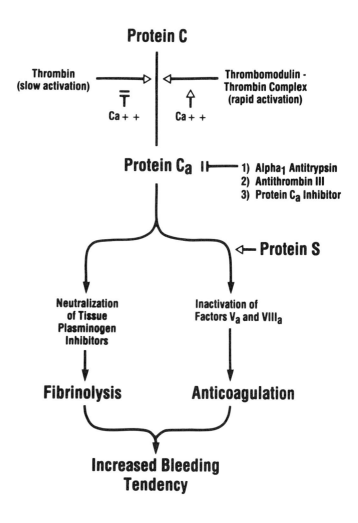

to heparin as an anticoagulant.[23] In addition, many investigators feel that patients with a deficiency of protein C are at increased risk for venous thromboembolic disease;[25–27] others do not.[28] An inherited heterozygous deficiency of protein C occurs with a prevalence rate of 1 in 300.

Not only does the vessel wall contain thrombomodulin for modulation of the protein C system but the vascular endothelial tissue also contains prostacyclin.[29] Unlike the platelet cyclo-oxygenase product of arachidonic acid (thromboxane A_2), prostacyclin acts as a potent vasodilator and inhibitor of platelet aggregation. Therefore, through the thromboxane A_2 and the prostacyclin systems, nature has set up another mechanism to balance normal hemostasis against overwhelming thrombosis. Obviously, imbalances in

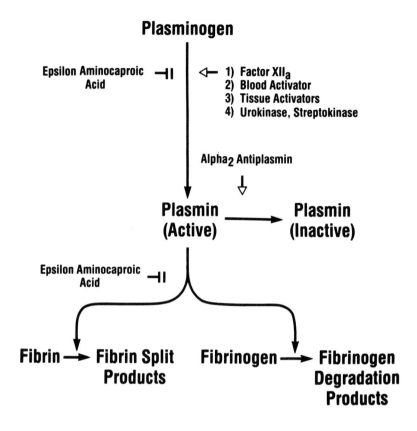

Figure 16–5. The fibrinolytic system acts as the primary balance to clot-promoting systems in the body. Inactive plasminogen is converted to plasmin by a variety of factors, including factor XIIa (the first step in clot formation through the intrinsic pathway). Plasmin actively destroys fibrin and fibrinogen, leading to clot dissolution. Epsilon aminocaproic acid acts through inhibition of plasmin formation as well as direct inhibition of active plasmin. Overwhelming fibrinolysis is prevented by alpha₂ antiplasmin's destruction of active plasmin.

either system from acquired or pharmacologic disruptions could lead to hemostatic problems.

Fibrinolysis

The primary system preventing clot formation from leading to overwhelming thrombosis is the fibrinolytic system. Induction of the fibrinolytic system occurs early in the initiation of clot formation (Fig. 16–5). The first step in the coagulation cascade of exposure of blood to vascular collagen is the conversion of factor XII to its active state, XIIa. Factor XIIa then initiates the coagulation cascade through the intrinsic pathway. However, factor XIIa has another important function—conversion of plasminogen to the nonspecific serine protease, plasmin.[30] Therefore, as soon as clot formation is stimulated, clot lysis is induced. Plasmin formation is also stimulated by a number of other tissue plasminogen activators.

Both plasmin and plasminogen have high chemical affinities for the fibrin molecule. As clot formation progresses, these factors are actively incorporated into the growing clot. The active plasmin molecule immediately begins enzymatically cleaving fibrin strands in the clot, leading to its dissolution and the release of fibrin split products. Only in the area of greatest stimulation for clot formation (at the wall of the severed vessel) can the clot-promoting systems overcome the clot-dissolving systems. The fibrin split products released during fibrin breakdown also act as substitute fibrin monomers during the polymerization of fibrin. Since fibrin split products are inadequate substitutes for fibrin monomers, the result is the formation of friable, abnormal, easily destroyed clots. Finally, plasmin also destroys other coagulation factors, including factors V and VIII and fibrinogen.[30, 31]

One can understand why an imbalance in the fibrinolytic system could lead to major derangements in the hemostatic process. Excessive plasmin production might rapidly lead to a fibrinolytic state in which all clot is dissolved and further clot formation impaired. The body's mechanism for preventing this situation is an additional plasma glycoprotein called alpha$_2$ antiplasmin, which rapidly inactivates serum plasmin.[1, 30] In spite of alpha$_2$ antiplasmin's presence, overstimulation of the fibrinolytic system can lead to clinical bleeding, whereas overinhibition increases the risk of widespread thromboses.

Thrombolysis

Manipulation of the fibrinolytic system via the use of pharmacologic agents has recently gained increased application as a method for destroying unwanted systemic thrombus. Both urokinase and streptokinase are fibrinolytic agents functioning in a manner similar to plasmin. Their primary clinical application has been to dissolve coronary thrombi during and after myocardial infarction. These agents have been shown to be effective in improving regional myocardial blood flow and left ventricular function during a myocardial infarction.[31–33] The primary disadvantage associated with the use of either of these agents is severe generalized fibrinolysis,[34] leading to significant bleeding complications[32] and prolonged derangement of coagulation (2 days or more). Emergency surgery in patients receiving thrombolytic therapy results in complex and difficult coagulation problems.[35]

A direct tissue plasminogen activator is presently available for clinical use, and it serves as an adequate substitute for the other kinases. The newer tissue plasminogen activator allows the destruction of clot by direct conversion of plasminogen to plasmin. Therefore, the body's natural defenses can destroy the resultant plasmin, leading to a short half-life for the drug (5–8 minutes) and the absence of prolonged derangements in hemostatic control.[30] Unfortunately, tissue plasminogen activator is expensive.

PHARMACOLOGY AND COAGULATION

Anticoagulants

Heparin

The initial intraoperative introduction of coagulation-monitoring devices was specifically aimed at evaluating the adequacy of anticoagulation during extracorporeal circulation. The variability of heparin's dose response–dose effect relationship negated the use of a predetermined dosage schedule for providing an accurate level of anticoagulation and mandated the development of intraoperative coagulation-monitoring devices allowing reliable, accurate, and reproducible assessment of the patient's state of anticoagulation.[36] Heparin is a mucopolysaccharide discovered by McLean in 1916.[37] The molecular weight of heparin varies between 15,000 and 18,000 daltons, depending upon the number of saccharide units in the chemical structure. The relatively large size of this molecule prevents it from crossing the blood-placental barrier and, for the most part, keeps it within the intravascular space.

Clinical use of a new, low–molecular weight heparin produced by digestion of the larger heparin molecule is under investigation. The main advantage of low–molecular weight heparin is its minimum effect on platelets.[38] However, potential disadvantages include weaker anticoagulant effect, longer half-life, and inability to easily reverse the anticoagulation with protamine. Its usefulness during open heart surgery is limited.

Structure-Activity Relationship

For the most part, only 25–30% of the heparin molecule is responsible for over 95% of the anticoagulant activity.[39] The portion of the heparin molecule most involved in producing anticoagulant is a specific tetrasaccharide sequence: L-iduronic acid, N-acetylated D-glucosamine-6 sulfate, D-glucuronic acid, and N-sulfated D-glucosamine-6 sulfate.[40] Part of the difficulty in predicting heparin's action in any individual patient is related to the varying amounts of specific tetrasaccharide in each heparin molecule. The amount of this tetrasaccharide can vary greatly, depending upon the mammalian source from which the heparin is extracted,[40] the organ system from which it is obtained,[41] and the pharmaceutic extraction process used for refining the heparin. In addition, different lots of heparin obtained from the same organ system and the same mammalian species can have widely variable anticoagulant activities based on a milligrams-per-milliliter sample. For these reasons, the pharmaceutic companies report heparin in units per milliliter rather than in milligrams per milliliter.

Also, a threefold variability can exist between patients' responses to a specific anticoagulant bolus dose of heparin.[36, 42] Individual variations in intravascular volume, age, sex,[43] and serum antithrombin III levels[41, 44] and previous exposure to heparin therapy[45] all contribute to the variability in individual patient responses to a specific dose of heparin. It is this variability that negates the use of heparin-dosing protocols as successful and acceptable mechanisms for providing reliable anticoagulation.[36] Another variable is the half-life of heparin, which can vary as much as fourfold among individuals.[36] Normally, the half-life of heparin is determined by first-order kinetics and is approximately 1.5 hours.[42, 44] However, since heparin inactivation occurs by reticuloendothelial system uptake,[46] differences in the activation and integrity of the reticuloendothelial system among patients also provide variability in the serum half-life for the drug. Finally, individuals with antiheparin antibodies and increased levels of platelet factor 4 (an antiheparin) have reduced efficacy from a dose of heparin.[47, 48]

Antithrombin III

If a bolus of heparin is placed in a test tube of clotted blood, the clot is not affected. Therefore, heparin's action occurs prior to clot formation. Heparin is not in and of itself an anticoagulant. Heparin produces anticoagulation through its interaction with a serum protein called antithrombin III. Antithrombin III's function in the body is to inactivate serine proteases in the coagulation cascade (activated coagulation factors XIa, IXa, Xa, and IIa).[38, 47, 49] By itself, antithrombin III is a fairly weak enzyme; but, in combination with heparin, a configurational change occurs in its structure, allowing a 2000–10,000-fold increase in activity.[40]

As might be expected, individuals with low levels of antithrombin III are more difficult to anticoagulate with heparin than are individuals with normal levels of antithrombin III.[44] Approximately 1 out of 2000 individuals have depressed antithrombin III levels on the basis of an inherited heterozygous defect. Patients homozygous for antithrombin III deficiency usually die prior to birth or in the early newborn period, owing to overwhelming thromboses. In addition, a variety of clinical conditions including liver disease, pregnancy, and debilitating illness depress serum levels of antithrombin III.[50] The antithrombin III not only affects the coagulation cascade but also neutralizes plasmin in the fibrinolytic system.[50] Antithrombin III deficiency may be responsible for as many as 2% of clinical cases of venous thrombosis.[50]

Dose

Owing to heparin's lack of effect on factor VII, low-dose heparin therapy primarily affects the intrinsic pathway with prolongation of the partial thromboplastin time (PTT) and maintenance of a relatively normal prothrombin time (PT). At higher doses, heparin's effect on factors in the final common pathway also leads to prolongation of the PT.

Coumarin

Coumarin, which inhibits the formation of vitamin K–dependent factors (II, VII, IX, and XII), primarily affects the extrinsic pathway in low doses with prolongation of the PT and little effect on the PTT.[5] As coumarin doses are increased, the PTT is also prolonged, owing to common final pathway effects.

Prostacyclin and Iloprost

Prostacyclin

Prostacyclin is a cyclo-oxygenase product of arachidonic acid metabolism found naturally in vascular endothelial walls (see Fig. 16–1). The chemical name for prostacyclin, (5Z)-9-deoxy-6,9α-epoxy-Δ^5-PGF$_{1\alpha}$, has the shorthand designation of PGI$_2$. The primary physiologic effects of PGI$_2$ are vascular dilatation and inhibition of platelet aggregation. Prostacyclin's effect on platelet aggregation is thought to occur through direct stimulation of platelet adenylate cyclase, leading to increased platelet adenosine monophosphate (cAMP). The increased cAMP inhibits Ca^{2+} mobilization, thereby preventing the calcium-dependent, platelet-dense granule release that causes platelet aggregation.[51] Of interest, unlike most prostaglandins, PGI$_2$ is not destroyed during passage through the lungs, and most of the PGI$_2$ activity is generated by lung tissue. The future importance of PGI$_2$ in medical therapy is its potential for use as a heparin substitute or at least to preserve platelets. During extracorporeal circulation[52, 53] and hemodialysis,[54] platelet activation and consumption can occur in spite of adequate anticoagulation. Unlike heparin, PGI$_2$ has an *in vitro* half-life of only a few minutes, inhibits platelets without affecting the coagulation cascade, and, when it is metabolized, allows the platelets to return to full active function. The primary problem associated with the clinical use of PGI$_2$ is vasodilatation, leading to systemic hypotension. PGI$_2$ has been used as a substitute for heparin in a safe and effective manner during hemodialysis, both experimentally[55] and clinically.[54]

Unlike with hemodialysis, use of PGI$_2$ as a sole substitute for heparin during extracorporeal circulation is not recommended. Although PGI$_2$ would preserve platelets during extracorporeal circulation, surface activation of other coagulation components could lead to a tragic thrombotic episode. The primary value of PGI$_2$ during extracorporeal circulation is as an adjunct to anticoagulation with heparin, in order to preserve platelet function after bypass. In spite of adequate anticoagulation, extracorporeal circulation leads to a significant release of platelet-dense granules causing platelet aggregation and consumption.[53, 56] An infusion of PGI$_2$ during bypass prevents dense granule release and preserves platelet function.[53]

Iloprost

During cardiac surgery, a prostacyclin analog called iloprost (ZK36374) has been effectively used.[56–58] Iloprost has a half-life of 15–30 minutes, is ten times more potent than PGI$_2$, and allows a complete return of platelet function once it is metabolized. In addition, iloprost has less of a hypotensive effect than that noted with PGI$_2$. Though iloprost can preserve postbypass platelet activity in the routine open heart surgical patient,[56] its primary clinical value has been the preservation of platelets in patients with heparin-induced thrombocytopenia.[57, 58] Heparin-induced thrombocytopenia is a relatively rare complication of heparin therapy. One to 5 days after initiation of heparin therapy, a sudden, severe drop in the platelet count and the occurrence of thrombotic episodes herald the onset of heparin-induced thrombocytopenia.[59, 60] If one of these patients receives a bolus of heparin prior to bypass, a sudden thrombotic episode secondary to massive platelet aggregation and the appearance of severe postbypass bleeding owing to the loss of platelets might be expected. An iloprost infusion started prior to giving the bolus of heparin effectively prevents the thrombocytopenic response and allows preservation of the patient's platelets throughout the bypass period.[57, 58]

Aspirin

Aspirin or acetylsalicylic acid was first introduced into clinical practice in 1899. Recently, aspirin has been recognized as an effective prophylactic agent to prevent myocardial infarction.[12] The beneficial effect of aspirin in atherosclerotic heart disease seems to be primarily mediated through its platelet-inhibitory action. Aspirin irreversibly inhibits the platelets' ability to release adenosine diphosphate.[11, 14, 61] By inhibiting adenosine diphosphate release, secondary aggregation is prevented. The aspirin-induced inhibition of adenosine diphosphate lasts for the life of the platelet. Therefore, a patient taking aspirin might have a normal platelet count but effectively have no platelet function. In addition, a second role of aspirin in preventing myocardial infarctions is the inhibition of thromboxane A_2 synthesis. Thromboxane A_2, by causing coronary constriction, may induce ischemic episodes that can be prevented by prophylactic pretreatment with aspirin.[11, 12]

For similar reasons, aspirin has been used following coronary artery bypass surgery as a method for improving postoperative graft patency.[62, 63] In spite of aspirin's beneficial effect for patients with ischemic heart disease, its preoperative use in patients without heart disease who are undergoing major surgical procedures may increase their risk for intraoperative hemorrhage.[64] For 5–7 days following a single dose of aspirin, normal platelet function may be compromised, but not all investigators have found that the resultant prolongation of the bleeding time necessarily leads to increased perioperative bleeding.[14] Since aspirin does cross the placental barrier and maternal ingestion of aspirin does induce neonatal hemostatic derangements, use of aspirin during pregnancy should be discouraged.[65]

Coagulants

Epsilon Aminocaproic Acid

Epsilon aminocaproic acid is a synthetic lysine analog that is effective in inhibiting the fibrinolytic system. Its mode of action is the occupation of the lysine binding sites on plasminogen and plasmin, preventing the esteric binding of these molecules with the lysine residues on fibrinogen and fibrin. At serum levels of 13 mg/dl, epsilon aminocaproic acid combines with both plasminogen activator and plasminogen, thereby preventing the formation of active plasmin. At higher serum levels of 130 mg/dl, epsilon aminocaproic acid causes direct inhibition of already formed plasmin. The drug is rapidly excreted by the kidneys, and approximately 80% of an intravenous dose is cleared within 3 hours. Owing to the small size of the molecule, epsilon aminocaproic acid penetrates the entire extravascular space, which slows complete elimination of the drug (total elimination can take 12–36 hours).[66]

The primary clinical indications for the use of epsilon aminocaproic acid include α_2 antiplasmin deficiency, fibrinolytic drug overdoses, and excessive plasminogen activation. Increased accumulation of serum plasmin in the body leads to a state in which adequate clot formation would be impossible. The mechanism for preventing this is a serum protein called α_2 antiplasmin. However, in patients with an inherited or acquired deficiency of α_2 antiplasmin, plasmin levels may be ten times normal. For these patients, epsilon aminocaproic acid effectively reduces the hyperfibrinolytic state and stabilizes the coagulation equilibrium.[67]

Another major use of epsilon aminocaproic acid is the reversal of hyperfibrinolytic states produced by fibrinolytic drugs. Increasingly, fibrinolytic drugs are being used during acute myocardial infarctions as a method for re-establishing coronary perfusion.[67–70] If a patient receives an overdose of an antifibrinolytic drug or requires emergency coronary artery bypass graft surgery,[35] the hyperfibrinolytic state can be controlled with the use of epsilon aminocaproic acid. Hopefully, the more recent use of shorter-acting tissue-type plasminogen activators in patients with evolving myocardial infarctions will decrease the need for pharmacologic intervention to reverse the heightened fibrinolytic state.[71]

More controversial is the use of epsilon aminocaproic acid at times of increased plasminogen activation. Patients with cyanotic congenital heart disease are known to have a heightened fibrinolytic state,[72–74] possibly owing to peripheral stasis and hypoxia leading to low-level activation of coagulation and fibrinolysis. Use of epsilon aminocaproic acid in the patient with cyanotic heart disease effectively corrects the hemostatic defect[72] and reduces perioperative bleeding during open heart surgery.[74] Prophylactic use of epsilon aminocaproic acid has been advocated as a means for reducing bleeding during all cardiopulmonary bypass operations, since an increased fibrinolytic state is frequently found following sternotomy and cardiopulmonary bypass.[75–77] An argument against the routine use of fibrinolytic inhibitors in the postbypass period is that the fibrinolysis is self-limited, lasting only 1–2 hours. More important, use of epsilon aminocaproic acid in patients with disseminated intravascular coagulation eliminates the body's natural defense for recanalization of thrombosed vessels.[78–80]

Another clinical condition in which the routine use of epsilon aminocaproic acid has been suggested is for patients with subarachnoid hemorrhage;[81] however, cerebral thrombosis is a known complication of this intervention.[82] The newest use for epsilon aminocaproic acid is for control of the severe fibrinolytic state occurring during liver transplant surgery.[83, 84] Unfortunately, no medical instrument is presently available that can rapidly and accurately direct the use of epsilon aminocaproic acid for balancing the fibrinolytic system. However, concentrations of fibrinogen and its degradation products can be measured, as described later.

Desmopressin Acetate

Desmopressin acetate is a synthetic vasopressin analog that differs from vasopressin in its lack of vasoactive responsiveness. Clinically, this drug has been used to improve the hemostatic state of patients with mild hemophilia or those with von Willebrand's disease. Although the exact mechanism through which desmopressin acetate works is unclear, the final result is the release of coagulation factor VIII, possibly from endothelial cell walls.[85] Of interest, desmopressin acetate has been used effectively following open heart surgical procedures as a means for decreasing blood loss.[85, 86] Since the usual cause of postoperative bleeding following open heart surgical procedures is platelet abnormalities, the mechanism for improved postoperative hemostasis with desmopressin acetate in these patients is unknown.

TECHNIQUES FOR INTRAOPERATIVE EVALUATION OF COAGULATION

Numerous instruments have been developed for the intraoperative evaluation of hemostasis. When these instruments are compared, specific characteristics that might increase a specific instrument's value include accuracy and usefulness of information provided, simplicity of use, reproducibility of results, compactness of size, quietness in function, quick availability of results, minimum operator's time or attention necessary, use of stable, long-lasting reagents, and cost-effectiveness in price and maintenance.[87]

Heparin Level Devices

Anticoagulation with heparin occurs in two stages. First, following a bolus dose of heparin, heparin is distributed throughout the intravascular space, producing a specific serum level. Second, the serum heparin interacts with antithrombin III to produce anticoagulation. This division of anticoagulation with heparin into these two stages may seem artificial, but, historically, the development of medical instrumentation for its evaluation has been directed along one of these stages. Devices aimed at the evaluation of the heparin level include the automated protamine titration system and the fluorometric substrate analysis system. Heparin effect is evaluated by automated, activated clotting time systems.

Protamine Titration

Protamine sulfate is a low–molecular weight protein extracted from the sperm of salmon and other fish. The strongly basic nature of protamine allows it to combine with the strongly acidic heparin to form a stable salt, thereby reversing the anticoagulant activity of heparin. The development of both manual and automated protamine titration tests is based on two primary characteristics of protamine sulfate. First, 1 mg of protamine sulfate completely neutralizes 100 U of heparin activity.[88] Second, *in vitro* protamine sulfate in excess acts as an anticoagulant and delays clot formation.

The earliest usage of protamine titration for evaluation of anticoagulation was performed by placing a series of test tubes in a 37°C heated block. Increasing concentrations of protamine sulfate were sequentially placed into the test tubes. By adding a specific volume of blood containing the unknown amount of heparin into each of the test tubes and observing which of the test tubes clotted first, a close approximation of heparin level in the unknown blood sample could be made. Test tubes containing excess protamine or excess heparin would be delayed in clot formation, whereas the test tube containing an amount of protamine most closely approximating the level of heparin in the unknown sample would undergo clot formation first. Unfortunately, in spite of the usefulness of this method, the attention of the anesthesiologist was required for adding the samples of protamine and blood as well as for constantly tipping the test tube to assess clot formation. Automation of this technique was a logical step.

Automated Protamine Titration

HemoTec, Inc. (Englewood, CO), has been the leader in the development of an automated system for protamine titration. Their newest system, the Hepcon/System B-10, was designed specifically for the evaluation of heparin level after extracorporeal circulation (Fig. 16–6). In addition to protamine titration, this system allows the evaluation of activated clotting times and the determination of heparin dose-response curves. Protamine titration with the Hepcon/System B-10 is performed by placing 0.8 ml of blood containing an unknown heparin level into four assay chambers containing increasing amounts of protamine in a premade cartridge (Fig. 16–7). Each assay chamber has a small "flag" mechanism attached to a plunger that fits inside the chamber. When a protamine titration is performed, the plunger is raised automatically and allowed to drop inside each chamber, causing the reagents and blood to mix. The plunger's drop rate slows as fibrin formation occurs, and this decrease in drop rate is detected by a photo-optical system.

HemoTec also produces the Hepcon/System A-10 for performance of protamine titrations during open heart surgical procedures. This system uses a disposable cartridge containing four assay chambers with increasing amounts of protamine in each chamber. A series of cartridges can be purchased containing different ranges of protamine levels. The choice of cartridge must be based on the anesthesiologist's expectation of the existing heparin level.

The technical approach used to perform protamine titration with the Hepcon/System A-10 is different than that used with the Hepcon/System B-10. After aliquots of heparinized blood are placed in each of the cartridge's assay chambers, the cartridge is placed within the machine and air is bubbled

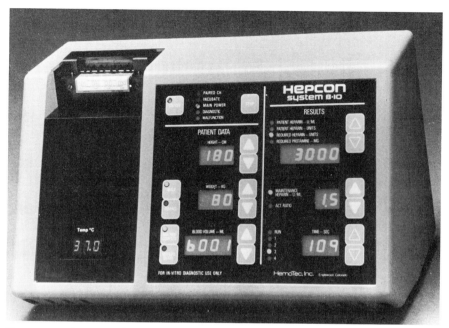

Figure 16–6. The Hepcon/System B-10. The primary purpose of this machine is to perform automated protamine titrations after open heart surgical procedures. When a protamine titration is performed, the amount of heparin within the patient as well as the amount of protamine necessary for reversal is computed based upon the test result and the patient's height and weight, which are entered prior to running the test. Activated clotting times, heparin dose-response curves, prothrombin times, and partial thromboplastin times can also be obtained. (From HemoTec, Inc., Englewood, CO. With permission.)

up through each of the chambers. The top of each assay chamber contains a silicon-coated fiber mesh that debubbles blood rising to the chamber's top while capturing any fibrin and clot. As more clot accumulates in the silicon mesh, the cartridge's blood level slowly falls until a photosensitive cell registers increased light transmission (the endpoint for clot formation) (Fig. 16–8). Based upon the amount of heparin within the assay chamber, the calculated blood volume of the patient using height and weight nomograms, and the pump prime volume (in the case of open heart surgical procedures), the Hepcon/System A-10 internally calculates the expected total amount of heparin within the patient.[89]

Advantages of both systems are simplicity of use, rapidity of results, reliability of information, and ease of intraoperative use. A disadvantage is the cost of the machine, both in initial capital outlay and in individual cartridge usage. Even with refrigeration, reagents within the cartridges outdate in only 60 days, requiring the constant replacement of unused cartridges.

Protamine Dose Assay. A device called a Hemochron Activated Clotting Time machine (described later) can also be used to determine the protamine dosages required to neutralize heparinization in the post–cardiopulmonary bypass period. Special tubes containing 0, 10, 30, and 40 μg of protamine as well as 12 mg of diatomaceous earth are used to conduct a modified protamine titration. On a special graph that plots protamine concentration

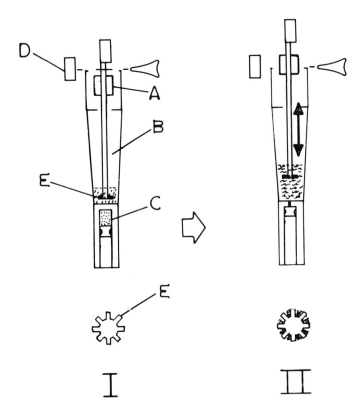

Figure 16–7. The Hepcon/System B-10 utilizes a four-chamber cartridge for evaluating protamine titration. A schematic representation of one of the plunger assay chambers is shown. *I,* An assay chamber is made up of (A) a small flange on the plunger shaft used by the optical system (D) to measure the drop rate of the plunger. In addition, there is a flange disk (E) at the bottom of the plunger shaft. The assay chamber is made up of a reaction chamber (B) containing the blood sample and a reagent chamber (C) containing the protamine. *II,* When a protamine titration is performed, protamine and blood are mixed by the plunger being elevated and dropped. Clot detection occurs when the drop rate of the plunger is slowed to a rate predetermined to indicate clot formation. (From Baugh R: Detection of whole blood coagulation. Am Clin Prod Rev 1984; 3:3. With permission.)

against activated clotting time (ACT), a plot is made of the patient's control ACT (ACT prior to heparinization), ACT at the time the patient is being evaluated ("status ACT"), and the ACT in one of the special tubes (tube chosen based on expected heparin concentration in the patient). Based upon the graph, a relatively accurate determination of the amount of protamine needed for complete heparin reversal can be calculated. An additional correction factor based on the potency of the protamine should also be applied (e.g., the correction factor is 1 if 100 U of heparin is neutralized by 1 mg of protamine). Weak protamines require a greater protamine dose and have a correction factor greater than 1. After the administration of protamine, the ACT is repeated, using a control tube (no protamine) and a tube containing 10 μg protamine. If both tubes demonstrate control ACTs, no additional protamine is necessary. If the ACT is prolonged in both tubes, a coagulopathy or protamine excess may be present. If the tube containing protamine demonstrates an ACT shorter than the control tube, additional protamine is necessary and can be calculated based on the graph described.

Usefulness of Intraoperative Heparin Level Devices

A proposed advantage for protamine titration devices is the ability to continuously and accurately assess heparin levels during cardiopulmonary bypass. However, as anesthesiologists, we must question whether a protamine titration device or any heparin level test provides us with the infor-

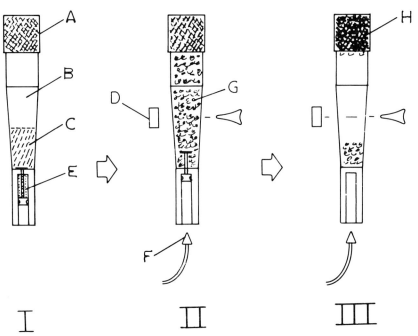

Figure 16–8. Cartridges for the Hepcon/System A-10 are made up of four assay chambers for the evaluation of automated protamine titrations. *I*, A single assay chamber in the cartridge consists of a foam mesh (A) located above a reaction chamber (B) into which the sample of blood is placed (C). Reagents including protamine are located in the reagent chamber (E). *II*, To run a protamine titration, the cartridge is placed within the Hepcon system detector module and air (F) is bubbled through the bottom of the chamber causing the protamine and blood (G) to mix. An optical detection system (D) evaluates light transmission through the chamber. *III*, The foam mesh (H) captures clotted blood, and nonclotted blood is defoamed and returned to the reaction chamber. As clot capture increases, a change in optical transmission signals which of the four assay chambers has undergone clot formation first. On the basis of this information, the amount of heparin in the unknown sample of blood can be estimated. (From Baugh R: Detection of whole blood coagulation. Am Clin Prod Rev 1984; 3:2. With permission.)

mation needed to make decisions throughout the period of open heart surgery. During open heart surgery, assessment of the patient's coagulation status is necessary (1) prior to heparin administration, (2) after heparin administration but before initiation of cardiopulmonary bypass, (3) after heparin administration during hypothermic cardiopulmonary bypass, and (4) immediately before and after reversal of heparin with protamine.

Prior to administration of heparin, protamine titration tests normally provide little information except in the occasional patient in whom either circulating natural heparin-like anticoagulants exist[5] or residual heparin from preoperative therapy is still present. Generally speaking, the protamine titration assay is of little value in assessing overall coagulation. In addition, the use of protamine titration tests for determining adequacy of anticoagulation prior to the initiation of cardiopulmonary bypass can be exceedingly dangerous.[90] In normal patients, serum levels of heparin of 4 u/ml are adequate for anticoagulation. However, the great variability in patients' responses to heparin, especially those patients with acquired or congenital antithrombin III deficiencies, can lead to intraoperative tragedies if the decision to initiate cardiopulmonary bypass is based upon serum heparin levels.[50] Antithrombin III–deficient patients may have serum heparin levels three or four times greater than the normal patient and still not have adequate inhibition of the coagulation cascade. In addition, a combination of patient variability and test variability leads to an overall inherent inaccuracy in protamine titration tests of 26% or more.[90, 91]

Following heparin administration and during hypothermic cardiopulmonary bypass, heparin level tests such as protamine titration are able to provide more accurate information on heparin levels than heparin effect–type tests. Normally, the initiation of cardiopulmonary bypass decreases serum heparin from 3–4 u/ml of blood to 1.5 – 2 u/ml. However, the anesthesiologist should not be concerned with the heparin *level* during hypothermia and hemodilution; rather the concern should be for the anticoagulant effect. As long as fibrin formation is inhibited, the actual heparin level is unimportant.

The major clinical value of an automated protamine titration analysis during open heart surgical procedures is for determining protamine reversal doses and deciding if inadequate heparin reversal is the cause for excessive postoperative bleeding.[87] In addition, protamine titration assays can assist in diagnosing postoperative bleeding secondary to heparin rebound.[92]

Fluorometric Substrate Analysis

Another medical device available for the intraoperative determination of heparin level is the fluorometric substrate analysis test or Protopath system (Dade Division of the American Hospital Supply Corp., Miami, FL).[93] This device allows the accurate intraoperative evaluation of heparin level, but performance of the test requires separation of plasma from the red blood cell fraction. A second instrument called the STATSEP plasma separator (Instrumentation Laboratories, Lexington, MA) allows rapid plasma separation such that both plasma separation and performance of the heparin level analysis can be performed in 5 minutes.[94]

Performance of a Protopath system evaluation depends upon the chemical interaction of heparin, antithrombin III, and thrombin (Fig. 16–9). A sample of plasma with an unknown heparin level is mixed with a diluted pool of normal plasma containing antithrombin III as a means of eliminating test inaccuracies from individual variations in antithrombin III levels. In addition, a known standard aliquot of thrombin is added to this mixture, thereby resulting in the formation of antithrombin III–heparin-thrombin complexes, plus excess thrombin remaining in solution. The amount of excess thrombin is inversely proportional to the amount of heparin in the unknown plasma sample. A thrombin-sensitive fibrinogen analog (D-phenylalanine-proline-arginine-5-amidoisophthalic acid, dimethyl ester, diacetate, or D-Phe-Pro-Arg-AIE) is added to this solution.[95] The excess thrombin remaining in solution enzymatically cleaves the fibrinogen analog and in doing so releases the fluorophore, AIE. Fluorometric analysis of the resulting fluorescence using the Protopath instrument allows a determination

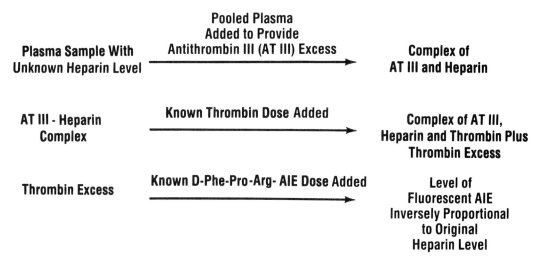

Figure 16–9. The fluorometric substrate analysis of heparin level, or Protopath technique, evaluates heparin level through a sequence of chemical interactions. The end result is the release of a fluorescent molecule in an amount inversely proportional to the original heparin level. Use of calibrated nomograms allows the heparin level to be accurately identified.

of the heparin level. The heparin level is inversely related to the excess thrombin remaining in solution and therefore inversely proportional to the amount of fluorescence. A comparison of fluorescence level with standardized curves allows determination of the heparin level with an accuracy of 0.02–0.05 U/ml.[96]

An advantage of the Protopath technique is that it provides an accurate determination of heparin level unaffected by the presence of intermediate procoagulants, fibrinogen, antithrombin III,[94] or hypothermia.[97] The disadvantages of the Protopath technique include the need to develop standardized curves for each set of fluorometric kits, each type of heparin, and each lot of heparin.[96] In addition, at least daily calibrations of the equipment are necessary in order to ensure continued accuracy. Finally, the meticulous aliquoting of chemicals as well as the strict attention to incubation times and other assay parameters distracts the anesthesiologist from direct patient care functions. Although the Protopath technique has been successfully used intraoperatively for the evaluation of residual heparinization,[94, 97] the primary objection to its routine use during open heart surgery is the same as for any heparin level test.

In spite of its disadvantages for evaluating heparinization, the Protopath assay may be extremely important for the evaluation of intraoperative hemostasis in the future. Through the use of different fluorometric kits, this system can also evaluate other components of coagulation, including plasminogen level[98] and antithrombin III level.[99] As more complete evaluations of intraoperative coagulation become necessary, the versatility and specificity of this system may allow it to have a greater clinical role in the intraoperative evaluation of total hemostasis.

Heparin Effect Devices

Rational conductance of open heart surgical procedures requires evaluation of anticoagulation on the basis of heparin effect rather than heparin level. Owing to heparin's effect on multiple serine proteases in the coagulation cascade, it is not surprising that a variety of heparin effect tests have been proposed and utilized for determination of adequate anticoagulation. Some of these tests include the whole blood clotting time,[87, 100] activated PTT,[95, 100–102] thrombin time,[103] and activated clotting time.[87, 100–102] For the purpose of intraoperative management of anticoagulation, the activated clotting time is the gold standard against which all other heparin effect tests are evaluated. Although the whole blood clotting time provides essentially the same information as the activated clotted time, the excessive time required to get information makes it of little practical value for procedures requiring extracorporeal circulatory techniques. An activated clotting time of 187 seconds corresponds to a whole blood clotting time of 30 minutes or more.[87]

The activated PTT has been advocated as a possible alternative to the activated clotting time for evaluation of heparin anticoagulation. However, interpretation of the results of activated PTTs is more difficult, because the reported results have a nonlinear relationship to the changing heparin blood levels.[100, 102] The nonlinearity of the activated PTT to serum heparin level is particularly striking at the higher levels of heparin necessary for cardiopulmonary bypass. Another disadvantage of the activated PTT is its lack of sensitivity compared with the activated clotting time in the presence of low heparin levels.[104]

The thrombin time has also been presented as a possible alternative to the activated clotting time for assessment of adequate heparinization. The thrombin time can be performed relatively easily, quantitatively, reproducibly, and comparatively rapidly (6–12 minutes).[103] The disadvantages of the thrombin time are a requirement for calibrated equipment and the need for a greater active involvement by the individual running the test.

Activated Clotting Time

Hattersley[105] was the first to describe a method for obtaining consistent reproducible clotting times at a rate much faster than whole blood clotting time by accelerating the clotting process with diatomite. This activated clotting time was found to be faster and more reliable than the Lee-White (whole blood) clotting time, and although it was temperature-sensitive (the sample had to be kept at 37°C), the results were not adversely affected by such variables as differing amounts of diatomaceous earth (4–46 mg), diameters of test tubes used for performing the test (10–20 mm), or volumes of blood used for the test procedure (1–3 ml).[105] Owing to the speed and reliability of the test result, the activated clotting time rapidly gained clinical acceptance; but it was cumbersome to perform in the operating room, since it required the anesthesiologist to constantly tilt tubes in order to assess clot formation.

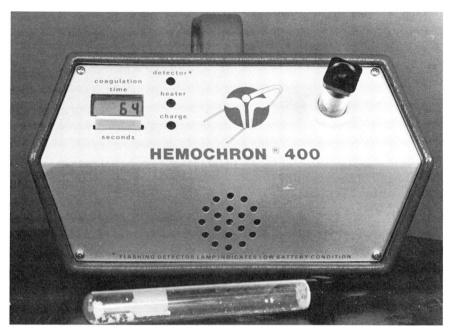

Figure 16–10. The Hemochron 400 System is a simple and reliable automated activated clotting time system. The test tube in the foreground contains diatomite for activation of the intrinsic coagulation pathway and a bar magnet for detection of fibrin formation.

Automation of the activated clotting time was clinically introduced in 1974 in the form of the Hemochron system (International Technidyne Corp., Edison, NJ). Although the automated test results were 10–15 seconds longer than manual methods, the delay was consistent at all levels of anticoagulation and provided excellent correlations with handheld methodology.[106] The Hemochron automated activated clotting system utilizes a disposable test tube containing diatomaceous earth and a bar magnet (Fig. 16–10). The fresh whole blood sample to be tested is immediately placed in the test tube and the tube inserted in the Hemochron machine while the coagulation timer is set to 0 seconds. The Hemochron machine heats the blood sample to 37°C while slowly rotating the test tube. As the test tube turns, the bar magnet retains its position at the bottom of the tube. As clot formation begins, fibrin strands bind the bar magnet, preventing it from maintaining its position at the bottom of the tube. As the magnet is displaced, a magnet sensor circuit is broken, resulting in stoppage of the timer. This automated system of activated clotting time fulfills nearly all the criteria needed in an intraoperative device for the evaluation of heparinization.[50]

HemoTec has also developed a machine for the evaluation of activated clotting times. The HemoTec activated clotting time system uses a disposable cartridge with a noncelite coagulation activator into which an aliquot of blood is placed. The mechanism for assessing clot formation is similar to the automated protamine titration Hepcon/System B-10. A small plunger is raised and dropped inside an assay cartridge, allowing the whole blood and activator to be mixed. Fibrin accumulation on the plunger and in the blood slows the drop rate to a point predetermined to indicate clot formation. The simplicity of use and reliability of information obtained with the HemoTec activated clotting time are similar to the Hemochron activated clotting time. However, the HemoTec device has the additional advantage of allowing the performance of PT, PTT recalcified clotting time, and other coagulation tests, depending upon the choice of cartridge. The versatility of this machine increases its value for the intraoperative evaluation of coagulation.

The primary advantage of the activated clotting time over other heparin effect tests is the constant linear relationship that exists between a plot of the activated clotting time and the milligram-per-kilogram heparin dose for any individual patient. In 1976, Bull and coworkers[102] studied this linear dose-response relationship in the context of anticoagulation for open heart surgery and suggested that a dose-response plot be made for each individual during the heparinization process. The slope of the dose-response plot is different for each patient and depends on such diverse factors as the patient's volume of distribution, antithrombin III level, platelet factor 4 level, and other variables. However, once the plot is formed, it can be used as a guide for providing additional heparin for that patient[102] as well as directing reversal of heparin with protamine after extracorporeal circulation.[107] The plot is produced by charting a baseline activated clotting time (preheparin) followed by a plot of a repeat activated clotting time once the patient is provided a specific milligram-per-kilogram dose of heparin (Fig. 16–11). A line is extended from the baseline point to the heparinized activated clotting time point, and the slope of this plot is specific for the patient receiving heparin.

A normal baseline activated clotting time is in the range of 110–130 seconds, using automated methods. A low baseline activated clotting time should alert the anesthesiologist to the presence of a hypercoagulable state,[108, 109] leading to possible heparin resistance.[110, 111] Initial studies indicated that an activated clotting time between 300 and 600 seconds was usually acceptable for initiation of extracorporeal bypass.[102] In their original paper, Bull and colleagues[36] suggested an optimal clotting time of 480 seconds, although adequate anticoagulation was achieved when the activated clotting time was over 300 seconds. As a result of this publication, heparin protocols based upon timed heparin doses were abandoned, and activated clotting times of over 300 seconds became the criteria for initiation and maintenance of cardiopulmonary bypass. In 1978, Young and coworkers[112] investigated fibrin monomer production (an indication of ongoing coagulation) at varying activated clotting times. They found that an activated clotting time of less than 400 seconds was not adequate, and their study led to the present recommendation that activated clotting times be kept over 400 seconds. Maintenance of an activated clotting time of 480 seconds as originally suggested by Bull[36] may still be optimal, since it provides not only adequate anticoagulation but also a safety margin.

Manufacturers of heparin level medical devices have criticized the use of activated clotting times as inaccurate and unreliable indicators of heparin level during hypothermia[113, 114] and hemodilution.[102, 114] At face value, this criticism is correct. However, it must be emphasized that during hypothermic cardiopulmonary bypass the objective is to provide a stable level of anticoagulation, not a stable heparin level. The activated clotting time during

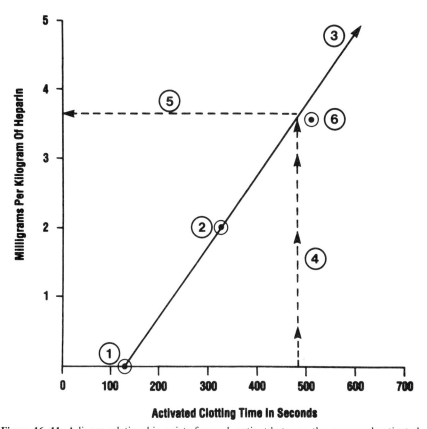

Figure 16–11. A linear relationship exists for each patient between the measured activated clotting time and the milligrams-per-kilogram dose of heparin. This relationship allows the prediction of additional heparin doses during anticoagulation and the amount of protamine necessary for heparin reversal. Generation of a heparin dose-activated clotting time plot is performed by (1) plotting the baseline activated clotting time on a graph of the activated clotting time versus milligrams-per-kilogram dose of heparin, (2) plotting a second activated clotting time performed after giving the patient a milligrams-per-kilogram dose of heparin, and (3) connecting a line between the two plotted points. (4) If a greater level of anticoagulation is desired, a line can be extended from the desired activated clotting time until it intersects the plot line (in the example shown an activated clotting time of 480 is desired). (5) By extending a second line (perpendicular to the ordinate) from the point of intersection, the additional milligrams-per-kilogram dose of heparin can be determined. (6) A repeat activated clotting time should be performed once the additional heparin is given to ensure that the original activated clotting time–milligrams-per-kilogram heparin dose plot was accurate.

both hypothermia and hemodilution continues to serve as an accurate indicator of the overall coagulation state. In addition, Cohen[115] has shown that the activated clotting time–heparin dose plot continues to be linear under hypothermic conditions for activated clotting times below 500 seconds. Therefore, during hypothermia, activated clotting times greater than 500 seconds indicate the presence of more than adequate anticoagulation.

One area in which heparin level tests may have an advantage over the activated clotting time is for determining the adequacy of protamine reversal. Although a heparin dose–activated clotting time plot can be used to determine the protamine reversal dose, difficulty occurs when the activated clotting time does not return to baseline following administration of protamine. In this situation, if a protamine titration device is not available, the typical clinical approach is to provide the patient with an additional dose of protamine and repeat the activated clotting time. If the activated clotting time at that point returns to baseline, the cause for the elevated activated clotting time was excess heparin. On the other hand, if the activated clotting time remains elevated or goes higher, then derangements in the coagulation system should be suspected.

In spite of the activated clotting time's value in evaluating heparinization, its use as an indicator of other hemostatic derangements is poor. Since normal clot formation depends upon only 20–50% of each component of the coagulation system, the activated clotting time does not tell us anything about relative deficiencies of specific coagulation factors. In addition, a total absence of factor VII would go unrecognized, since diatomaceous earth stimulates only the intrinsic pathway. The activated clotting time is also an inadequate indicator of platelet function. Normal activated clotting times can be observed even in the presence of severe thrombocytopenia, although there is evidence that prostacyclin inhibition of platelet function does prolong activated clotting time.[116] Finally, the activated clotting time only provides information on coagulation up to the time of fibrin formation. Coagulation events occurring after fibrin formation, such as clot retraction, cross-linkage (factor XIII), and fibrinolysis, are not evaluated. In spite of the inadequacies of the automated activated clotting time, this test continues to be the most valuable intraoperative medical device for ensuring adequate anticoagulation and avoiding catastrophic thrombotic episodes during cardiac surgery.[117]

Viscokinetic Devices

Medical instrumentation for evaluating anticoagulation was a direct result of the development of extracorporeal circulatory techniques. It is not surprising that recent developments in coagulation-monitoring devices have also been stimulated by the development of new surgical interventions. Recent advances in transplant surgery, particularly liver transplantation, emphasized the need for intraoperative evaluation of the rapidly changing coagulation states of these patients.[83] Heparin-monitoring devices are of little value for these patients, so two new coagulation-monitoring devices have recently been brought into the operating room. These instruments are the Thromboelastograph (Haemoscope Corp., Morton Grove, IL) and the Sonoclot Coagulation Analyzer (Sienco, Inc., Morrison, CO). Both of these machines evaluate viscokinetic changes in blood during the clotting process in order to indicate abnormalities in coagulation.

Thromboelastograph

Although its appearance in the operating room is relatively recent, thromboelastography was developed during World War II[118] and was used

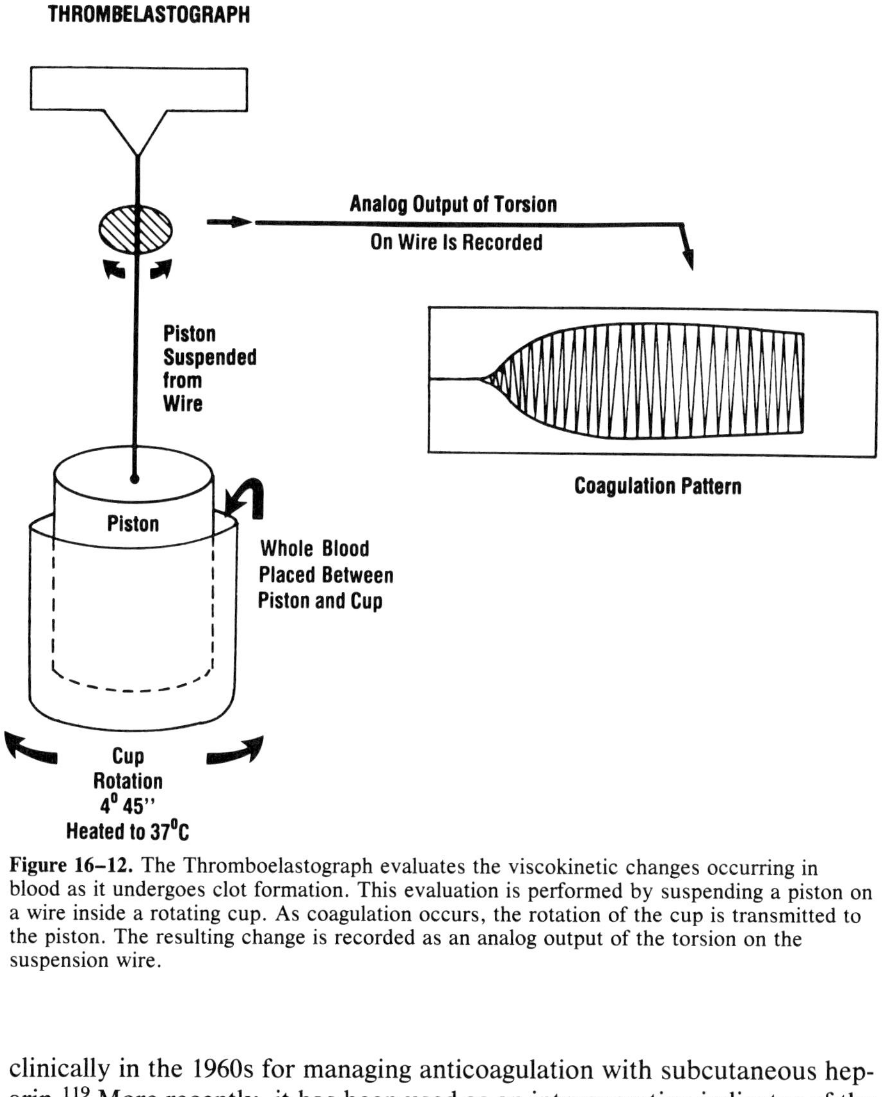

THROMBELASTOGRAPH

Figure 16–12. The Thromboelastograph evaluates the viscokinetic changes occurring in blood as it undergoes clot formation. This evaluation is performed by suspending a piston on a wire inside a rotating cup. As coagulation occurs, the rotation of the cup is transmitted to the piston. The resulting change is recorded as an analog output of the torsion on the suspension wire.

clinically in the 1960s for managing anticoagulation with subcutaneous heparin.[119] More recently, it has been used as an intraoperative indicator of the rapidly changing coagulation state during liver transplant surgery,[83] as an indicator of post–cardiopulmonary bypass coagulopathies,[120, 121] and for the evaluation of coagulation during massive blood loss.[122] The basic principle behind the operation of the Thromboelastograph is the evaluation of changes in blood viscosity as it undergoes coagulation. The core of the machine is a cylindric stainless steel cup into which a blood sample is placed (Fig. 16–12). A piston is suspended into the cup from a wire so that torque placed on the wire is electrically amplified through a recorder-printer. The cup is heated to 37°C and undergoes horizontal, oscillatory rotations of 4°45′ at 9-second intervals.[123] When the blood is in its liquid state, the cup's rotation is not transmitted to the piston and the recorder-printer indicates no deviation. As coagulation begins to occur, the increase in viscosity of the blood as well as the deposition of fibrin strands between the cup and the piston leads to incremental increases in piston deviation, increased

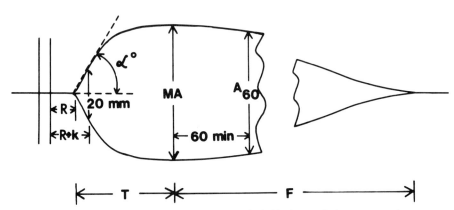

Figure 16–13. The Thromboelastograph generates individual coagulation patterns that are specific for a variety of clotting disorders. The characteristics of a normal coagulation pattern are represented schematically (R = reaction time, R + k = coagulation time, alpha slope = clot formation rate, MA = maximum amplitude, A_{60} = amplitude 60 minutes after MA, T = whole blood clotting time, F = whole blood lysis time). (Reprinted with permission from the International Anesthesia Research Society from Intraoperative changes in blood coagulation and thromboelastographic monitoring in liver transplantation by Kang YG, Martin DJ, Marquez J, et al., Anesthesia and Analgesia, 1985; 64:891.)

torque on the suspension wire, and recording of the changing viscokinetic pattern of blood.[123]

A representative example of the Thromboelastograph pattern generated during normal coagulation is shown in Figure 16–13. The R time (reaction time) corresponds to the time between the taking of the sample of blood and the occurrence of the first oscillatory movements. In a patient with normal coagulation, this is usually between 6 and 8 minutes. The k time is the period between onset of clot formation and a point at which the oscillatory amplitude is 20 mm. The combination of R and k times gives a value called the coagulation time, which is normally between 10 and 12 minutes. The angle generated by the slope of the line drawn between the time oscillatory movement first begins and the clot formation rate is designated the alpha angle, which is normally greater than 50°. The maximum amplitude (MA) is the point of greatest oscillatory deviation and is normally between 50 and 70 mm. Finally, the amplitude of oscillation 60 minutes after the MA is called the A_{60}. A whole blood clot lysis index indicating the rate of fibrinolysis can be calculated by dividing the A_{60} by the product of the MA and 100. Normally, this value is greater than 85% and decreases in the presence of active fibrinolysis.[83] Another indicator of fibrinolysis is the time following the MA for clot dissolution to occur, and this is called the F time, which is usually greater than 300 minutes. All values discussed are for nonactivated Thromboelastograph evaluations. Parameters of coagulation may be obtained more rapidly with the use of coagulation activators.

The advantage of the Thromboelastograph compared with heparin-monitoring instruments is that more information is obtained concerning clot integrity, including rate of formation, strength, and long-term stability.[124] In addition, indirect evidence is obtained concerning coagulation factor levels, platelet integrity, and the occurrence of fibrinolysis. Clinical decision making for liver transplant patients based on the Thromboelastograph has been successful in reducing both blood and coagulation factor transfusions.[83] The Thromboelastograph R time has been found to have a positive correlation with the activated PTT, and the MA correlates with both the functional platelet count and the fibrinogen level. In addition, the whole blood lysis time (F) is positively correlated with the euglobulin lysis time (ELT).[83]

Aside from liver transplant surgery, the Thromboelastograph has been used to monitor both the hypercoagulable and the fibrinolytic states after thrombotic episodes[119] and during the postpartum period.[125] Use of the Thromboelastograph for assessment of heparinization prior to open heart surgery is questionable, but it has been used to assess postbypass coagulopathies.[120, 121] Its major value has been for the direction of epsilon aminocaproic acid and blood component therapy for liver transplantation patients.[83, 84] Future uses of the Thromboelastograph may well include monitoring plasminogen activator therapy for patients with acute myocardial infarction[34, 126] and the resultant fibrinolytic state during emergency myocardial revascularization.[35]

Sonoclot

The Sonoclot system evaluates the viscokinetic changes occurring during clot formation and provides information similar to that obtained with the Thromboelastograph. The Sonoclot system was developed in response to perceived disadvantages of the early Thromboelastograph system, including nonportability, lack of ruggedness, complexity of use, and lack of computerization.[127] The Sonoclot analyzer records the changing mechanical impedance of clotting blood against a vibrating, oscillating probe. The probe has an oscillatory amplitude less than 1 μ and an oscillatory frequency of less than 200 Hz, and the sample of blood is warmed to 37°C (Fig. 16–14).[128] As the blood undergoes coagulation, a record of the changing mechanical impedance is converted to an analog output and recorded on a chart.[129] The resultant pattern or "signature" resembles one half of the Thromboelastograph pattern (Fig. 16–15). The T_1 time, or onset of clot formation time (normal 80–130 seconds in the activated cuvette), corresponds to the Thromboelastograph R time. The Sonoclot rate of coagulation slope (normal 15–30 U/minute) corresponds to the Thromboelastograph alpha slope. One difference in the Sonoclot signature is the presence of an inflection or hump on the upward slope indicating initial platelet activation and the presence of a peak and downward slope (normal greater than 2 U/minute) indicating clot retraction. Both the Thromboelastograph and the Sonoclot require the recognition of characteristic clotting patterns in order to identify the coagulation disorders.

The Sonoclot analyzer has been proposed as an effective instrument for the qualitative evaluation of platelet function.[129] In the presence of either thrombocytopenia or dysfunctional platelets, changes in the Sonoclot signature include a lag in the coagulation onset time, a decrease in slope (rate), loss of the upward slope inflection (thought to correspond to initial platelet-induced contraction of fibrin strands), and dampening of the primary peak as well as the resultant downslope (from platelet-mediated clot contraction).

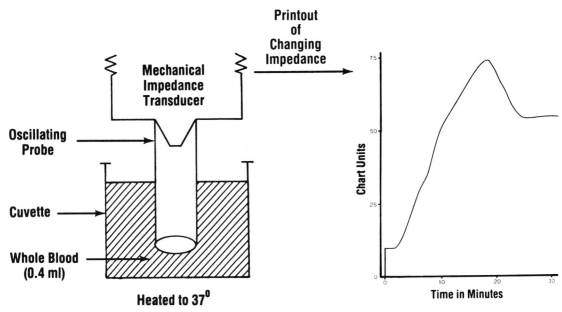

Figure 16-14. The Sonoclot coagulation analyzer evaluates the viscokinetic changes in blood as it undergoes coagulation through the use of an oscillating probe. A mechanical impedance transducer translates the changing impedance into a pattern (signature) of the blood as it undergoes clot formation.

As with the Thromboelastograph, the Sonoclot pattern does not indicate the exact cause of a coagulation abnormality. Delays in onset time, depression of the upward slope, and dampening of the inflection occur with decreased levels of factors II, V, VIII, IX, X, and XI.[129] These changes also occur in the presence of heparin. Clinically, the Sonoclot analyzer has been used for predicting patients at increased risk for thromboembolic episodes following surgery[130] and for evaluating coagulation during hypothermic cardiopulmonary bypass.[131] As a way of increasing the versatility, specificity, and usefulness of the Sonoclot, additional cuvettes to evaluate activated clotting time, heparin level, and other coagulation parameters are being prepared.

Other Tests

Although the results are not usually immediately available, intraoperative determinations of PT, PTT, and fibrinogen are helpful in the management of patients receiving massive transfusions or undergoing hepatic transplantation or who have disseminated intravascular coagulation or have received thrombolytic therapy. The HemoTec automated system for PT and PTT makes these tests more readily available in the operating room.

PTT

The PTT measures coagulation in the intrinsic system and final common pathway. Heparin effect is easily demonstrated. Citrated blood is centrifuged and the plasma added to tubes containing calcium and partial thromboplastin

Figure 16–15. The Sonoclot signature is generated by the changing impedance on a vibrating probe placed in blood as it undergoes coagulation. The *initiation time* corresponds to the time the probe is immersed in the blood sample. The *onset time* indicates the initial formation of fibrin. *Upsloping rates* correspond to the rate of fibrin formation and platelet activation. The *inflection* seen on the upslope is a function of both platelet aggregation and contraction of the first fibrin strands. The *peak* corresponds to completion of fibrin formation, and the *downsloping rate* is produced by platelet-induced contraction of the fibrin clot. (Modified from Sienco, Inc., product literature.)

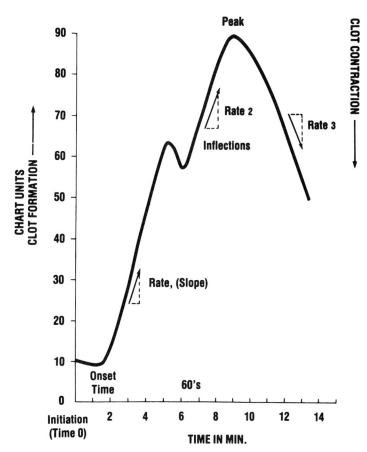

reagent. After incubation for 30 seconds, the tube is tilted until clotting occurs (normally in 73–84 seconds). A "partial" thromboplastin cannot compensate for deficiencies of factors VIII, IX, X, XI, and XII, resulting in prolonged values. Activation with kaolin or diatomaceous earth shortens the PTT.

PT

A "complete" thromboplastin is used in determining the PT. The one-stage method of Quick is used to determine defects in the extrinsic system. In this test, the plasma obtained from centrifugation of citrated blood is added to calcium, and thromboplastin and clotting time are determined. Reference values are 11–15 seconds, or the value may be given as a percentage of control.

Fibrinogen

Fibrinogen is converted to fibrin, which is measured using a standard biochemical protein assay. Normal values are 170–370 mg/dl. The presence of fibrinolysis (spontaneous lysis of clot normally occurs over 24–48 hours) caused by thrombolytic agents or endogenously in primary or secondary fibrinolysis is determined using the ELT. The ELT is significantly shortened when fibrinolytic activity is present. Latex agglutination tests detect fibrinogen degradation product fragments D and E.

SPECIAL CONCERNS IN COAGULATION MONITORING

Massive Blood Loss—Liver Transplant Surgery

Recent advances in the development of devices for the intraoperative evaluation of coagulation have been a direct result of the need to monitor the severe coagulation derangements occurring during liver transplant surgery.[83, 84] The combination of a need for massive blood component therapy during these operative procedures and the recent recommendations concerning curtailment and caution in blood component usage[132] emphasizes the necessity for having an accurate method to assess coagulation. Most of the recent interest in avoidance of homologous blood product transfusion has arisen from the fear of acquired immunodeficiency syndrome (AIDS) virus.[133, 134] This fear may not be entirely rational, since the incidence of AIDS virus in donor blood with the use of newer screening techniques is extremely rare. However, recipients of blood provided by an AIDS virus–positive donor have a 70% or greater risk of becoming seropositive for this disease.[135] In addition, avoidance of homologous blood products decreases the transmission of hepatitis, malaria, and cytomegalovirus as well as the risk of alloimmunization reactions.[134]

The patient undergoing a liver transplant is of particular interest for coagulation monitoring owing to the wide range of coagulation derangements occurring during the perioperative period. These patients frequently come to the operating room with coagulation defects due to the inadequate generation of liver-dependent coagulation factors and to deficiencies in platelet activity from both endogenous abnormalities and preoperative medications. During the operative procedure, major swings in fibrinolysis, platelet activity, and coagulation factor levels also occur, necessitating intervention for normalization of the coagulation process. Overstimulation of the fibrinolytic system can become a major problem, owing to increases in serum tissue plasminogen activator levels during dissection and removal of the diseased liver.

Aside from the coagulation problems directly associated with the diseased liver, a major problem during liver transplant surgery is massive blood loss.[83] Previous studies have defined massive blood loss as the loss of one to one and one-half times a patient's blood volume.[136, 137] However, during the course of liver transplant procedures, the patient may have his or her estimated blood volume replaced 12 or more times. Problems associated with massive transfusion encompass a variety of metabolic abnormalities including increased serum potassium, free hemoglobin, and pH[136, 138, 139] and decreased 2,3-diphosphoglycerate and ionized calcium. Platelets and coagulation factors decrease during massive transfusions. Platelet counts decrease more slowly than expected, owing to maintenance of platelet levels through release of splenic and bone marrow reserves.[137] However, in some patients a single estimated blood volume exchange decreases platelet count well below 50,000/μl.[140] Depletions of the labile clotting factors, particularly factors V and VIII, also occur during massive transfusion.[136]

Autologous Blood Use and Intraoperative Salvage

Autotransfusion

In conjunction with the recommendations for decreased use of homologous red blood cell and component therapy,[132] a resurgence in preoperative collection of autologous blood and intraoperative salvage of blood from the surgical field has occurred. The collection of autologous blood preoperatively, as a method of supplying blood for surgery when major blood losses are expected, is not new.[141–143] Normal, healthy volunteers with phlebotomies of 3–5 U of blood/week for as many as 23 weeks can maintain a stable hemoglobin by using intravenous iron dextran supplementation to increase erythropoiesis.[144] In nonhealthy patients, preoperative phlebotomy of up to 4 U of blood (1 U every 48 hours) during the 10 days prior to a scheduled surgical procedure has been performed with resultant hematocrits of over 30% when iron dextran is provided.[145] Use of autologous blood not only avoids the risks associated with homologous blood transfusion but also has the advantage of being richer in 2,3-diphosphoglycerate, platelets, and labile clotting factors.[146] The fresher the blood, the greater the amount of available clotting factors V and VIII. One method of autologous blood use is removal of blood immediately prior to the surgical procedure through the use of hemodilution techniques.[141, 142, 146, 147] By reinfusing the freshly taken blood during the surgical procedure, total blood loss can be decreased 25–95%.[141, 142, 146]

Intraoperative salvage techniques aimed at saving blood lost during the surgical procedure have also decreased the need for homologous blood transfusions. Intraoperative blood salvage dates back to the late 1800s,[134] but it was not until the Vietnam War that a device was developed specifically for the rapid intraoperative autotransfusion of lost blood (Bentley Laboratories, Inc., Santa Ana, CA). The Bentley autotransfusion machine was a simple device consisting of a roller-head pump attached to tubing leading from the surgical field. Blood was aspirated from the surgical field into a reservoir, where it was defoamed and filtered prior to reinfusion back to the patient.[134, 148, 149] With this technique, patients had as much as 40 L of blood reinfused during the course of a surgical procedure. A disadvantage of this system was the requirement for anticoagulation, of either the scavenged blood or the patient. Another major disadvantage was the risk for inadvertent infusion of large air emboli during the course of blood reinfusion. These difficulties led to the elimination of the Bentley system as a modern method for autotransfusion.

The Bentley system was superseded by devices for rapid red blood cell washing and reinfusion of scavenged blood[149] including commercially available devices from Haemonetics Corp., Braintree, MA, and Electromedics, Englewood, CO. The early cell washing systems required a long duration between the wash cycles and reinfusion, but with the newer systems, reinfusion can be accomplished in as little as 3 minutes. The washing process accomplishes the removal of non–red blood cell debris suctioned from the surgical field; also removed are activated clotting factors, free hemoglobin, pharmaceutic agents including heparin, and normal clotting factors. Unfortunately, bacteria, cancer cells,[134] and microfibrillar collagen hemostat[150] are not removed with the washing cycles. Although the scavenging systems do allow return of red blood cells, the blood reinfused is depleted of platelets and coagulation factors. Therefore, increased usage of these devices necessitates improved intraoperative coagulation-monitoring devices to evaluate whether coagulation component infusions are required.

Blood Substitutes

Artificial blood substitutes have also been evaluated as possible methods for avoiding homologous blood transfusions. The primary blood substitute investigated is Fluosol-DA, but the clinical application of this product is extremely limited.[151] These agents improve only the oxygen-carrying capacity while they dilute serum coagulation factors. Under these circumstances, constant evaluation of the integrity of the coagulation system is necessary.

FUTURE DEVELOPMENTS

The need for specific, reliable, and rapid intraoperative evaluation of all components leading to hemostasis will increase in the coming years. Pharmacologic advancements in the development of medications that inhibit and promote various components of hemostasis continue to occur. In addition, the development of new transplant surgical techniques as well as other therapeutic modalities will necessitate an accurate evaluation of the hemostatic state as a method of guiding therapeutic intervention.

Future development of medical instrumentation for the evaluation of intraoperative hemostasis will most likely occur along two lines. First, present medical instrumentation will be refined and expanded to allow more specific and accurate evaluations of particular components of the hemostatic system. This is already being seen in the expansion of the HemoTec activated clotting time machine and the Sonoclot viscokinetic analyzer. The use of specifically prepared cuvettes or cartridges will allow the evaluation of specific components of the coagulation system as well as other factors involved in the hemostatic process. The second major route in the development of coagulation monitoring devices will be immunobiologic assays. The expansion of monoclonal antibody research will most likely lead to the development of simple immunobiologic assays that can rapidly, specifically, and accurately evaluate derangements in coagulation. As the cost of monoclonal antibody production decreases and the intraoperative need for such specific evaluation increases, availability of such assays should increase. However, in spite of expected advances in the intraoperative evaluation of hemostasis, maintaining the intricate balance of all hemostatic factors remains a challenge.

References

1. Ellison N: What the anesthesiologist should know about coagulation. International Anesthesia Research Society Review Course Lectures. Cleveland: International Anesthesia Research Society, 1986; 127–132.
2. Hoffman WS, Tomasello DN, MacVaugh H: Control of postcardiotomy bleeding with PEEP. Ann Thorac Surg 1982; 34:71–73.
3. Thompson GE, Miller RD, Stevens WC, Murray WR: Hypotensive anesthesia for total hip arthroplasty: A study of blood loss and organ function (brain, heart, liver, and kidney). Anesthesiology 1978; 48:91–96.
4. Lawson NW, Thompson DS, Nelson CL, et al: Sodium nitroprusside–induced hypotension for supine total hip replacement. Anesth Analg 1976; 55:654–662.
5. Ellison N: Diagnosis and management of bleeding disorders. Anesthesiology 1977; 47:171–180.
6. Rizza CR: Coagulation factor therapy. Clinics in Haematology 1976; 5:113–133.
7. Richard LC, Buller HR, Bovill J, Ten Cate JW: Influence of anaesthesia on coagulation and fibrinolytic proteins. Br J Anaesth 1983; 55:869–872.
8. Barrier MJ, Ellison N: Platelet function. Anesthesiology 1977;46:202–211.
9. Mustard JF: Anesthetics and platelets. (Editorial.) Anesthesiology 1971; 34:401–402.
10. Davies MJ, Thomas A: Thrombosis and acute coronary-artery lesions in sudden cardiac ischemic death. N Engl J Med 1984; 310:1137–1140.
11. Weksler BB, Pett SB, Alonso D, et al: Differential inhibition by aspirin of vascular and platelet prostaglandin synthesis in atherosclerotic patients. N Engl J Med 1983; 308:800–805.
12. Cairns JA, Gent M, Singer J, et al: Aspirin, sulfinpyrazone, or both in unstable angina. N Engl J Med 1985; 313:1369–1375.
13. Harker LA, Slichter SJ: The bleeding time as a screening test for evaluation of platelet function. N Engl J Med 1972; 287:155–159.
14. Amrein PC, Ellman L, Harris WH: Aspirin-induced prolongation of bleeding time and perioperative blood loss. JAMA 1981; 245:1825–1828.
15. Hindman BJ, Koka BV: Usefulness of the post-aspirin bleeding time. Anesthesiology 1986; 64:368–370.
16. Hicks GL, Jensen LA, Norsen LH, et al: Platelet inhibitors and hydroxyethyl starch: Safe and cost-effective interventions in coronary artery surgery. Ann Thorac Surg 1985; 39:422–425.
17. Lichtenfeld KM, Schiffer CA, Helrich M: Platelet aggregation during and after general anesthesia and surgery. Anesth Analg 1979; 59:293–296.
18. Dalsgaard-Nielsen J, Risbo A, Simmelkjaer P, Gormsen J: Impaired platelet

aggregation and increased bleeding time during general anaesthesia with halothane. Br J Anaesth 1981; 53:1039–1041.

19. Walter F, Vulliemoz Y, Verosky M, Triner L: Effects of halothane on the cyclic 3',5'-adenosine monophosphate enzyme system in human platelets. Anesth Analg 1980; 59:856–861.

20. Fauss BG, Meadows JC, Bruni CY, Qureshi GD: The *in vitro* and *in vivo* effects of isoflurane and nitrous oxide on platelet aggregation. Anesth Analg 1986; 65:1170–1174.

21. Ueda I: The effects of volatile general anesthetics on adenosine diphosphate-induced platelet aggregation. Anesthesiology 1971; 34:405–408.

22. Kazmier FJ: Thromboembolism, coumarin necrosis, and protein C. Mayo Clin Proc 1985; 60:673–674.

23. Clouse LH, Comp PC: The regulation of hemostasis: The protein C system. N Engl J Med 1986; 314:1298–1304.

24. Knobl PN, Zilla P, Fasol R, et al: The protein C system in patients undergoing cardiopulmonary bypass. J Thorac Cardiovasc Surg 1987; 94:600–605.

25. Griffin JH, Evatt B, Zimmerman TS, et al: Deficiency of protein C in congenital thrombotic disease. J Clin Invest 1981; 68:1370–1373.

26. Broekmans AW, van der Linden IK, VeltKamp JJ, Bertina RM: Prevalence of isolated protein C deficiency in patients with venous thrombotic disease and in the population. (Abstract.) Thromb Haemost 1983; 50:350.

27. Pabinger-Fasching I, Bertina RM, Lechner K, et al: Protein C deficiency in two Austrian families. Thromb Haemost 1983; 50:810–813.

28. Miletich J, Sherman L, Broze G Jr: Absence of thrombosis in subjects with heterozygous protein C deficiency. N Engl J Med 1987; 317:991–996.

29. Fitzgerald DJ, Roy L, Catella F, FitzGerald GA: Platelet activation in unstable coronary disease. N Engl J Med 1986; 315:983–998.

30. Jaffe AS, Sobel BE: Thrombolysis with tissue-type plasminogen activator in acute myocardial infarction. JAMA 1986; 255:237–239.

31. Laffel GL, Braunwald E: Thrombolytic therapy: A new strategy for the treatment of acute myocardial infarction. N Engl J Med 1984; 311:710–717.

32. ISAM Study Group: A prospective trial of intravenous streptokinase in acute myocardial infarction (I.S.A.M.). N Engl J Med 1986; 314:1465–1471.

33. Kennedy JW, Ritchie JL, Davis KB, et al: The western Washington randomized trial of intracoronary streptokinase in acute myocardial infarction. A 12-month follow-up report. N Engl J Med 1985; 312:1073–1078.

34. Cowley MJ, Hastillo A, Vetrovec GW, et al: Fibrinolytic effects of intracoronary streptokinase administration in patients with acute myocardial infarction and coronary insufficiency. Circulation 1983; 67:1031–1038.

35. Goldberg M, Colonna-Romano P, Babins NA: Emergency coronary artery bypass surgery following intracoronary streptokinase. Anesthesiology 1984; 61:601–604.

36. Bull BS, Korpman RA, Huse WM, Briggs BD: Heparin therapy during extracorporeal circulation. I. Problems inherent in existing heparin protocols. J Thorac Cardiovasc Surg 1975; 69:674–684.

37. McLean J: The thromboplastic action of cephalin. Am J Physiol 1916; 16:250–207.

38. Salzman EW: Low-molecular-weight heparin. Is small beautiful? N Engl J Med 1986; 315:957–959.

39. Lam LH, Silbert JE, Rosenberg RD: The separation of active and inactive forms of heparin. Biochem Biophys Res Commun 1976; 69:570–577.

40. Rosenberg RD, Lam L: Correlation between structure and function of heparin (mucopolysaccharide/anticoagulant function). Proc Natl Acad Sci USA 1979; 76:1218–1222.

41. Novak E, Sekhar NC, Dunham NW, Coleman LL: A comparative study of the effect of lung and gut heparins on platelet aggregation and protamine neutralization in man. Clinical Medicine 1972; July:22–27.
42. Estes JW, Poulin PF: Pharmacokinetics of heparin. Thromb Diath Haemorrh 1974; 33:26–37.
43. Jick H, Slone D, Borda IT, Shapiro S: Efficacy and toxicity of heparin in relation to age and sex. N Engl J Med 1968; 279:284–286.
44. Blauhut B, Nacek S, Kramar H, et al: Activity of antithrombin III and effect of heparin on coagulation in shock. Thromb Res 1980; 19:775–782.
45. Cloyd GM, D'Ambra MN, Akins CW: Diminished anticoagulant response to heparin in patients undergoing coronary artery bypass grafting. J Thorac Cardiovasc Surg 1987; 94:535–538.
46. Perry MO, Horton J: Kinetics of heparin administration. Arch Surg 1976; 111:403–409.
47. Anderson EF: Heparin resistance prior to cardiopulmonary bypass. Anesthesiology 1986; 64:504–507.
48. Palmer NR, Rick ME, Rick PD, et al: Circulating heparin sulfate anticoagulant in a patient with a fatal bleeding disorder. N Engl J Med 1984; 310:1696–1699.
49. Ellison N: Heparin: New information on an old drug. (Editorial.) J Cardiothorac Anesth 1987; 1:377–378.
50. Rosenberg RD: Actions and interactions of antithrombin and heparin. N Engl J Med 1975; 292:146–151.
51. Gorman RR: Modulation of human platelet function by prostacyclin and thromboxane A_2. Federation Proceedings 1979; 38:83–88.
52. Coppe D, Wonders T, Snider M, Salzman EW: Preservation of platelet number and function during extracorporeal membrane oxygenation by regional infusion of prostacyclin. *In* Vane JR, Bergstrom S (eds): Prostacyclin. New York: Raven, 1979; 371–383.
53. Malpass TW, Hanson SR, Savage B, et al: Prevention of acquired transient defect in platelet plug formation by infused prostacyclin. Blood 1981; 57:736–740.
54. Zusman RM, Rubin RH, Cato AE, et al: Hemodialysis using prostacyclin instead of heparin as the sole antithrombotic agent. N Engl J Med 1981; 304:934–939.
55. Woods HF, Ash G, Weston MJ, et al: Prostacyclin can replace heparin in haemodialysis in dogs. Lancet 1978; 2:1075–1077.
56. Kappa JR, Horn MK III, Fisher CA, et al: Efficacy of iloprost (ZK36374) versus aspirin in preventing heparin-induced platelet activation during cardiac operations. J Thorac Cardiovasc Surg 1987; 94:405–413.
57. Ellison N, Kappa JR, Fisher CA, Addonizio VP Jr: Extracorporeal circulation in a patient with heparin-induced thrombocytopenia. Anesthesiology 1985; 63:336–337.
58. Kappa JR, Ellison N, Fisher CA, Addonizio VP: The use of iloprost (ZK36374) to permit cardiopulmonary bypass in 2 patients with heparin-induced thrombocytopenia. (Abstract.) Anesthesiology 1985; 63:A32.
59. Smith JP, Walls JT, Muscato MS, et al: Extracorporeal circulation in a patient with heparin-induced thrombocytopenia. Anesthesiology 1985; 62:363–365.
60. Bell WR, Tomasulo PA, Alving BM, Duffy TP: Thrombocytopenia occurring during the administration of heparin. Ann Intern Med 1976; 85:155–160.
61. Weiss HJ, Aledort LM, Kochwa S: The effect of salicylates on the hemostatic properties of platelets in man. J Clin Invest 1968; 47:2169–2180.
62. Chesebro JH, Clements IP, Fuster V, et al: A platelet-inhibitor-drug trial in coronary-artery bypass operations. Benefit of perioperative dipyridamole and

aspirin therapy on early postoperative vein-graft patency. N Engl J Med 1982; 307:73–78.

63. Chesebro JH, Fuster V, Elveback LR, et al: Effect of dipyridamole and aspirin on late vein-graft patency after coronary bypass operations. N Engl J Med 1984; 310:209–214.

64. Rubin RN: Aspirin and postsurgery bleeding. Ann Intern Med 1978; 89:1006.

65. Stuart MJ, Gross SJ, Elrad H, Graeber JE: Effects of acetylsalicylic-acid ingestion on maternal and neonatal hemostasis. N Engl J Med 1982; 307:909–912.

66. McNicol GP, Fletcher AP, Alkaersig N, Sherry S: The absorption, distribution, and excretion of epsilon-aminocaproic acid following oral or intravenous administration to man. J Lab Clin Med 1962; 59:15–24.

67. Aoki N, Sakata Y, Matsuda M, Tateno K: Fibrinolytic states in a patient with congenital deficiency of $alpha_2$-plasmin inhibitor. Blood 1980; 55:483–488.

68. Kennedy JW, Ritchie JL, Davis KB, Fritz JK: Western Washington randomized trial of intracoronary streptokinase in acute myocardial infarction. N Engl J Med 1983; 309:1477–1482.

69. Markis JE, Malagold M, Parker JA, et al: Myocardial salvage after intracoronary thrombolysis with streptokinase in acute myocardial infarction. Assessment by intracoronary thallium-201. N Engl J Med 1981; 305;777–782.

70. Khaja F, Walton JA, Brymer JF, et al: Intracoronary fibrinolytic therapy in acute myocardial infarction. Report of a prospective randomized trial. N Engl J Med 1983; 308:1306–1318.

71. Van der werf F, Ludbrook PA, Bergmann SR, et al: Coronary thrombolysis with tissue-type plasminogen activator in patients with evolving myocardial infarction. N Engl J Med 1984; 310:609–614.

72. Gralnick HR: Aminocaproic acid in preoperative correction of haemostatic defect in cyanotic congenital heart disease. Lancet 1970; 2:1204–1205.

73. Brodsky I, Gill DN, Lusch CJ: Fibrinolysis in congenital heart disease. Preoperative treatment with aminocaproic acid. Am J Clin Pathol 1969; 51:51–57.

74. McClure PD, Izsak J: the use of epsilon-aminocaproic acid to reduce bleeding during cardiac bypass in children with congenital heart disease. Anesthesiology 1974; 40:604–608.

75. Midell AI, Hallman GL, Bloodwell RD, et al: Epsilon-aminocaproic acid for bleeding after cardiopulmonary bypass. Ann Thorac Surg 1971; 11:577–582.

76. Lambert CJ, Marengo-Rowe AJ, Leveson JE, et al: The treatment of postperfusion bleeding using aminocaproic acid, cryoprecipitate, fresh-frozen plasma, and protamine sulfate. Ann Thorac Surg 1979; 28:440–441.

77. Sterns LP, Lillehei CW: Effect of epsilon aminocaproic acid upon blood loss following open-heart surgery: An analysis of 340 patients. Can J Surg 1967; 10:304–307.

78. Naeye RL: Thrombotic state after a hemorrhagic diathesis, a possible complication of therapy with epsilon-aminocaproic acid. Blood 1962; 19:694–701.

79. Charytan C, Purtilo D: Glomerular capillary thrombosis and acute renal failure after epsilon aminocaproic acid therapy. N Engl J Med 1969; 280:1102–1104.

80. Gibbon JH, Camishion RC: Problems with hemostasis with extracorporeal apparatus. Ann NY Acad Sci 1964; 115:195–198.

81. Adams HP, Nibbelink DW, Torner JC, Sahs AL: Antifibrinolytic therapy in patients with aneurysmal subarachnoid hemorrhage. A report of the cooperative aneurysm study. Arch Neurol 1981; 38:25–29.

82. Hoffman EP, Koo AH: Cerebral thrombosis associated with amicar therapy. Radiology 1979; 131:687–689.

83. Kang YG, Martin DJ, Marquez J, et al: Intraoperative changes in blood co-

agulation and thromboelastographic monitoring in liver transplantation. Anesth Analg 1985; 64:888–896.

84. Kang YG, Navalgund A, Russell M, Starzl TE: Antifibrinolytic therapy during liver transplantation. Anesthesiology 1985; 63:A92.

85. Salzman EW, Weinstein MJ, Weintraub RM, et al: Treatment with desmopressin acetate to reduce blood loss after cardiac surgery. A double-blind randomized trial. N Engl J Med 1986; 314:1402–1406.

86. Czer L, Bateman T, Gran R, et al: Prospective trial of DDAVP in treatment of severe platelet dysfunction and hemorrhage after cardiopulmonary bypass. Circulation 1985; 72 (Suppl 3):III130.

87. Jobes DR, Schwartz AJ, Ellison N, et al: Monitoring heparin anticoagulation and its neutralization. Ann Thorac Surg 1981; 31:161–166.

88. Chargaff E, Olson KB: Studies on the chemistry of blood coagulation. Studies on the action of heparin and other anticoagulants. The influence of protamine on the anticoagulant effect in vivo. J Biol Chem 1937; 122:153–167.

89. Hill AG, Lefrak EA: Monitoring heparin and protamine therapy during cardiopulmonary bypass procedures. Pro Am Sect 1978; 6:10–13.

90. Bull MH, Huse WM, Bull BS: Evaluation of tests used to monitor heparin therapy during extracorporeal circulation. Anesthesiology 1975; 43:346–353.

91. Gravlee GP, Brauer SD, Roy RC, et al: Predicting the pharmacodynamics of heparin: A clinical evaluation of the Hepcon System 4. J Cardiothorac Anesth 1987; 1:379–387.

92. Pifarre R, Babka R, Sullivan HJ, et al: Management of postoperative heparin rebound following cardiopulmonary bypass. J Thorac Cardiovasc Surg 1981; 81:378–381.

93. Mitchell GA, Gargiulo RJ, Huseby RM, et al: Assay for plasma heparin using a synthetic peptide substrate for thrombin. Thromb Res 1978; 13:47–52.

94. Umlas J, Taff RH, Gauvin G, Swierk P: Anticoagulant monitoring and neutralization during open heart surgery—a rapid method for measuring heparin and calculating safe reduced protamine doses. Anesth Analg 1983; 62:1095–1099.

95. Choo IHF, Didisheim P, Doerge ML, et al: Evaluation of a heparin assay method using a fluorogenic synthetic peptide substrate for thrombin. Thromb Res 1982; 25:115–123.

96. Anido G, Freeman DJ: Heparin assay and protamine titration. Am J Clin Pathol 1981; 76:410–415.

97. Hughes DR, Faust RJ, Didisheim P, Tinker JH: Heparin monitoring during cardiopulmonary bypass in man: Use of fluorogenic heparin assay to validate activated clotting time. Anesth Analg 1982; 61:189–190.

98. Pochron SP, Mitchell GA, Albareda I, et al: A fluorescent substrate assay for plasminogen. Thromb Res 1978; 13:733–739.

99. Mitchell GA, Hudson PM, Huseby RM, et al: Fluorescent substrate assay for antithrombin III. Thromb Res 1977; 12:219–225.

100. Schriever HG, Epstein SE, Mintz MD: Statistical correlation and heparin sensitivity of activated partial thromboplastin time, whole blood coagulation time, and automated coagulation time. Am J Clin Pathol 1973; 60:323–329.

101. Dauchot PJ, Berzina-Moettus L, Rabinovitch A, Ankeney JL: Activated coagulation and activated partial thromboplastin times in assessment and reversal of heparin-induced anticoagulation for cardiopulmonary bypass. Anesth Analg 1983; 62:710–719.

102. Bull BS, Huse WM, Brauer FS, Korpman RA: Heparin therapy during extracorporeal circulation. II. The use of a dose-response curve to individualize heparin and protamine dosage. J Thorac Cardiovasc Surg 1975; 69:685–689.

103. Cohen JA, Frederickson EL, Kaplan JA. Plasma heparin activity and antagonism during cardiopulmonary bypass with hypothermia. Anesth Analg 1977; 56:564–570.

104. Donahoo KM, Taylor CA, Baugh RF, Soloway HB: A promising new multifunction instrument for monitoring heparin therapy. Advances in Therapy 1985; 2:150–159.

105. Hattersley PG: Activated coagulation time of whole blood. JAMA 1966; 196:436–440.

106. Hill JD, Dontigny L, de Leval M, Mielke C: A simple method of heparin management during prolonged extracorporeal circulation. Ann Thorac Surg 1974; 17:129–134.

107. Esposito RA, Culliford AT, Colvin SB, et al: The role of the activated clotting time in heparin administration and neutralization for cardiopulmonary bypass. J Thorac Cardiovasc Surg 1983; 85:174–185.

108. Weinberg S, Phillips L, Twersky R, et al: Hypercoagulability in a patient with a brain tumor. Anesthesiology 1984; 61:200–202.

109. Fyman PN, Gotta A, Casthely PA, et al: Factor IX–induced hypercoagulable state. Anesthesiology 1985; 62:515–516.

110. Hanowell ST, Kim YUD, Rattan V, MacNamara TE: Increased heparin requirement with hypereosinophilic syndrome. Anesthesiology 1981; 55:450–452.

111. Esposito RA, Culliford AT, Colvin SB, et al: Heparin resistance during cardiopulmonary bypass. The role of heparin pretreatment. J Thorac Cardiovasc Surg 1983; 85:346–353.

112. Young JA, Kisker CT, Doty DB: Adequate anticoagulation during cardiopulmonary bypass determined by activated clotting time and the appearance of fibrin monomer. Ann Thorac Surg 1978; 26:231–240.

113. Culliford AT, Gitel SN, Starr N, et al: Lack of correlation between activated clotting time and plasma heparin during cardiopulmonary bypass. Ann Surg 1981; 193:105–111.

114. Thomas SJ, Gitel SN, Starr NJ, et al: Activated clotting time and heparin levels during hypothermic cardiopulmonary bypass. Anesthesiology 1980; 53:S115.

115. Cohen JA: Activated coagulation time method for control of heparin is reliable during cardiopulmonary bypass. Anesthesiology 1984; 60:121–124.

116. Moorehead MT, Westengard JC, Bull BS: Platelet involvement in the activated coagulation time of heparinized blood. Anesth Analg 1984; 63:394–398.

117. King DO, Kane PB: Blood clot formation during multiple cardiopulmonary bypass procedures necessitated by massive hemorrhage. Anesth Analg 1978; 57:273–276.

118. Franz RC, Coetzee WJC: The thromboelastographic diagnosis of hemostatic defects. Surg Annu 1981; 13:75–107.

119. Eliot RS, von Kaulla KN, Blount SG: Thromboelastographic studies with a twenty-four-hour schedule for subcutaneous heparin. Circulation 1961; 24:1206–1214.

120. Spiess BD, Tuman KJ, McCarthy RJ, et al: Thromboelastography as an indicator of post–cardiopulmonary bypass coagulopathies. J Clin Monit 1987; 3:25–30.

121. Tuman KJ, Spiess BD, Schoen RE, Ivankovich AD: Use of thromboelastography in the management of von Willebrand's disease during cardiopulmonary bypass. J Cardiothorac Anesth 1987; 1:321–324.

122. Tuman KJ, Spiess BD, McCarthy RJ, Ivankovich AD: Effects of progressive blood loss on coagulation as measured by thrombelastography. Anesth Analg 1987; 66:856–863.

123. von Kaulla KN: Continuous automatic recording of fibrin formation and fibri-

nolysis: A valuable tool for coagulation research. J Lab Clin Med 1957; 49:304–312.

124. Zuckerman L, Cohen E, Vagher JP, et al: Comparison of thrombelastography with common coagulation tests. Thromb Haemost 1981; 46:752–756.

125. Kang YG, Abouleish E: Thrombelastography in obstetrics. Anesthesiology 1981; 55:A304.

126. Koren G, Weiss AT, Hasin Y, et al: Prevention of myocardial damage in acute myocardial ischemia by early treatment with intravenous streptokinase. N Engl J Med 1985; 313:1384–1389.

127. von Kaulla KN, Ostendorf P, von Kaulla E: The impedance machine: A new bedside coagulation recording device. J Med 1975; 6:73–87.

128. Chandler WL, Schmer G: Evaluation of a new dynamic viscometer for measuring the viscosity of whole blood and plasma. Clin Chem 1986; 32:505–507.

129. Saleem A, Blifeld C, Saleh SA, et al: Viscoelastic measurement of clot formation: A new test of platelet function. Ann Clin Lab Sci 1983; 13:115–124.

130. Kurica K, Holmes J, Peck S, et al: Hypercoagulation and predictability of thromboembolic phenomena in total hip and total knee surgery. Thromb Haemost 1981; 46:17.

131. Goto H, Nonami R, Hamasaki Y, et al: Effect of hypothermia on coagulation. Anesthesiology 1985; 63:A107.

132. Committee on Blood and Blood Products: Questions and Answers about Transfusion Practices. Park Ridge, IL: American Society of Anesthesiologists, 1987; 1–44.

133. Miller RD, Bove JR: Acquired immunodeficiency syndrome (AIDS) and the blood products. Anesthesiology 1983; 58:493–494.

134. Council on Scientific Affairs: Autologous blood transfusions. JAMA 1986; 256:2378–2380.

135. Menitove JE: Status of recipients of blood from donors subsequently found to have antibody to HIV. N Engl J Med 1986; 315:1095–1096.

136. Zauder HL: Massive transfusion. Int Anesthesiol Clin 1982; 20:157–170.

137. Miller RD, Robbins TO, Tong MJ, Barton SL: Coagulation defects associated with massive blood transfusions. Ann Surg 1971; 174:794–801.

138. Abbott TR: Changes in serum calcium fractions and citrate concentrations during massive blood transfusions and cardiopulmonary bypass. Br J Anaesth 1983; 55:753–759.

139. Kahn RC, Jascott D, Carlon GC, et al: Massive blood replacement: Correlation of ionized calcium, citrate, and hydrogen ion concentration. Anesth Analg 1979; 58:274–278.

140. Coté CJ, Liu LMP, Szyfelbein SK, et al: Changes in serial platelet counts following massive blood transfusion in pediatric patients. Anesthesiology 1985; 62:197–201.

141. Hallowell P, Bland JHL, Buckley MJ, Lowenstein E: Transfusion of fresh autologous blood in open-heart surgery. J Thorac Cardiovasc Surg 1972; 64:941–948.

142. Ochsner JL, Mills NL, Leonard GL, Lawson N: Fresh autologous blood transfusions with extracorporeal circulation. Ann Surg 1973; 177:811–817.

143. Barbier-Bohm G, Desmonts JM, Couderc E, et al: Comparative effects of induced hypotension and normovolaemic haemodilution on blood loss in total hip arthroplasty. Br J Anaesth 1980; 52:1039–1043.

144. Hamstra RD, Block MH: Erythropoiesis in response to blood loss in man. J Appl Physiol 1969; 27:503–507.

145. Newman MM, Hamstra R, Block M: Use of banked autologous blood in elective surgery. JAMA 1971; 218:861–863.

146. Kramer AH, Hertzer NR, Beven EG: Intraoperative hemodilution during elective vascular reconstruction. Surg Gynecol Obstet 1979; 149:831–836.
147. Jobes DR, Gallagher J: Acute normovolemic hemodilution. Int Anesthesiol Clin 1982; 20:77–95.
148. Stehling LC, Zauder HL, Rogers W: Intraoperative autotransfusion. Anesthesiology 1975; 43:337–345.
149. Rosenblatt R, Dennis P, Draper LD: A new method for massive fluid resuscitation in the trauma patient. Anesth Analg 1983; 62:613–616.
150. Robicsek F, Duncan GD, Born GVR, et al: Inherent dangers of simultaneous application of microfibrillar collagen hemostat and blood-saving devices. J Thorac Cardiovasc Surg 1986; 92:766–770.
151. Gould SA, Rosen AL, Sehgal LR, et al: Fluosol-DA as a red-cell substitute in acute anemia. N Engl J Med 1986; 314:1653–1656.

chapter seventeen

Monitoring Arterial Blood Gases and Acid-Base Balance

■ CHARLES G. DURBIN, JR., M.D.

Since the discovery of oxygen in the air, humans have been fascinated by the function of this gas in biologic systems. The prevailing view that the universe was made up of the four primary elements—earth, water, air, and fire—was gradually replaced in the nineteenth century by the more general theories of chemistry. The existence of oxygen and carbon dioxide in the blood was discovered in the early 1800s, but it was not until the middle of the twentieth century that the full significance of these discoveries was apparent.

The value of chemical measurements has depended in large part on the equipment used to make the measurements. The clinical use of blood gases and acid-base information has depended on the reliability of available methods of measurement. The use of blood gases and acid-base data discussed in this chapter is shaped by the equipment and technology that are being used to obtain the values of these variables. It is essential that the capabilities and limitations of the equipment be kept foremost in mind when using the measured data for clinical applications and decisions. Limitations of methods and techniques are discussed in detail.

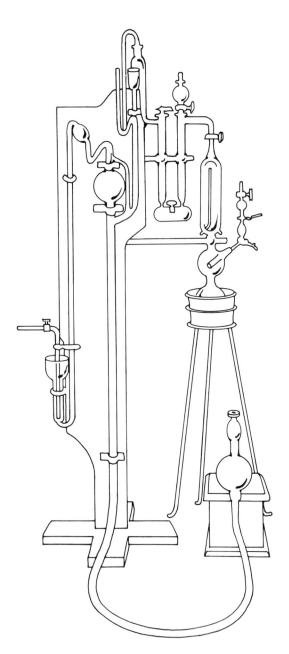

Figure 17–1. A vacuum extraction device for measuring gases dissolved in blood. It was designed and built by Nathan Zuntz, of Bonn, Germany, in the 1880s. (Modified from Astrup P, Severinghaus JW: The History of Blood Gases, Acids and Bases. Copenhagen: Munksgaard, 1986; 164.)

HISTORY

Credit for discovering the elemental gas, oxygen, is given to Priestley, who in 1774 collected the gas over water in a closed vessel. He also discovered that it was produced by green plants and was necessary to sustain animal life or a candle flame. Davy succeeded in proving that both oxygen and carbon dioxide were present in blood by using vacuum extraction tech-

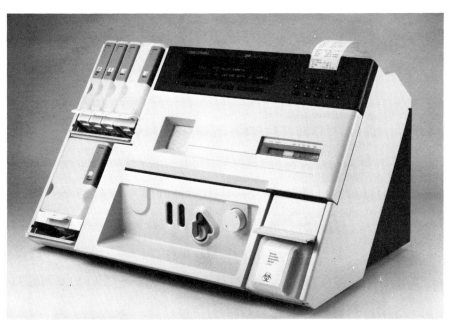

Figure 17-2. The 288 Blood Gas System, produced by Ciba Corning Diagnostics, rapidly analyzes a blood sample for blood gas partial pressures. It is microprocessor-driven, automatically calibrated, and very accurate.

niques. One such device was built and used by Zuntz in the 1880s (Fig. 17–1). It was remarkably accurate. Even today, the industry standard for blood gas analysis is dependent on such a technique. The time required to perform the measurement as well as the amount of blood required makes this technique impractical for frequent use. Modern methods of analysis depend on

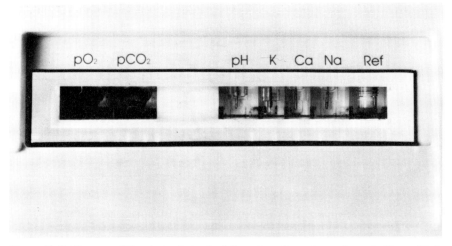

Figure 17-3. Close-up of the electrode bank of the automatic analyzer shown in Figure 17–2 illustrates the fact that analysis for calcium, sodium, and potassium is also available.

selectively permeable membranes and the electrochemical activity of the gases present.

Clark, in 1953, covered a platinum oxygen electrode with cellophane and created a way of accurately and rapidly measuring P_{O_2} in blood. The Clark electrode remains the basis of the electrochemical measurement of oxygen today.

Modern measurement devices, such as the one shown in Figure 17–2, combine analysis of oxygen, carbon dioxide (CO_2), and blood pH in a rapid and accurate manner. This device (produced by Ciba Corning Diagnostics) includes the automatic measurement of sodium, potassium, and calcium levels as well as blood gas analysis, as seen in Figure 17–3. Maintenance is streamlined, and calibration checks are automatic. Most equipment provides data that have an accuracy of ±2–3% of the measured variables.

INDICATIONS FOR P_{O_2} MONITORING

Arterial P_{O_2} is usually measured in an intermittent fashion. The goal of this form of monitoring is to direct changes in inspired O_2 and ventilatory support. Continuous measurement of transcutaneous P_{O_2} (tco_2) is available and has been used extensively, especially in newborns. Long warm-up time,

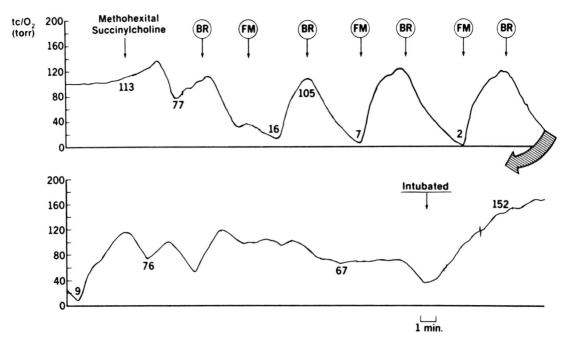

Figure 17–4. The changes in transcutaneous P_{O_2} (tco_2) occurring during fiberoptic bronchoscopy. (BR = during bronchoscopy, FM = while the patient is being ventilated with oxygen by a face mask.) Note the rapid and precipitous falls in tco_2 that occur throughout the procedure. (Reprinted with permission from the International Anesthesia Research Society from Transcutaneous oxygen monitoring during bronchoscopy and washout for cystic fibrosis, by Harnik E, Kulcycki L, Gomes MN. Anesthesia and Analgesia, 1983; 62:358.)

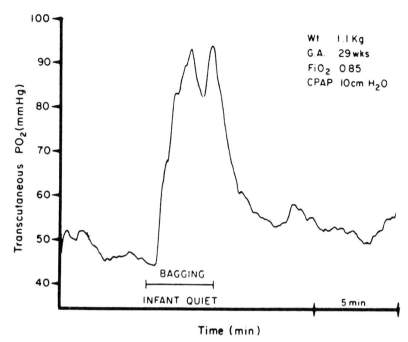

Figure 17–5. Transcutaneous P_{O_2} monitoring in an infant during manual hyperventilation. (From Okken A, Rubin IL, Martin RJ: Intermittent bag ventilation of preterm infants on continuous positive airway pressure: The effect on transcutaneous P_{O_2}. Pediatrics 1978; 93:281. With permission.)

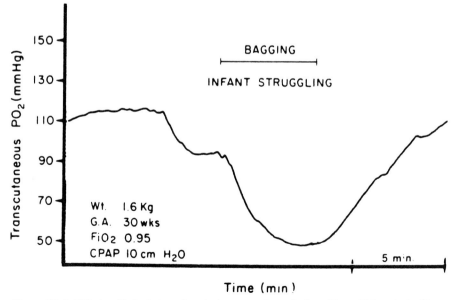

Figure 17–6. Effects of infant struggling during manual ventilation. (From Okken A, Rubin IL, Martin RJ: Intermittent bag ventilation of preterm infants on continuous positive airway pressure: The effect on transcutaneous P_{O_2}. Pediatrics 1978; 93:281. With permission.)

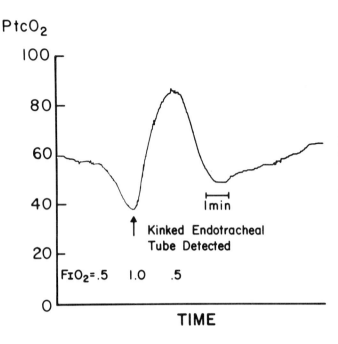

Figure 17-7. The effect of kinking of the endotracheal tube on tco_2 is demonstrated in this record obtained during anesthesia in a small child. (From Marshall TA, Kattwinkel J, Berry FA, Shaw A: Transcutaneous monitoring of neonates during surgery. J Pediatr Surg 1980; 15:800. With permission.)

the need to change sensor site, and the technical difficulty in preparing and calibrating sensors have made the use of this form of monitoring less acceptable in many clinical settings (see Chapter 8).

The value of continuous Po_2 monitoring is illustrated by transcutaneous monitoring in Figure 17-4. Changes in tco_2 produced by bronchoscopic maneuvers are reflected in rapid changes in the monitor output. The response to changes in respiratory support maneuvers is also rapidly seen, as demonstrated in infants in Figures 17-5, 17-6, and 17-7. Other factors such as volume status and cardiac output also affect this monitor (Fig. 17-8). In each of these examples, the cause of decreased tco_2 was different. The change in the monitor output initiated further investigations in order to diagnose the cause of the change. Since several clinical conditions may have caused the "hypoxia," this monitor is not very specific; however, it is useful in preventing the brain from experiencing hypoxic damage. An excellent review of the technical aspects of this form of monitoring has been published.[1]

ARTERIAL BLOOD GAS SAMPLING

Sample Collection

Samples for intermittent blood gas measurement are collected by direct arterial puncture with a small-gauge, sterile needle or from an indwelling arterial catheter. Indwelling continuous arterial blood gas–monitoring devices have been developed and are becoming commercially available.[2, 3]

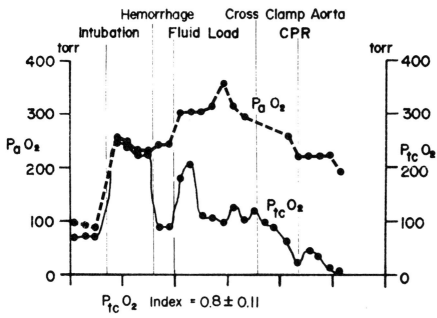

Figure 17–8. Occurrences besides airway compromise can cause changes in Ptco$_2$. In this example, both Ptco$_2$ and arterial oxygen partial pressure (Pao$_2$) are being monitored. The difference between arterial and transcutaneous values reflects the change in cutaneous perfusion occurring with changes in volume status and cardiac output. (From Tremper KJ, Shoemaker WC: Transcutaneous oxygen monitoring of critically ill adults, with and without low flow shock. Crit Care Med 1981; 9(10):706–709, © by The Williams & Wilkins Company, 1981.)

Indications for insertion, techniques for placement, and complications from arterial catheters are discussed in Chapter 4. Direct arterial puncture is usually carried out after infiltrating the skin with a small amount of local anesthetic without a vasoconstrictor. A small metal needle that has been flushed with a solution containing 0.1 or 1.0 mg of heparin/L is inserted into a palpable artery after use of sterilizing skin preparation. A butterfly needle or a hypodermic needle attached to a small (1–3 ml) syringe is used, and pulsatile flow is confirmed. After an adequate sample is withdrawn (0.2–1.5 ml, depending on the specific analyzer), the needle is removed and manual pressure applied for several minutes. The site should be examined again after several minutes for the development of a hematoma. Infection from a single arterial puncture is rare; pain from hematoma formation is common. Spasm, clot, and ischemia may occur and must be treated in order to prevent permanent disability. This technique is contraindicated in patients who are anticoagulated. An indwelling arterial catheter may be of less risk under this circumstance.

When a blood sample is obtained from an arterial catheter, care must be taken to avoid contamination of the sample with the flushing solution. Three times the dead space amount of fluid must be withdrawn and discarded to produce an uncontaminated sample. A simple way to do this is to note the volume that is withdrawn until blood just appears in the aspirating sy-

Table 17–1. EFFECT OF HEPARIN SOLUTION CONTAMINATION ON BLOOD GAS VALUES

Blood Heparin	100% 0%	50% 50%	0% 100%
With Normal Blood Gases*			
P_{CO_2}	44.9	18.8	3.2
P_{O_2}	143.5	152.4	171.4
pH	7.41	7.44	6.11
HCO_3^-	28.2	12.7	0.1
With Low Oxygen and Bicarbonate*			
P_{CO_2}	16.2	7.2	3.2
P_{O_2}	45.1	48.1	171.4
pH	7.25	7.25	6.11
HCO_3^-	16.2	7.2	0.1

* The top section illustrates the effect on a relatively normal sample; the bottom section shows the effect on a hypoxic sample with metabolic acidosis. The principal effect is on the P_{CO_2} measurement and bicarbonate calculation.

ringe; this is approximately 80% of the dead space volume. Removing three to four times this volume guarantees an adequate sample.[4]

Sample Handling

The syringe should be capped and sealed and immediately processed in a blood gas machine. If there is to be a delay before performing the analysis (longer than 20–30 minutes), the sample should be placed on ice in order to reduce the metabolic activity of the white blood cells. In the case of a patient with leukemia, this metabolic change in the sample may be quite significant.[5]

The effects of dilution with heparin flush are indicated in Table 17–1. The primary abnormality induced by this type of contamination is in the Pa_{CO_2} measurement. Because the CO_2 content is directly proportional to the P_{CO_2} of the blood and very little CO_2 is present in the heparin solution, the Pa_{CO_2} is markedly reduced in the contaminated sample. The calculated bicarbonate concentration is similarly affected. There are commercially prepared heparin-coated syringes in both glass and plastic that obviate the problem of contamination by heparin.

The use of glass syringes for blood gas sampling has been debated, because plastic is semipermeable to O_2 and CO_2. The rate of change in these values is rather slow and not clinically important, if samples are analyzed in a reasonably short time.

Temperature Correction of Arterial Blood Gases

Solubility of oxygen and carbon dioxide in blood is dependent on the temperature. Blood gas analyzers are maintained at 37°C. Whether to correct

---

Table 17–2. TEMPERATURE CORRECTION
OF ARTERIAL BLOOD GASES

Pco₂

Pco_2 (at patient temperature, T°C)

$$= Pco_2 \text{ (measured)} \times 10^{(0.019 \times [T - 37])}$$

pH

pH (at patient temperature, T°C)

$$= pH \text{ (measured)} + (-0.0147 \times [T - 37])$$

Po₂

Po_2 (at patient temperature, T°C)

$$= Po_2 \text{ (measured)} \times 10f(T - 37)$$

$$f = 0.0052 + \{0.0268 \times [1 - e^{-0.3(100 - \%O2sat)}]\}$$

Temperature correction formulas are derived empirically. The values obtained at 37°C are "corrected" to the
patient's actual body temperature. See the text for a description of the use of these equations.

the values obtained from patients with abnormal body temperatures to 37°C
has been debated for many years. Temperature-correction formulas are
listed in Table 17–2. These have been obtained by cooling or heating anaerobically treated blood samples (or plasma samples) and measuring blood
gases in analyzers maintained at the same temperature as the sample. Reference or "normal" values are those obtained from samples having normal
blood gas values at 37 degrees; the mathematic formulas "correct" them to
this normal range.[6] Deviations are assumed to indicate a disease process.

Clinical and experimental data suggest that this approach of tempera-
ture-correcting blood gases may actually be incorrect. Study of several poi-
kilothermic animals indicates that if their blood is obtained at several different temperatures and analyzed in a machine at 37 degrees, the values
obtained are identical to the "normal" values obtained and analyzed at 37
degrees. In humans in cold environments, blood obtained from cold distal
arteries has the same values as blood obtained from warm central arteries
when both are analyzed at 37 degrees. If the values were temperature-corrected, the cold sample would be alkalotic (lower $Paco_2$) and have a lower
Pao_2.

The effects of temperature change on enzyme system activities parallel
changes in hydrogen ion activity. To maintain neutrality, that is, the same
relative activity of $[H^+]$ and $[OH^-]$, the solution must become slightly alkalotic as temperature decreases. The increased solubility of CO_2 accomplishes this change. A "normal" value should be obtained when the sample
is warmed. No artificial test-tube correction is necessary or appropriate.[7]
These concepts are well discussed by Rahn and colleagues.[8]

Clinical evidence also refutes temperature correction of blood gases.

Profoundly hypothermic animals given sodium bicarbonate to normalize temperature-corrected blood gases invariably develop profound alkalemia and suffer myocardial damage on rewarming.[9] Hypothermic patients given little or no bicarbonate have normal acid-base balance when returned to normothermia.[10]

Temperature correction of Pa_{O_2} is usually done, because O_2 solubility is affected by temperature. The same considerations of chemical activity changes affecting Pa_{CO_2} should apply to the transportation and utilization of oxygen. Since oxygen is more soluble in cold blood, the temperature-correction formula reduces the measured Pa_{O_2} value. Therefore, temperature corrections may indicate the need for increased FI_{O_2}. However, the risks of administration of extra oxygen for a short period of time (increasing the FI_{O_2}) are minimal, and the extra margin of safety is probably justified.

Variability of Oxygen Measurements

When deciding to make an intervention based on a measurement of Pa_{O_2}, it is important to keep in mind the variability of this value as determined in the analyzer. If laboratory or commercially prepared standards are used for quality control, the variability of P_{O_2} on repeated measurements on the same machine is very small, 1–4 torr standard deviation at clinical levels of Pa_{O_2}. This variability is dependent on the composition of the standard and its temperature. Warm fluorocarbon solutions demonstrate the least variation, and cool aqueous solutions, the most.[11] Failure to meet these accuracy levels should initiate machine repair. Variation between different analyzers is much greater, however. As much as 10–15 torr difference in Pa_{O_2} around a "true" Pa_{O_2} of 60 torr may occur between different analyzers.[11]

Another source of variability in Pa_{O_2} results from patient variability. As seen previously, with continuous monitoring, often the tc_{O_2} varies quite widely in response to clinical interventions. Occasionally, wide variations are seen without discernible causes. Arterial blood gases in clinically stable patients often reflect a wide range of variability.[12] When a Pa_{O_2} value is interpreted, this large variability must be borne in mind. Interpretation must be based on trends rather than on absolute values.

INDEXES OF OXYGENATION

Alveolar-Arterial Oxygen Partial Pressure Difference (A-a Gradient)

The expected arterial partial pressure of oxygen varies with the inspired fraction of oxygen. The relationship between the ideal alveolar concentration of oxygen and the inspired oxygen fraction is shown in the alveolar air equation:

$$PA_{O_2} = FI_{O_2}(Pb - 47) - Pa_{CO_2}/R$$

where PA_{O_2} = the ideal alveolar partial pressure of oxygen, FI_{O_2} = the inspired oxygen fraction, Pb = the barometric pressure in torr, 47 = the vapor pressure of water in torr at 37°C, Pa_{CO_2} = the partial pressure of carbon dioxide in the blood, and R = the respiratory quotient (the volume of CO_2 produced for each volume of oxygen consumed). There is a small (5%) underestimation of Pa_{O_2} when R = 0.8. If R = 1.0, the error is eliminated. The term Pa_{CO_2}/R is a measure of the oxygen that is being removed by the blood flowing through the lungs in relation to the amount of oxygen being brought into the lungs by ventilation. The difference between this ideal value for oxygen and the actual measured value is called the alveolar-arterial oxygen difference or the A-a gradient for oxygen ($A\text{-}aP_{O_2}$).

Calculating and following the A-a gradient is a clinical tool to monitor deficits in oxygenation. Changes in this number are produced by several mechanisms. $A\text{-}aP_{O_2}$ is very much affected by the inspired oxygen fraction as indicated in the previous equation. A "normal" gradient is about 5–10 torr on room air, but it increases to 50–70 torr on an FI_{O_2} of 1.0. Other causes of an increased gradient include poor cardiac function with a decreased cardiac output, lung disease with increased resistance to diffusion of oxygen, ventilation-perfusion mismatching, or intrapulmonary or intracardiac shunting. Decreased $A\text{-}aP_{O_2}$ is seen with increased cardiac output, systemic sepsis, left to right intracardiac shunts, and failure to utilize oxygen in the tissues as occurs in cyanide or carbon monoxide poisoning.

Calculation of $A\text{-}aP_{O_2}$ is useful when changing the FI_{O_2} on a mechanical ventilator. For example, Pa_{O_2} of 246 torr is obtained from an intubated, ventilated patient. The FI_{O_2} is 1.0. The $A\text{-}aP_{O_2}$ is calculated

$$PA_{O_2} = 1.0(760 - 47) - 40/0.8$$

assuming the barometric pressure is 760 torr, the PA_{CO_2} is normal (40 torr), and the respiratory quotient is 0.8.

$$Pa_{O_2} = 663$$
$$A\text{-}aP_{O_2} = 663 - 246 = 417$$

To change the FI_{O_2} to produce a Pa_{O_2} of 100 torr, the same equation is solved for FI_{O_2}:

$$PA_{O_2} - Pa_{O_2} = 417$$
$$\text{Setting } Pa_{O_2} = 100$$
$$PA_{O_2} = 517$$
$$517 = FI_{O_2}(760 - 47) - 40/0.8$$
$$FI_{O_2} = (517 + 40/0.8)/(760 - 47) = 0.80$$

The assumptions made in this calculation are that equilibration had taken place before the first blood sample was obtained and that no change occurred in A-aPo$_2$. As implied previously, the A-aPo$_2$ changes with changes in FIo$_2$. Since, in the example, the new FIo$_2$ was lower than the previous setting, the gradient would also be lower, thus providing a margin of safety.

Oxygenation Ratio

A method to eliminate the effects of changes in A-aPo$_2$ caused by changes in FIo$_2$ is to divide the Pao$_2$ by the FIo$_2$ or by the PAo$_2$.[13] This is referred to as the oxygenation ratio. To use this parameter in the example shown previously:

$$Pao_2/FIo_2 = 246/1.0 = 246$$

to obtain a Pao$_2$ = 100, then

$$100/FIo_2 = 246$$
$$FIo_2 = 100/246 = 0.41$$

This result differs significantly from the previous method and reflects the fact that the A-aPo$_2$ is smaller as the FIo$_2$ is reduced.

Arterial-Alveolar Oxygen Ratio

Another index of gas exchange is the ratio of arterial to alveolar O$_2$ (a/A Po$_2$).[14] This index is less affected by FIo$_2$, more constant than A-aPo$_2$, and most constant above alveolar oxygen values of 200 mmHg.[13] Normal a/A Po$_2$ values are 0.7–0.8.

MONITORING OF OXYHEMOGLOBIN

Oxyhemoglobin Dissociation Curve

The discussion up to this point has been about the partial pressure of oxygen in the blood. The amount of oxygen dissolved in blood is quite small, however, and would be quickly exhausted if it were not for the large amount of hemoglobin present in red blood cells. Hemoglobin reversibly binds large quantities of oxygen and acts as a reservoir for this gas. The biochemical basis of this process is the tertiary structure of hemoglobin and its ferrous core.

Hemoglobin consists of four heme subunit proteins clustered around a ferrous ion. There are four binding sites in each molecule of hemoglobin (one on each heme subunit). As the first O$_2$ molecule is bound, the other chains rotate and the binding of the next O$_2$ molecule is easier (more tightly bound). This configurational change occurs with the addition of each suc-

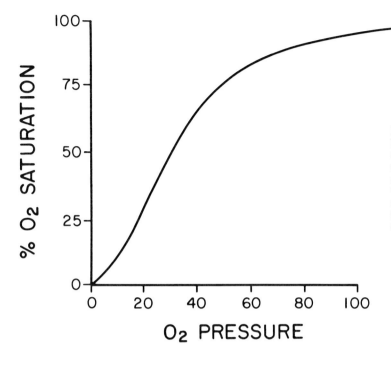

Figure 17–9. The relationship between the Po_2 and the percentage saturation of hemoglobin is demonstrated. The position of this curve is affected by many factors, which are explained in the text. The sigmoid shape of the curve is due to facilitated binding of successive oxygen molecules.

cessive O_2 molecule, until all four binding sites are occupied.[15, 16] This allosteric cooperation accounts for the shape of the oxyhemoglobin dissociation curve (Fig. 17–9).

The relationship between oxygen saturation and Po_2 is important to remember in clinical practice. A simple rule of thumb is that at a Po_2 of 40 torr, hemoglobin is about 70% saturated; at 60 torr, it is about 90% saturated. The 40, 50, 60; 70, 80, 90 rule is illustrated in the following easy-to-recall form:

Po_2 40 50 60
                  \   \   \
% Saturation 70 80 90

In 1904, Bohr discovered the sigmoid shape of the oxyhemoglobin dissociation curve of whole blood. He also described the effect of carbon dioxide tension on the position of this curve. This leftward shift of the curve that occurs when CO_2 is released in the lungs is termed the Bohr effect.

Measurement

Measurement of hemoglobin saturation is easily carried out by determining the light absorbance in the visual and infrared spectral range in a co-oximeter. Oxygenated blood absorbs light differently than deoxygenated blood. The absorbance spectra for these species are illustrated in Figure 17–10. By comparing the absorbance at several wave lengths, the percentage saturation can be calculated. Current co-oximeters use at least four different

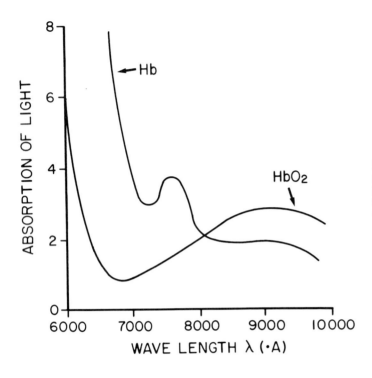

Figure 17–10. Absorption of light of oxygenated and deoxygenated hemoglobin. Comparing the absorption at several wavelengths allows calculation of the percentage saturation.

wave lengths and calculate carboxyhemoglobin and methemoglobin percentages as well as the percentage of oxygen saturation of normal hemoglobin.

Alterations in Oxyhemoglobin Dissociation

Various conditions listed in Table 17–3 affect the position of the oxyhemoglobin dissociation curve. Major factors shifting the curve to the right (reducing hemoglobin affinity for oxygen) are acidosis (respiratory or metabolic), fever, and increased 2,3-diphosphoglycerate (2,3-DPG). Minor factors include increased hemoglobin, exogenous cortisol, hyperaldosteronism, and hyperthyroidism. Factors that shift the curve to the left (producing more avid binding of oxygen) are cold, alkalosis, reduced 2,3-DPG, anemia, hypothyroidism, carboxyhemoglobin, and methemoglobin.[17] Genetic hemoglobin variants have differing effects on the curve. The clinical effects of shifts in the oxyhemoglobin dissociation curve have not been established.[18]

P_{50}

A useful way to describe the amount of shift in the oxyhemoglobin dissociation curve is to calculate or determine experimentally the P_{O_2} at which the blood sample is 50% saturated. This is called the P_{50} value. A normal value for this number is about 27 torr. If the P_{50} is greater, the curve is shifted to the right. If it is less, the curve is shifted to the left. The mag-

---

Table 17–3. FACTORS AFFECTING
HEMOGLOBIN-OXYGEN AFFINITY

Causes of Increased Oxygen Affinity
  Hypothermia
  Respiratory alkalosis
  Metabolic alkalosis
  Decreased 2,3-diphosphoglycerate (2,3-DPG)
  Decreased serum phosphate
  Anemia
  Hypothyroidism

Factors That Decrease Oxygen Affinity
  Fever
  Respiratory acidosis
  Metabolic acidosis
  Increased 2,3-DPG
  Steroid administration
  Hyperaldosteronism
  Hyperthyroidism
  Polycythemia

---

nitude of the shift is indicated by the degree of deviation from this normal value.

Oxygen Content

The oxyhemoglobin dissociation curve is useful in that it describes the amount of oxygen carried by hemoglobin, and hemoglobin is the major reservoir of oxygen for tissue metabolic needs. The actual amount of molecular oxygen dissolved in blood or plasma is related to the partial pressure of oxygen and is quite small in relation to the amount bound to hemoglobin. The following equation describes the amount of oxygen in arterial blood:

$$Cao_2 = (Hbg \times 1.36 \times Sao_2) + 0.0031 \times Pao_2$$

$$\text{Content} = \text{Bound} \qquad + \text{Dissolved}$$

Cao_2 = the oxygen content in ml of oxygen/100 ml of whole blood; Hbg = the hemoglobin content in gm/100 ml of blood; 1.36 = the milliliters of oxygen in a fully saturated gram of hemoglobin; Sao_2 = arterial saturation; and 0.0031 = the amount of oxygen dissolved in plasma per torr of oxygen partial pressure.

Oxygen Transport

When describing the amount of oxygen that is available to the body, the concept of oxygen transport (Cao_2 times 10 to convert oxygen content to liters multiplied by the cardiac output) is frequently used. More appropriately called oxygen availability, this product estimates the total available arterial oxygen. In states in which oxygen transport is inadequate, this concept allows a rational therapeutic approach to be taken by addressing each of the components of the delivery system independently.

Although this oxygen transport variable is useful in a conceptual sense, there are several problems in using it clinically. The tissues are able to extract only some of the available oxygen, and this fraction varies among different tissues. The heart is efficient at removing the available oxygen and removes as much as 90% of the oxygen delivered (coronary sinus hemoglobin saturation of 5%).[19] Other organs may begin to fail at much higher oxygen contents, such as the brain, which begins to fail at a Pa_{O_2} of about 30 torr (venous blood about 50% saturated).

A-V Oxygen Difference

Comparing the oxygen content of the venous blood with the amount available in the arterial blood gives a measure of the utilization of oxygen by the whole body. $C(a-v)_{O_2}$, or the arteriovenous oxygen content difference, is easily calculated if a mixed venous blood sample can be obtained (usually from a pulmonary artery or central venous catheter). $C(a-v)_{O_2}$ is usually 5–6 vol% but it may increase to 8–10 vol% in stress states. A problem with this parameter, as well as the oxygen availability parameter described previously, is that the entire body is averaged in the calculations. Regional differences in supply and demand are not reflected in these overall indexes. The monitoring of tissue oxygenation is discussed in Chapter 8. Mixed venous P_{O_2} (Pv_{O_2}) gives some indication of total body oxygen supply and demand balance.

ARTERIAL OXYGENATION

Hypoxia

Physiologic Effects

Oxygen is essential to all tissues for energy generation through oxidative phosphorylation in the Krebs cycle. Oxygen is transported by the blood (bound to hemoglobin and freely dissolved) and must diffuse to the mitochondria from the capillaries. There are almost no tissue or blood stores of oxygen in the body. Oxygen must be continually delivered in order to maintain organ function and prevent cellular death. The driving force for oxygen delivery is diffusion down a partial pressure gradient. The partial pressure of oxygen in the mitochondrion is probably less than 2 torr.[20] Oxygen extraction from blood by the brain seems to fail when venous blood reaches a P_{O_2} of about 20 torr.[20] This may occur at P_{O_2} of 25–35 torr, depending on the hemoglobin type, concentration, and blood flow. Other organs may tolerate lower venous (and arterial) oxygen partial pressures.

Table 17-4. EFFECT OF HYPERCARBIA ON
Pa_{O_2}

Pa_{CO_2} Room Air (torr)	Pa_{O_2} Room Air (torr)	Pa_{O_2} 30% FI_{O_2} (torr)
40	92	156
50	80	144
60	68	132
70	56	120
80	44	108
90	32	96
100	20	84

The predicted Pa_{O_2} due to a rise in Pa_{CO_2} on room air (21% FI_{O_2}) and on 30%. A normal, unchanging alveolar-to-arterial gradient is assumed in performing the calculations.

Complete interruption of oxygen delivery, anoxia, results in rapid disruption of organ function and, if it persists for a short period, organ death. The tolerance to anoxia varies from organ to organ. Irreversible brain injury occurs after only 3–5 minutes of total anoxia. The heart may resume normal function after several hours without perfusion.

When Pa_{O_2} is monitored in the clinical arena, there are two conditions that need to be avoided, hypoxia and hyperoxia. Although the definition of hypoxia varies from organ to organ, a Pa_{O_2} of 55 torr or less or a saturation of 88% is usually considered to be hypoxia.[21] At this point on the oxyhemoglobin dissociation curve, there is still a large quantity of bound oxygen. The use of high inspired concentrations of oxygen to achieve this desired level of Pa_{O_2} is associated with development of pulmonary oxygen toxicity. Abnormalities of gas exchange and pathologic anatomic changes in lung structure occur. In extreme cases, the adult respiratory distress syndrome follows high inspired oxygen concentrations.[22]

Causes of Hypoxia

Hypoventilation

The simplest cause of low Pa_{O_2} is hypoventilation on room air. It can be seen from the alveolar gas equation described earlier in this chapter that a high Pa_{CO_2} (hypoventilation) results in a low Pa_{O_2} when the FI_{O_2} is low, even with normal pulmonary function. The effect of increasing Pa_{CO_2} is shown in Table 17-4. By simply increasing the FI_{O_2}, this cause of hypoxia can be overcome. For example, the Pa_{O_2} of a patient with a Pa_{CO_2} of 80 torr would only be 44 torr on room air; this would improve dramatically to 108 torr by increasing the FI_{O_2} slightly to 0.30. Hypoventilation is often seen as a consequence of general anesthesia, especially when narcotics are employed. The practice of administering an increased inspired O_2 to the recovering patient is based on this consideration.[23]

Table 17–5. EFFECT OF INCREASED ALTITUDE AND DECREASED FI_{O_2} ON P_{O_2}

Altitude (Feet)	Barometric Pressure	Alveolar P_{O_2}	Arterial P_{O_2}
0	760	149	99[1]
2000	707	138	88[1]
4000	656	127	77[1]
6000	609	118	68[1]
8000	564	108	58[1]
10000	523	100	50[1]
12000	483	91	41[1]
14000	446	83	41[2]
16000	412	76	34[2]
18000	379	69	27[2]
20000	349	63	21[2]
30000	226	37	0[2]

The fall in barometric pressure is shown as altitude increases. The alveolar partial pressure and estimated arterial partial pressure of oxygen are illustrated. The (A-a)P_{O_2} is assumed to be 0, the Pa_{CO_2} is assumed to be 40 torr[1] or 25 torr[2], and the respiratory quotient is assumed to be 0.8.

Decreased Inspired Oxygen

A second cause of low Pa_{O_2} that can be entirely explained by the alveolar gas equation is the effect of decreased FI_{O_2}, such as occurs at high altitude. Table 17–5 illustrates the effect on Pa_{O_2} of increased height above sea level. Once again, this cause of hypoxia can be overcome by increasing the inspired oxygen fraction. This is the reason that mountain climbers and pilots employ oxygen masks at high altitudes.

Diffusion Defects

Several years ago, the idea of a diffusion defect for oxygen was suggested. Since oxygen is more limited by diffusion than CO_2 and several other gases are, an increase in the thickness of the alveolar-capillary membrane could decrease Pa_{O_2}. A pulmonary function test, the carbon monoxide diffusion capacity, was purported to correlate with an increase in the thickness of this membrane (Chapter 9). This led to the concept of alveolar-capillary block, which was used to explain the hypoxia seen in a wide variety of pulmonary diseases. The clinical significance of this pathophysiologic mechanism has been questioned. In Figure 17–11, it can be seen that during transit through the pulmonary circulation the average red cell is fully saturated in less than 0.25 second, one third the time spent in contact with the gas exchange membrane. Even in those patients in disease states with massive thickening of this membrane (interstitial fibrosis, alveolar proteinosis), oxygenation is complete during the normal red cell transit time. It is only during periods when transit time is reduced (such as with increased cardiac output from exercise or fever) that desaturation occurs. This cause of arterial hy-

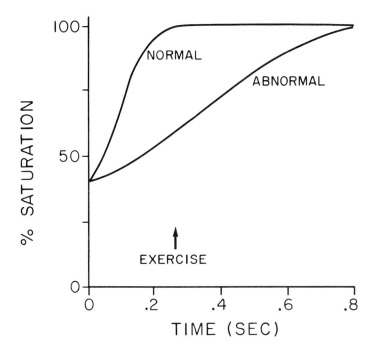

Figure 17–11. The time spent in transit through the pulmonary bed. Full saturation with oxygen is obtained in about one third of this time. Even in extremely abnormal alveoli with thickened walls, saturation is complete during the normal passage. Exercise shortens transit time and may cause desaturation in the extremely diseased lung by this mechanism. See the text for details.

poxia can be easily overcome by slight increases in the FIo_2. The use of portable, low-flow oxygen delivery devices has markedly improved the lifestyle of patients suffering from diseases causing this form of oxygenation failure.

Ventilation-Perfusion Mismatching

The most important cause of oxygenation failure is ventilation to perfusion mismatching ($\dot{V}/\dot{Q}$ mismatching). The extreme example of this problem is shunt, in which there is perfusion of areas that have no ventilation. Unlike the causes of hypoxia discussed in the preceding paragraphs, this cause of hypoxia is not overcome by simply increasing the FIo_2. To separate the effects of $\dot{V}/\dot{Q}$ mismatching from true shunt, 100% O_2 may be administered; any residual oxygenation deficit is due to true shunt. The series of curves in Figure 17–12 illustrate the relationship of FIo_2 to Pao_2 with various degrees of intrapulmonary shunt (extrapulmonary venous to systemic shunts behave in an analogous manner). Thirty percent inspired oxygen fails to correct the hypoxia caused by a shunt greater than 15%.

Therapeutic Approaches to Hypoxia

Diseases that lead to $\dot{V}/\dot{Q}$ mismatching and shunt include cardiogenic pulmonary edema, adult respiratory distress syndrome, pneumonia, pulmonary embolism, volume overload, inhalation burn injury, respiratory distress syndrome of the newborn, use of antineoplastic agents, and other diverse conditions. The therapeutic goal is treatment of the primary problem;

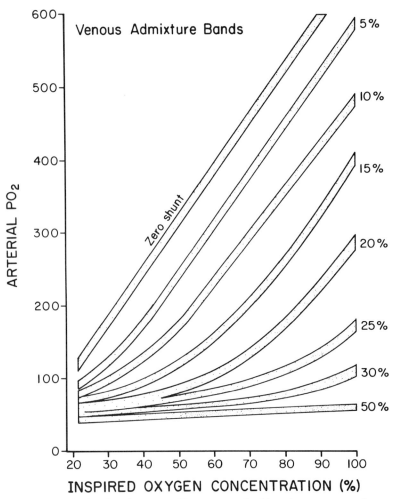

Figure 17–12. Bands showing the range of Pa_{O_2} expected with various amounts of venous admixture or shunt. Knowing the Pa_{O_2} and the inspired oxygen allows a guess at the amount of shunt present. (Modified from Nunn JF: Applied Respiratory Physiology. Cambridge: Butterworth, 1987; 371.)

however, maintenance of an appropriate Pa_{O_2} is essential for recovery. The main therapies used to increase Pa_{O_2} are increased FI_{O_2} and raised airway pressure. The goal in treatment of this class of disease is to maintain oxygenation on a nontoxic FI_{O_2}. Pulmonary oxygen toxicity occurs in less than 24 hours at an FI_{O_2} of 100%.[24] FI_{O_2} levels of 40–60% are probably acceptable at sea level.

Positive end-expiratory pressure (PEEP) is a useful and popular method of raising airway pressure. PEEP decreases shunt and increases lung volume (functional residual capacity).[25] The effectiveness of this form of therapy is increased if the lung pathology is uniformly distributed throughout both lungs. Since cardiac output may decrease with the application of PEEP, the actual Pa_{O_2} may decrease owing to a lower mixed venous P_{O_2} despite improvement in lung function and reduction of intrapulmonary shunt.

Table 17–6. METHODS PROPOSED TO
DETERMINE THE IDEAL LEVEL OF PEEP

Pa_{O_2} is acceptable
Static lung compliance is maximum[a]
Intrapulmonary shunt is 15% or less[b]
PEEP is lowest, and FI_{O_2} is up to 80%[c]
FI_{O_2} is less than or equal to 40%
Smallest end-tidal to arterial carbon dioxide gradient[d]

---

[a] Suter PM, Fairley HB, Isenberg MC: Optimum end-expiratory pressure in patients with acute pulmonary failure. N Engl J Med 1975; 292:284–289.
[b] Gallagher J, Civetta JM: Goal-directed therapy of acute respiratory failure. Anesth Analg 1980; 59:831–834.
[c] Petty TL, Fowler AA: Another look at ARDS. Chest 1982; 82:98–104.
[d] Murray IP, Modell JH, Gallagher TJ, Banner MJ: Titration of PEEP by the arterial minus end-tidal carbon dioxide gradient. Chest 1984; 85:100–104.

Table 17–6 lists several methods that have been suggested in order to decide on the "best" PEEP level. On one extreme is the group headed by Kirby and coworkers, who believe that PEEP is therapeutic and should be used to maximum effect regardless of the cardiovascular or barotraumatic effects.[26] The other side of the debate is illustrated by Petty and Fowler, who suggest that PEEP is toxic and should be employed only if high levels of FI_{O_2} are ineffective in preventing severe hypoxia (Petty and Fowler's work is done at an altitude over 5000 feet, and an FI_{O_2} of 100% is equivalent to an FI_{O_2} of only 78% at sea level).[27] Early use of some low level of end-expiratory pressure (10–12 cm of water pressure) in patients at risk for developing hypoxic lung disease is practiced by most clinicians, and it appears that the syndrome of adult respiratory distress syndrome is waning in incidence or its severity is decreasing.

Because the side effects of positive pressure ventilation and PEEP are significant and always affect the cardiovascular system,[28] monitoring of cardiac function is usually indicated when these modalities are employed. This is often assisted by use of a flow-directed pulmonary artery catheter, which may be used to optimize cardiac filling, cardiac output, and shunt fraction ($\dot{Q}s/\dot{Q}t$). The insertion techniques, use, and complications of this device are described in Chapter 5. Calculation of $\dot{Q}s/\dot{Q}t$ is performed with the following equation:

$$\dot{Q}s/\dot{Q}t = (Ca_{O_2} - Cc_{O_2})/(Cv_{O_2} - Cc_{O_2})$$

where Ca_{O_2}, arterial content of oxygen, is calculated from arterial saturation and measured hemoglobin, and Cv_{O_2}, mixed venous content of oxygen, is calculated from a mixed venous sample obtained from the distal port of the pulmonary artery catheter. Care must be taken to aspirate this sample slowly (usually over 20–30 seconds) in order to avoid arterializing the blood. The pulmonary capillary oxygen content, Cc_{O_2}, is estimated from the following equation:

$$Cc_{O_2} = 1.36 \times Hbg \times 100\% + 0.0031 \times Pa_{O_2}$$

This calculation is performed assuming that pulmonary capillary blood is fully saturated and that there is no alveolar-pulmonary capillary gradient for oxygen. These assumptions are incorrect, but the errors introduced are small and inconsequential for clinical management decisions.

The usefulness of the shunt calculation is that it removes the effect of changes in cardiac output from the intrapulmonary effects of airway pressure therapy. Although there is no *a priori* reason to believe that shunt is the pathologic problem in adult respiratory distress syndrome, those clinicians who monitor changes in shunting report the lowest mortality in this condition.[29] The use of PEEP to improve pulmonary compliance makes physiologic sense. However, difficulties in measuring pulmonary compliance and conflicting results by various investigators have made it a less useful parameter to optimize PEEP. All authors agree that PEEP should be used to avoid high concentrations of inspired oxygen.

The cardiac effects of PEEP (and positive airway pressure) include reduced venous return, increased right ventricular afterload, decreased left ventricular afterload,[30] and leftward shift of the intraventricular septum.[31] Possible effects of PEEP are reduced cardiac compliance[32] and reduced contractility.[33] Some authors have actually shown an increase in contractility with elevated airway pressure.[34] Since airway pressure may be reflected in vascular pressures, the absolute values of filling pressure are in doubt when increased airway pressures are employed. As much as half of the PEEP may be reflected in the ventricular filling pressure and should be subtracted from the measured value.[35] Cardiac status should be assessed by observing the changes in filling pressures and cardiac output occurring after volume challenges and not on the actual values seen during monitoring.

The effects of changes in the level of PEEP on the cardiovascular system are rapid and occur in several minutes. The effects on arterial blood gases are more gradual, requiring at least 10–15 minutes to reach a new steady state. The same is true for changes in FI_{O_2}, although evidence suggests that a shorter equilibration time period may be acceptable.[36]

Hyperoxia

Hyperoxia (Pa_{O_2} greater than 75 torr) in the premature infant is associated with the development of blindness due to retrolental fibroplasia.[37] Hyperoxia (at greater than 1.5 atm as seen in divers or in patients in hyperbaric chambers) stimulates the central nervous system and causes seizures.

However, there are several short-term therapeutic uses of hyperoxia (Table 17–7). Administration of 100% oxygen is therapeutic in carbon monoxide poisoning. Hyperbaric oxygen may also be employed in this circumstance (if a hyperbaric chamber is readily available). Systemic or venous air embolism is an indication for high FI_{O_2} in order to reduce the size of the bubble. Denitrogenation of the blood creates a pressure gradient for nitrogen to leave the bubble. Tension pneumocephalus[38] or pneumothorax may be

Table 17–7. THERAPEUTIC USES OF INCREASED FI_{O_2}

> Carbon monoxide poisoning
> Venous air embolism
> Arterial air (or other gas) embolism
> Fetal distress (maternal hyperoxia)
> Acute myocardial ischemia
> Cerebral ischemia
> Pneumothorax
> Pneumocephalus
> Fluorocarbon blood substitute
> Anaerobic infections

improved by a high Pa_{O_2}, but direct removal of the trapped air is the normal therapeutic approach. In obstetric delivery, fetal metabolic status may be improved when maternal Pa_{O_2} is elevated above 200 torr. When a fluorocarbon blood substitute is used to replace red cells, 100% oxygen must be used to raise the amount of dissolved oxygen to acceptable levels (5 vol%).[39] Administration of high FI_{O_2} is practiced in patients with chest pain presumably due to myocardial infarction or ischemia in order to prevent hypoxia from pulmonary edema and to improve cardiac oxygenation. Hyperoxia has been shown to improve cerebral function in patients after cerebral artery occlusion,[40] but the risks from oxygen toxicity have not made this a standard practice for long-term treatment.

CARBON DIOXIDE AND pH

Investigations into pH and CO_2 measurements originated with concerns over fermentation processes in the 1800s. Pasteur demonstrated that control of acidity was essential for proper brewing and creation of wine from grapes. Nernst developed the theory of electrochemical activity, which led Oswald to the development of the hydrogen electrode capable of measuring pH. The equipment was refined and used on blood by Hasselbalch, Belcher, Astrup, and others. Gasometric techniques developed by Van Slyke enabled researchers and clinicians to determine the P_{CO_2} accurately. Today, the measurement of P_{CO_2}, pH, and P_{O_2} is combined in a single machine capable of analyzing as little as 50–100 μl of blood.

Transport of Carbon Dioxide

The end products of cellular respiration are carbon dioxide and water. The human body produces about 12,000 mEq of acid in the form of CO_2 every 24 hours. This tremendous load is excreted by the lungs in the form of volatile acid (CO_2), and body pH is closely regulated. A smaller amount of fixed acid is excreted by the kidneys. This amounts to about 1 mEq/kg

Table 17–8. FORMS AND AMOUNT OF CO_2 CARRIED IN WHOLE VENOUS BLOOD

Dissolved CO_2	1.27 mmol/L
Carbonic acid (undissociated)	0.0012 mmol/L
Bicarbonate ion	20.3 mmol/L
Carbamino compounds (hemoglobin)	1.7 mmol/L
Total	23.3 mmol/L

O_2 saturation is 70%, hemoglobin is 12–14 gm/100 ml.

of body mass/day. These two systems are responsible for the control of body acid-base balance and maintenance of optimal pH for metabolic function of individual organs and the whole body.

In order for ventilation to be efficient in acid removal, metabolic CO_2 must be transported to the lungs. CO_2 is relatively insoluble in blood and is predominantly carried as bicarbonate, which is produced by reaction with water as shown in the following chemical equation:

$$CO_2 + H_2O \rightleftharpoons H_2CO_3 \rightleftharpoons H^+ + HCO_3^-$$

In order for this system of CO_2 transport to work, the normally slow conversion of CO_2 to bicarbonate is facilitated by the enzyme carbonic anhydrase in the red blood cells. Hemoglobin and other proteins serve as carriers for some of the CO_2 produced. The relative amounts of CO_2 carried in each of these forms is indicated in Table 17–8.

Hemoglobin acts as a buffer when oxygen is released at the tissue level. This allows some of the H^+ produced from carbonic acid to be neutralized by hemoglobin. This is referred to as the Haldane effect. As illustrated in Figure 17–13, when a solution of oxygenated free hemoglobin at pH 7.3 is deoxygenated, the solution pH increases to 7.5. As oxygen is released at the tissues, the buffering effect of hemoglobin allows less pH change than would otherwise occur with the production of carbonic acid.

Most of the important parts of the CO_2 transport system occur inside red cells. Major ion and chemical shifts are indicated in Figure 17–14. In order to maintain electrical neutrality inside the red cell, chloride ion is exchanged for bicarbonate. This is termed the chloride shift. Potassium ion is excreted from the cell as well. The total number of particles in the red cell increases as a result of these events, and water passively enters the cell along an osmotic gradient. The red cell swells, resulting in a venous hematocrit level that is slightly greater than the arterial (6–10%) change. Venous potassium levels are similarly elevated. These differences should be kept in mind when analyzing blood drawn from arterial catheters and comparing the results with normal venous values.

Buffer systems consist of a weak acid or base and its salt. These systems change in pH by increasing or decreasing the amount of their dissociated form when a stronger acid or base is added to the system. The general behavior of such buffers is illustrated for a theoretic buffer system in Figure

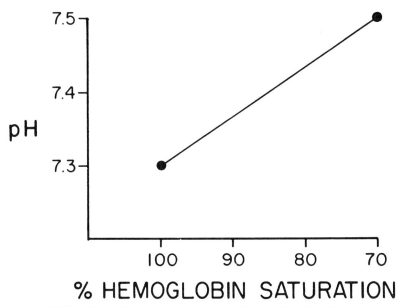

Figure 17–13. The effect of desaturating a solution of hemoglobin. The pH increases as the saturation decreases. This is referred to as the Haldane effect.

17–15. As acid or base is added to the system, the pH tends to remain unchanged. A buffer system is most resistant to changes in pH and is most efficient at buffering around its pK. The pK is the pH at which the weak acid or base is half dissociated.

The general chemical dissociation formula for a weak base is shown in the following equation:

$$BOH \rightleftharpoons OH^- + B^+$$

where BOH = a weak base, OH^- = the hydrogen ion accepter, and B^+ is available to form a salt. When a strong acid is combined with a weak base, the following equation describes the buffer system formed:

$$strong\ base\ +\ weak\ base \rightleftharpoons weak\ acid\ +\ neutral\ salt$$

pH is defined as the negative logarithm of the hydrogen ion concentration of an aqueous solution. K is the ionization constant for an acid or a base. K can be defined in the following way for a weak acid:

$$K[HA] = [H^+] \times [A^-]$$

where [HA] = the concentration of the un-ionized acid, $[H^+]$ = the concentration of the hydrogen ion, and $[A^-]$ = the concentration of the salt-forming radical (or base). Rearranging this equation yields

$$[H^+] = K[HA]/[A^-]$$

Taking the negative logarithm of both sides yields

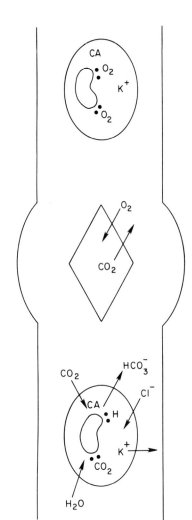

ARTERIAL

	Blood	Red Cells
pCO_2 (torr)	40	42
pO_2 (torr)	100	100
pH	7.40	7.14
HCO_3^- (meq/L)	24	10
K^+ (meq/L)	4.0	140
Cl^- (meq/L)	105	5
Hematocrit	40	

CAPILLARY BED

VENOUS

	Blood	Red Cells
pCO_2 (Torr)	46	50
PO_2 (Torr)	40	40
pH	7.36	7.04
HCO_3^- (meq/L)	28	14
K^+ (meq/L)	4.5	137
CL^- (meq/L)	103	7
Hematocrit	43	

Figure 17–14. The transition of blood from arterial to venous. (CA = carbonic anhydrase.) The chemical composition and blood gas changes are illustrated. An important change is the increase in levels of hematocrit and potassium. Other details are explained in the text.

$$-Log\ [H^+] = pH = -LogK + Log\ \{[A^-]/[HA]\}$$

By convention, pK is the negative logarithm of K. pH can be defined in terms of any of its buffer pairs as suggested by the following general formula:

$$pH = pK + Log\ \{[base]/[acid]\}$$

Since bicarbonate is present in the blood in large quantities, the use of carbonic acid in this equation yields the following description of blood pH:

$$pH = pK + Log\ \{[HCO_3^-]/[H_2CO_3]\}$$

The pK for this reaction is 3.5, far from the usual blood pH.[41] By expressing this equation in terms of CO_2 (since there is approximately 600

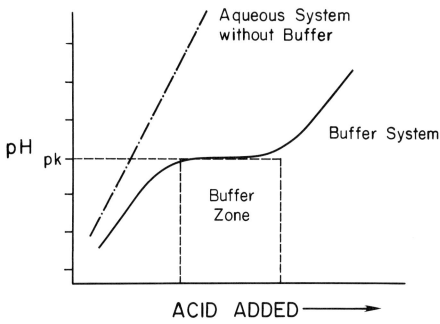

Figure 17–15. The performance of a "typical" buffer system. A buffer system resists change best around its pK. The effect on pH of an aqueous system without buffer is contrasted.

times more CO_2 than H_2CO_3 present in blood), the apparent pK becomes 6.1, and the classic Henderson-Hasselbalch form of the equation is

$$pH = 6.1 + Log \{[HCO_3^-]/(s \cdot PCO_2)\}$$

where s = the solubility factor for CO_2. Even with this pK, this buffer would not be a very satisfactory one to maintain a pH of 7.40. However, since the CO_2 can be continually removed from the system, the pH can be regulated. This is called an open system. The importance of respiration in the maintenance of acid-base balance is demonstrated during apnea when the blood pH rapidly falls to very low levels in several minutes. This is illustrated in Figure 17–16. To change the pH by an equivalent amount using renal compensatory mechanisms takes several days.

Use of the term pH is somewhat confusing in clinical practice because it represents logarithmic changes in hydrogen ion concentrations. As seen in Figure 17–17, the hydrogen ion concentration changes 10 times between pH of 7.00 and 8.00. At a normal pH of 7.40, the hydrogen ion concentration is about 40 mEq/L. When we consider how tightly controlled most body chemicals are (such as potassium or sodium), it is surprising to see that hydrogen ion is normally allowed to vary between 32 and 45 mEq/L (pH 7.35–7.45).

Clinical Acid-Base Management

Respiratory disorders are determined from the value of the Pa_{CO_2}. If the Pa_{CO_2} is greater than 45 torr, then a respiratory acidosis is present. This

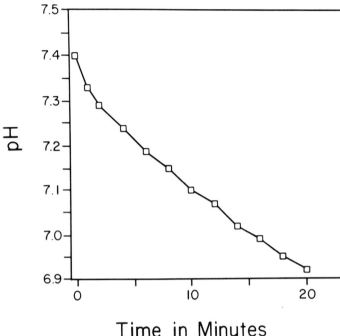

Figure 17–16. pH changes over time during apnea. The importance of the respiratory system to acid-base balance is discussed in the text.

is often called hypoventilation; however, this term carries the connotation of a patient who is breathing slowly and shallowly. Patients may, in fact, be hyperventilating in a clinical sense (breathing rapidly or deeply with an elevated minute ventilation). In order to avoid confusion, increased Pa_{CO_2} is called "respiratory acidosis" or "hypercapnia" throughout the remainder of this chapter. Respiratory alkalosis is defined as a Pa_{CO_2} less than 35 torr. This is not referred to as "hyperventilation" but as "hypocapnia" or "respiratory alkalosis." In referring to the various components of a respiratory or metabolic derangement, processes are identified with the suffix "osis" regardless of the blood pH. The pH of the blood is referred to as "emia." For example, a patient with a low pH due to metabolic acidosis may have partial respiratory compensation (pH < 7.35 and $Pa_{CO_2} < 35$); this would be described as acidemia (low blood pH) from metabolic acidosis (the metabolic process) with respiratory alkalosis or hypocapnia (the respiratory process).

The major problem in dealing with the interpretation of acid-base information is separation of the metabolic and respiratory components. For every primary disorder, there is a partial or complete compensatory response in the other component. When a disorder is treated, it is essential to identify the initiating disturbance, as this may require therapy. Treatment must not be applied to the compensatory changes. Many systems of analysis have been developed to deal with the problem of identifying the primary disorder and secondary response. Several of these approaches are described later in this chapter. None of the systems is totally effective or always produces the correct answer. Whenever there is more than a single primary disorder, no

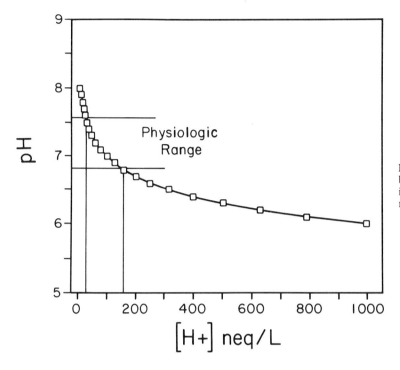

Figure 17–17. The relationship between pH and actual hydrogen ion concentration. The normal range is quite wide.

system is capable of sorting out the issues and directing therapy. The clinical status of the patient and her or his response to attempted correction of a disturbance provide the information needed to correctly proceed in diagnosis and treatment.

When blood gas results are reported from an automated analyzer, the P_{CO_2} and the pH are measured with electrodes having accuracies of 2–3%. The values for bicarbonate, standard bicarbonate, or base excess are calculated from nomograms based on the Henderson-Hasselbalch equation or other nomograms based on the behavior of blood or plasma in a test tube (*in vitro*). These derived parameters were devised in attempts to separate the metabolic or fixed component (renal) from the respiratory component (Pa_{CO_2}) of the acid-base status. Table 17–9 lists the normal values for some of these proposed parameters. Some of these indexes attempt to remove the

Table 17–9. METABOLIC INDEXES OF ACID-BASE BALANCE

Parameter	Range of Normal
Plasma bicarbonate	22–26 mEq/L
Total CO_2	23–27 mEq/L
CO_2 combining power	21–27 mEq/L
Standard bicarbonate	21–25 mEq/L
Whole buffer base	45–50 mEq/L
Base excess	−3 to +3 mEq/L

respiratory component of the disorder. This is done by equilibrating the sample with a gas mixture having a P_{CO_2} of 40 torr and a P_{O_2} of 100 torr under standard conditions at normal body temperature (37°C).

Total CO_2 includes bicarbonate and dissolved CO_2. It is based on extraction techniques and is not very different from plasma bicarbonate[42] (CO_2 dissolved is only $\frac{1}{20}$ the amount of bicarbonate). No correction is made for the respiratory system contribution in either of these indexes.

CO_2 combining power was suggested as a way to account for the respiratory contribution to the disorder. Plasma is equilibrated with gas having a P_{CO_2} of 40 torr. The total CO_2 (and bicarbonate) is determined and should approximate the "corrected" metabolic contribution to acid-base balance. Theoretic problems with this variable are that it is based only on the plasma component of blood (as indicated previously, hemoglobin plays a significant buffering role clinically), and it is an *in vitro* correction.

Standard bicarbonate, proposed by Astrup, is the bicarbonate of whole blood equilibrated under standard conditions of P_{CO_2} and temperature and includes the *in vitro* buffering contribution of hemoglobin.[43]

Whole buffer base includes the addition of the "unmeasured" buffers (amino acid protein components) to plasma bicarbonate. It does not take into account the contribution from changes in hemoglobin oxygenation, which may buffer pH at the tissue level. Whole buffer base is normally 45–50 mEq/L. It is not measured under standard conditions and is subject to influence by hemoglobin level.

Base excess is the amount of acid (or base) needed to return a sample of whole blood to normal pH under standard conditions of P_{CO_2}, P_{O_2}, and temperature.[44] It is also an *in vitro* method for estimating the body's metabolic attempt to correct for abnormalities in acid-base status. The normal value for base excess is 0.

All these methods describe *in vitro* techniques to define the metabolic components of an acid-base disorder. Deviations from normal values are proposed to indicate a metabolic derangement. A problem of interpretation of these parameters is caused by the fact that compensation does occur and "normal" values are not necessarily appropriate.[45]

DISORDERS OF ACID-BASE EQUILIBRIUM

The use of "significance bands" as described by Arbus and associates[46] helps identify the primary disorder and the expected compensatory response range. As seen in Figure 17–18,[47] the six primary disorders can be identified in graphic form. These disorders, described later in this chapter, are acute respiratory alkalosis, chronic respiratory alkalosis, metabolic alkalosis, acute respiratory acidosis, chronic respiratory acidosis, and metabolic acidosis.

To use the graphic method to identify the types of derangements present, plot the pH and Pa_{CO_2}. The intersection identifies the type of problem. For example, a pH of 7.54 with a Pa_{CO_2} of 25 indicates "acute respiratory al-

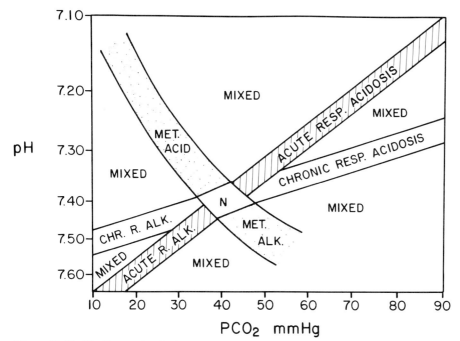

Figure 17–18. Significance bands describing the expected range of compensation for the primary disorders. See text for details. (Reprinted [modified] with permission from the International Anesthesia Research Society from Acid-base disorders: Application of total body carbon dioxide titration in anesthesia, by Levesque RP, Anesthesia and Analgesia, 1975; 54:307.)

kalosis'' with appropriate metabolic compensation. The areas marked "mixed" identify situations in which more than one primary disorder are present or the degree of compensation is inappropriate. There is no system available to separate the components when more than a single primary disorder is present. The clinical situation must be known in order to appropriately diagnose the problem. Further information can be obtained by making interventions and repeating measurements. Only primary derangements should be treated, and then only if certain limits are exceeded and symptoms are present.

The data used to design the "significance bands" in Figure 17–18 were obtained by observing groups of patients with only one primary disorder and recording their range of compensation. These data have been collected and summarized.[48] Table 17–10 summarizes the *in vivo* compensation that occurs in response to a primary disorder. To use this information, simply use the correction factor to predict the corrected value. Any deviation from this value indicates a second disorder and may require treatment.

Arterial versus Venous Acid-Base Balance

Because there is very little difference between arterial and venous P_{CO_2}, usually only 4–5 torr, a venous sample can be used to evaluate acid-base

Table 17–10. COMPENSATORY RESPONSES TO THE SIX PRIMARY DISORDERS

Primary Disorder	Compensatory Response (Expected)	Magnitude of Response (Predicted)
Respiratory alkalosis (acute)	Decreased bicarbonate	$[HCO_3{}^-]$ decreases 2 mEq/L for each 10 torr decrease in $Paco_2$
Respiratory alkalosis (chronic)	Decreased bicarbonate	$[HCO_3{}^-]$ decreases 5 mEq/L for each 10 torr decrease in $Paco_2$
Metabolic alkalosis	Increased $Paco_2$	$Paco_2 = 0.9 \times [HCO_3{}^-] + 9$ $Paco_2 = 0.9 \times [HCO_3{}^-] + 15.6$ $Paco_2 = $ base excess $ + 40.6$
Respiratory acidosis (acute)	Increased bicarbonate	$[HCO_3{}^-]$ increases 1 mEq/L for each 10 torr increase in $Paco_2$
Respiratory acidosis (chronic)	Increased bicarbonate	$[HCO_3{}^-]$ increases 3.5 mEq/L for each 10 torr increase in $Paco_2$
Metabolic acidosis	Decreased $Paco_2$	$Paco_2 = 1.5 \times [HCO_3{}^-] + 8$ $Paco_2 = 1.8 \times $ (base excess $- 24) + 8$ $Paco_2 = $ Last 2 digits pH

The direction of the expected response is indicated as well as several rules of thumb for determining the magnitude of the response.

status. Bicarbonate is calculated from the pH and is also only slightly lower in venous samples. This is a useful fact to remember in the operating theater when the diagnosis of malignant hyperthermia is being entertained. Since this hypermetabolic state is characterized by early development of a mixed metabolic and respiratory acidosis, venous acid-base balance is an excellent monitor for this syndrome.[49] In the case of a patient with cardiorespiratory arrest when external chest compressions are being performed, a large discrepancy between arterial and venous blood gases may exist.[50] The venous Pco_2 may reflect the adequacy or inadequacy of the artificial circulation and tissue acid-base status. The end-tidal Pco_2 may be a useful monitor of tissue acidosis, as it reflects venous and tissue Pco_2 in this circumstance.[51]

Acute Respiratory Alkalosis

The $Paco_2$ decreases when alveolar ventilation exceeds carbon dioxide production (Table 17–11). This results in a rise in pH. An immediate change in total CO_2 and base excess follows the change in $Paco_2$. This amounts to a decrease of 2 mEq/L of bicarbonate (1.8 base excess units) for each 10 torr change in $Paco_2$. This immediate compensation is not due to renal mechanisms; it is most likely due to local tissue factors. After several hours, renal retention of acid increases this fall in the metabolic component and the disorder becomes chronic.

As seen in Table 17–11, many of the causes of hypocapnia have no

Table 17–11. CAUSES OF RESPIRATORY ALKALOSIS

Hypoxemia
Decreased pulmonary compliance
  Pulmonary edema
  Adult respiratory distress syndrome
  Pulmonary fibrosis
Infection
  Septic syndrome
  Pneumonia
  Fever
Bronchospasm (early)
Pulmonary embolism
Drugs
  Doxapram hydrochloride
  Theophylline
  Progesterone
  Salicylates
Pregnancy
Central nervous system disorders
Cirrhosis
Excessive mechanical ventilation
Anxiety
Psychogenesis

Some of these may require primary treatment; however, the low Pa_{CO_2} is usually never itself treated.

specific therapy. Respiratory alkalosis reduces cerebral blood flow and may improve intracranial compliance in patients with brain injury or tumor. No treatment would be appropriate because this is a normal protective response. Anxiety can often be treated with anxiolytic agents or reassuring discussions with the patient. Hypoxia (Pa_{O_2} less than 55 torr) affects the peripheral chemoreceptors (aortic and carotid bodies) and increases minute ventilation. Other disorders may be treated, but therapy is not appropriate for the hypocapnia *per se*.

Chronic Respiratory Alkalosis

When hypocapnia persists for several hours or longer, renal mechanisms are activated and further compensation occurs. Renal compensation occurs naturally in inhabitants of high altitudes. Respiratory alkalosis can be completely compensated with a normal pH, which is unusual in other disorders. For every 10 torr fall in Pa_{CO_2}, there is up to a 5 mEq/L decrease in bicarbonate (4 base excess units) as seen in Table 17–10.[52] It may take several weeks to normalize pH in this condition.

Metabolic Alkalosis

Because metabolic disorders develop slowly and respiratory compensation occurs rapidly, there is no chronic or acute differentiation. Despite

Table 17–12. CAUSES OF METABOLIC ALKALOSIS

Diuretic use
Nasogastric suction
Vomiting
Diarrhea (containing chloride)
Antacid administration
Transfusions (citrate)
Drugs
  Carbenicillin
  Penicillin
Hypokalemia
Hypercalcemia
Primary hyperaldosteronism

this fact, the respiratory response elicited may be quite variable. No definite reasons for this variability have been identified. A normal or low $Paco_2$ implies a coexisting respiratory alkalosis. Several formulas have been proposed to predict the respiratory compensation seen in metabolic alkalosis. The $Paco_2$ was equal to $0.9 \times$ [bicarbonate] $+ 12$ (range, 9–16) in a group of patients in whom alkalosis was induced by a variety of methods.[53] Other authors have found less of a compensatory respiratory acidosis, as indicated in Table 17–10.[54]

There are many causes of this common abnormality of acid-base balance. Some are listed in Table 17–12. Diuretic use with hypokalemia and hypochloremia is a common cause. Acid and chloride loss from the gastrointestinal tract, antacid administration, certain antibiotics, and some endocrine abnormalities are also implicated. Some causes are treatable by replacement of chloride and potassium. There are several undesired side effects of metabolic alkalosis. These include increased oxygen consumption, myocardial depression, increased cardiac arrhythmias, desensitized respiratory center, and hypoxia on room air (see causes of low Pao_2, given previously).

Acute Respiratory Acidosis

Disorders that decrease the efficiency of pulmonary carbon dioxide excretion may increase $Paco_2$. Acute changes in the metabolic component result in pH being returned toward normal. Normal people with acute elevation in $Paco_2$ show about 1 mEq/L increase in bicarbonate for each 10 torr increase in $Paco_2$ (0.8 base excess units) owing to tissue and hemoglobin buffers.[55] Renal regulation takes much longer but is far more complete, as described later.

The causes of acute respiratory acidosis include drug effects on the respiratory center or neuromuscular transmission and upper or lower airway obstruction. Narcotics and sedatives, general anesthetics, bronchospasm, upper airway occlusion, and rebreathing of exhaled CO_2 are causes of acute CO_2 retention (Table 17–13).

Table 17–13. CAUSES OF RESPIRATORY ACIDOSIS

Chronic obstructive pulmonary disease
Acute bronchospasm
Primary alveolar hypoventilation syndrome
  Ondine's curse
  Pickwickian syndrome
High-level spinal cord injury
Myasthenia gravis
Multiple sclerosis
Muscular dystrophies
Bulbar polio
Guillain-Barré syndrome
Narcotic drug effects
Neuromuscular-blocking drugs
Airway obstruction
General anesthetics
Mechanical ventilation
Rebreathing
  Intentional
  Equipment failure

The effects of acute hypercapnia are fairly benign. If hypoxia is avoided, hypercapnia increases heart rate and blood pressure. It shifts the hemoglobin saturation curve to the right. Dysrhythmias and enhanced cardiac contractility result. Serum potassium increases. If the $Paco_2$ increases above 80–90 torr, anesthesia or CO_2 narcosis usually results.

Treatment of acute hypercapnia is directed at relief of the underlying cause rather than the pH change. Occasionally, it is necessary to correct the pH with exogenous base. The use of bicarbonate is controversial in that more CO_2 is produced and the pH may remain unchanged. Also, since the CO_2 can freely diffuse into cells, the intercellular pH may actually fall further. Nonbicarbonate buffers such as THAM (tris[hydroxymethyl]aminomethane) have been suggested for this use.[56, 57]

Chronic Respiratory Acidosis

When an elevated $Paco_2$ persists for longer than 6–10 hours, the metabolic response is more complete. Hypercapnia causing acidemia stimulates retention of bicarbonate. Compensation does not return blood pH to normal if $Paco_2$ is greater than 55 torr. An increase of 3.5 mEq/L bicarbonate (3 base excess units) for every 10 torr rise in $Paco_2$ is seen in response to this primary disorder.[58] CO_2 retention is a result of ventilation-perfusion mismatch in chronic lung disease.[59] End-stage restrictive lung disease (such as kyphoscoliosis) may also result in hypercapnia. Ondine's curse and the pickwickian syndrome are conditions in which the central nervous system center controlling respiratory drive becomes less sensitive to changes in pH, with a resultant elevation in $Paco_2$. As a consequence of this abnormality, pulmonary hypertension and right heart failure frequently follow prolonged elevations of Pa_{CO_2}. Hypoxia on room air (described previously) also occurs as a consequence of elevated Pa_{CO_2}.

The treatment of the elevated CO_2 should be directed at the underlying cause. Ventilatory muscle weakness, fatigue,[60] and malnourishment[61] contribute to elevated CO_2 in chronic pulmonary disease. Diaphragm rest and nutritional improvement can favorably affect gas exchange. Conditioning exercises may also improve muscle strength and endurance.[62] High glucose loads during parenteral feeding can increase CO_2 production by stimulating fat synthesis and may worsen respiratory failure.[63] Drugs that have been used to reduce Pa_{CO_2} include estrogens, caffeine, aminophylline, and doxapram hydrochloride.[64] Surgical procedures to correct airway obstruction and obesity have been successful in treating the pickwickian syndrome. Positive pressure ventilation reverses the CO_2 retention, but this may mean indefinite commitment to artificial ventilation. The use of a ventilator during sleep may improve function and prolong life in those terminal patients with very high Pa_{CO_2} levels.

Metabolic Acidosis

When metabolic acid products decrease the serum bicarbonate, the respiratory center is stimulated and ventilation increases. This response is proportional to the degree of change in bicarbonate and is delayed 12–24 hours. This delay is due to the resistance to transfer of bicarbonate across the blood-brain barrier. Central nervous system pH changes are slower than blood pH changes. When the brain is involved in the process, causing metabolic acidosis, this delay is absent. The expected Pa_{CO_2} in compensation for a decreased bicarbonate[65] is about 1.5 × [bicarbonate] + 8. Another rule of thumb is that the Pa_{CO_2} should be equal to the first two decimal point digits of the pH (a pH of 7.25 should have a Pa_{CO_2} of about 25) (see Table 17–10).

The causes of metabolic acidosis are listed in Table 17–14. These are divided into two groups; those with acid accumulation, called "high anion gap"; and those with bicarbonate loss, "normal anion gap." The anion gap is defined as the serum sodium minus the sum of the chloride and bicarbonate. This accounts for unmeasured anions, such as proteins, phosphate, sulfate, and others. The anion gap is usually 10–12. An increase in the anion gap means an accumulation of acid products such as lactic acid.

The underlying cause of the acidosis should be treated if possible. The following formula is useful to calculate the required amount of bicarbonate if correction of a deficit is deemed desirable:

Bicarbonate dose (mEq) = − base excess × 0.2 × weight (kg) or

Bicarbonate dose (mEq) = (24 − [HCO_3^-]) × 0.2 weight (kg)

These approximations allow about half the deficit in plasma to be corrected. The effect of treatment on acid-base parameters should be closely monitored. Recent data suggest that aggressive correction of the deficit in

Table 17–14. CAUSES OF METABOLIC ACIDOSIS

Normal Anion Gap	Elevated Anion Gap
Renal tubular acidosis	Renal failure
Diarrhea	Ketoacidosis
Carbonic anhydrase inhibitors	Starvation
	Ethanol ingestion
Ureteral diversions	Methanol ingestion
Hyperalimentation (chloride)	Ethylene glycol ingestion
	Salicylates
Renal failure (early)	Lactic acidosis
Acid ingestion	Nephrotic syndrome
Hyperchloremia	Seizures
	Circulatory failure
	Cyanide poisoning
	Carbon monoxide poisoning

metabolic acidosis may be associated with paradoxical central nervous system depression and respiratory arrest.[66] Concern for the levels of potassium, phosphate, and ionized calcium should also be considered in these disorders and during therapy. Complications often result from these other electrolyte imbalances.

Combined Acid-Base Disorders

The disorders described in the preceding sections were single primary disorders with the appropriate expected compensatory responses. More than one primary disorder may be present. This is indicated when the expected response to the first disorder is not seen. For a detailed description of these combined disorders, which are beyond the scope of this chapter, the reader should consult the excellent review by Narins and Emmett.[48]

OTHER MONITORS

The discussion about acid-base monitoring and clinical implications is based on the fact that the total body's contribution to metabolic activity is averaged in the blood. This sample only approximates what is happening in each separate tissue. Monitors of tissue pH, Pco_2, K^+, and Po_2 are being developed in laboratories and used in animals and some humans. Tissue probes are closer to the intracellular environment where the abnormalities originate and have their most significant effects. Other technologies, such as magnetic resonance imaging, identify intracellular metabolic derangements and may lead to the development of monitoring at the cellular level.

References

1. Severinghaus JW: Transcutaneous blood gas analysis. Respir Care 1982; 27:152–159.
2. Peterson JI, Fitzgerald RV, Buckhold DK: Fiberoptic probe for measurement of oxygen partial pressure. Anal Chem 1984; 56:62–67.
3. Eberhart RC: Indwelling blood compatible chemical sensors. Surg Clin North Am 1985; 65:1025–1040.
4. Bourke DL: Errors in intraoperative hematocrit determination. Anesthesiology 1976; 45:357–359.
5. Fox MJ, Brody JS, Weintraub LR et al: Leukocyte larceny: A cause of spurious hypoxemia. Am J Med 1979; 67:742–746.
6. Andritsch RF, Muravchick S, Gold MI: Temperature correction of arterial blood-gas parameters: A comparative review of methodology. Anesthesiology 1981; 55:311–316.
7. Ream AK, Reitz BA, Silverberg G: Temperature correction of P_{CO_2} and pH in estimating acid-base: An example of the emperor's new clothes? Anesthesiology 1982; 56:41–44.
8. Rahn H, Reeves RB, Howell BJ: Hydrogen ion regulation, temperature, and evolution. Am Rev Respir Dis 1975; 112:162–165.
9. Becker H, Vinten-Johansen J, Buckberg GD, et al: Myocardial damage caused by keeping pH 7.40 during deep systemic hypothermia. J Thorac Cardiovasc Surg 1981; 82:810–820.
10. Blayo MC, LeCompte Y, Pocidalo JJ: Control of acid-base status during hypothermia in man. Respir Physiol 1980; 42:287–298.
11. Ong ST, David D, Snow M, Hanson JE: Effect of variations in room temperature on measured values of blood gas quality-control materials. Clin Chem 1983; 29:502–505.
12. Thorson SH, Marini JJ, Pierson DJ, Hudson LD: Variability of arterial blood gas values in stable patients in the ICU. Chest 1983; 84:14–18.
13. Gilbert R, Auchincloss JH, Kuppinger M, Thomas MV: Stability of the arterial/alveolar oxygen partial pressure ratio. Crit Care Med 1979; 7:267–272.
14. Gilbert R, Keighley JF: The arterial-alveolar oxygen tension ratio. An index of gas exchange applicable to varying inspired oxygen concentrations. Am Rev Respir Dis 1974; 109:142–145.
15. Perutz NF: Stereochemistry of cooperative effects in hemoglobin. Nature 1970; 228:726–739.
16. Perutz NF: Hemoglobin structure and respiratory transport. Sci Am 1978; 239:92–125.
17. Shappell SD, Lenfant CJM: Adaptive, genetic, and iatrogenic alterations of the oxyhemoglobin-dissociation curve. Anesthesiology 1972; 37:127–139.
18. Schumacker PT, Long GR, Wood LDH: Tissue oxygen extraction during hypovolemia: Role of hemoglobin P_{50}. J Appl Physiol 1987; 62:1801–1807.
19. Rubio R, Berne RM: Regulation of coronary blood flow. Prog Cardiovasc Dis 1975; 43:105–122.
20. Nunn JF: Applied Respiratory Physiology. London: Butterworth, 1987; 241, 473.
21. Block AJ, Cherniac RM, Christopher KL, et al: Problems in prescribing and supplying oxygen for medicare patients. Am Rev Respir Dis 1986; 134:340–341.
22. Deneke SM, Fanburg BL: Normobaric oxygen toxicity of the lung. N Engl J Med 1980; 303:76–86.
23. Marshall BE, Wyche MQ: Hypoxemia during and after anesthesia. Anesthesiology 1972; 37:178–209.
24. Davis WB, Rennard SI, Bitterman PB, Crystal RG: Pulmonary oxygen toxicity,

early reversible changes in human alveolar structures induced by hyperoxia. N Engl J Med 1983; 309:878–883.

25. Roes DM, Downes JB, Heenan TJ: Temporal responses of functional residual capacity and oxygen tension to changes in positive end-expiratory pressure. Crit Care Med 1981; 9:79–82.

26. Kirby RR, Downs JB, Civetta JM, et al: High level end expiratory pressure (PEEP) in acute respiratory failure. Chest 1975; 67:156–163.

27. Petty TL, Fowler AA: Another look at ARDS. Chest 1982; 82:98–104.

28. Dorinsky PM, Whitcomb ME: The effect of PEEP on cardiac output. Chest 1983; 84:210–216.

29. Gallagher J, Civetta JM: Goal-directed therapy of acute respiratory failure. Anesth Analg 1980; 59:831–834.

30. Luce JM: The cardiovascular effects of mechanical ventilation and positive end-expiratory pressure. JAMA 1984; 252:807–811.

31. Jardin F, Farcot JC, Boisante L, et al: Influence of positive end-expiratory pressure on left ventricular performance. N Engl J Med 1981; 304:387–392.

32. Haynes JB, Carson SD, Whitney WP, et al: Positive end-expiratory pressure shifts left ventricular pressure-area curves. J Appl Physiol 1980; 48:670–676.

33. Prewitt RM, Wood LDH: The effect of positive end-expiratory pressure on ventricular function in dogs. Am J Physiol 1979; 236:H534–544.

34. Buda AJ, Pinsky MR, Ingels NB, et al: Effects of intrathoracic pressure on left ventricular performance. N Engl J Med 1979; 301:453–459.

35. Chapin JC, Downs JB, Douglas ME, et al: Lung expansion, airway pressure transmission, and positive end-expiratory pressure. Arch Surg 1979; 114:1193–1197.

36. Mathews PJ: The validity of Pa_{O_2} values 3, 6, and 9 minutes after an FI_{O_2} change in mechanically ventilated heart-surgery patients. Respir Care 1987; 32:1029–1034.

37. Lucey JF, Dangman B: A reexamination of the role of oxygen in retrolental fibroplasia. Pediatrics 1984; 73:82–96.

38. Kitahata LM, Katz JD: Tension pneumocephalus after posterior fossa craniotomy: A complication of the sitting position. Anesthesiology 1976; 44:448–450.

39. Faithfull NS: Fluorocarbons: Current status and future applications. Anaesthesia 1987; 42:234–242.

40. Kapp JR: Neurological response to hyperbaric oxygen—a criterion for cerebral revascularization. Surg Neurol 1981; 15:43–46.

41. Roughton JWF: Transport of oxygen and carbon dioxide. *In* Fenn WO, Rahn H (eds): Handbook of Physiology, Section 3, Respiration, Vol 1. Washington, DC: American Physiological Society, 1964; 800.

42. Van Slyke DD, Cullen GE: Studies of acidosis. I. Bicarbonate concentration of blood plasma: Its significance and its determination as measure of acidosis. J Biol Chem 1917; 30:289–346.

43. Astrup P: New approach to acid-base metabolism. Clin Chem 1961; 7:1–15.

44. Astrup P, Jorgensen K, Siggaard Andersen O, Engle K: Acid-base metabolism: A new approach. Lancet 1960; 1:1035–1039.

45. Schwartz WB, Relman AS: A critique of the parameters used in the evaluation of acid-base disorders. N Engl J Med 1963; 268:1382–1388.

46. Arbus CS, Hebert LA, Levesque PR, et al: Characterization and clinical application of the "significance band" for acute respiratory alkalosis. N Engl J Med 1969; 280:117–123.

47. Levesque PR: Acid-base disorders: Application of total body carbon dioxide titration in anesthesia. Anesth Analg 1975; 54:299–307.

48. Narins RG, Emmett M: Simple and mixed acid-base disorders: A practical approach. Medicine 1980; 59:161–187.

49. Durbin CG: Malignant hyperthermia syndrome: Identification and management. *In* Berry FA (ed): Anesthetic management of difficult and routine pediatric patients. New York: Churchill Livingstone, 1986; 414–415.

50. Grundler W, Weil MH, Rackow EC, et al: Selective acidosis in venous blood during human cardiopulmonary resuscitation: A preliminary report. Crit Care Med 1985; 13:886–887.

51. Garnett AR, Ornato JP, Gonzalez ER, Johnson EB: End-tidal carbon dioxide monitoring during cardiopulmonary resuscitation. JAMA 1987; 257:512–515.

52. Lahiri S, Milledge JS: Acid-base in Sherpa altitude residents and lowlanders at 4880 M. Respir Physiol 1967; 2:323–334.

53. Fulop M: Hypercapnia in metabolic alkalosis. NY State J Med 1976; 76:19–22.

54. Goldring RM, Cannon PJ, Heinemann HO, Fishman AP: Respiratory adjustment to chronic metabolic alkalosis in man. J Clin Invest 1968; 47:188–202.

55. Brackett NC, Cohn JJ, Schwartz WB: Carbon dioxide titration curve of normal man: Effect of increasing degrees of acute hypercapnia on acid-base equilibrium. N Engl J Med 1965; 272:6–12.

56. Minuck M, Sharma GP: Comparison of THAM and sodium bicarbonate in resuscitation of the heart after ventricular fibrillation in dogs. Anesth Analg 1977; 56:38–45.

57. Manfredi F, Sieker HO, Spoto AP, Saltzman HA: Severe carbon dioxide intoxication: Treatment with organic buffer (trishydroxymethyl aminomethane). JAMA 1960; 173:999–1003.

58. Brackett NC, Wingo CF, Muren O, Solano JT: Acid-base response to chronic hypercapnia in man. N Engl J Med 1969; 280:124–130.

59. West JB: Causes of carbon dioxide retention in lung disease. N Engl J Med 1971; 284:1232–1236.

60. Arora NS, Rochester DF: Respiratory muscle strength and maximal voluntary ventilation in undernourished patients. Am Rev Respir Dis 1982; 126:5–8.

61. Hunter MAB, Cary MA, Larsh HW: The nutritional status of patients with chronic obstructive pulmonary disease. Am Rev Respir Dis 1981; 124:376–381.

62. Sonnes LJ, Davis JA: Increased exercise performance in patients with severe COPD following inspiratory resistive training. Chest 1982; 82:436–439.

63. Covelli HD, Black JW, Olsen MS, Beekman JF: Respiratory failure precipitated by high carbohydrate loads. Ann Intern Med 1981; 95:579–581.

64. Aubier M, De Troyer A, Sampson M, et al: Aminophylline improves diaphragm contractility. N Engl J Med 1981; 305:249–277.

65. Albert MS, Dell RB, Winters RW: Quantitative displacement acid-base equilibrium in metabolic acidosis. Ann Intern Med 1967; 66:312–322.

66. Morris LR, Murphy MB, Kitabchi AE: Bicarbonate therapy in severe diabetic ketoacidosis. Ann Intern Med 1986; 105:836–840.

chapter eighteen

Perioperative Biochemical Monitors

■ WILLIAM P. ARNOLD III, M.D.

The anesthesiologist depends on many biochemical analyses to gather information not available from either physical examination or other monitors. In recent years, reliance on intraoperative laboratory data has become routine, especially in more extensive surgical procedures. Although the relevance of laboratory data is usually well understood by the clinician, the nuts and bolts of the assays that produce these data are less clear. The purpose of this chapter is to review the basis of biochemical tests commonly used during the perioperative period, while highlighting the role of the acute or "stat" clinical laboratory. Emphasis will be placed on the details of the assay rather than on the myriad of clinical implications discussed in general textbooks of anesthesiology. Included are reasons for inaccuracies, errors in sample handling by those obtaining blood for analyses (e.g., effects of anticoagulants, sample volume), the importance of understanding the various methods employed by the clinical chemist, and the effects of different assay methods on interpretation of results (e.g., serum sodium, pseudohyponatremia). For a detailed discussion of the gamut of determinations performed by the clinical chemist, the reader is encouraged to consult a comprehensive textbook of clinical chemistry.[1]

615

THE ACUTE LABORATORY

Our ability to provide intensive perioperative care has been significantly advanced by improvements in the methods employed by clinical chemistry laboratories and especially by the creation of satellite facilities, called acute or stat laboratories, located in close proximity to acute care areas.

An acute laboratory, dedicated only to those assays required for the perioperative management of critically ill patients and those undergoing extensive surgical procedures, is an essential part of many hospitals. Although these laboratories are physically separated from the main clinical laboratory, they usually remain under the administrative and operational control of the clinical chemist.[2] This is extremely important since personnel involved full-time are more aware of the need for quality control and maintenance of analytic equipment than are those to whom the laboratory is only a means to an end.[3, 4]

The proximity of the laboratory to the ward or operating room permits a positive, ongoing interaction between the clinician and the clinical chemist. A close relationship between the disciplines is important because it encourages discussion of a variety of factors that may affect results. These include such things as the time that a sample is obtained, the effects of various anticoagulants, the patient's condition, and the source of the sample (whether it is central or peripheral venous, arterial, or capillary).[4] It also instills a sense of active participation on the part of the clinical chemist, which would otherwise be absent owing to the remoteness of the main laboratory.[5]

ASSAY METHODS IN THE ACUTE LABORATORY

Flame Photometry

Flame photometry is still used by some clinical laboratories to determine the concentrations of various ions, including sodium, potassium, and lithium, in body fluids. Certain ions emit colors when heated. The wavelength of the color produced by a given ion is characteristic of that ion, for example, 589 and 766 nm (yellow and red-violet) for sodium and potassium, respectively. In practice, a salt-containing solution is injected into a flame. After the water in the sample has been evaporated, the molecules of the salt are dissociated into an atomic vapor. A small number of the atoms are subsequently excited by the heat, resulting in the displacement of electrons into higher orbitals. Almost immediately, these atoms return to their ground state and, in doing so, release light of a specific wavelength that identifies that ion. The intensity of the color is directly proportional to the concentration of the ion in question. It is measured by a phototube, the output of which is displayed as a concentration. Sodium and potassium may be measured simultaneously with this method. Lithium is usually added to the sample as an internal standard to compensate for variables that otherwise might result in quantitative inaccuracies. A separate phototube is used for each ion. Standard solutions of the ions in question must be used to calibrate the instrument, since it is impossible to calculate the light intensity emitted by a given concentration of sodium or potassium.[6]

Flame photometry used to be an important method in the acute laboratory, but it has been displaced by newer methods. One of the main objections to the technique was the need to have explosive gas (propane) in the laboratory in order to provide a source for the flame.[1]

Ion-Selective Electrodes

The ion-selective electrode (ISE) has become the mainstay for assaying electrolytes in the modern acute laboratory. Although it is not important for the clinician to understand all of the nuances of these devices, a basic understanding of their operation aids in interpretation of results and in understanding the occasional differences between results determined with ISEs and results from other methods used in central clinical chemistry laboratories.

ISEs are basically batteries that develop a voltage or potential between two electrodes in contact with the sample. The potential is proportional to the concentration of the specific ion being assayed (Fig. 18–1). The potential is mathematically related to the concentration by the Nernst equation:

$$E = E_0 + \frac{RT}{nF} \ln (fC)$$

where E = electrical potential, E_0 = constant potential, R = universal gas constant, T = temperature, n = charge of the ion being measured, F = Faraday's constant (96,500 coulombs), f = activity coefficient of the ion being measured, C = concentration of that ion.

Because ISEs respond to a difference in potential, they are referred to as potentiometric sensors. Some measuring devices respond to current instead of voltage and are thus amperometric sensors. An example of the latter is the Clark oxygen electrode, a modification of which is used in some glucose analyzers.[1]

All ISEs are composed of a reference electrode and a measuring electrode, each of which may be thought of as a half-cell.[1] The voltage between the two electrodes is displayed as the activity of ion being assayed. The reference electrode is usually composed of either a silver wire covered with a coating of silver chloride or mercury in contact with calomel ($HgCl_2$). The electrode is immersed in an internal filling solution of potassium chloride or other constituents of known concentration that in turn, via a liquid-liquid junction, forms a salt bridge with the solution being measured. The measuring electrode is a metallic conductor that is immersed in an internal solution containing a known concentration of the ion in question. This solution is separated from the sample in question by a membrane that is selectively responsive to the ion. A potential develops across the membrane as the result

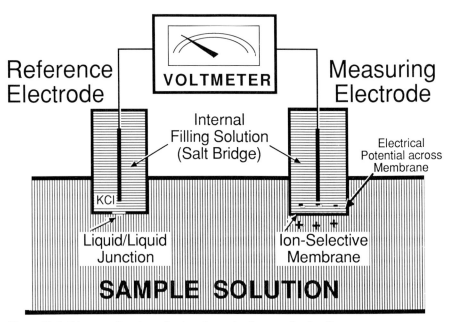

Figure 18–1. Diagram of an ion-selective electrode. See text for details.

of an exchange of ions in the outer layers of the membrane. The potential difference between the measuring and the reference electrodes is proportional to the concentration of the ion being assayed. This difference is detected by a sensitive voltmeter, converted to the appropriate units, and displayed as a concentration.

Some ISEs require that the sample be diluted prior to assay (indirect potentiometry), whereas others detect ions in undiluted samples (direct potentiometry). Results from diluted samples are reported in units of concentration of an ion, and those from undiluted samples are reported as activities of that ion.[1] Although this distinction may seem arcane, it becomes important when interpreting results (see Activity versus Concentration).

The prototype of the ISE is the pH electrode. It consists of a calomel reference electrode and a measuring electrode containing a solution of 0.1 N hydrogen chloride that is separated from the sample by a thin membrane made of glass composed of oxides of sodium, silicon, and calcium. This glass membrane is selective for hydrogen ions. When the electrode is placed into a sample, a potential develops across the membrane. Hydrogen ions in the sample cause the oxides on the outer surface of the glass to become charged. Similarly, the hydrogen chloride in contact with the inner surface of the membrane induces a charge in the oxides on that surface. An electrical potential develops across the glass membrane that is proportional to the number of hydrogen ions in the sample. The potential that develops between the reference and the measuring electrodes is converted to pH units. All other ISEs work by essentially the same principle.[1]

ISEs have been developed to measure Na^+, K^+, Ca^{2+}, F^-, Cl^-, and others. All are potentiometric sensors. The keys to the function of these various electrodes are the membranes that make each electrode selective for only the ion being measured. Like the pH electrode, the membrane in the sodium electrode is made of glass. The glass is composed of a mixture of oxides of silicon, sodium, and aluminum that is selective for sodium.

The membrane in widespread use for determining potassium consists of a collodion sheet impregnated with valinomycin, a cyclic antibiotic that is a highly selective binder of potassium ions.[7] The selectivity results, in part, from the conformation of the valinomycin molecule, the central cavity of which is about the size of the potassium ion. Glass electrodes have been developed to measure potassium, but they have proved to be less selective for the ion.[7]

A membrane composed of a liquid ion exchanger was developed in 1967 for the detection of ionized (or free) calcium.[8] The membrane contains the calcium salt of a disubstituted phosphoric acid. When the electrode and its reference half-cell come into contact with a sample, an electrical potential proportional to the concentration of ionized calcium in the sample develops across the membrane. Ionized calcium may be measured in serum, plasma, or whole blood. When whole blood is assayed, erythrocytes may alter the liquid junction potential of the reference electrode, resulting in artifactual increases in calcium activities (and sodium and potassium activities to a lesser extent). This problem has been eliminated by substituting sodium formate for potassium chloride in the salt bridge of the electrode.[9]

In practice, these membranes are not absolutely selective. Sodium electrodes in common use are a thousand times more selective for sodium than for potassium. Potassium electrodes have about ten thousand times greater affinity for potassium than for sodium.[6] The calcium electrode is capable of measuring free calcium in solutions containing a 1000-fold greater concentration of sodium or potassium ions.[9] Thus, at clinical concentrations of these ions, interference is unlikely. Clinically important details regarding interference with the output of electrodes are discussed in the sections dealing with specific ions.

ACTIVITY VERSUS CONCENTRATION

Most assay methods, including flame photometry and indirect potentiometry, determine the concentration of the total amount of ion in plasma or serum. In contrast, direct potentiometry measures only the concentration of the free unbound ion in plasma water, a value more accurately termed activity. Activity refers to the amount of ion that is physiologically active rather than to the total amount of ion (see Osmolality). It must be stressed that activities are determined in plasma water rather than in the entire plasma volume. This is an important distinction when considering the significance of reported values since physiologic control mechanisms regulate the concentrations of ions in the water phase rather than in the entire plasma volume.[10] Even though ISEs respond to activity rather than concentration, results are usually reported in units of concentration. Activity is related to concentration by the following formula:

$$A = \gamma c$$

where A = activity, γ = the activity coefficient, and c = the concentration of the ion.[11]

The difference between activity and concentration becomes important in certain diseases, such as hyperlipidemia or hyperproteinemia. In these diseases, lipids or proteins displace water from the portion of the plasma that they occupy and similarly displace all material dissolved in the water phase. Thus, the volume occupied by ions is significantly smaller than the total volume of the plasma. An example of this phenomenon is the pseudohyponatremia associated with hyperlipidemia. It is an artifactual occurrence solely dependent on the method used to measure sodium. Assays requiring dilution of the sample, such as flame photometry and indirect potentiometry, are inaccurate when used to assay sodium in lipemic serum, since the differences between activity and concentration diminish if the sample is diluted prior to assay.[10, 12] With lipemic serum, either of these methods produces results that may be as much as 15–25 mmol/L lower than the physiologically correct value as determined by direct potentiometry, which does not involve dilution of the sample.[12] Values determined by indirect potentiometry in hyperlipemic plasma may also be incorrect.[12] Perfluorocarbon emulsions, used experimentally as blood substitutes, also displace water in plasma. As expected, these compounds have a similar effect on laboratory values.[13]

SAMPLE HANDLING

Laboratory results may sometimes be changed significantly by improper methods of sample collection and transportation. Details that may seem insignificant have the potential to alter results enough to modify clinical decisions. The specific factors that are relevant to individual analytes are discussed in the sections on these compounds. This section covers some of the general aspects of sample handling that affect results but may be overlooked, especially during the intensive management of critically ill patients.[1, 3]

Sample Collection

Variability

Arterial or venous blood samples obtained in the operating room or intensive care unit are usually anticoagulated with heparin and sent to the acute laboratory in a syringe immediately after collection. Results from these specimens may not be identical to those determined in a central laboratory on samples sent from the ward. A variety of things may unknowingly cause differences between routine and stat samples leading to confusion or misinterpretation. Some of the more common factors affecting the routine samples are discussed in the following sections.

Position

Changes in body position alter the concentrations of many blood constituents. It is widely recommended that patients should be seated or supine for at least 15 minutes prior to phlebotomy. The increase in hydrostatic pressure from standing causes significant shifts of the filterable components of blood into cells, resulting in hemoconcentration and a decrease in plasma volume ranging from 12% in healthy individuals to as much as 30% in those who are ill.[14] Standing increases serum potassium, calcium, total protein, albumin, and some enzyme activities when compared with the supine position.[15] The Scandinavian Committee on Reference Values suggests that persons at bed rest and ambulatory individuals who have been seated for 15 minutes represent different reference populations (see Reference Values versus ''Normal'' Values).[16] Thus, patient position during phlebotomy for preoperative laboratory values affects the reported results.

Venipuncture

The technique of venipuncture used by the phlebotomist may alter test values. Tourniquets cause venous stasis, resulting in increased protein concentration, concomitantly increased protein-bound constituents, release of certain intracellular chemicals, and decreased pH as lactate accumulates.[1] If the fist is pumped during phlebotomy, increases in plasma potassium of more than 1 mmol/L have been observed,[17] and further increases in lactate are likely. The decrease in pH increases the concentration of ionized calcium.[18] Some authors, however, have reported that a tourniquet decreases[15] or has no effect on the concentration of serum potassium.[19]

Vacuum Tubes

Both vacuum tubes that aspirate blood through a needle and vigorous manual aspiration may artificially increase the plasma concentration of intracellular constituents by causing hemolysis.[1, 20] An erroneous increase in potassium concentration is the most common result of hemolysis seen in the acute laboratory (see Potassium). The activities of many enzymes, including lactate dehydrogenase, aspartate aminotransferase, acid phosphatase, creatine kinase, and alanine aminotransferase, are fallaciously increased if hemolysis is present.[20] In contrast, hemolysis has no effect on observed concentrations of albumin, total protein, calcium, chloride, creatinine, glucose, sodium, urea, and many other constituents.[21]

Tube Filling Order. The order in which tubes are filled should be indicated, since it may affect certain constituents. The notable effect is on potassium, the concentration of which is slightly higher (0.1 mmol/L) in the initial few milliliters of blood removed during phlebotomy.[20]

Tube Composition. Glass tubes made of soda lime release trace ele-

Table 18–1. CODING OF STOPPER COLOR

Color	Additive	Use
Gray	Oxalate, fluoride and iodoacetate	To inhibit glycolysis in plasma or whole blood
Yellow	None	To collect sterile samples
Green	Heparin	To collect plasma or whole blood
Red	None	To collect serum
Blue	Citrate	To collect plasma or whole blood
Lavender	Ethylenediaminetetra-acetic acid	To collect plasma or whole blood

Modified from Young DS, Bermes EW Jr: Specimen collection and processing; sources of biological variation. *In* Tietz NW (ed): Textbook of Clinical Chemistry. Philadelphia: WB Saunders, 1986; 482.

ments, such as magnesium and calcium, into the sample and may spuriously increase the observed values. Tubes composed of borosilicate do not have this effect.[1]

Anticoagulant

Commercially prepared tubes containing known quantities of specific anticoagulants are commonly used if whole blood or plasma is required for testing. The anticoagulant in the tube is indicated by the color of the stopper (Table 18–1).[1] By convention, tubes with either red or yellow tops contain no anticoagulant and are thus used to collect serum after the blood has been allowed to clot. The values for certain analytes, including calcium, glucose, inorganic phosphorus, potassium, and total protein, vary considerably between serum and plasma. Occasionally, the differences are great enough to influence clinical decisions (see Potassium). Therefore, it is important to consider which anticoagulant has been used when interpreting results.[22]

Heparin is the most common anticoagulant in specimens assayed in the acute laboratory. It is an acidic, heterogeneous polymer of D-glucuronic acid and D-glucosamine containing sulfuric acid ester groups. Heparin readily forms salts and is commonly supplied as the sodium salt, although preparations containing lithium or other cations are also available. Heparin is prepared commercially from bovine lung and porcine intestinal mucosa. It functions immediately by neutralizing several activated clotting factors.[23]

Final concentrations of heparin needed to anticoagulate samples of blood are said to be 1 u of heparin/ml of sample,[23] 2 u/ml,[1] and 20 u/ml.[1] The dead space volume of a 3-ml disposable syringe is about 60 μl.[24] Commercially prepared heparin is usually supplied in a concentration of 1000 u/ml. If a 3-ml syringe, the dead space of which contains heparin, is filled completely with blood, the concentration of heparin in the blood will be approximately 15 u of heparin/ml of blood. For most assays, this concentration should have minimum effect on laboratory results. However, heparin may alter certain values if more than the recommended amount is added to the sample. For example, 10–50 u of sodium heparin/ml of blood increases the observed value for sodium by 0.5–2 mmol/L.[1, 25] In contrast to these small changes, heparin significantly decreases the observed values for ionized calcium (see Calcium).

Although anticoagulants other than heparin are not normally used for perioperative chemical analyses, they are frequently used for routine analyses (Table 18–1). If an improper anticoagulant is used, results may be significantly altered. Fluoride, a preservative for glucose, is a potent inhibitor of many enzymes. Ethylenediaminetetra-acetic acid (EDTA) interferes with methods used to determine chloride. Both citrate and EDTA, used in coagulation and hematologic studies, decrease calcium activities by chelation. Oxalates also bind calcium. Iodoacetate inhibits creatine kinase.[1, 3]

Sampling from Catheters and Tubing

Most samples are obtained intraoperatively from indwelling catheters. For results of these assays to be correct, the samples must be drawn properly. A volume nearly that of the tubing must be withdrawn from an arterial catheter before blood-tinged fluid appears, and accurate results can be assured only after withdrawing six times the volume of the tubing.[26] Similar recommendations hold true for samples drawn from central venous catheters.[27] Dilutions of the sample by the flush solution in the line alter results significantly and must be avoided.

Risk of Infection

Any biologic sample may contain pathogens. Human immunodeficiency virus (HIV), discovered in 1983 to be the etiologic agent in acquired immunodeficiency syndrome (AIDS), has recently become a topic for discussion, debate, and controversy among many specialties, including anesthesiology.[27–31] Hepatitis is far more common and also of concern.

HIV may be transmitted by parenteral inoculation, with likelihood of transmission usually being related to the volume of the inoculum. Although transfusion of blood containing HIV carries a high risk, a small inoculum, such as that from a needle stick (the volume of which is less than 2 μl),[32] is associated with a low incidence of transmission of the virus. However, at least one case may have resulted from merely compressing a puncture site following an unsuccessful attempt to cannulate a radial artery.[33] The minimum dose required to infect humans is unknown. The reported incidence of HIV infection in health care workers having a history of parenteral contact with the virus is 1.3–3.9/1000 exposures.[34] The upper 95% confidence limit for the risk of acquiring the disease at this writing is 0.76%.[34] The most common preventable exposures are from needle sticks during attempts to recap needles and from improperly discarded objects. Nearly 10% of the exposures occur in laboratories.[35]

The overall incidence of AIDS in health care workers as of July 1987 was identical to that in the general population. In both groups, the disease is common only in those individuals who have exhibited high-risk behavior.[36] In contrast to AIDS, the likelihood of health care workers developing hepatitis from contact with infected patients or specimens is much higher. The incidence of seropositivity following parenteral inoculation with hepatitis B ranges from 19% to 27%. The risk of infection strongly correlates with the extent of blood contact and the frequency of needle accidents.[37]

Because every patient may be infected with communicable pathogens, not all of which can be identified preoperatively, the Centers for Disease Control have recommended that all patients be treated as if they are infective. Similarly, all laboratory specimens should be considered to be infective. Gloves should be worn while obtaining and processing samples. Needles should be handled with extreme caution and should not be recapped. Containers should be sturdy and covered in order to prevent leakage during transport. Blood that is discarded following analysis should be either incinerated or poured into a sanitary sewer. Warning labels are not needed if all specimens are treated with the same precautions.[36]

Transportation of Samples

Transportation may have an adverse effect on laboratory results. Factors such as cellular metabolism[38] and pH changes[18] may occur during delays in forwarding samples. It is critically important that certain specimens be kept on ice, especially if there are delays between collection and analysis. Pneumatic transport systems may subject samples to harmful vibration and forces of acceleration if they are rapidly propelled. Cells may rupture during transport and may release intracellular contents, especially if specimen containers are inadequately cushioned or are only partially filled with blood. Although most tube systems are capable of transporting samples safely, such systems should be evaluated before they are used for this purpose.[39] Messengers need to be aware of the critical importance of their role in providing rapid, safe transport of hand-carried samples.

SPECIFIC ANALYTES

The following sections discuss specifics regarding the analytes (the sample being analyzed) commonly measured in the acute laboratory, with emphasis on those factors that may affect results. Although each section contains brief discussions of the physiologic role of each analyte, the reader should refer to other texts for more extensive discussions of these functions.

Glucose

Specimen Collection

Both arterial and venous blood may be obtained in the perioperative period, but for many analytes, including glucose, the results from these two sources are not strictly comparable. Arterial and capillary blood may contain significantly higher concentrations of glucose than does venous blood.[40, 41] There is little difference between arterial and venous values in fasti tients. However, during infusion of solutions containing glucose, arterial values may be as much as 70 mg/dl greater than venous values in samples drawn simultaneously.[42]

Precautions must be taken to prevent glycolysis by the cellular components of blood after a sample has been obtained. In the absence of a metabolic inhibitor, blood with normal hematologic values undergoes a decrease in glucose concentration of about 10 mg/dl (0.56 mmol/L) of blood per hour when stored at 25°C.[1] Erythrocytes at 37°C metabolize glucose at a rate of up to 18 mg/dl (1 mmol/L) of blood per hour,[43] and leukocytes metabolize about half this amount over the same period.[44] Leukocytosis may decrease the concentration of glucose as much as 65 mg/dl over 1–2 hours if no glycolytic agent has been added to the sample.[45] The most effective antiglycolytic agents are fluoride and iodoacetate (gray-colored stopper). Samples that are analyzed immediately after being drawn need not contain these agents. The clinician must be aware, however, that results may be affected significantly if processing is delayed.[38]

Methods of Analysis

Glucose is usually measured in plasma or serum rather than in whole blood. It is also measured in urine as a screening test for diabetes and also to guide perioperative glucose control in diabetic patients. Values for glucose in whole blood are about 10% lower than values in plasma. The explanation follows, and it is similar to that for pseudohyponatremia (see Activity versus Concentration). Glucose is limited to the water phase of blood. Its concentration in the aqueous phases of both red cells and plasma is identical.[46] However, erythrocytes contain 20% less water than does an equivalent volume of plasma. Thus, there is less glucose per unit volume of red cells, since the portion of the red cell that is nonaqueous excludes glucose. Consequently, a given volume of blood contains less glucose than does the same volume of plasma.

Immobilized enzymes are used as reagents in the assay of glucose. The enzyme glucose oxidase is immobilized or bonded to an adsorbent such as cellulose or agarose. It then participates in but is not consumed by the following chemical reaction:

$$glucose + O_2 \xrightarrow{glucose\ oxidase} gluconic\ acid + H_2O_2$$

The change in oxygen concentration with respect to time as measured with a Clark oxygen electrode reflects the glucose concentration in the sample. Since the Clark oxygen electrode is used to detect the disappearance of oxygen, some mention of its operation is warranted before discussing the use of immobilized enzymes in the assay for glucose.

The Clark method for detecting oxygen is an amperometric, or current-measuring, assay. In amperometric assays, a constant voltage is applied to two electrodes in an electrochemical cell. The analyte, which must be capable of being oxidized or reduced, is brought into contact with the cell. It is ionized by the voltage, and a current proportional to its concentration through the cell. The current is measured and displayed as the con-

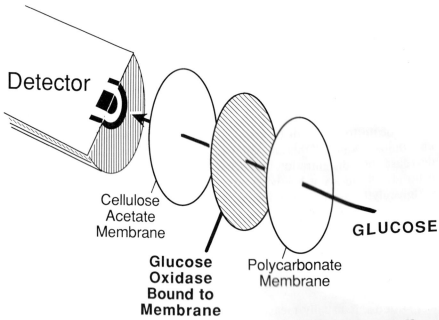

Figure 18–2. Diagram of a glucose analyzer that employs immobilized enzyme. Glucose oxidase is bound to the membrane in the center. Depending on the specific analyzer, the amperometric detector, shown on the left, measures either the decrease in oxygen or the increase in hydrogen peroxide produced during the conversion of glucose to gluconic acid. A similar method may be used to assay lactate by substituting lactate oxidase for glucose oxidase and measuring hydrogen peroxide. (Modified from Clark LC Jr, Noyes LK, Grooms TA, Moore MS: Rapid micromeasurement of lactate in whole blood. Crit Care Med 12(5):461–464, © by Williams & Wilkins, 1984.)

centration of the analyte in question. The Clark electrode works by this principle. It consists of a platinum cathode maintained at a potential of -0.65 V and a silver–silver chloride anode in phosphate buffer containing potassium chloride. The electrode is separated from the solution being tested by a membrane permeable to oxygen. Oxygen diffuses across the membrane and is reduced at the cathode; current proportional to the amount of oxygen in the sample flows through the electrode.[47]

A multitude of time-consuming, complex methods have been developed for assaying glucose.[6] Rapid methods such as the amperometric glucose oxidase method are used in acute laboratories. The glucose analyzer contains a membrane to which glucose oxidase has been bound (Fig. 18–2). The catalytic ability of the enzyme is not altered by the membrane. The enzyme may be used for multiple assays and is stable for months.[48] As with all assays involving enzymes, temperature and other reaction conditions must be painstakingly controlled. To perform the assay, the operator injects a precisely measured sample into the analyzer. It is assumed that all the glucose in the sample is oxidized to gluconic acid. The P_{O_2} in the reaction mixture is continuously measured by a Clark oxygen electrode as the reaction proceeds. The amount of oxygen consumed during the reaction, which is proportional to the concentration of glucose in the sample, is recorded by an el circuit. Results are displayed as the concentration of glucose in the sample and are available within 20 seconds.[49] Similar amperometric methods for glucose have been developed to measure the appearance of hydrogen peroxide rather than the disappearance of oxygen.[50]

The glucose oxidase method is also used for urinary glucose determinations. Reagents are impregnated into filter paper, making a convenient paper strip for urine testing.

Reference Ranges*

To some extent, reference ranges for glucose are dependent upon the assay method used. They also are influenced by the techniques of the individual laboratory. For the glucose oxidase–oxygen method, the range is 65–110 mg/dl.[6] Normally, glucose is absent in the urine until the plasma levels exceed 150–300 mg/dl. This variability results from variation in the rate of delivery of glucose to the proximal tubule and tubular reabsorption efficiency.

Sources of Inaccuracy

As discussed previously, results of glucose assays are affected by the source of the sample (arterial or venous) and the length of time between collection and analysis if inhibitors of glycolysis have not been added to the sample. Results may also be influenced by drugs that a patient is taking preoperatively. Acetylsalicylic acid and indomethacin increase, caffeine has a variable effect, and ibuprofen has no effect on apparent values for glucose when assayed by a variety of methods.[51] Ascorbic acid at high therapeutic levels decreases glucose slightly.[52] None of these changes is of a major magnitude. In contrast, acetaminophen, which has become a drug of abuse, significantly interferes with the amperometric-H_2O_2 method of glucose analysis when large amounts of the drug are ingested. Thus, falsely elevated values for glucose occur after ingestion of large quantities of acetaminophen.[53]

Physiologic Role

Glucose is an essential source of energy. It is the primary substrate for the phosphorylation of adenosine to adenosine triphosphate. It is converted to glycogen for storage in the liver and may also be converted to fat. It may be formed from sources other than carbohydrates by gluconeogenesis. Its concentration in blood is regulated by insulin, which enhances the transfer of glucose into cells, and by several other hormones, including glucagon, epinephrine, and cortisol, which increase its concentration. Glucose is an absolute requirement for proper function of the central nervous system, which is incapable of storing glucose.[1]

---

* See pages 648–649 for a discussion of the differences between reference ranges and normal values. The former is the more acceptable terminology.

Lactate

Specimen Collection

Lactate concentrations were measured during anesthesia well before the development of rapid measurement techniques.[54] The significance of isolated lactate analyses in anesthetized patients was questioned decades ago, but the ratio of lactate to pyruvate (L/P) was felt to be a marker of oxygenation in these patients and thus of some importance.[55] Later work demonstrated that L/P is not always an accurate indicator of oxygenation at the cellular level.[56] Although changes in lactate concentration occur in the anesthetized patient, the perioperative utility of the information is still somewhat unclear, especially if examined without regard to other physiologic and biochemical data.[57]

Method of Analysis

An analyzer has been developed that measures lactate in less than 1 minute in either whole blood or plasma.[58] The method is identical in principle to the amperometric-H_2O_2 technique for glucose. Immobilized lactic oxidase catalyzes the following reaction:

$$\text{lactate} + O_2 \xrightarrow{\text{lactic oxidase}} \text{pyruvate} + H_2O_2$$

Hydrogen peroxide is detected amperometrically. The rapidity of the method makes it suitable for both acute and research laboratories.

Reference Ranges

Normal arterial blood lactate concentrations are 9.7–16.3 mg/100 ml at rest. Lactate concentrations increase with physical exercise.

The clinical significance of these measurements in the perioperative period is currently being investigated. Plasma lactate levels have been measured in conjunction with other tests during hepatic transplantation. In one report, lactate increased at a rate of 2.6 mmol/L/hour prior to hepatectomy in 12 recipients. Lactate increased less rapidly during the anhepatic phase but increased acutely and then decreased when the allograft was perfused after vascular anastomosis. The magnitude of the decrease in plasma lactate concentrations after reperfusion may predict subsequent hepatic function.[59]

OSMOMETRY

Biologic fluids contain dissolved particles of widely differing sizes, ranging from ions such as hydrogen, sodium, and chloride to proteins. Semipermeable membranes permit some small particles to cross while inhibiting the passage of others. The particles are distributed across cell membranes in part by osmosis, a measurable phenomenon. Since water freely crosses biologic membranes, there is osmotic equilibrium throughout the body.

Osmometry is the measurement of the concentration of solute particles in a solvent such as water, without regard to the identity of the particles. It is based on the measurement of any one of four related physical properties, also known as colligative properties, that are common to all solutions containing particles. These properties are osmotic pressure, boiling point, vapor pressure, and freezing point. Changes in these variables are related to the collective concentrations of all the particles in solution. The first two increase and the latter two decrease as the solute concentration is increased. Osmosis refers to the flow of water across a semipermeable membrane. The direction that water travels is governed by the difference in concentrations of the solutions on the two sides of the membrane. Generally, the flow of water is toward the side containing the greater number of solute particles. That is, water flows down its concentration gradient. An example of osmosis is the swelling and lysis of red cells when placed in distilled water. Osmotic pressure is strictly defined as the hydrostatic pressure required to prevent changes in volume when solutions containing solutes of differing concentrations are separated by a semipermeable membrane. The contribution of small molecules is determined by measuring the osmolality of a solution. The effect of large molecules is assessed by measuring colloid osmotic pressure.[1, 6]

Osmolality

The molarity of a solution is the number of moles of a compound per liter of water. Molality is the number of moles per kilogram of water. Concentrations are usually reported in moles per liter; that is, with respect to the *volume* of water rather than to its mass. In contrast, molality is applied to osmometry because the calculations are simpler with respect to mass than to volume.

Osmolality is the number of moles of particles per kilogram of water. It is directly related to the molal concentration of all the solutes in a liquid. If a solution contains only noncharged particles, then the numeric values for molality and osmolality are identical. Solutions of salts composed of monovalent ions, such as sodium chloride, yield 2 moles of particles/mole of salt (assuming complete dissociation), making the osmolality twice the molality. Calcium chloride dissociates into three particles, so its osmolality is three times its molality. Actually, most salts are not completely dissociated in solution. For example, sodium chloride is only about 93% dissociated in physiologic solutions, making its actual osmolality only 1.86 times its molality. The true osmolality is equal to the molal activity of the compound, which reflects the biologically effective concentration of the ions in solution (see Activity versus Concentration).[6]

Specimen Collection

Osmolality may be measured in either serum or plasma. If plasma is analyzed, heparin is the appropriate anticoagulant, since others increase the observed osmolality.[60]

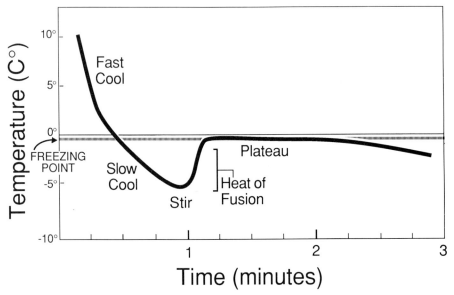

Figure 18–3. Temperature changes in a freezing point osmometer. See text for details.

Method of Analysis

Osmolality is determined by measuring any of the four colligative properties of solutions. In practice, only decreases in freezing point and vapor pressure are used routinely. Freezing point depression is most commonly used because of its ease and relative simplicity. The change in freezing point is directly related to the number of particles in a solution. This principle is used "therapeutically" by road maintenance engineers to melt ice and snow by increasing the osmolality of the precipitate and thus decreasing its freezing point. Each mole of particles added to pure water lowers the freezing point of the solution by 1.858°C. The freezing point of a solution containing 285 mOsm/L is thus −0.53°C.

By definition, the freezing point of liquid is the temperature at which the liquid and crystalline phases of a substance are in equilibrium. It is this temperature that is determined by a freezing point osmometer (Fig. 18–3). In practice, a small sample, typically 25–250 μl, is injected into the osmometer. The sample is first supercooled to −5°C to −7°C, a temperature well below its freezing point. Crystallization is then induced by vigorous stirring. As freezing proceeds, the heat of fusion released by the developing ice crystals warms the sample. After rapid freezing has stopped, an equilibrium temperature is attained between crystals and liquid. This plateau temperature is measured with a thermistor and is reported as the osmolal concentration of the sample.[1, 6]

Changes in vapor pressure also reflect the osmolality of a solution. The vapor pressure or dew point of an aqueous solution at 25°C is decreased by 0.3 mmHg/mole of particles. The vapor pressure osmometer measures the dew point temperature of a sample and converts the observed decrease into milliosmoles per liter. The volume sampled is less than 10 μl, making the technique attractive for use in pediatrics.[1, 6] Drawbacks of the method include the inability to detect volatile solutes that contribute to the osmolality of plasma, such as ethanol and other compounds of interest in acute poisoning.[61] It also gives erroneously high readings with lipemic sera.[62]

Reference Ranges

The normal osmolality of blood is 300 mOsm/kg with a range of 278–305 mOsm/kg. Urinary osmolality varies from 40 to 1350 mOsm/kg.

Physiologic Role

Serum osmolality alone does not permit an accurate assessment of the state of hydration. Evaluation of osmolality is important primarily to determine major deviations in serum water content and to screen for exogenous substances such as alcohol.[63] To do either, the observed and calculated osmolalities must be compared. The primary solutes contributing to the osmolality of serum are sodium, glucose, and blood urea nitrogen (BUN). Several empirical equations, each utilizing the observed values for these analytes, have been proposed for use in calculating serum osmolality.[63–65] One of these follows:

$$\text{Calculated osmolality} = 2 \times \text{sodium} + \text{glucose}/18 + \text{BUN}/2.8$$

where sodium is in mmol/L and glucose and BUN are in mg/dl.[63] Differences between observed and calculated values, referred to as the osmolal gap, result primarily from decreased serum water content as in hyperlipidemia and hyperproteinemia or from the presence of low-molecular substances such as ethanol, mannitol, and toxins. An osmolal gap of greater than 10 mOsm/kg suggests that one or more of these compounds are present.[63] Glycine may also contribute to the osmolal gap during transurethral resection of the prostate. Urine osmolality of greater than 600 mOsm/L demonstrates that the kidney is able to concentrate urine. Lower values are nondiagnostic.[6]

Colloid Osmotic Pressure

Colloid osmotic pressure (COP, or oncotic pressure) is osmotic pressure produced by large molecules in solution. In plasma it is generated primarily by albumin and to a lesser extent by globulins. Owing to their large molecular weights (30,000 daltons and more), the molal concentration of proteins in plasma is small. These macromolecules contribute less than 2 mOsm/kg of water to the osmolality of plasma, as determined by freezing point depression.

Method of Measurement

COP may be calculated if the concentrations of plasma proteins are known, although the calculated values are inaccurate in patients receiving intravenous colloid solutions and in critically ill patients.[30, 31]

COP is measured with a colloid osmometer. This device consists of a chamber divided into two compartments by a membrane permeable to molecules smaller than 30,000 daltons. The membrane separates the sample from physiologic saline, which is in contact with a pressure transducer. When serum or plasma from either arterial or central venous blood is injected into the osmometer, saline crosses the membrane by osmosis and enters the sample. After equilibrium has been reached, the pressure in the saline compartment has decreased by a value equal to the COP of the sample.[66] This value is presented on a digital display in millimeters of mercury.

Reference Range

COP in normal human plasma averages about 25 mmHg. It decreases with age and bed rest and is lower in females.

Sources of Inaccuracy

Peripheral venous blood should not be used for analysis, since stasis induced by a tourniquet drives intravascular water into tissues and artifactually increases the COP in the sample.[66] Dextran increases COP significantly in plasma, since it develops several fold greater pressure than do equimolar solutions of proteins.[1]

Physiologic Role

COP, in combination with pulmonary capillary wedge pressure, is felt by some authors to be of clinical importance in the diagnosis and treatment of pulmonary edema caused by left ventricular failure (see Chapter 5).[66] The gradient between COP and wedge pressure is normally about 10 mmHg. In patients with pulmonary edema, it is significantly lower.[67] Other authors question the clinical utility of the measurement, especially in patients with chronic hypoproteinemia.[68]

Sodium

Specimen Collection

Sodium may be determined in whole blood, serum, or plasma. Hemolysis, unless severe, has little effect on determined values for sodium, because its concentration in red cells is only 10% of its plasma concentration. Sodium values are minimally affected by venous stasis, time of sampling, postural changes, prolonged bed rest, eating, and exercise. Values are increased by 1–20 mmol/L if sodium heparin is used to anticoagulate the sample.[3, 25]

Method of Analysis

Sodium is most commonly determined with an ISE. Flame photometry may also be used, but the risk of explosion makes it less attractive.[1]

Reference Range

The reference range for serum sodium is 136–146 mmol/L. It is applicable from infancy through old age.[1]

Sources of Inaccuracy

Spuriously low values for sodium result when the analyte is assayed by flame photometry or indirect potentiometry in sera from patients with hyperlipidemia or hyperproteinemia (see Activity versus Concentration).[12]

Physiologic Role

Sodium is the major cation in extracellular water. Dietary intake and renal excretion of sodium are equal in the absence of pathology. Since sodium salts make up more than 90% of the solutes in plasma, they are responsible for most of its osmolality. The volume of the extracellular fluid is directly related to the quantity of sodium in the fluid. It is closely regulated by renal mechanisms involving the renin-angiotensin-aldosterone system and other hormones.[69]

Measurement of plasma sodium concentrations in the perioperative period is done routinely. Some authors, however, believe that plasma sodium measurements are unhelpful except to diagnose such things as primary aldosteronism and causes for the alteration in neurologic state seen with acute water overload. The decrease in sodium commonly seen postoperatively usually results from water overload rather than from lack of sodium, especially since the stress of surgery causes secretion of antidiuretic hormone. At times, the results are misinterpreted. For example, unless results are evaluated in conjunction with serum osmolality, the differentiation of postoperative fluid overload from sodium loss cannot be made with certainty.[70]

Potassium

Specimen Collection

Because the intracellular concentration of potassium is nearly 40-fold greater than its plasma concentration, and its concentration in red blood cells is 25 times greater than plasma, great care must be exercised during phlebotomy and subsequent analysis to avoid contaminating the sample with potassium of cellular origin (see Sources of Inaccuracy, in this section). Preferably, an anticoagulant should be added when the sample is obtained.[3, 71]

Method of Analysis

In the acute laboratory, potassium is usually assayed with an ISE. This method is rapid and accurate, and it avoids the dangers imposed by flame photometers (see Assay Methods in the Acute Laboratory).

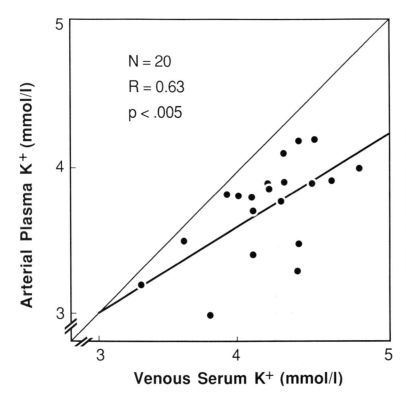

Figure 18–4. Arterial plasma versus venous serum potassium. The line running from the lower left corner to the upper right corner represents the line of identity. All venous values are below the line. (Modified from Ward CF, Arkin DB, Benumof J, Saidman LJ: Arterial versus venous potassium: Clinical implications. Crit Care Med 6(5):335–336, © by Williams & Wilkins, 1978.)

Reference Range

The reference range for potassium is 3.5–5.0 mmol/L.

Sources of Inaccuracy

Determined concentrations for potassium vary greatly between serum and plasma. Although samples referred to the acute laboratory are usually anticoagulated, the routine samples assayed in a central laboratory are frequently not. This may result in confusion if results from different laboratories are compared. The average concentration in serum is 0.4 mmol/L higher than plasma, but the range is quite wide: −0.6 to +1.4 mmol/L.[22, 50, 71] Similar differences have been observed between venous serum and arterial plasma (Fig. 18–4), the latter values being comparable with venous plasma.[72] These differences result from the release of potassium from platelets during clotting. Although there is a positive correlation between higher platelet counts and increases in serum versus plasma potassium in the same patient, there is such great variability between patients that prediction of the quantitative effect of thrombocytosis on potassium is impossible.[73] Potassium may also be released from white blood cells during the process of clotting, although this source is only important with extreme leukocytosis.[74]

Potassium values are increased by hemolysis, because of the great disparity between its intra- and its extracellular concentrations. A hemoglobin concentration of at least 20 mg/dl is required for one to recognize hemolysis

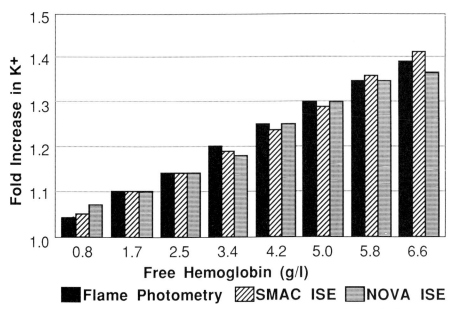

Figure 18–5. Effect of hemolysis on potassium. Free hemoglobin was obtained by freeze-fracturing red cells from the sample prior to assay. Results were determined on the sample by flame photometry and indirect and direct potentiometry (SMAC [Technicon] and NOVA I [Nova] ion-selective electrodes, respectively). Significant increases do not occur below the visual threshold for hemolysis. (Data from Sonntag O: Haemolysis as an interference factor in clinical chemistry. J. Clin Chem Clin Biochem 1986; 24:127–139.)

visually.[1] Plasma potassium increases linearly with increases in free hemoglobin (Fig. 18–5). Eighty mg/dl of free hemoglobin, a concentration easily detected by inspection, increases potassium concentrations by only 1.04-fold when assayed by either flame photometry or ISE. In contrast, 660 mg/dl produces a 1.4-fold increase.[21] Thus, although hemolysis causes significant increases in the observed concentrations of potassium, the visual threshold for detecting free hemoglobin in serum or plasma corresponds to only a slight increase in potassium.

If an anticoagulated sample of blood is not analyzed rapidly, then the plasma should be removed from the cellular components, since glucose metabolism by the cells has been shown to affect the concentration of potassium. Potassium in plasma is very stable after the cells have been removed.[3]

Physiologic Roles

Potassium, whose concentration in cells approximates 150 mmol/L, is the predominant intracellular cation. About 98% of the roughly 3500 mmol of potassium found in the hypothetic 70-kg person is intracellular. In contrast, extracellular fluid potassium concentration ranges from 3.5 to 5 mmol/L in healthy individuals. Maintenance of the appropriate ratio of intra- to extracellular potassium is essential to the proper functioning of the cardiovascular and neuromuscular systems. Alterations in the delicate internal harmony may be caused by such things as metabolic acidosis and hypertonicity of body fluids (including infusion of hypertonic solutions), both of which cause hyperkalemia; catecholamines, which have a biphasic effect; and insulin, which decreases plasma potassium.[75] A major external influence on potassium homeostasis is diuretic use. In a study of over two thousand nonrandomly selected ambulatory patients older than 65 years, 40% of women and 30% of men were on at least one diuretic drug. Serum potassium concentrations were most influenced by thiazides and averaged 0.44 mmol/L lower than those of age-matched controls.[76]

Chloride

Specimen Collection

Concentrations of chloride are commonly measured in serum, urine, and cerebrospinal fluid. However, chloride concentrations provide the least useful information of the four measured electrolytes, sodium, potassium, and bicarbonate. Samples should be separated from cellular constituents to prevent shifts in ionic equilibrium secondary to metabolism and pH alterations. Under aerobic conditions, loss of carbon dioxide changes the distribution between plasma and cells. However, chloride is stable for long periods of time in plasma, serum, and other acellular fluids at room temperatures or below.

Method of Analysis

Chloride in serum or cerebrospinal fluid is measured with an ISE, by quantitative displacement of thiocyanate by chloride from mercuric thiocyanate with subsequent formation of a red ferric thiocyanate complex, or with a semiautomated coulometric-amperometric technique. The mercuric-ferric thiocyanate method is most frequently used and is quite accurate and precise. ISEs are being increasingly used and are also precise and accurate.

Reference Range

The normal serum chloride range is 98–110 mmol/L. In the cerebrospinal fluid, the concentration is 120–132 mmol/L. Because urinary chloride varies with diet, the average chloride excretion ranges from 110 to 250 mmol/day. Chloride does not vary with age or gender.

Sources of Inaccuracy

With the ferric thiocyanate method, the chemical reaction is very temperature-sensitive, and temperature must be carefully controlled in order to assure accuracy. All the analysis methods for chloride demonstrate positive interference from other halides.

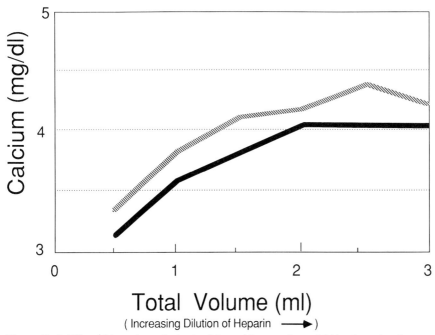

Figure 18–6. Effect of heparin on ionized calcium. Aliquots of arterial blood ranging from 0.5 to 3 ml were drawn into syringes the dead spaces of which contained heparin (1000 units/ml of heparin). All samples were analyzed for ionized calcium with a NOVA ion-selective analyzer. The data shown are from two patients. (Protocol approved by committee.)

Physiologic Role

Decreased serum chloride concentrations are present in patients with metabolic acidosis (uncontrolled diabetes), addisonian crisis, prolonged vomiting (pyloric stenosis, nasogastric suction, or high intestinal obstruction), salt-losing nephritis, and metabolic alkalosis (increased bicarbonate causes reciprocal decreases in chloride). Increased chloride concentrations are present in respiratory alkalosis, renal tubular acidosis, and dehydration.

Calcium

Specimen Collection

One must exercise caution when obtaining whole blood for calcium assay. Although heparin is the only suitable anticoagulant, it binds free calcium and may produce major decreases in the reported values for ionized calcium (Fig. 18–6). The decrease is directly related to the concentration of heparin in the sample and is reported to range from 0.002[11] to 0.01 mmol/L[77] for each unit of heparin per milliliter of sample. Some recommend that the heparin concentration be less than 10 U/ml of blood.[24] These data suggest that if less than 2 ml of blood is added to heparin contained in the dead space of a 3-ml disposable syringe, the observed value will be significantly less than the actual calcium activity.

The observed value for ionized calcium is inversely related to the pH of the specimen. As pH increases, protein binding of free calcium also increases, thus decreasing the ionized fraction of calcium. If the sample is exposed to air or transported in a tube that is only partially filled with blood, its pH increases as CO_2 is lost, and reported values are artifactually low. To avoid these changes, samples should be collected anaerobically, as they are for the determination of blood gases.[1, 18] Perioperative samples for analysis of ionized calcium are usually obtained from indwelling catheters, which avoids the problems induced by stasis from the use of a tourniquet (see Venipuncture).

Method of Analysis

Historically, ionized calcium was first assayed in biologic and clinical fluids in 1934 by exposing hearts from "healthy, full-blooded frogs of medium size" to the sample in question. The resulting amplitude of contraction of the heart, as recorded on a smoked kymograph drum, was a function of the concentration of ionized calcium in the specimen. Unknown values were quantified by comparing the resulting contractions with those produced by reference solutions.[78]

Several instruments incorporating ISEs are now available for assaying ionized calcium. The technology has been progressively refined since the development of the first calcium electrode in 1967,[8] but it is still evolving as experience with the technique accumulates. For example, although whole blood rather than plasma or serum is preferred for assay,[79] erythrocytes may falsely increase the observed value for ionized calcium by as much as 11%. This results from a positive voltage created by red cells at the junction between the sample and the reference electrode (see Fig. 18–1). This has been eliminated by altering the electrolyte solution in the reference electrode.[9] Values determined with instruments from different manufacturers may differ as much as 8%, in part owing to differences in electrode design. However, the reproducibility of the individual instruments is excellent.[80]

Reference Ranges

Reference intervals for ionized calcium in the absence of disease are 1.05–1.30 mmol/L or 4.2–5.2 mg/dl.[11] Even though clinical research on ionized calcium was first reported as long ago as 1935,[81] appropriate reference ranges for the analyte are still being disputed. In question is exactly what is being measured, the activity or the concentration of ionized calcium (see Activity versus Concentration).[82] The activity of calcium ion in the plasma of healthy individuals is about 0.38 mmol/L. Most analyzers divide the observed activity by an activity coefficient of 0.304 to give a substance concentration of about 1.25 mmol/L or 5.0 mg/dl.[82] However, certain disease states alter this activity coefficient. It is lower with severe hypernatremia and higher with hyperlipidemia or hyperproteinemia, making the true substance concentration higher or lower, respectively.[82]

Sources of Inaccuracy

Inaccuracies in the reported values for ionized calcium may be caused by errors in sample collection, by transportation, by delays between collection and analysis, and by the method used for assay. Already discussed are such things as the amount of heparin in the sample, the effects of increases in pH resulting from loss of CO_2, and certain technical features. Temperature-dependent increases in ionized calcium occur with storage of heparinized whole blood. At 4°C, 20°C, and 37°C, the increases are 0.02, 0.04, and 0.08 mmol/L, respectively, over 4 hours. These changes are due to glycolysis and lactic acid formation.[18] If the concentrations of electrolytes in the specimen differ significantly from their reference ranges, the observed value for ionized calcium will be affected. At sodium concentrations of 112 and 168 mmol/L, ionized calcium is respectively 4% less than and 4% greater than its value when the sodium concentration is normal. In contrast, potassium has no effect on the assay.[11] These effects vary in magnitude between analyzers depending upon the manufacturer.[83]

Physiologic Role

Calcium, the fifth most abundant element (and most abundant mineral element) in the human body, is incredibly important to both anatomic structure and physiologic function. More than 99% of the 1–2 kg of calcium in the adult is in bone. The remainder is found in cells, blood, and extracellular fluid. Extraskeletal calcium is involved in a myriad of regulatory and metabolic functions. Some of these include the release of central and peripheral neurotransmitters, contraction of cardiac and skeletal muscle, secretion of hormones (including insulin, adrenocorticotropic hormone, corticosteroids, prolactin, luteinizing hormone, oxytocin, and vasopressin), and a vital role in blood coagulation. Calcium is the major inorganic second messenger for the regulation of cellular function.

Circulating calcium accounts for less than 1% of total body calcium. It exists in three states: protein-bound (45%), ionized (45%), and complexed to small anions including citrate, phosphate, and bicarbonate (10%). Ionized or free calcium is the only fraction of physiologic importance and is responsible for calcium's regulatory effects.[1, 84] The cardiovascular effects of ionized calcium have been detailed by Drop.[85]

Proteins

Hematocrit

Specimen Collection

Hematocrit is determined in whole blood containing an anticoagulant that does not affect the size of erythrocytes.

Method of Analysis

The blood sample is centrifuged in a tube of uniform bore. After centrifugation, the hematocrit percentage is determined as the height of the red cell column in millimeters divided by the total height of the column in millimeters times 100.

Reference Ranges

The reference range for hematocrit in males is 41–53%, and in females it is 36–46% of the packed red cell volume.

Sources of Inaccuracy

A single determination is usually accurate enough for routine work. However, hematocrit levels determined in capillary tubes are often performed in duplicate. Errors arise if the sample is not centrifuged adequately enough to assure complete packing of the cells. About 5% of the packed cell volume is actually trapped plasma. The hematocrit is usually more accurate than either erythrocyte count or hemoglobin.

Physiologic Role

The concentration of erythrocytes and their content of oxygen-carrying hemoglobin are factors affecting tissue oxygen delivery. However, in many clinical conditions, the actual hematocrit is more useful as an indicator of whether to administer blood or crystalloid to a given patient (i.e., is the patient anemic?) than is the timing of blood administration. Acute hemorrhage causes concomitant loss of plasma and erythrocytes, so that hematocrit may remain normal, although total erythrocyte mass is severely decreased. Similar problems occur with acute shifts of fluids between intra- and extravascular space in patients in shock or acute cardiac failure.

Myoglobin

Myoglobin is an oxygen-binding protein found in skeletal and cardiac muscle.

Specimen Collection

Myoglobin is analyzed in either serum or urine. Nonlipemic, nonhemolyzed serum is preferred. Urine samples should be collected without preservative. If either serum or urine cannot be analyzed within 24 hours, serum specimens should be frozen, and urine specimens should be refrigerated at 2–8°C.

Method of Analysis

Although there are many methods available for analyzing serum or urine myoglobin, most are either lacking in sensitivity or difficult to control qualitatively. The most commonly used are the latex agglutination and radioimmunoassay methods. Neither of these methods is commonly offered by "acute" laboratories. Latex agglutination is easy to perform, because latex beads coated with antibody to myoglobin readily agglutinate in the presence of myoglobin. A visual reading of the extent of agglutination provides qualitative evidence of the presence of myoglobin.[6]

The radioimmunoassay method is more sensitive and detects concentrations as low as 15 ng/ml.[6] It can also be performed with shortened incubation times as a stat procedure with results available in 1 hour.

Reference Ranges

Normally, very low levels of myoglobin are found in serum; 20–60 ng/ml in females and 20–70 ng/ml in males. Myoglobin concentrations increase with age, so children have lower myoglobin concentrations than adults. Myoglobin level also varies with race.

Sources of Inaccuracy

Myoglobin concentrations exhibit circadian variation, with the highest levels in the morning and the lowest occurring between 6:00 and 11:00 P.M.[86]

Significance of Positive Assay

Myoglobin must be differentiated from hemoglobin in the urine, since both yield positive results for protein and occult blood. The two substances can be differentiated by electrophoresis, ultrafiltration, gel filtration, absorption spectra, or solubility. In addition, red cells are absent on microscopic examination of the urine when myoglobinemia is present.

Increases in serum myoglobin occur after myocardial infarction, shock, crush injuries, vigorous exercise, or other skeletal muscle trauma. Myoglobin levels can be used as early indicators of myocardial infarction and of reinfarction, since they decrease more rapidly than do creatine kinase levels.[6] Evaluation of muscle damage in muscular dystrophy or myopathies or after malignant hyperthermia or administration of succinylcholine is facilitated by myoglobin assay. The released myoglobin is excreted in the urine, causing it to become cola- or coffee-colored. Copious amounts of myoglobin in the urine may occlude renal tubules, causing impairment of renal function.

PSEUDOCHOLINESTERASE AND DIBUCAINE NUMBER

The enzyme pseudocholinesterase (PCE) is of interest to anesthesiologists because it biotransforms succinylcholine. About 1 in 1500–2500 patients has an atypical variant of PCE that is incapable of metabolizing succinylcholine, although it retains the ability to metabolize other substrates. Thus, its ability to inactivate succinylcholine is not predictable with methods commonly used to assay its activity but may be determined by assaying the enzyme with and without dibucaine and comparing the respective activities. Because of its lack of substrate specificity, PCE has been given a variety of names including cholinesterase, nonspecific cholinesterase, and butyrylcholinesterase.[87]

Specimen Collection

PCE activity may be assayed in either serum or plasma. Conventionally, it is determined in serum removed from a red-topped tube after clot retraction has occurred. Heparin is a suitable anticoagulant if the activity of the enzyme is desired in plasma, although the differences in PCE activity between serum and plasma are usually of no clinical significance. Five milliliters of blood provides an abundant amount of serum for assay. Many methods use less than 100 μL of sample, but the excess is important should the assay need to be repeated. The enzyme is extremely stable in serum and may be stored in a refrigerator for weeks with little change in activity. Samples used for quality control may be frozen and stored for months to years, although repeated freezing and thawing decrease the activity.

Method of Analysis

PCE is an enzyme capable of biotransforming a host of substrates. For this reason, a multitude of methods using many different substrates have been developed. Substrates that are frequently used to assay the enzyme include benzoylcholine, butyrylthiocholine, and propionylthiocholine. The first of these requires the use of a recording ultraviolet spectrophotometer, and it is more cumbersome than the latter two, which are colorimetric methods that can be performed easily by automated analyzers.

By assaying PCE in the absence and presence of a given concentration of dibucaine, the ability of the enzyme to metabolize succinylcholine may be predicted. The extent of the inhibition of PCE activity by dibucaine is reported as the dibucaine number, as shown in the following formula:

$$\text{Dibucaine number} = \left\{ 1 - \left(\frac{\text{activity with dibucaine}}{\text{activity without dibucaine}} \right) \right\} \times 100$$

Classically, benzoylcholine was used as the substrate in this determination. A dibucaine concentration of 1×10^{-5} M inhibited the normal enzyme by about 80%, whereas the abnormal enzyme, which is incapable of biotransforming succinylcholine, was inhibited by only about 25%.[88] A 10-fold greater concentration of dibucaine produces the same differential inhibition of normal versus atypical PCE if butyrylcholinesterase is used as the substrate. The advantage of the latter method is that it has been modified for use on an automated analyzer, with results available within 30 minutes of sample collection.[89]

Reference Range

The lack of substrate specificity of PCE has resulted in the development of many assays for the enzyme, each of which has its own reference range.

Table 18–2. DIBUCAINE NUMBERS

Patient	PCE Activity (reference range 7–17 iu)	PCE + Dibucaine	DN	Duration of Succinylcholine
A	10	2	80	5 minutes
B	4	1	75	15 minutes
C	4	3	25	3 hours

iu = international units, PCE = pseudocholinesterase, DN = dibucaine number.

Thus, it is imperative that a given activity be compared with the reference range for the specific method used to determine that activity.

In contrast, the reference ranges for dibucaine numbers are independent of the method of assay. For these, values for the normal, heterozygous, and atypical variants are 75 or greater, 40–70, and 30 or less, respectively.

Sources of Inaccuracy

At very low activities of PCE, dibucaine numbers may be unreliable if the activity determined in the presence of dibucaine is less than the lower linear limit of the assay. In this case, the apparent extent of inhibition of activity of genetically normal enzyme by dibucaine may be less than the actual inhibition, leading to the incorrect interpretation that the enzyme is other than genetically normal. This is usually of academic rather than clinical interest, because the duration of action of succinylcholine is frequently prolonged regardless of its phenotype if the enzyme activity is extremely low.

Physiologic Role

PCE is important in the elimination of succinylcholine. The ability of genetically normal PCE to metabolize succinylcholine is so great that the duration of action of the drug is usually not significantly prolonged in patients with activities far below the lower end of the reference range, as long as the enzyme is genetically normal. In contrast, the activity of genetically atypical enzyme may fall within the reference range of the assay and yet be completely incapable of metabolizing succinylcholine. Thus, enzyme activity alone cannot be used to predict the duration of action of succinylcholine unless the drug itself is used as the substrate in the assay. Although this method has been used as a research tool, it is too cumbersome for use in the clinical laboratory.

The dibucaine number can be used to predict the duration of action of succinylcholine, whereas reference to PCE activity alone may be misleading, as shown in Table 18–2. Patients A and B have genetically normal enzyme, and patient C has the dibucaine-resistant variant. Patient B has decreased PCE activity.

Atypical enzymes other than the dibucaine-resistant variant have been identified using other inhibitors of the enzyme, such as fluoride, chloride, formaldehyde, and urea. Of these, the most well evaluated compound is fluoride. The fluoride-resistant variant has an incidence of about 1 in 155,000.[90] The incidence of the other variants is less well documented.

The role of PCE, other than its ability to metabolize succinylcholine and other ester-containing drugs such as tetracaine and 2-chloroprocaine hydrochloride, is still in question. It may be involved in the metabolism of certain steroids and fatty acids.

RENAL FUNCTION

Tests of renal function including blood urea nitrogen (BUN), creatinine, and urinalysis are performed preoperatively as well as perioperatively. Pre-operative assessments of renal function permit alterations in intraoperative management in order to enhance perfusion and glomerular filtration. In the postoperative period, determinations of quality and quantity of urine are diagnostic in the differentiation of prerenal, renal, or postrenal azotemia.

BUN

Urea is the major end product of nitrogen metabolism, so production depends upon dietary intake. In the kidney, urea is excreted and partially reabsorbed. During dehydration, more urea is reabsorbed, resulting in increased BUN.

Specimen Collection

The urease–glutamate dehydrogenase assay described here requires serum or heparinized plasma. Because fluoride inhibits urease, fluoride-preserved serum cannot be used. Serum and urine samples should be kept at 4–8°C in order to avoid bacterial degradation of urea.

Method of Analysis

The most commonly used method for measurement of BUN is a coupled enzymatic spectrophotometric assay. In the assay, urease catalyzes the formation of ammonia from urea. The amount of ammonia formed is detected in a NAD/NADH (nicotinamide adenine dinucleotide/nicotinamide-adenine dinucleotide [reduced form]) indicator reaction involving glutamate dehydrogenase that is monitored at 340 nm. Such reactions can be performed in automated analyzers.

Reference Ranges

Serum levels vary with diet, age, and analytic method. Reference ranges for adults using the urease–glutamate dehydrogenase method are 50–170 mg/L or 1.8–6.1 mmol/L. Higher values are found in males and the elderly.

Sources of Inaccuracy

Both endogenous and exogenous ammonia may affect results. If the sample is diluted prior to assay, no significant interference from bilirubin, lipemia, hemoglobin, or other nitrogenous substances occurs.

Physiologic Role

Urea is the endpoint of protein catabolism in the liver. Because BUN varies with dietary intake and state of hydration as well as renal and hepatic function, the metabolic situation must always be considered in evaluating BUN. However, since it is filtered at the glomerulus and passively reabsorbed in the proximal tubules, it does provide a semiquantitative assessment of renal function.

Creatinine

Creatinine is more reliable than BUN as a measure of glomerular filtration rate. If creatinine production is constant, plasma creatinine is inversely related to the glomerular filtration rate.

Specimen Collection

Creatinine is measured in plasma, serum, or urine. With the exception of the ammonium salt of heparin, the anticoagulants heparin and fluoride do not interfere in enzymatic methods of analysis.[6] When the Jaffé reaction is used, specimens are stable for 7 days at refrigerated temperatures, but enzymatic methods require immediate separation of serum from erythrocytes.

Method of Analysis

Creatinine is determined using the Jaffé reaction in which creatinine reacts with sodium picrate to form a red Janovsky complex whose absorbance is measured spectrophotometrically at 510–520 nm. Enzymatic methods that hydrolyze creatinine to creatine before its spectrophotometric measurement with creatine kinase are used in automated analyses.

Reference Ranges

Serum creatinine depends upon concentration, rate of production, and excretion. The reference range is 0.6–1.3 mg/dl. Muscular individuals may have concentrations as high as 1.6 mg/dl.

Sources of Inaccuracy

Fuller's earth is used to adsorb the creatinine and isolate it from potential interferents. Substances known to interfere in the Jaffé reaction include uric acid, protein, pyruvate, acetoacetate, glucose, aminohippurate, ascorbic acid, and cephalosporin antibiotics.[6]

Physiologic Role

The principal source of creatinine is muscle metabolism, since creatinine in blood is derived from muscle creatine. Normally, there is a fairly constant turnover of 1–2% of muscle creatine, depending upon the individual's age, sex, and size. Renal excretion by filtration removes creatinine from the serum, making serum creatine a good indicator of glomerular filtration.

Because the reference range is large owing to considerable individual variation, glomerular filtration can be severely impaired before creatinine concentrations exceed the reference range. Plasma creatinine concentrations may not increase significantly for hours to days after complete cessation of glomerular filtration, because the level rarely increases more than 1.5 mg/dl/day. The clearance of creatinine, an indicator of glomerular filtration rate superior to either BUN or creatinine level, can be measured with the following equation using either 2-hour or 24-hour samples:

Creatinine clearance (ml/minute)

$$= \text{Urine creatinine} \times \text{Urine volume/Plasma creatinine}$$

Creatinine clearance is corrected for surface area by multiplying by 1.73/body surface area. Reference ranges are 90–120 ml/minute when corrected for surface area.

Urine

Sample Collection

Urine output is determined perioperatively by collection of urine in a graduated vessel connected to an indwelling urethral catheter. Most patients requiring continuous evaluation of urinary output need indwelling catheters despite the risk of urinary tract infection. Voided specimens are used for preoperative evaluation of renal function. Fresh specimens can be examined at any time for glucose and specific gravity and microscopically for casts, erythrocytes, leukocytes, and microorganisms.

Obstruction of the lower urinary tract or external urinary drainage system should always be corrected prior to assuming that decreased urine output is from renal causes. Likewise, adequacy of extracellular fluid volume and hemodynamic function must be present in order to exclude prerenal causes.

Methods of Analysis

Various tests are performed on urine. Specific gravity is measured, even though it correlates only roughly with urine osmolality. A calibrated hydrometer designed for urine specific gravity determinations is used. The

Table 18–3. URINALYSIS

Test	Reference Range of Normal Urine Findings
pH	4.6–8.0
Specific gravity	1.015–1.025
Glucose	negative on dipstick (<0.5 gm/24 hours)
Sodium	130–260 mmol/24 hours
Potassium	25–100 mmol/24 hours
Protein	negative on dipstick (40–150 mg/24 hours)
Osmolality	38–1400 mOsm/kg
Urine sediment	3–5 white blood count/ high-power field occasional red blood count occasional mucus occasional bacteria

hydrometer is allowed to float freely in the specimen, and the scale on the stem is read at the meniscus. Correction factors should be applied to the hydrometer reading for temperature, glucose, and protein as follows:

Add or subtract 0.001 to or from the reading for each 3°C that the temperature is above or below the calibration temperature of the hydrometer.
Subtract 0.003 for each 1 gm/dl of protein present.
Subtract 0.004 for each 1 gm/dl of glucose.[1]

Glucose is determined as indicated previously. Urine protein is determined by the benzethonium chloride turbidimetric method.

Microscopic analysis of the urine is usually performed in a qualitative rather than a quantitative fashion. A drop of centrifuged urine sediment suspended in a known volume of urine is examined under a microscope, and the number of the various elements per high-power field are reported. Supravital staining of the sediment further facilitates identification of specific elements. Casts are cylindrical bodies formed in the distal and collecting tubules from erythrocytes (red cell casts), epithelial cells (epithelial casts), or cells and cellular debris with protein (hyaline casts). They indicate the presence of glomerular or tubular disease.

Because the rate of urinary sodium excretion depends upon intake, the fractional excretion of sodium is a more useful indicator of renal function. Fractional excretion of sodium is calculated by dividing the urinary:plasma sodium concentration ratio by the urinary:plasma creatine concentration ratio. Values of less than 1% indicate prerenal dysfunction, whereas values over 2–3% indicate compromised tubular function.

Reference Ranges

The reference range for urine protein, sugar, electrolytes, specific gravity, pH, and other substances are in Table 18–3. Microscopic examination of the urine should reveal few erythrocytes or leukocytes and no casts in healthy humans. The presence of pus cells indicates urinary tract infection. Erythrocytes and red cell casts indicate glomerulonephritis. Epithelial or hyaline casts are present in patients with nephrotic syndrome or chronic renal insufficiency.

Sources of Inaccuracy

Measurement of specific gravity using a urinometer gives erroneous values if the urinometer is not allowed to float freely in the specimen or if correction factors for temperature are overlooked. Gross proteinuria or glucosuria also affects specific gravity determinations as indicated previously.

Physiologic Changes

Glomerular filtration and tubular reabsorption rates determine urine output. In the perioperative period, urine output should be 0.5–1 ml/kg/hour. Complete bladder emptying must be assured by insertion of an indwelling catheter together with suprapubic compression, positional changes, and flushing of the catheter with saline or air to avoid intraluminal obstruction.

Proteinuria occurs because of increased glomerular permeability, defective tubular reabsorption, abnormal secretion of protein into the urinary tract, and abnormal proteins causing protein overload owing to increased plasma proteins. Benign types of proteinuria include those caused by exercise, pyrexia, or posture. Proteinuria due to defective glomerular permeability indicates the presence of serious conditions such as primary renal disease, diabetes, or immune complex disorders.

Acute renal failure is defined as a rapid, progressive decrease of renal function associated with azotemia and oliguria. Oliguria lasts about 7–10 days, with ranges from a few hours to several weeks. Even after urine volume begins to increase, BUN may continue to rise.

However, in certain phases of renal failure in some patients, urine output is increased. Polyuric renal failure is present when urine output exceeds 2.5 L/day, whereas in nonoliguric renal failure the output is 0.4–2.5 L/day. Urine volume increases after administration of mannitol in patients with prerenal azotemia but not in those with acute tubular necrosis or renal failure. The differentiation of etiology of renal failure is facilitated by results of plasma and urine tests. (Table 18–4).

PRESENTATION OF RESULTS

Reference Values versus "Normal" Values

To interpret laboratory values, we frequently compare an observed value with published values that may loosely be referred to as being "normal." If the value in question falls between the upper and the lower values, we assume that the result is "within normal limits," without, per-

Table 18–4. RENAL FAILURE: PLASMA AND URINE TESTS

Test	Acute Renal Failure	Acute Tubular Necrosis	Prerenal Azotemia
BUN (mg/dl)	>20	>20	>20
Serum creatinine (mg/dl)	>1.5	>1.5	>1.5
Urine/plasma creatinine	>20:1	<10:1	>40:1
Urine osmolality (mOsm)	<350	<350	>500
Urine/plasma osmolality	<1.1:1	<1.2:1	>1.5:1
Urine specific gravity	1.010	1.010–1.015	>1.015
Urine sodium (mmol/L)	>40	>25	<10–20
Fractional excretion of sodium	>1	>1	<1
Urine sediment	Granular and tubular casts, tubular cells	Tubular cell casts	Hyaline casts or normal sediment

haps, considering what normal means. In the strict sense of the word, normal assumes that the results are those of a healthy population and that the distribution of values is gaussian, with the normal range falling within two standard deviations of the mean. In most cases, the normal distribution for a specific assay is rarely this ideal.[91]

Instead, clinical laboratories report results as those given in this chapter with respect to reference ranges of values. The concept of reference values, recommended by the International Federation of Clinical Chemistry, circumvents the difficulties caused by the use of the term normal.[1] Reference values are reported for specific populations, with selection criteria based on such things as age, sex, race, physical condition, and socioeconomic factors. Some values may also be influenced by a variety of factors including the time of day that the sample is collected and body posture at the time of collection.

The observed value for a specific patient must be interpreted with respect to the reference range appropriate for that patient. The result is usual if it falls within the reference range and low or high if it is outside the range. For detailed discussions of reference values, the interested reader should consult a standard textbook of clinical chemistry.

Units of Measure

At this writing, the majority of the world has adopted the use of Système International (SI) units for reporting data. Conversion to these units in the United States is now occurring gradually and is being encouraged by the American National Metric Council and the American Medical Association, among other organizations.[92, 93] Although the system may appear somewhat

Table 18–5. CONVENTIONAL AND SYSTÈME INTERNATIONAL UNITS

	Conventional		Conversion Factors		Système International	
Analyte	*Reference Ranges*	*Units*	*Conventional to SI*	*SI to Conventional*	*Reference Ranges*	*Units*
Calcium, ionized	4.2–5.2	mg/dl	0.25	4	1.05–1.30	mmol/L
Chloride	100–109	mEq/dl	1	1	100–109	mmol/L
Glucose	70–110	mg/dl	0.055	18	3.8–6.1	mmol/L
Magnesium	1.8–3.0	mg/dl	0.41	2.43	0.8–1.2	mmol/L
Potassium	3.5–5.0	mEq/L	1	1	3.5–5.0	mmol/L
Sodium	135–147	mEq/L	1	1	135–147	mmol/L
Urea nitrogen	12–20	mg/dl	0.356	2.81	3.00–6.5	mmol/L
Osmolality	280–300	mOsm/kg	1	1	280–300	mmol/L

Data from Lundberg GD, Iverson C, Radulescu G: Now read this: The SI units are here. JAMA 1986; 255:2329–2339.

cumbersome at the outset, many feel it will make the integration of laboratory values with patient care more scientific. The goals are to improve communication between the clinician and the clinical chemist and to clarify the interpretation of laboratory data.

There is a scientific basis for making the transition. Concentrations of analytes and drugs in the SI are expressed as moles of compound rather than in more conventional units of mass, i.e., glucose is reported as 5.5 mmol/L rather than as 100 mg/dl. The reasoning for this becomes apparent when one considers that substances interact physiologically based on the relative numbers of molecules rather than on the masses of the individual molecules. Consider ionized calcium as an example. Conventionally, Ca^{2+} is reported in milligrams per deciliter rather than in moles or millimoles per liter. Although it is unfamiliar, the latter, when added to the concentrations of other cations, provides a more precise quantification of the ionic balance of plasma. By reporting all measured cations and anions in these units, one may be able to quantitate accurately such things as the concentrations of the normally unmeasured compounds responsible for the anion gap.[94] Table 18–5 compares conventional units with SI units for some analytes.

Total adoption of SI in the United States remains controversial. Whereas one faction suggests its scientific validity, another feels that the system leads to confusion that could contribute to errors in patient care. Other grounds for resistance range from economic to the feelings of some that it is un-American.[95] The change from milliequivalent to millimole for univalent ions has proceeded without opposition, since the numeric values are identical. Further change is being resisted, including the conversion of units of pressure from millimeters of mercury to kilopascals,[96] although it may become necessary if only to make the data reported in European journals more understandable.[93, 95]

THE FUTURE

Rapid analysis of biochemical substances in the perioperative period has become a reality. On the horizon are implantable electrodes capable of continually analyzing pH, oxygen, carbon dioxide, sodium, potassium, calcium, glucose, hormones, enzymes, and even drugs.[97] Although miniaturized sensors for a variety of analytes have been developed over the past 2 decades, none has yet become important clinically. Problems still to be overcome include drift, interference, inadequate structural integrity, and slow response times. To date, incorporation of an implantable reference electrode near the sensor remains an unsolved technical challenge in the development of intravascular ISEs. Development of suitable membranes and encapsulants for long-term electrodes also poses a significant technical challenge. Miniaturization of colorimetric assays using implantable fiberoptic bundles is an additional technique currently under development.[97] Another major hurdle is the problem of the biocompatibility of materials used in implantable sensors. Development of this technology, currently in its early stages, is essential to the future of continuous biochemical analysis in the perioperative period.[98]

Whether this technology will become commonplace is open to speculation at present. Should it happen, it will provide even more on-line data than is currently available. But will it lead to improved management of patients or will it provide yet another distraction from the direct patient contact that is essential to patient monitoring?

References

1. Tietz NW (ed): Textbook of Clinical Chemistry. Philadelphia: WB Saunders, 1986.
2. Berger RL, Rutenberg AM, Hechtman HB, Egdahl RH: The intensive-care laboratory. Surgery 1973; 73:159–160.
3. Sonnenwirth AC, Jarett L (eds): Gradwohl's Clinical Laboratory Methods and Diagnosis, 8th Ed. St Louis: CV Mosby, 1980; 149–209.
4. Willatts SM, Myerson K: Electrolyte measurement by clinicians. Intensive Care Med 1987; 13:411–415.
5. Evans SE, Buckley BM: Biochemists nearer the patient? Br Med J 1983; 287:1399–1400.
6. Kaplan LA, Pesce AJ (eds): Clinical Chemistry: Theory, Analysis, and Correlation. St Louis: CV Mosby, 1984; 51–73, 232–239, 917–921, 1032–1043, 1075–1078.
7. Pioda LAR, Simon W: Determination of potassium ion concentration in serum using a highly selective liquid-membrane electrode. Clin Chim Acta 1970; 29:289–293.
8. Ross JW: Calcium-selective electrode with liquid ion exchanger. Science 1967; 156:1378–1379.
9. Siggaard-Andersen O, Fogh-Andersen N, Thode J: Elimination of the erythrocyte effect on the liquid junction potential in potentiometric measurements on whole blood using mixed salt bridge solutions. Scand J Clin Lab Invest [Suppl] 1983; 165:43–46.
10. Worth HGJ: Plasma sodium concentration: Bearer of false prophecies? Br Med J 1983; 287:567–568.
11. Ladenson JH, Bowers GN Jr: Free calcium in serum. I. Determination with the ion-specific electrode, and factors affecting the results. Clin Chem 1973; 19:565–574.
12. Ladenson JH, Apple FS, Koch DD: Misleading hyponatremia due to hyperlipidemia: A method-dependent error. Ann Intern Med 1981; 95:707–708.

13. Mullins RE, Hutton PS, Conn RB: Effects of Fluosol-DA (artificial blood) on clinical chemistry tests and instruments. Am J Clin Pathol 1983; 80:478–483.
14. Fawcett JK, Wynn V: Effects of posture on plasma volume and some blood constituents. J Clin Pathol 1960; 13:304–310.
15. Statland BE, Bokelund H, Winkel P: Factors contributing to intra-individual variation of serum constituents. 4. Effects of posture and tourniquet application on variation of serum constituents in healthy subjects. Clin Chem 1974; 20:1513–1519.
16. Felding P, Tryding N, Hyltoft Petersen P, Hørder M: Effects of posture on concentrations of blood constituents in healthy adults: Practical application of blood specimen collection procedures recommended by the Scandinavian Committee on Reference Values. Scand J Clin Lab Invest 1980; 40:615–621.
17. Romano AT, Young GW Jr: Mild forearm exercise during venipuncture, and its effect on potassium determinations. Clin Chem 1977; 23:303–304.
18. Thode J, Fogh-Andersen N, Aas F, Siggaard-Andersen O: Sampling and storage of blood for determination of ionized calcium. Scand J Clin Lab Invest 1985; 45:131–138.
19. Hill AB, Nahrwold ML, Noonan D, Northrop P: A comparison of methods of blood withdrawal and sample preparation for potassium measurements. Anesthesiology 1980; 53:60–63.
20. Leppänen E, Gräsbeck R: The effect of the order of filling tubes after venipuncture on serum potassium, total protein, and aspartate and alanine aminotransferases. Scand J Clin Lab Invest 1986; 46:189–191.
21. Sonntag O: Haemolysis as an interference factor in clinical chemistry. J Clin Chem Clin Biochem 1986; 24:127–139.
22. Ladenson JH, Tsai LM, Michael JM, et al: Serum versus heparinized plasma for eighteen common chemistry tests: Is serum the appropriate specimen? Am J Clin Pathol 1974; 62:545–552.
23. O'Reilly RA: Anticoagulant, antithrombotic, and thrombolytic drugs. *In* Gilman AG, Goodman LS, Rall TW, Murad F (eds): Goodman and Gilman's The Pharmacological Basis of Therapeutics, 7th Ed. New York: Macmillan, 1985; 1338–1359.
24. Heining MPD, Jordan WS: Heparinization of samples for plasma ionized calcium measurement. Crit Care Med 1988; 16:67–68.
25. Shek CC, Swaminathan R: Errors due to heparin in the estimation of plasma sodium and potassium concentrations. Intensive Care Med 1985; 11:309–311.
26. Bourke DL: Errors in intraoperative hematocrit determination. Anesthesiology 1976; 45:357–359.
27. Jackson EF: The reliability of blood tests drawn from intravenous lines. Ohio Med 1972; 68:32–35.
28. Kunkel SE, Warner MA: Human T-cell lymphotropic virus type III (HTLV-III) infection: How it can affect you, your patients, and your anesthesia practice. Anesthesiology 1987; 66:195–207.
29. Bazaral M: Preoperative testing for human immunodeficiency virus infection. Anesthesiology 1987; 67:278.
30. Berry AJ: Prevention of blood-borne infections in anesthesia personnel. Anesthesiology 1988; 68:164.
31. Arden J: Managing patients with AIDS—update. Anesthesiology 1988; 68:164–165.
32. Napoli VM, McGowan JE: How much blood is in a needle stick? J Infect Dis 1987; 155:828.
33. Centers for Disease Control. Update: Human immunodeficiency virus infections in health-care workers exposed to blood of infected patients. MMWR 1987; 36:285–289.

34. Friedland GH, Klein RS: Transmission of the human immunodeficiency virus. N Engl J Med 1987; 317:1125–1135.
35. McCray E: Occupational risk of the acquired immunodeficiency syndrome among health care workers. N Engl J Med 1986; 314:1127–1132.
36. Centers for Disease Control: Recommendations for prevention of HIV transmission in health-care settings. MMWR 1987; 36 (Suppl 2S):3S–18S.
37. Hadler SC, Doto IL, Maynard JE, et al: Occupational risk of hepatitis B infection in hospital workers. Infect Control 1985; 6:24–31.
38. Weissman M, Klein B: Evaluation of glucose determinations in untreated samples. Clin Chem 1958; 4:420–422.
39. Steige H, Jones JD: Evaluation of pneumatic-tube system for delivery of blood specimens. Clin Chem 1971; 17:1160–1164.
40. Gibbs EL, Lennox WG, Nims LF, Gibbs FA: Arterial and cerebral venous blood: Arterial-venous differences in man. J Biol Chem 1942; 144:325–332.
41. Larsson-Cohn U: Differences between capillary and venous blood glucose during oral glucose tolerance tests. Scand J Clin Lab Invest 1976; 36:805–808.
42. Duffy T, Phillips N, Pelligrin F: Review of glucose tolerance—a problem in methodology. Am J Med Sci 1973; 265:117–133.
43. Phillips GB, Mendershausen PB: Glucose consumption by red cells of diabetic patients and normal subjects. Effect of ethanol. Clin Chim Acta 1975; 61:175–182.
44. Stjernholm RL, Manak RC: Carbohydrate metabolism in leukocytes. XIV. Regulation of pentose cycle activity and glycogen metabolism during phagocytosis. J Reticuloendothel Soc 1970; 8:550–560.
45. Schwartz MK: Interferences in diagnostic biochemical procedures. Adv Clin Chem 1973; 16:1–45.
46. Holtkamp HC, Verhoef NJ, Leijnse B: The difference between the glucose concentrations in plasma and whole blood. Clin Chim Acta 1975; 59:41–49.
47. Clark LC Jr, Clark EW: A personalized history of the Clark oxygen electrode. In Tremper KK, Barker SJ (eds): Advances in Oxygen Monitoring. Int Anesthesiol Clin 1987; 25:1–29.
48. Kunz HJ, Stasny M: Immobilized glucose oxidase used to measure glucose in serum. Clin Chem 1974; 20:1018–1022.
49. Kadish AH, Litle RL, Sternberg JC: A new and rapid method for the determination of glucose by measurement of rate of oxygen consumption. Clin Chem 1968; 14:116–131.
50. Chua KS, Tan IK: Plasma glucose measurement with the Yellow Springs glucose analyzer. Clin Chem 1978; 24:150–152.
51. Jelić-Ivanović Z, Majkić-Singh N, Spasić P, et al: Interference by analgesic and antirheumatic drugs in 25 common laboratory assays. J Clin Chem Clin Biochem 1985; 23:287–292.
52. Wright LA, Foster MG: Effect of some commonly prescribed drugs on certain chemistry tests. Clin Biochem 1980; 6:249–252.
53. Farrance I, Aldons J: Paracetamol interference with YSI glucose analyzer. Clin Chem 1981; 27:782–783.
54. Ronzoni E, Koechig I, Eaton EP: Ether anesthesia. III. Role of lactic acid in the acidosis of ether anesthesia. J Biol Chem 1924; 61:465–492.
55. Greene NM: Lactate, pyruvate and excess lactate production in anesthetized man. Anesthesiology 1961; 22:404–412.
56. Cohen RD, Simpson R: Lactate metabolism. Anesthesiology 1975; 43:661–673.
57. Waxman K, Nolan LS, Shoemaker WC: Sequential perioperative lactate determination: Physiological and clinical implications. Crit Care Med 1982; 10:96–99.

58. Clark LC Jr, Noyes LK, Grooms TA, Moore MS: Rapid micromeasurement of lactate in whole blood. Crit Care Med 1984; 12:461–464.

59. Fath JJ, Ascher NL, Konstantinides BS, et al: Metabolism during hepatic transplantation: Indicators of allograft function. Surgery 1984; 96:664–673.

60. Smith JC Jr, Lewis S, Holbrook J, et al: Effect of heparin and citrate on measured concentrations of various analytes in plasma. Clin Chem 1987; 33:814–816.

61. Epstein FB: Osmolality. Emerg Med Clin North Am 1986; 4:253–261.

62. Mercier DE, Feld RD, Witte DL: Comparison of dewpoint and freezing point osmometry. Am J Med Technol 1978; 44:1066–1069.

63. Gennari FJ: Serum osmolality: Uses and limitations. N Engl J Med 1984; 310:102–105.

64. Dowart WV, Chalmers L: Comparison of methods for calculating serum osmolality from chemical concentrations, and the prognostic value of such calculations. Clin Chem 1975; 21:190–194.

65. Bhagat CI, Garcia-Webb P, Fletcher E, Beilby JP: Calculated vs measured plasma osmolalities revisited. Clin Chem 1984; 30:1703–1705.

66. Morissette MP: Colloid osmotic pressure: Its measurement and clinical value. Can Med Assoc J 1977; 116:897–900.

67. Luz PL, Shubin H, Weil MH, et al: Pulmonary edema related to changes in colloid osmotic and pulmonary artery wedge pressure in patients after acute myocardial infarction. Circulation 1975; 51:350–357.

68. Duncan A, Young DS: Measurements of serum colloid osmotic pressure are of limited usefulness. Clin Chem 1982; 28:141–145.

69. Fernandez P, Cox M: Basic concepts of renal physiology. *In* Priebe HJ (ed): The Kidney in Anesthesia. Int Anesthesiol Clin 1984; 22:1–33.

70. Morgan DB: Why plasma electrolytes? Ann Clin Biochem 1981; 18:275–280.

71. Lum G, Gambino SR: A comparison of serum versus heparinized plasma for routine chemistry tests. Am J Clin Pathol 1974; 61:108–113.

72. Ward CF, Arkin DB, Benumof J, Saidman LJ: Arterial versus venous potassium: Clinical implications. Crit Care Med 1978; 6:335–336.

73. Hartmann RC, Auditore JV, Jackson DP: Studies on thrombocytosis. I. Hyperkalemia due to release of potassium from platelets during coagulation. J Clin Invest 1958; 37:699–707.

74. Bronson WR, Devita VT, Carbone PP, Cotlove E: Pseudohyperkalemia due to release of potassium from white blood cells during clotting. N Engl J Med 1966; 274:369–375.

75. Cox M: Potassium homeostasis. Med Clin North Am 1981; 65:363–384.

76. Stewart RB, Hale WE, Marks RG: Diuretic use in an ambulatory elderly population. Am J Hosp Pharm 1983; 40:409–413.

77. Biswas CK, Ramos JM, Kerr DNS: Heparin effect on ionised calcium concentration. Clin Chim Acta 1981; 116:343–347.

78. McLean FC, Hastings AB: A biological method for the estimation of calcium ion concentration. J Biol Chem 1934; 107:337–350.

79. Wandrup J, Kancir C: The concentration of free calcium ions in whole blood. Scand J Clin Lab Invest [Suppl] 1983; 165:47–48.

80. Brauman J, Delvigne CH, DeConinck I, Willems D: Factors affecting the determination of ionized calcium in blood. Scand J Clin Lab Invest [Suppl] 1983; 165:27–31.

81. McLean FC, Hastings AB: Clinical estimation and significance of calcium-ion concentrations in the blood. Am J Med Sci 1935; 189:601–613.

82. Siggaard-Andersen O, Thode J, Fogh-Andersen N: What is "ionized calcium"? Scand J Clin Lab Invest [Suppl] 1983; 165:11–16.

83. Grima JM, Brand MJD: Activity and interference effects in measurement of ionized calcium with ion-selective electrodes. Clin Chem 1977; 23:2048–2054.

84. Bringhurst FR, Potts JT Jr: Calcium and phosphate turnover, and metabolic actions. *In* DeGroot LJ, Cahill GF Jr, Odell WD, et al (eds): Endocrinology, vol 2. New York: Grune & Stratton, 1979; 551–585.

85. Drop LJ: Ionized calcium, the heart, and hemodynamic function. Anesth Analg 1985; 64:43–51.

86. Bombardieri S, Clerico A, Riente L, et al: Circadian variations of serum myoglobin levels in normal subjects and patients with polymyositis. Arthritis Rheum 1982; 25:1419–1424.

87. Brown SS, Kalow W, Pilz W, et al: The plasma cholinesterases: A new perspective. *In* Latner AL, Schwartz MK (eds): Advances in Clinical Chemistry, vol 22. New York: Academic, 1981; 1–123.

88. Kalow W, Genest K: A method for the detection of atypical forms of human serum cholinesterase. Determination of dibucaine numbers. Can J Biochem 1957; 35:339–346.

89. Arnold WP: A rapid, semi-automated method for determining dibucaine numbers. Anesthesiology 1981; 55:676–679.

90. Whittaker M: Plasma cholinesterase variants and the anesthetist. Anaesthesia 1980; 35:174–197.

91. Jones JD: Factors that affect clinical laboratory values. J Occup Med 1980; 22:316–320.

92. Lundberg GD, Iverson C, Radulescu G: Now read this: The SI units are here. JAMA 1986; 255:2329–2339.

93. Council on Scientific Affairs: SI units for clinical laboratory data. JAMA 1985; 253:2553–2554.

94. Young DS: Standardized reporting of laboratory data: The desirability of using SI units. N Engl J Med 1974; 290:368–373.

95. Powsner ER: SI quantities and units for American medicine. JAMA 1984; 252:1737–1741.

96. Michenfelder JD: Who's afraid of Blaise Pascal? Anesthesiology 1982; 56:245–246.

97. Kazacos M, Skalsky M, Skyllas-Kazacos M: A review of developments in implantable selective chemical sensors. Life Support Syst 1985; 3:189–205.

98. Galletti PM, and Members of the Consensus Development Panel: Consensus conference: Clinical applications of biomaterials. JAMA 1983; 249:1050–1054.

Monitoring the Central and Peripheral Nervous System

chapter nineteen

Intracranial Pressure

■ WAYNE K. MARSHALL, M.D.

Brain function is directly dependent upon oxygen supply and blood flow. Cerebral blood flow (CBF) and metabolism are affected by intracranial pressure (ICP), anesthesia concentration, and blood partial pressures of oxygen, carbon dioxide, and hydrogen ion. Preoperative neurologic function can be determined with a routine neurologic examination including level of consciousness, memory, cognition, sensation, motor strength, cranial nerve evaluation, and cerebellar tests. Except during certain forms of regional anesthesia, such tests are impossible intraoperatively and in the early portions of the recovery period.

Various methods to monitor intraoperative cerebral function, such as measurement of ICP or regional CBF and recording of cellular electrical activity using electroencephalography (see Chapter 20) or evoked potentials (see Chapter 22), have therefore evolved. Of these techniques, intraoperative measurement of regional CBF using [133]xenon washout is limited to only a few medical centers because it is invasive (inhalation, intravenous or intracarotid administration of radioactive tracer required), requires radiation exposure, and provides only an intermittent measurement of blood flow. ICP, however, is more easily evaluated. The origin and importance of normal cerebrospinal fluid (CSF) pressure and intracranial hypertension, the effects of commonly used drugs and anesthetics on ICP, the rationale for clinical measurement of ICP, and the common devices used for measurement of ICP are discussed.

659

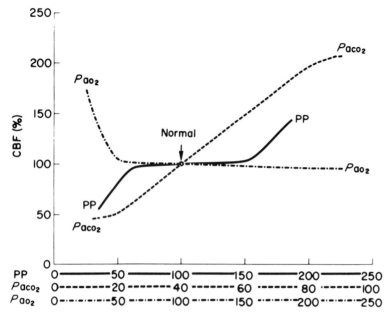

Figure 19–1. The effects on cerebral blood flow (CBF) of arterial oxygen tension (Pao$_2$ [torr]), arterial carbon dioxide tension (Paco$_2$ [torr]), as a percentage of control, and cerebral perfusion pressure (PP [torr]) are demonstrated. CBF is little affected by Po$_2$ except during hypoxia. Autoregulation of CBF occurs between perfusion pressures of about 60–150 torr. CBF is quite sensitive to changes in Paco$_2$. (From Michenfelder JD: The cerebral circulation. *In* Prys-Roberts C [ed]: The Circulation in Anesthesia. London: Blackwell Scientific, 1980; 212. With permission.)

PHYSIOLOGY OF CEREBRAL CIRCULATION

Normal CBF

Normal CBF in awake humans averages 50 ml/100 gm/min for whole brain.[1, 2] Blood flow to the brain provides nutrients (glucose) and oxygen and removes the waste products of cellular metabolism (carbon dioxide, lactic acid, and so on). Brain cells are acutely dependent upon adequate blood flow to accomplish these tasks. As CBF decreases, both the delivery of glucose and oxygen and the removal of waste products decrease.

At levels of CBF under 25 ml/100 gm/min, early changes in cerebral electrical activity become apparent.[3] These electroencephalographic changes represent evidence of ischemia of brain cells. CBF of 25 ml/100 gm/min corresponds to a cerebral perfusion pressure (CPP) of 45 torr (Fig. 19–1).[4] This correlation of CPP to level of CBF provides a readily available, objective clinical indication of adequacy of cerebral perfusion.

CBF is directly responsible for delivery of glucose and oxygen to, and removal of carbon dioxide, lactic acid, and other waste products from, the actively metabolizing cells of the brain. In normal individuals, blood flow is regulated by several factors broadly categorized as either metabolic or neurogenic.[5] These various factors interact to produce an effect known as autoregulation of CBF. Cerebral autoregulation is the maintenance of CBF over a pressure range of 50–150 torr. Metabolic, neurogenic, and auto-regulatory effects are all ultimately mediated through changes in cerebral vessel size and, therefore, changes in the relative resistance to blood flow.

Table 19–1. SUBSTANCES AFFECTING CEREBRAL VASCULATURE

Substance Affecting [H$^+$]	Effect on pH	Effect on Cerebral Vessels
Increased arterial P_{CO_2}	Acidosis	Vasodilatation
Decreased arterial P_{CO_2}	Alkalosis	Vasoconstriction
Increased bicarbonate ion	Alkalosis	Vasoconstriction
Decreased bicarbonate ion	Acidosis	Vasodilatation
Increased metabolic acid (lactic, pyruvic)	Acidosis	Vasodilatation
Decreased metabolic acid	Alkalosis	Vasoconstriction

Metabolic Control

Four metabolic mechanisms affect CBF: hydrogen ion concentration, oxygen, carbon dioxide, and basic cerebral metabolic rate.

pH Effect

The concentration of hydrogen ions in the tissues surrounding the vessels in the brain affects blood flow. This is known as the pH effect. The relationship of pH to hydrogen ion concentration is illustrated in the following equation:

$$pH = -\log [H^+]$$

Therefore, increased hydrogen ion concentration produces a lower pH (acidosis), and decreased hydrogen ion concentration produces a higher pH (alkalosis).[6] An increased extracellular fluid hydrogen ion concentration decreases pH, and the resulting acidosis produces vasodilatation and increases blood flow.[7] Likewise, decreased extracellular fluid hydrogen ion concentration increases pH, and this alkalosis produces vasoconstriction and a decrease in blood flow.[7] Substances that affect pH by changing the hydrogen ion concentration are given in Table 19–1. The pH effect, although functional, usually plays a secondary role in regulation of CBF when compared with other factors.[8]

Oxygen and Carbon Dioxide Effects

The effects of the respiratory gases oxygen and carbon dioxide are usually considered in relation to the arterial partial pressure of each gas (Pa_{O_2} and Pa_{CO_2}).

Pa_{O_2} Effect. Insufficient oxygen supply to the brain, whether by inadequate volume of blood or by inadequate oxygen tension in the blood, increases CBF through vasodilatation of the cerebral vessels.[9] This occurs when the Pa_{O_2} falls below 60 torr (Fig. 19–1).[9] High arterial oxygen tensions only minimally affect the cerebral vessels by vasoconstriction (Fig. 19–1).[10]

Pa_{CO_2} Effect. The arterial tension of carbon dioxide exerts a vasoactive effect through two mechanisms. The direct effect of Pa_{CO_2} causes progressive vasoconstriction and decreases blood flow in response to a decreased Pa_{CO_2}[11] and progressive vasodilatation and increased blood flow in response to an increased Pa_{CO_2} (Fig. 19–1).[12] This effect is independent of changes in hydrogen ion concentration.[13–15]

The indirect effect of Pa_{CO_2} operates through the pH effect. Both arterial and tissue carbon dioxide combine with water to produce carbonic acid, which in turn dissociates to increase hydrogen ion concentration.[7] Therefore, increased Pa_{CO_2} produces increased hydrogen ion concentration, decreased pH, and resultant vasodilatation and increased blood flow;[7, 9] decreased Pa_{CO_2} produces decreased hydrogen ion concentration, increased pH, and resultant vasoconstriction and decreased CBF.[16]

The duration of the vasoconstrictive effect of decreased Pa_{CO_2} through hyperventilation may also be limited. After an unpredictable period of time (as long as 72 hours), the effect of continuous hyperventilation begins to decrease. This is thought to be due to the buffering of the induced pH changes by the CSF and renal compensatory mechanisms.

Metabolic Rate Effect

Finally, the overall basic rate of metabolism of brain cells also affects blood flow.[17] An increase in cerebral metabolic rate results in vasodilatation and increased blood flow.[18, 19] A decrease in cerebral metabolic rate results in vasoconstriction and decreased blood flow.[19]

Neurogenic Control

Cerebral vessels are also under the control of the autonomic nervous system. The effects of neurogenic influences on CBF are usually masked by the powerful metabolic mechanisms previously described.[7] However, the intracranial vessels are innervated by both sympathetic and parasympathetic fibers.[20] Under certain circumstances (i.e., severe exercise, intracranial hemorrhage, stroke), strong sympathetic outflow produces cerebral vasoconstriction and decreased CBF.[7, 21]

Autoregulation

The multiple mechanisms described previously interact through control of cerebral vessel size to produce CBF levels that closely match the metabolic needs of the brain. Normally, this system of autoregulation operates over a range of mean CPPs from 60 to 150 torr (see Fig. 19–1).[4] Pressures below a mean of 60 torr decrease blood flow because vessels are maximally dilated and flow is directly dependent upon pressure (Fig. 19–1).[4] Conversely, at mean pressures above 150 torr, blood flow is again pressure-dependent, owing to maximum vessel constriction, and flow increases with pressure (Fig. 19–1).[4] Within the normal range of mean CPP (60–150 torr), blood flow is held constant (Fig. 19–1).[4]

The effects of the respiratory gases oxygen and carbon dioxide can defeat normal autoregulation.[10, 22] Thus, at any given perfusion pressure, a

Pao$_2$ less than 60 torr or an increase in Paco$_2$ produces vasodilatation and increases CBF; a decrease in Paco$_2$ produces vasoconstriction and decreases blood flow.[4]

PHYSIOLOGY OF ICP

CSF Physiology

CSF is the body's shock absorber for the central nervous system. It bathes and surrounds the entire brain and spinal cord to act as a natural cushion for those very delicate structures.

The normal intracranial-intraspinal volume of the central nervous system is approximately 1650 ml, of which 150 ml is CSF.[7] The normal rate of CSF production is approximately 500 ml/day.[23]

CSF is mainly produced by the choroid plexus in all four ventricles of the brain,[7, 23, 24] with the major portion coming from the lateral ventricles. It flows from the lateral ventricles through the foramen of Monro to the third ventricle, through the aqueduct of Sylvius to the fourth ventricle, through the foramen of Luschka and foramen of Magendie to the cisterna magna, and thence to the subarachnoid space surrounding the brain and spinal cord (Fig. 19–2).[7] Absorption occurs (into the venous blood) through the arachnoid villi in the sagittal venous sinus. In the absence of pathology, the rate of absorption is equal to the rate of production.[7] The fact that production is largely active (pressure-independent) and absorption is largely passive (pressure-dependent) produces a measurable CSF pressure (ICP) that is normally less than 15 torr.[7, 22]

Determinants of ICP

The intracranial cavity is bordered by the cranium, a rigid structure of bone with only one real outlet for the intracranial contents, the foramen magnum. CSF is only one of several substances contained in this cavity, the normal contents of which are listed in Figure 19–3.[25]

An increase in the volume of one or more of the normal constituents of the intracranial cavity produces a concomitant and compensating decrease in the volume of other intracranial contents in order to partially maintain volume and pressure at a constant level.[25] Glial cells, neurons, and extracellular fluid are noncompressible, have no ready avenue to exit the cranial vault, and are usually not part of this compensatory mechanism.[25] Thus, volume compensation results from the decrease of either intracranial intravascular blood volume or CSF volume, or both.[25] An overwhelming pathologic increase in intracranial volume exhausts this mechanism for compliance compensation, and ICP increases.[25] Any further increase in intracranial volume produces a concomitant increase in ICP.[25] The pressure/volume (intracranial compliance) relationship is illustrated in Figure 19–4.[26]

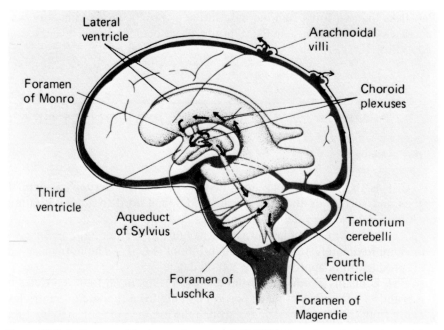

Figure 19–2. In the normal brain, cerebrospinal fluid (CSF) flows from the lateral ventricles through the foramen of Monro to the third ventricle, through the aqueduct of Sylvius to the fourth ventricle, through the foramina of Magendie and Luschka to the cisterna magna and finally to the cerebral and spinal subarachnoid spaces. (From Guyton AC: Textbook of Medical Physiology, 7th Ed. Philadelphia: WB Saunders, 1986; 374.)

Intracranial Pressure/Volume Curve

Utilizing this pressure/volume relationship another way allows for the determination of intracranial pressure/volume status in individual patients. With very small increments (0.1 ml—0.5 ml—1.0 ml) of sterile preservative-free saline solution injected into the CSF space and the concomitant change in CSF pressure produced measured, relatively accurate determinations can be made about the position of an individual patient on the pressure/volume curve. The higher on the sharp limb of the curve, the tighter the brain is, and the more dramatic the increase in ICP with each increment in intracranial volume (Fig. 19–4).

The effect of intracranial volume on ICP also depends upon the rate of volume increase. Compensatory mechanisms respond more readily to slower increases in intracranial volume, and in this circumstance, acute changes in ICP in response to volume changes are less profound.[27] A very rapid increase in volume rapidly increases ICP.[27] However, there is an absolute limit to the volume compensatory mechanisms, and when that limit is exceeded, the rate of volume expansion becomes irrelevant.[27]

Causes of Intracranial Hypertension

Abnormal increases in ICP are produced by many different pathologic conditions.[7] The mechanisms of production of increased ICP include an

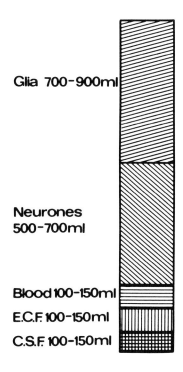

Figure 19–3. Intracranial contents and volume in an average adult human. Total intracranial volume is 1500–2050 ml. (ECF = extracellular fluid.) (From Jennett B, Teasdale G: Management of Head Injuries. Philadelphia: FA Davis, 1981; 60. With permission.)

expanding intracranial mass, cerebral edema, intracranial CSF volume increase, and intracranial blood volume increase.[7] Some conditions are caused by more than one mechanism.

Intracranial Masses

Expanding intracranial masses include intracranial tumors and intracranial hematomas. These are conditions in which an abnormal constituent of increasing size is added to the intracranial contents. Although intravascular blood is a normal intracranial substance, extravascular collections of blood are not.

Cerebral Edema

Cerebral edema represents an increase in cellular volume and possibly an increase in extracellular fluid volume as well. Cerebral edema may be classified as either global or regional. Conditions producing global edema include closed head injury, cerebral anoxic damage, Reye's syndrome,[28] and severe systemic hypertension. Some examples of conditions producing regional cerebral edema are edema surrounding an intracranial tumor,[29] localized cerebral trauma, and stroke.

Increased CSF Volume

Intracranial CSF volume increases owing to decreased absorption of CSF or obstruction of venous outflow from the head. Decreased absorption

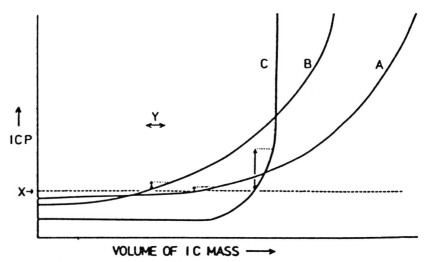

Figure 19–4. Three possible intracranial pressure/volume curves. The most widely accepted is curve C. As the volume of intracranial mass (IC) increases, the intracranial pressure (ICP) increases. In curve C, the flat portion represents the volume compensation of normal brain. Once this compensation is exhausted, further increases in volume produce greater and greater increases in ICP. A patient with an elevation of ICP to point X is on the steep portion of the curve. Any further increase in volume (Y) produces a large increase in ICP in curve C but smaller increases in curves A and B. The relative position of any patient on the curve (intracranial compliance) can be determined by injecting small increments of volume into the CSF (*arrows*) and observing the concomitant change in pressure (see text). (From Leech P, Miller JD: Intracranial volume-pressure relationships during experimental brain compression in primates. Pressure responses to changes in ventricular volume. J Neurol Neurosurg Psychiatry 1974; 37:1093–1098. With permission.)

of CSF produces hydrocephalus. Communicating hydrocephalus occurs when the CSF is not normally absorbed through the arachnoid villi. Noncommunicating hydrocephalus is produced by an obstruction to CSF flow through the ventricles to the subarachnoid space. Usually, this obstruction occurs in the aqueduct of Sylvius between the third and the fourth ventricles.

Venous outflow obstruction decreases CSF absorption probably by increasing the passive filtration pressure across the arachnoid villi through an increase in sagittal sinus venous pressure. Venous outflow obstruction can occur intracranially secondary to traumatic disruption of the venous sinus tract or extracranially from jugular venous compression or even assumption of the supine position, which removes the negative venous hydrostatic pressure gradient present in the upright position.

Increased Intracranial Blood Volume

Increased intracranial blood volume is also a consequence of venous outflow obstruction as well as of cerebral vasodilatation. Cerebral vasodilatation in turn can be caused by severe systemic hypertension, direct vasodilator drugs, and acute respiratory failure. It is also produced by a decrease in PaO_2 (hypoxia), an increase in $PaCO_2$ (hypercapnia) and a decrease in arterial pH (acidosis). Cerebral vasodilatation increases cerebral blood volume.[7, 9, 11–15]

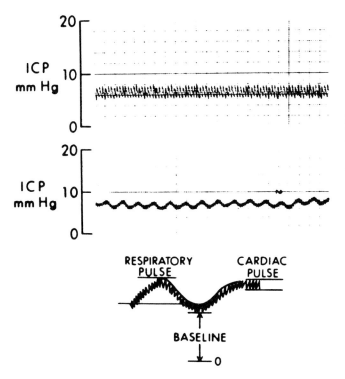

Figure 19–5. Normal ICP is a pulsatile waveform with pressures of 5–7 torr. On this pressure are superimposed the effects of the cardiac and respiratory cycles. The top graph is at high paper speed in order to illustrate the cardiac effect, the middle graph represents the respiratory effect, and the bottom graph illustrates the basic components of an ICP waveform during one respiratory cycle. (From Marmarou A, Tabaddor K: Intracranial pressure: Physiology and pathophysiology. *In* Cooper PR [ed]: Head Injury, 115–127, © 1982, the Williams & Wilkins Co., Baltimore.)

ICP Waveforms

When it is measured and displayed on an oscilloscope, the CSF pressure normally exhibits a characteristic pulsatile waveform.[27] The amplitude varies with the cardiac cycle, owing to transient changes in blood volume, and with respiration, probably owing to transient changes in intrathoracic pressure, which are transmitted via the venous system to the venous sinus in the cranium. These pulsatile variations are superimposed on a steady-state volume level of CSF (Fig. 19–5).

Normal CSF pressures are less than 15 torr. In patients with abnormally increased ICP, the amplitude of the pulsatile component increases. Abnormal waveforms seen in cases of pathologically increased ICP are usually intermittent and of two basic types: A waves or plateau waves, lasting for several minutes, acutely exhibit ICP of 50–100 torr and usually denote very poor neurologic outcome; B waves are of lower amplitude with shorter duration than A waves (Fig. 19–6).[30]

Anesthetic Effects on ICP

The effects of various drugs on the ICP are summarized in Table 19–2. The potent anesthetic agents halothane, enflurane, and isoflurane increase ICP primarily by direct cerebral vasodilatation and resultant increased cerebral blood volume.[31–39] Uncompensated respiratory depression from these agents may also cause cerebral vasodilatation secondary to an increase in Pa_{CO_2}.[12]

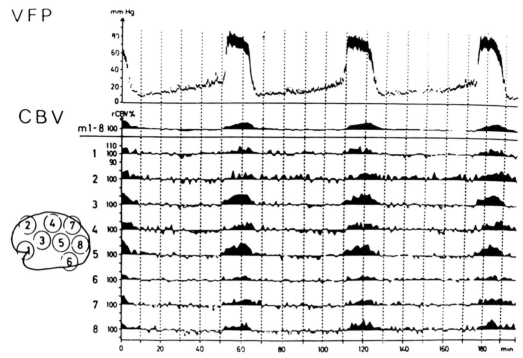

Figure 19–6. Simultaneous recordings of intracranial pressure ([ICP] ventricular fluid pressure [VFP]) and cerebral blood volume (CBV) regionally in eight separate areas of the left hemisphere in a single patient. The Y-axis represents time in minutes during the measurement. The top graph illustrates VFP (ICP) A waves or plateau waves. The second graph represents average CBV from the eight areas. Note the similar course of VFP (ICP) and CBV; the A waves are accompanied by increases in CBV. (From Risberg J, Lundberg N, Ingvar DH: Regional cerebral blood volume during acute transient rises of the intracranial pressure [plateau waves]. J Neurosurg 1969; 31:303–310. With permission.)

Although nitrous oxide (N_2O) does not clinically affect ICP, there is some evidence that it increases ICP under certain circumstances.[40–43] However, N_2O is still very widely used in patients with intracranial hypertension without deleterious effects. The one exception to this occurs in patients in whom air is present inside the cranium, as after pneumoencephalography.

The barbiturate drugs, of which thiopental sodium is commonly used in anesthesia, decrease ICP by direct cerebral vasoconstriction and decreased cerebral blood volume.[44, 45] Narcotic agents such as morphine and fentanyl citrate either do not affect CSF pressure or may even decrease ICP by primarily decreasing cerebral metabolic rate and CBF.[46–50] However, like the potent anesthetic agents, narcotics also depress respiration, and unless ventilation is supported when necessary, increased Pa_{CO_2} may increase ICP.[12]

Ketamine hydrochloride produces an increase in ICP owing to an increase in CBF from cerebral vasodilatation.[51–53] The benzodiazepines (diazepam, lorazepam, midazolam) decrease ICP by cerebral vasoconstriction.[54–56] A relatively new agent, etomidate, decreases ICP by decreasing CBF.[57]

The muscle relaxants commonly used in anesthesia vary in their effects on ICP. Pancuronium bromide, vecuronium bromide, and atracurium be-

Table 19–2. DRUG EFFECTS ON INTRACRANIAL PRESSURE

Drug	Primary	Secondary	Reference
Potent anesthetic agents			
Halothane	+ +		31–33
Enflurane	+ +		34–36
Isoflurane	+ +		37–39
Barbiturates			
Thiopental sodium	– –		44, 45
Narcotics			
Morphine	0	+	46–50
Fentanyl citrate	0	+	46–50
Ketamine hydrochloride	+		51–53
Benzodiazepines			
Diazepam	–		54–56
Lorazepam	–		54–56
Midazolam	–		54–56
Neuromuscular-blocking drugs			
Succinylcholine chloride	+	0	64–66
d-tubocurarine	0	+	58
Pancuronium bromide	0		58, 59
Vecuronium bromide	0		60, 61
Atracurium besylate	0		62, 63
Etomidate	–		57
Diuretics			
Mannitol	–		68, 69
Furosemide	–		67
Vasodilators			
Sodium nitroprusside	+		70
Hydralazine hydrochloride	+		71
Nitroglycerin	+		72
Trimethaphan camsylate	0	+	70, 73
Beta-adrenergic blockers			
Propranolol	0		74
Labetalol	0		75
Esmolol	0		76
Nitrous oxide	0	+	40–43

+ + = Major increase; + = Moderate increase; 0 = No effect; – – = Major decrease;
– = Moderate decrease

sylate have all been shown to have no effect on ICP.[58–63] D-Tubocurarine, however, may increase ICP secondary to histamine release and cerebral vasodilatation.[58] Succinylcholine chloride is the most controversial member of this group in that there is evidence that, although the drug causes increases in ICP, this effect may be attenuated by pretreatment with a nondepolarizing relaxant drug.[64–66]

Diuretic agents, including furosemide and mannitol, are commonly used to treat intracranial hypertension. Furosemide is a loop diuretic that decreases ICP by producing a fluid diuresis through the kidney.[67] The resultant fluid shifts effectively reduce cerebral edema. Mannitol, an osmotic diuretic, also produces this effect through diuresis; however, it may also increase ICP transiently through an osmotic effect on brain water.[68, 69] Both drugs depend ultimately upon normal renal function for their effect.

Hypotensive agents such as primary vasodilators, trimethaphan camsylate, or beta-adrenergic blockers are occasionally needed to control systemic hypertension or to produce deliberate hypotension (e.g., in cerebral aneurysm surgery). The primary vasodilator agents, sodium nitroprusside, hydralazine hydrochloride, and nitroglycerin, produce dose-related increases in ICP by dilating cerebral vessels and increasing CBF and volume.[70–72] Trimethaphan camsylate, a ganglionic blocking agent, may also increase ICP through vasodilatation secondary to histamine release; however, this effect is still debated.[70, 73] The beta-adrenergic blocking drugs, propranolol, labetalol, and esmolol, do not primarily affect ICP.[74–76]

PATHOPHYSIOLOGY OF INTRACRANIAL HYPERTENSION

CPP

To understand why increased ICP is deleterious and of concern, it is necessary to understand the concept of cerebral perfusion pressure (CPP).[25] CPP is defined as the pressure gradient across the cerebral capillary bed, which perfuses blood through the brain. The CPP is calculated according to the following formula:

$$CPP = MAP - ICP$$

where MAP = mean arterial inflow pressure and ICP = the mean resistance to outflow of blood. For accuracy, the MAP should be measured at the level of the external auditory meatus. Under some circumstances, the central venous pressure measured at the level of the external auditory meatus may be used in place of the ICP.

Intracranial hypertension produces pathologic insults through two basic mechanisms: ischemia of brain tissue and mechanical damage due to bulk shifts of brain tissue.

Cerebral Ischemia

The final common pathway leading to cell damage from intracranial hypertension is ischemia of the cells in the brain.[77] As stated previously, CBF delivers oxygen and glucose to and removes carbon dioxide and waste products from metabolizing brain cells. Ischemia of these cells produces hypoxia and acidosis of brain tissue. When CPP decreases below approximately 45 torr, CBF decreases to ischemic levels (see Fig. 19–1).[3]

From the preceding formula, it can be seen that CPP decreases as the MAP decreases or ICP increases, or both. Normal CPP is between 60 and 150 torr. This corresponds to a CBF of 50 ml/100 gm/min (Fig. 19–1). As the CPP decreases below 60 torr, autoregulation is defeated, and CBF decreases with pressure. At a CPP of 45 torr, CBF is approximately 50% of normal, i.e., 25 ml/100 gm/min (Fig. 19–1). At this point, the first electrical evidence of ischemia appears.[3] Further reduction in CBF produces more profound changes. An absolutely safe level of CBF during low-flow states that does not produce permanent cell damage is not known. However, in addition to the level of CBF achieved, the duration of time spent at that level also plays an important role in determining the survival of cells. Pre-existing abnormal cerebral vessels reduce the margin for decreased CBF (as in chronic hypertension).[78] Therefore, when possible every attempt should be made to maintain CPP at or near normal levels.

Herniation

In addition to brain cell ischemia, bulk shifts of brain tissue can produce mechanical damage to brain cells through the process known as herniation.[25, 27] Although herniation through a craniotomy is possible, brain herniation in the intact cranium occurs through the foramen magnum (cerebellum), the tentorium, (temporal lobe or uncus), and the falx (cingulate gyrus and cerebral hemisphere). Herniation occurs with increases in ICP owing to mass effects from intracranial tumor or hematoma. The type of herniation that occurs depends upon the location of the mass.[27] Supratentorial masses include temporal masses, which produce severe midbrain herniation, and frontal or occipital masses, which affect the brain stem less severely for the same size mass and same ICP level.[27] In addition to location, rapidly increasing masses produce a greater effect on the ICP and herniation than do more slowly growing masses.[27]

ICP MONITORING TECHNIQUES

General Considerations

Historically, many different techniques and devices have been used to measure ICP. Several are in common clinical use at present. In deciding which technique or device to use in a given clinical situation, several aspects of placement should be taken into consideration.[79] First, an ICP monitor should be reliable and stable during long-term use. In general, the simpler the device the more reliable it is.[79] Second, the placement procedure should be as innocuous to the patient and the patient's central nervous system as possible. The risks of bleeding and infection should be minimum.[79] Third, the technique should allow for continuous measurement and recording of ICP while at the same time allowing adequate comfort and nursing care for the patient.[79] Finally, the technique chosen should be within the realm of expertise of the operator and as inexpensive as possible.

Monitoring Indications

Indications for monitoring ICP clinically, then, are based on the fact that ischemia or a decrease in CBF owing to a decrease in CPP is the primary common pathway for secondary brain injury after the initial insult has occurred.[77] Prevention of this secondary injury is the area in which therapy may be beneficial, as no therapy can reverse the damage already produced by the primary insult.

ICP should be monitored whenever secondary injury is of concern:

1. In patients with head injuries with a Glasgow coma score of 7 or less.[72]
2. In patients with Reye's syndrome, as uncontrolled increases in ICP are a major factor in mortality.[28]
3. In patients with intracranial tumors, especially during induction of anesthesia when peritumoral edema is present.[29]
4. In any patient with intracranial pathology when the clinical neurologic exam cannot be followed—i.e., (a) intraoperatively (this becomes ineffective once the dura is opened); (b) during barbiturate-induced coma; and (c) during the use of neuromuscular-blocking agents in neurosurgical patients in the intensive care unit.
5. In any circumstance in which therapeutic maneuvers are made that adversely affect CPP and ICP.[77]

Classification of Devices

The devices and techniques now available for monitoring ICP can be classified into groups by geographic location of the device in the central nervous system, inherent invasiveness of the device, and method of measuring ICP. All the devices outlined in this chapter require placement through surgical entry into the skull and, therefore, should be inserted only by an experienced operator.

The geographic location of the device can vary among the lumbar spine, the cervical spine, the posterior fossa, and the supratentorial area of the cranium. Supratentorial placement is almost always preferred because of pathologically decreased flow of CSF around the tentorium in the subarachnoid space and subsequent intracranial herniation.[79] In patients with increased ICP, invasion of the subarachnoid space in the spinal canal and subsequent loss of CSF below the tentorium or the foramen magnum, or both, may even produce herniation.

Another means of describing ICP monitoring devices is by method of measurement. Devices that place the pressure-measuring transducer at a site remote from the patient utilize a column of fluid in tubing to transmit the pressure wave from the CSF to the transducer. These devices are said to be fluid-coupled. The fluid and fluid path must be sterile, nonirritating to tissues, and free of leaks and air bubbles. The transducer should usually be placed at the level of the external auditory meatus for accuracy. Care must be taken to prevent any inadvertent injection of drugs or volume into this system. This has been a problem and is a continuing risk owing to the close resemblance of this system to other physiologic pressure–monitoring equipment, i.e., arterial pressure apparatus. Another precaution that is necessary is to prevent the use of continuous flush systems in this setting. Nursing personnel and physicians caring for patients with fluid-coupled monitoring devices must be trained in the differences between other physiologic-monitoring equipment and ICP monitors. Experienced operators, however, can safely perform clinical intracranial pressure/volume determinations on patients with this apparatus.

Newer devices utilize light transmission (fiberoptics) or a column of gas (pneumatics) instead of fluid-coupling to transmit the CSF pressure wave to the pressure-measuring electronic device. At least one device places the transducer directly in contact with the dura. There are also several experimental devices that attempt to implant the pressure transducer directly into the CSF. The major problems with newer devices are reliability and miniaturization of the electronics or power supplies.

Intraventricular Devices

Classification according to the invasive nature of the device distinguishes among intraventricular devices, subarachnoid devices, epidural devices, and surface devices.

The intraventricular catheter is one of the oldest and one of the simplest devices used to measure ICP.[80–82] It is classified as a fluid-coupled device; ICP waves are transmitted via an uninterrupted fluid path to a pressure sensor, usually a strain-gauge transducer outside of the cranium. This is accomplished by placing a hollow, fluid-filled catheter directly into one of the lateral ventricles through a cranial burr hole and intact brain tissue. A typical arrangement of the tubing and transducer is shown in Figure 19–7. With this device, although it is very invasive, long-term ICP measurements can be made, pressure/volume determinations can be performed, intrathecal drugs (antibiotics) can be injected, and CSF can be withdrawn for both diagnostic studies and therapeutic needs (e.g., to decrease ICP). In order to achieve accurate ICP measurements with this device, the external transducer should be located at the level of the external auditory meatus (see Chapter 3).

Since the tubing arrangement for this device closely resembles that of other intravascular pressure-monitoring devices, care must be taken to remove any continuous flush system from the apparatus. Flushing of the tubing and catheter are occasionally necessary but should be done carefully, only with preservative-free saline solution and only by an experienced operator. Because this technique requires invasion of tissue and violation of the dura, the potential for infection exists and has been estimated at less than 6.3%.[83–85] Likewise, if the ventricular system is collapsed or relatively small, the operator may be unable to accurately place a catheter into the lateral ventricle (Fig. 19–8). Computed tomography facilitates location of the lateral ventricles and intraventricular catheter placement.

Subarachnoid Devices

Subarachnoid Bolt

In an effort to circumvent the necessity of perforating brain tissue, as with a ventricular catheter, yet still directly interface with CSF, the sub-

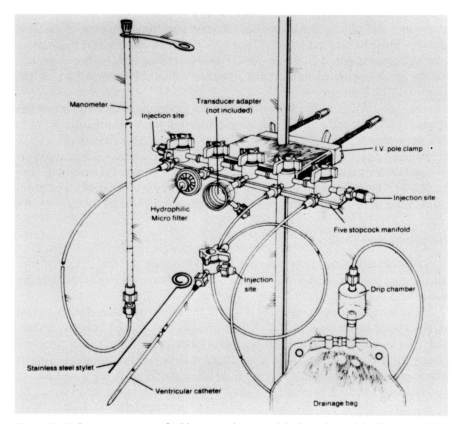

Figure 19–7. One arrangement of tubing, transducer, and drainage bag originally proposed by Becker. Note the transducer dome in the center, the absence of a continuous flush system, and ports for injection and drainage of CSF. The transducer should be positioned at the level of the external auditory meatus. This apparatus may be used for measurement of either intraventricular or subarachnoid pressures. (From Wilkinson HA: Intracranial pressure monitoring: Techniques and pitfalls. *In* Cooper PR [ed]: Head Injury, 155, © 1982, the Williams & Wilkins Co., Baltimore.)

arachnoid bolt was developed (Fig. 19–9). Sometimes referred to as the Richmond bolt because of pioneering work done by Becker, Vries, Young, and others at the Medical College of Virginia, this device is also placed via a burr hole in the supratentorial area of the skull, with the tip placed below the arachnoid membrane.[80, 86] Figure 19–10 compares optimum insertion sites with undesirable locations. Like the intraventricular catheter, the bolt is fluid-coupled to an external pressure transducer, which should be placed at the level of the external meatus. Continuous flushing systems should be excluded from the fluid path (see Fig. 19–7). Regular flushing of the bolt should be performed manually but only with very small amounts of preservative-free saline solution. Because the tip of the bolt actually rests close to or on the brain surface, withdrawal of CSF is impossible. Pressure/volume determinations are possible; however, drugs cannot be reliably injected. Potential for infection does exist but is considered to be less likely than with a ventricular catheter.[85, 86] Because of the relative ease of placement and

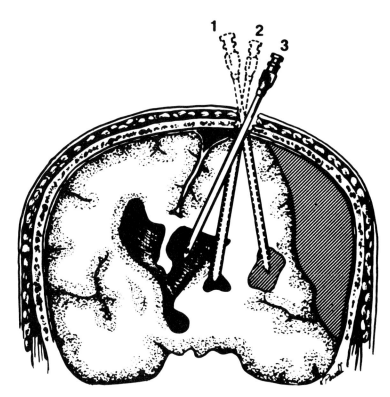

Figure 19–8. Potential problems encountered in placing an intraventricular catheter. The subdural hematoma has shifted the brain to the contralateral side and compressed the ipsilateral ventricle. Needle position 3 is the appropriate placement in this case and was achieved after blind passage, as in 1 and 2. With the ready availability of computed tomography, needle placement is much more precise. (From Wilkinson HA: Intracranial pressure monitoring: Techniques and pitfalls. *In* Cooper PR [ed]: Head Injury, 158, © 1982, the Williams & Wilkins Co., Baltimore.)

the relative accuracy of the pressure measurement, the subarachnoid bolt is a device widely used for measuring ICP.[86]

Cup Catheter

Another subarachnoid device available is the cup catheter, which operates similarly to the subarachnoid bolt (Fig. 19–11). This device is a ribbon-shaped catheter passed into the cerebral subarachnoid space through a burr hole, with the skin incision remote from the craniotomy site, thus possibly decreasing the incidence of infection.[87] The cup catheter is also fluid-coupled in order to ensure filling of the cup. This catheter is somewhat more difficult to place than the bolt and is less widely used.

Epidural Devices

Three devices are currently available for epidural ICP measurement: epidural transducer, fiberoptic transducer, and pneumatic transducer. All three devices measure ICP through the intact dura and avoid the use of a fluid path (i.e., are not fluid-coupled). Because the dura is not opened, the risk of infection is felt to be less than it is with intraventricular or subarachnoid devices.

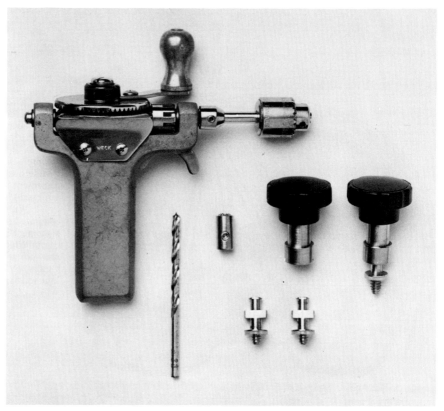

Figure 19–9. A subarachnoid bolt and the equipment for its insertion. The twist drill has a movable collar that produces a well in the outer table of the skull to allow accurate depth of placement. The black handles are for inserting the bolt itself.

Epidural Transducer

The epidural transducer is produced and marketed by NV Phillips, The Netherlands. It is a device designed to be threaded into a burr hole in the skull far enough to stretch the intact dura across the flat sensor at the tip (Fig. 19–12).[88] The measurement of ICP with this device depends on the principle of coplanarity,[89] that is, the flat sensor must be exactly parallel to the plane of the dura and in intimate contact with it. The CSF pressure waves are transmitted across the intact dura to the transducer surface. Therefore, accuracy of placement is critical. When the device is properly placed, however, the pressure measurements correspond well with those obtained with an intraventricular catheter.[88] Because there is no fluid coupling, injection of drugs is impossible and intracranial pressure/volume measurement cannot be performed. The device does not need to be flushed periodically, as do fluid-coupled devices. However, the transducer is nondisposable and relatively expensive.[88]

Fiberoptic Epidural Monitor

The Ladd fiberoptic sensor and monitor (Ladd Research Industries, Burlington, VT) constitute a dedicated system designed for epidural use,

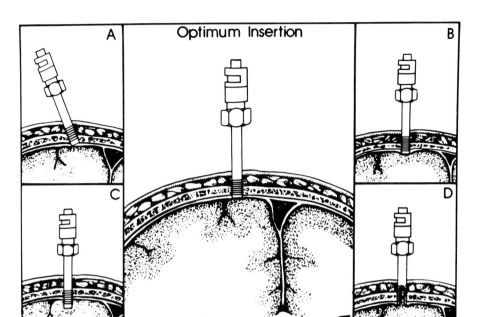

Figure 19–10. Optimum placement of the subarachnoid bolt is seen in the center of the figure. Potential problems with bolt placement: *A*, Oblique placement does not allow full approximation to the subarachnoid space; *B*, A thin cranium allows movement of the bolt and occlusion; *C*, The bolt is placed too deep and damages brain tissue; *D*, Brain tissue has herniated into the bolt and produced occlusion. (From Wilkinson HA: Intracranial pressure monitoring: Techniques and pitfalls. *In* Cooper PR [ed]: Head Injury, 161, © 1982, the Williams & Wilkins Co., Baltimore.)

although it can be used subdurally as well (Fig. 19–13).[90] The fiberoptic sensor is designed so that light produced in the base unit is transmitted over one fiber bundle into the sensor. This light beam strikes the mirror attached to the membrane by a solid pillar and is reflected into the two return fiber bundles. When the membrane is at a neutral position, the amount of light returning to the photo cells in the base unit is the same in each return fiber bundle. When the membrane moves in response to pressure on the outside surface, the mirror reflects more light into one return fiber bundle than the other. This is interpreted by the base unit, and air is pumped into the sensor chamber through the air inlet tube until the pressure inside the sensor returns the membrane to the neutral position, and the light returning to the base unit is again equal in both fiber bundles. This pressure in the sensor chamber is interpreted as the ICP and displayed. The pressure transducer, pump, light source, and photo-sensitive cells are all contained within the base unit (Fig. 19–14).

The sensor is designed to minimize zero-drift and recalibration problems, and it produces a stable and reliable pressure waveform during clinical use.[90] Proper placement is illustrated in Figure 19–15. The sensor has no fluid couple; therefore, CSF withdrawal, drug injection, and pressure/volume determinations are not possible. When the sensor is used in the epidural space, the infection rate is less than that resulting from subdural techniques.

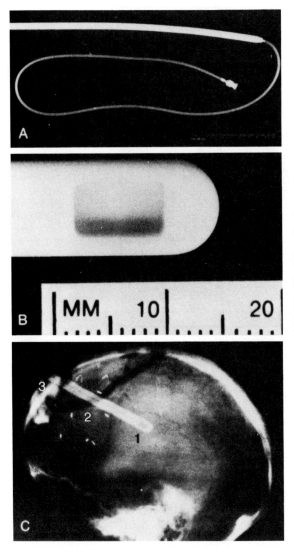

Figure 19–11. The cup catheter (*A*) is ribbon-shaped, made of rubber, and has a cup formed in its end (*B*). It is designed as a surface-monitoring device to be placed so that the open cup rests on the brain surface (*C*). This device is also fluid-coupled and must be flushed periodically. Point 1 is the end of the catheter on intact brain. Point 2 is the device penetrating the dura. Point 3 is the skin exit site. (From Wilkinson HA: Intracranial pressure monitoring: Techniques and pitfalls. *In* Cooper PR [ed]. Head Injury, 215, © 1987, the Williams & Wilkins Co., Baltimore.)

The sensor is placed under the inner table of the skull through a burr hole with the dura resting against the underside of the sensor. The sensor itself is very delicate, nondisposable, and expensive. The sensor only functions when connected to the Ladd ICP Monitor. This system can only be used for ICP monitoring and only on one patient at a time, leading to a relatively high cost per patient.[90] This device has also been used in infants with open fontanelles for noninvasive measurement of ICP.[91]

Pneumatic Epidural Monitor

The Ladd-Steritek ICP monitoring system is a new approach to the epidural transducer concept. This device utilizes a disposable pneumatic sensor, which is placed the same way as the fiberoptic sensor (Fig. 19–15).

679

INTRACRANIAL PRESSURE

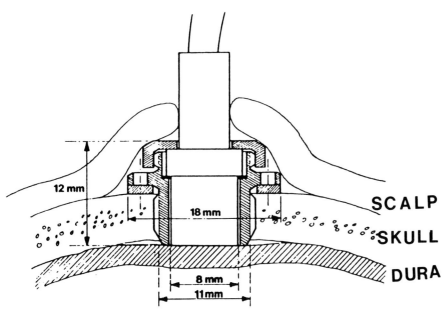

Figure 19–12. A schematic diagram of the epidural transducer. The clear layer overlapping the top edge of the device is scalp. The transducer is threaded into a burr hole in the skull, and the transducer surface is directly adherent to the dura. (From Koster WG, Kuypers MH: Intracranial pressure and its epidural measurement. Med Prog Technol 1980; 7:21–27. With permission.)

The Ladd-Steritek base unit (containing an air pump, transducer, and microprocessor) provides a constant flow of air at 40 cc/minute into the sensor chamber through the air inlet tube (Figs. 19–16 and 19–17). The metal disk membrane occludes the air exhaust port when acted upon by pressure outside the sensor. The pressure inside the chamber is measured constantly by the transducer. Air is pumped into the chamber until the pressure is sufficient to lift the membrane and open the exhaust port again. This pressure is the ICP. Advantages of the Ladd-Steritek are disposability, lower cost, and less fragile sensors. However, it is a dedicated monitor that can be used on only one patient at a time and has no other uses.

All the epidural devices presented here eliminate the need for fluid couples and the inherent problems of fluid systems; e.g., leakage and sterility.

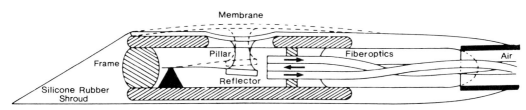

Figure 19–13. Schematic diagram of Ladd fiberoptic ICP monitor sensor. The top layer is a flexible membrane attached to a reflector mirror. There are three fiber bundles and one pneumatic tube connected to the sensor. The membrane surface is placed against the dura under the skull (see text). (From Levin AB: The use of a fiberoptic intracranial pressure monitor in clinical practice. Neurosurgery 1977; 1:266–271. With permission.)

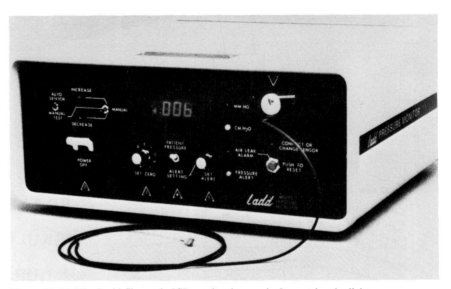

Figure 19–14. The Ladd fiberoptic ICP monitor base unit. It contains the light source, pneumatic pump, transducer, and electronics. This unit can be used for only one purpose and on only one patient at a time. (From Ladd Research Industries, Burlington, VT. With permission.)

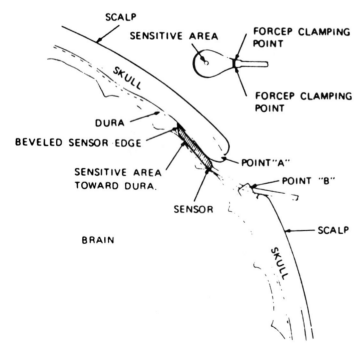

Figure 19–15. The placement of the Ladd fiberoptic sensor. The membrane surface is placed against the dura through a burr hole in the skull. The beveled edge of the sensor aids insertion. The sensor should rest securely between the dura and the inner table of the skull. The scalp may be placed at a distant site from the burr hole. (From Levin AB: The use of a fiberoptic intracranial pressure monitor in clinical practice. Neurosurgery 1977; 1:266–271. With permission.)

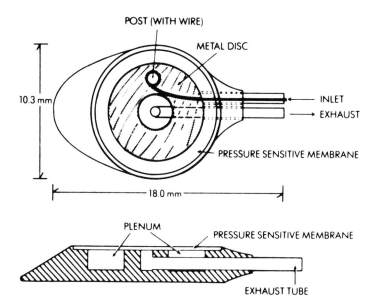

Figure 19–16. The disposable sensor for the new Ladd-Steritek ICP monitoring system. The pressure-sensitive membrane is a thin metal disk that can occlude the exhaust gas port. Gas enters the sensor through the inlet port at 40 cc/minute. (From Ladd Research Industries, Burlington, VT. With permission.)

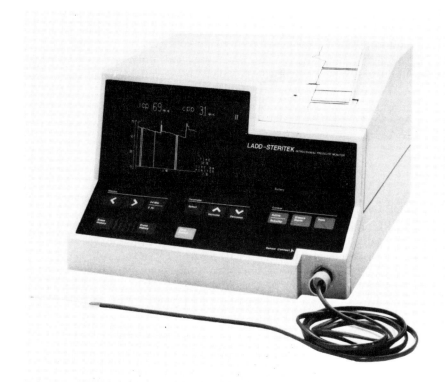

Figure 19–17. The microprocessor-based Ladd-Steritek ICP monitor base unit. The unit houses the microprocessor, transducer, and pneumatic pump. This device can be used for only one purpose on only one patient at a time. (From Ladd Research Industries, Burlington, VT. With permission.)

They are, however, more expensive and more difficult to place and are dedicated instruments with only one use.

Therapy of Increased ICP

The therapy of increased ICP is based on the contents of the intracranial cavity. Of the various structures and substances contained in the cranial vault, only the blood and CSF volumes can be readily affected by common therapeutic modalities.

Therefore, a decrease in ICP can be achieved by (1) decreasing the volume of CSF through ventriculostomy drainage; (2) decreasing intracranial blood volume through hyperventilation, administering barbiturate therapy, preventing hypoxia, improving venous drainage (head-up position), avoiding jugular venous compression, maintaining normal CPP by avoiding hypotension, and avoiding cerebral vasodilator drugs; (3) decreasing cerebral edema and extracellular fluid by the use of diuretics and avoidance of fluid overload; and (4) surgically removing any existing intracranial mass such as a hematoma or tumor.[25, 77]

The need to measure ICP in order to guide therapy in pathologic conditions and the significance of elevated ICP in those circumstances stem from a sound knowledge base of the physiology of the cerebral circulation and the dynamics of the CSF. All the clinical monitoring techniques available today require surgical procedures for placement. Of the various types of systems available, the older techniques of intraventricular and subarachnoid, fluid-coupled devices are still the simplest, most reliable, and most cost-effective. The choice of technique depends upon many factors, one of the most important of which is the expertise and preference of the operator.

References

1. Lassen NA, Ingvar DH: Radioisotopic assessment of regional cerebral blood flow. Prog Nucl Med 1972; 1:376–409.
2. Obrist WD, Thompson HK, Wand HS, Wilkinson WE: Regional cerebral blood flow estimated by ^{133}xenon inhalation. Stroke 1975; 6:245–256.
3. McKay RD, Sundt TM, Michenfelder JD: Internal carotid artery stump pressure and cerebral blood flow during carotid endarterectomy: Modification by halothane, enflurane and innovar. Anesthesiology 1976; 45:390–399.
4. Michenfelder JD: The cerebral circulation. *In* Prys-Roberts C (ed): The Circulation in Anesthesia. London: Blackwell Scientific, 1980; 212.
5. Halsey JH, McFarland S: Oxygen cycles and metabolic autoregulation. Stroke 1974; 5:219–225.
6. Shapiro BA, Harrison RD, Walton JR: Clinical Application of Blood Gases, 3rd Ed. Chicago: Year Book Medical, 1982; 14.
7. Guyton AC: Textbook of Medical Physiology, 7th Ed. Philadelphia: WB Saunders, 1986; 339.
8. Siesjo BK: Cerebral circulation and metabolism. J Neurosurg 1984; 60:883–908.
9. Seymour SS, Kety S, Schmidt CF: The effects of altered arterial tensions of

carbon dioxide and oxygen on cerebral blood flow and cerebral oxygen consumption of normal young men. J Clin Invest 1948; 27:484–492.

10. Turner J, Lambertsen CJ, Owen SG, et al: Effects of .08 and .8 atmospheres of inspired P_{O_2} upon cerebral hemodynamics at a constant alveolar P_{CO_2} of 43 mmHg. (Abstract.) Fed Proc 1967; 16:130.

11. Raichle ME, Posner JB, Plum F: Cerebral blood flow during and after hyperventilation. Arch Neurol 1970; 23:394–403.

12. Raichle ME, Stone HL: Cerebral blood flow autoregulation and graded hypercapnia. Eur Neurol 1971-72; 6:1–5.

13. Lambertsen CJ, Smyth SM, Gelfand R: H^+ and P_{CO_2} as chemical factors in respiratory and cerebral circulatory control. J Appl Physiol 1961; 16:473–484.

14. Harper AM, Bell RA: The effect of metabolic acidosis and alkalosis on the blood flow through the cerebral cortex. J Neurol Neurosurg Psychiatry 1963; 26:341–344.

15. Sokoloff L: The effect of carbon dioxide on the cerebral circulation. Anesthesiology 1960; 21:664–673.

16. Reivich M: Arterial P_{CO_2} and cerebral hemodynamics. Am J Physiol 1964; 206:25–35.

17. Lassen NA: Control of cerebral circulation in health and disease. Circ Res 1974; 34:749–760.

18. Olesen J: Contralateral focal increase of cerebral blood flow in man during arm work. Brain 1971; 94:635–646.

19. Lassen NA, Christensen MS: Physiology of cerebral blood flow. Br J Anaesth 1976; 48:719–734.

20. Wolfgang K, Wahl M: Local chemical and neurogenic regulation of cerebral vascular resistance. Physiol Rev 1978; 58:656–689.

21. Bevegard BS, Shepherd JT: Regulation of the circulation during exercise in man. Physiol Rev 1967; 47:178–213.

22. Michenfelder JD, Gronert GA, Rehder K: Neuroanesthesia. Anesthesiology 1969; 30:65–100.

23. Cutler RWP, Page L, Galicich J, Watters JV: Formation and absorption of cerebrospinal fluid in man. Brain 1968; 91:707–720.

24. Cserr HF: Physiology of the choroid plexus. Physiol Rev 1971; 51:273–311.

25. Jennett B, Teasdale G: Management of Head Injuries. Philadelphia: FA Davis, 1981.

26. Leech P, Miller JD: Intracranial volume-pressure relationships during experimental brain compression in primates. Pressure responses to changes in ventricular volume. J Neurol Neurosurg Psychiatr 1974; 37:1093–1098.

27. Marmarou A, Tabaddor K: Intracranial pressure: Physiology and pathophysiology. *In* Cooper PR (ed): Head Injury. Baltimore: Williams & Wilkins, 1982; 115–127.

28. Venes JL, Shaywitz BA, Spender DD: Management of severe cerebral edema in the metabolic encephalopathy of Reye-Johnson syndrome. J Neurosurg 1978; 48:903–915.

29. Bedford RF, Morris L, Jane JA: Intracranial hypertension during surgery for supratentorial tumor: Correlation with preoperative computed tomography scans. Anesth Analg 1982; 61:430–433.

30. Risberg J, Lundberg N, Ingvar DH: Regional cerebral blood volume during acute transient rises of the intracranial pressure (plateau waves). J Neurosurg 1969; 31:303–310.

31. McDowall DG: The effects of clinical concentrations of halothane on the blood flow and oxygen uptake of the cerebral cortex. Br J Anaesth 1967; 39:186–196.

32. Marx GF, Andrews IC, Orkin JR: Cerebrospinal fluid pressures during halothane anaesthesia. Can Anaesth Soc J 1962; 9:239–245.

33. Alexander SC, Wollman H, Cohen PJ, et al: Cerebrovascular response to Pa_{CO_2} during halothane anesthesia in man. J Appl Physiol 1964; 19:561–565.

34. Manohar M, Parks CM: Porcine brain and myocardial perfusion during enflurane anesthesia without and with nitrous oxide. J Cardiovasc Pharmacol 1984; 6:1092–1101.

35. Artru AA: Relationship between cerebral blood volume and CSF pressure during anesthesia with halothane or enflurane in dogs. Anesthesiology 1983; 58:533–539.

36. Miletich DJ, Ivankovich AD, Albrecht RF, et al: Absence of autoregulation of cerebral blood flow during halothane and enflurane anesthesia. Anesth Analg 1976; 55:100–109.

37. Cucchiara RF, Theye RA, Michenfelder JD: The effects of isoflurane on canine cerebral metabolism and blood flow. Anesthesiology 1974; 40:571–574.

38. Artru AA: Relationship between cerebral blood volume and CSF pressure during anesthesia with isoflurane or fentanyl in dogs. Anesthesiology 1984; 60:575–579.

39. Eger EI: Isoflurane: A review. Anesthesiology 1981; 55:559–576.

40. Henriksen HT, Jorgensen PB: The effect of nitrous oxide on intracranial pressure in patients with intracranial disorders. Br J Anaesth 1973; 45:486–492.

41. Laitinen LV, Johansson GG, Tarkkanen L: The effect of nitrous oxide on pulsatile cerebral impedance and cerebral blood flow. Br J Anaesth 1967; 39:781–785.

42. Sokoloff L: The action of drugs on the cerebral circulation. Pharmacol Rev 1959; 11:1–85.

43. Smith AL, Wollman H: Cerebral blood flow and metabolism: Effects of anesthetic drugs and techniques. Anesthesiology 1972; 36:378–400.

44. Pierce ED, Lambertsen CJ, Deutsch S, et al: Cerebral circulation and metabolism during thiopental anesthesia and hyperventilation in man. J Clin Invest 1962; 41:1664–1671.

45. Shapiro HM, Galindo A, Wyte SR, Harris AB: Rapid intraoperative reduction of intracranial pressure with thiopentone. Br J Anaesth 1973; 45:1057–1062.

46. Jobes DR, Kennell E, Bitner R, et al: Effects of morphine–nitrous oxide anesthesia on cerebral autoregulation. Anesthesiology 1975; 42:30–34.

47. Jobes DR, Kennell EM, Bush GL, et al: Cerebral blood flow and metabolism during morphine–nitrous oxide anesthesia in man. Anesthesiology 1977; 47:16–18.

48. Keats AS, Mithoefer JC: The mechanism of increased intracranial pressure induced by morphine. N Engl J Med 1955; 30:1110–1113.

49. Moss E, Powell D, Gibson RM, McDowall DG: Effects of fentanyl on intracranial pressure and cerebral perfusion pressure during hypocapnia. Br J Anaesth 1978; 59:779–784.

50. Carlsson C, Smith DS, Keykhah MM, et al: The effects of high-dose fentanyl on cerebral circulation and metabolism in rats. Anesthesiology 1985; 57:375–380.

51. Gibbs JM: The effect of intravenous ketamine on cerebrospinal fluid pressure. Br J Anaesth 1971; 44:1298–1302.

52. Shapiro HM, Wyte SR, Harris AB: Ketamine anaesthesia in patients with intracranial pathology. Br J Anaesth 1972; 44:1200–1204.

53. Sari A, Okuda Y, Takeshita H: The effect of ketamine on cerebrospinal fluid pressure. Anesth Analg 1972; 51:560–565.

54. Carlsson C, Chapman AG: The effect of diazepam on the cerebral metabolic state in rats and its interaction with nitrous oxide. Anesthesiology 1981; 54:488–495.

55. Foster A, Juge O, Morel D: Effects of midazolam on cerebral blood flow in human volunteers. Anesthesiology 1982; 56:453–455.

56. Rockoff MA, Naughton KVH, Shapiro HM, et al: Cerebral circulatory and metabolic responses to intravenously administered lorazepam. Anesthesiology 1980; 53:215–218.
57. Milde LN, Milde JH, Michenfelder JD: Cerebral functional, metabolic, and hemodynamic effects of etomidate in dogs. Anesthesiology 1985; 63:371–377.
58. Varma YS, Sharma PL, Minocha KB: Comparative evaluation of cerebral and hepatic blood flow under d-tubocurarine and pancuronium in dogs. Indian J Med Res 1977; 66:317–322.
59. Belik J, Wagerle LC, Delivoria-Papadopoulos M: Cerebral blood flow and metabolism following pancuronium bromide in newborn lambs. Pediatr Res 1984; 18:1305–1308.
60. Griffin JP, Hartung J, Cottrell JE, et al: Effect of vecuronium on intracranial pressure, mean arterial pressure and heart rate in cats. Br J Anaesth 1986; 58:441–443.
61. Rosa G, Sanfilippo M, Vilardi M, et al: Effects of vecuronium bromide on intracranial pressure and cerebral perfusion pressure. Br J Anaesth 1986; 58:437–440.
62. Minton MD, Stirt JA, Bedford RF, Haworth C: Intracranial pressure after atracurium in neurosurgical patients. Anesth Analg 1985; 64:1113–1116.
63. Lanier WL, Milde JH, Michenfelder JD: The cerebral effects of pancuronium and atracurium in halothane-anesthetized dogs. Anesthesiology 1985; 63:589–597.
64. Lanier WL, Milde JM, Michenfelder JD: Cerebral stimulation following succinylcholine in dogs. Anesthesiology 1986; 64:551–559.
65. Minton MD, Grosslight K, Stirt JA, Bedford RF: Increases in intracranial pressure from succinylcholine: Prevention by prior nondepolarizing blockade. Anesthesiology 1986; 65:165–169.
66. Stirt JA, Grosslight KR, Bedford RF, Vollmer D: "Defasciculation" with metocurine prevents succinylcholine-induced increases in intracranial pressure. Anesthesiology 1987; 67:50–53.
67. Cottrell JE, Robustelli A, Post K, Turndorf H: Furosemide- and mannitol-induced changes in intracranial pressure and serum osmolality and electrolytes. Anesthesiology 1977; 47:28–30.
68. Leech P, Miller JD: Intracranial volume-pressure relationships during experimental brain compression in primates. J Neurol Neurosurg Psychiat 1974; 37:1105–1111.
69. Johnston IH, Harper AM: The effect of mannitol on cerebral blood flow: An experimental study. J Neurosurg 1973; 38:461–471.
70. Turner JM, Powell D, Gibson RM, McDowall DG: Intracranial pressure changes in neurosurgical patients during hypotension induced with sodium nitroprusside or trimetaphan. Br J Anaesth 1977; 49:419–424.
71. James DJ, Bedford RF: Hydralazine for controlled hypotension during neurosurgical operations. Anesth Analg 1982; 61:1016–1019.
72. Ghani GA, Sung YF, Weinstein MS, et al: Effects of intravenous nitroglycerin on the intracranial pressure and volume pressure response. J Neurosurg 1983; 58:562–565.
73. Fahmy NR, Soter NA: Effects of trimethaphan on arterial blood histamine and systemic hemodynamics in humans. Anesthesiology 1985; 62:562–566.
74. Berntman L, Carlsson C, Siesjo BK: Influence of propranolol on cerebral metabolism and blood flow in the rat brain. Brain Res 1978; 151:220–224.
75. Aken HV, Puchstein C, Schweppe ML, Heinecke A: Effect of labetalol on intracranial pressure in dogs with and without intrancranial hypertension. Acta Anaesthiol Scand 1982; 26:615–619.

76. Benfield P, Sorkin EM: Esmolol. A preliminary review of pharmacodynamic and pharmacokinetic properties, and therapeutic efficacy. Drugs 1987; 33:392–412.

77. Marshall LF, Bowers SA: Medical management of intracranial pressure. *In* Cooper PR (ed): Head Injury. Baltimore: Williams & Wilkins, 1982; 129–146.

78. Strandgaard S: Autoregulation of cerebral blood flow in hypertensive patients. Circulation 1975; 53:720–727.

79. Wilkinson HA: Intracranial pressure monitoring: Techniques and pitfalls. *In* Cooper PR (ed): Head Injury. Baltimore: Williams & Wilkins, 1982; 147–184.

80. Mendelow AD, Rowan JO, Murray L, Kerr AE: A clinical comparison of subdural screw pressure measurements with ventricular pressure. J Neurosurg 1983; 58:45–50.

81. Jorgensen PB, Riishede J: Comparative clinical studies of epidural and ventricular pressure. *In* Brock M, Dietz H (eds): Intracranial Pressure: Experimental and Clinical Aspects. Berlin: Springer-Verlag, 1972; 41–45.

82. Friedman WA, Vries JK: Percutaneous tunnel ventriculostomy. J Neurosurg 1980; 53:662–665.

83. Narayan RK, Kishore PR, Becker DP, et al: Intracranial pressure: To monitor or not to monitor? J Neurosurg 1982; 56:650–659.

84. Langfitt TW: Clinical methods for monitoring intracranial pressure and measuring cerebral blood flow. Clin Neurosurg 1976; 23:302–320.

85. Rosner MJ, Becker DP: ICP monitoring: Complications and associated factors. Clin Neurosurg 1976; 23:494–519.

86. Vries JK, Becker DP, Young HF: A subarachnoid screw for monitoring intracranial pressure. J Neurosurg 1973; 39:416–419.

87. Wilkinson HA: The intracranial pressure-monitoring cup catheter: Technical note. Neurosurgery 1977; 1:139–141.

88. Koster WG, Kuypers MH: Intracranial pressure and its epidural measurement. Med Prog Technol 1980; 7:21–27.

89. Kleiber M: Physical instruments for the biologist. Rev Scient Instruments 1945; 16:79–81.

90. Levin AB: The use of a fiberoptic intracranial pressure monitor in clinical practice. Neurosurgery 1977; 1:266–271.

91. Hill A, Volpe JJ: Measurement of intracranial pressure using the Ladd intracranial pressure monitor. J Pediatr 1981; 98:974–976.

chapter twenty

Electro-
encephalography

■ WARREN J. LEVY, M.D.

In 1987, intraoperative electroencephalography reached a milestone—50 years had passed since the initial report[1] of the effects of various drugs on the electroencephalogram (EEG). Although the role of most monitoring techniques becomes well defined after such a time span, this has not been the case for intraoperative electroencephalography. The history of EEG monitoring can easily be divided into two periods, the early analog period, when strip-chart display of the raw signal was used, and the current, processed period, when a number of processing techniques have been used in order to facilitate the use of electroencephalography as a monitor. Although this is an accurate description, historically speaking, it may give the impression that analog EEG is passé, that anesthesiologists do not need to understand or interpret it, and that the output of the next EEG processing system will provide the definitive answer to all problems of anesthetic depth, brain perfusion, and neurologic well-being. Nothing could be less accurate, for no EEG processor is better than the analog signal it receives, and no processed EEG contains information not in the original signal. Understanding the origin of the EEG is mandatory in order to record the signal, categorize its character, and interpret it for intraoperative monitoring.

ORIGINS OF THE EEG

It is generally accepted that the electrical activity ultimately recorded as the EEG originates spontaneously in the most superficial layers of the cerebral cortex.[2] In these layers, the pyramidal cells have many dendrites oriented perpendicular to the surface, and the spread of the postsynaptic potentials along these structures produces electric fields, called dipoles, which summate over adjacent neurons because of their common orientation. Ionic flow secondary to excitatory stimuli causes negativity in the extracellular space around the dendrite compared with the area near the cell body. This electrical summation process is quite complex, since the polarity, timing, and depth of various postsynaptic potentials differ. In addition, there are dendrites that are not perpendicularly oriented to the surface, and these also generate postsynaptic potentials and correspondingly oriented dipoles.

Studies of the time course of EEG activity have demonstrated that cortical action potentials do not play a major direct role in the generation of the EEG. Obviously, if there were no action potentials at all, there would be no synaptic transmission and thus no postsynaptic potentials to summate into the EEG. Many of the axons whose terminal synapses are responsible for cortical postsynaptic potentials originate in subcortical tissues. An alteration in the function of these subcortical neurons changes the pattern of postsynaptic activity and thus influences the EEG. However, not all subcortical structures have cortical projections, and many studies of intracerebral electrical activity have demonstrated the absence of associations of EEG with underlying subcortical structures. For this reason, it is common to utilize EEG monitoring as if the EEG were derived purely from cortical activity.

Cortical EEG

The EEG recorded at the cortical surface differs in many ways from that recorded on the scalp.[3] These differences arise during the passage of the electrical activity through the skull and soft tissue. The skull is fairly resistant to the transmission of electrical signals and considerably reduces their amplitude. Abrupt changes in skull thickness, such as after craniectomy, cause distortion or asymmetry of the EEG, as compared with recordings made over contralateral, intact structures. In most cases, however, EEG monitoring is performed over areas of relatively uniform bone density, and transmission through the skull does not excessively distort EEG activity. The most important change in electrical activity that occurs during the transmission process is that averaging of nearby dipoles into a more uniform electrical gradient. Thus, even though areas of cortex only 1–2 mm apart can show different activity (recorded on the surface of the cortex), the EEG, recorded from the scalp, only reflects a composite of nearby activity.

The process by which these signals are averaged strongly influences the distance at which a signal may be recorded, particularly in the presence of other activity originating at sites closer to the recording electrode. Studies using cortical evoked potentials[4] suggest that the amplitude of the recording decreases dramatically when the recording electrode is more than a few centimeters from the site of the activity. Thus, even though EEG activity can be recorded at a greatly reduced amplitude many centimeters away from its origin, it is likely to be masked by the presence of higher-amplitude activity generated closer to the recording electrode.

RECORDING OF THE EEG

The limited dispersion of the EEG signal has created several characteristics of the EEG recording process. First, there is the need to record from many electrodes (8–16 or more) simultaneously in order to examine different areas of the brain. Also, there is the need for careful measurement of electrode positions in order to place the electrodes in reproducible relationships to the underlying cortical structures. Third, consistent and logical electrode montages must be used, since different combinations of electrodes may make the recording appear different, even though the underlying electrical activity is unchanged.

Technical Considerations

Although these issues cover many of the technical considerations of EEG monitoring, issues of artifact identification and elimination and the basic electronics of biologic amplifiers must be considered as well. In fact, the technology of EEG recording is probably the single factor most responsible for the success (or failure) of efforts to monitor the EEG during anesthesia and surgery.

In order to appreciate the technical problems of recording the intraoperative EEG, it is only necessary to consider the characteristics of this signal in comparison with other signals recorded from the patient. The EEG is a signal of a few microvolts in amplitude (perhaps as high as 100 μv) with an irregular pattern of oscillation a few times per second (1–30 Hz). Muscle artifact, generated by frontalis or extraocular muscles, can be several hundred microvolts in amplitude, and the normal electrocardiogram (ECG), at 2–4 mV, is nearly one thousand times the amplitude of the desynchronized EEG recorded during some normal mental states. Finally, electrical equipment, including the ubiquitous electrocautery, can create electrical gradients of many volts across the patient. Obviously, if the EEG is to be extracted from all this extraneous electrical noise, considerable attention to detail is required.

Electrodes

The recording electrode is the single most important part of the recording system, the easiest to misuse, and the part that yields the greatest improvement in performance for the expenditure of effort. The scalp is a difficult location from which to record electrical activity, with hair impeding mechanical contact, oil and cornified skin impeding electrical contact, and a dense subcutaneous plexus of blood vessels that bleed profusely if punctured by an intradermal electrode. The type of electrode selected depends, in large measure, on which characteristics are compromised in order to optimize others.

Traditionally, anesthesiologists have opted for needle electrodes, perhaps because their biggest disadvantage, patient discomfort, was eliminated by the administration of anesthesia. Additionally, these electrodes can be applied much more quickly than can metal and collodion systems, and they can be placed within a sterile field if necessary. Unfortunately, the electrical characteristics of needle electrodes are suboptimal, and their small surface area results in relatively high electrode impedances, even when properly placed. The electrodes are mechanically unstable, coming out as easily as they are inserted; and sterile technique (including needle sterilization between patients) is mandatory. Perhaps most important, when EEG monitoring is used to ensure cerebral perfusion during cerebrovascular procedures, the monitoring should begin before the induction of anesthesia, necessitating the discomfort of multiple needle insertions in an awake patient. Placement within a sterile field is probably the only situation in which needle electrodes are truly preferable.

Metal surface electrodes come in many shapes, sizes, and compositions, including gold, silver, and tin. Silver electrodes must be coated with silver chloride in order to reduce their electrode impedance, but this can be accomplished easily by soaking them in household bleach. Although there are subtle differences among the metals, these factors do not appear to be significant for routine intraoperative monitoring. Nor does the choice of conductive agent, although the duration of some procedures allows drying of the conductive paste or jelly. This is undesirable, since it increases the electrode impedance, often in an erratic fashion. Taping over the electrode with plastic tape is often performed in order to reduce the drying and thus eliminate the need to refresh the conductive agent intraoperatively.

Another approach to electrode selection (and placement) is a cap, not unlike a bathing cap, that has electrodes fastened to it (Electrocap [Electrocap International, Inc., Dallas TX]). Such a system greatly simplifies proper placement of electrodes; however, for best results, a chin or chest strap is suggested in order to maintain the position of the cap, and this strap can interfere with access to the surgical field or airway.[5]

Prepackaged adhesive EEG electrodes are also available, although these are rarely recommended by EEG technologists. In general, these electrodes cannot be placed over the scalp in close proximity to neural tissue at risk for hypoperfusion, although an occasional balding patient does permit correct placement. Their use is recommended largely by manufacturers who are responding to the desires of individuals who value simplicity over precision or who are concerned only with global EEG effects that can be assessed from frontal electrodes. For those who wish to perform multichannel recordings in hirsute individuals, prepackaged adhesive electrodes are not a satisfactory option.

The impedance, the interface between the electrode and the subject's skin, must be minimized for good EEG recordings. Recommended imped-

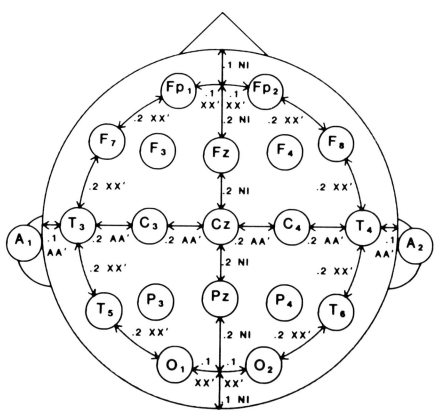

Figure 20–1. This schematic describes the measurements necessary to identify the 21 scalp electrodes of the International 10–20 system of electrode placement. Measurements are either 10% (0.1) or 20% (0.2) of a circumferential measurement. (NI = the distance from the nasion to the inion, measured over the vertex of the head.) The preauricular distance (AA′) is measured from tragus to tragus over the vertex.

ances are less than 3000–5000 Ω. Impedance reduction is achieved by meticulous skin preparation and careful electrode application.

Standard Electrode Positions

The positioning of electrodes is another area in which anesthesiologists often attempt to achieve shortcuts, usually by "eyeballing" positions or placing electrodes at symmetric but ill-defined locations. There are several standard systems for determining electrode placement, the International 10–20 system[6] being one of the most commonly used.

International 10–20 System. In the 10–20 system, electrode positions are defined in relation to cranial dimensions (Fig. 20–1), and the electrodes are positioned in reproducible relationships with cortical structures. Occasionally, additional nonstandard electrode positions are desirable, although these are more frequently used to optimize the amplitude of evoked potentials rather than to record spontaneous EEG. The advantages of anatomically reproducible electrode positions are obvious, and they include both the abil-

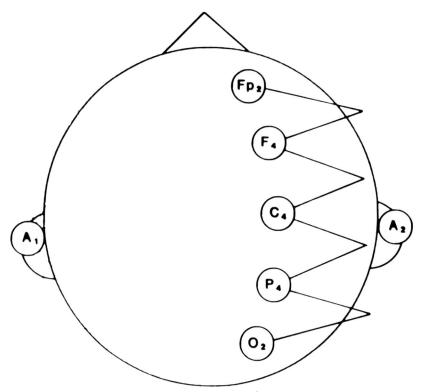

Figure 20–2. A bipolar montage is created by recording from pairs of electrodes as shown. Only the ground electrode (A_2) is common to all channels.

ity to generalize and discuss the findings of one patient relative to another and the ability to correlate the EEG findings and the underlying neuropathology.

The International 10–20 system comprises 21 surface electrodes that can be connected in many thousands of different ways. Although most of these possibilities have no logical rationale, three patterns of electrode connections are commonly used that influence the appearance of the EEG. The bipolar montage is created by recording multiple channels of EEG, each of which is derived from two active electrodes placed at any of the defined electrode positions (Fig. 20–2). A third electrode is required as an electrical ground, and the ipsilateral ear is often used. Most commonly, these electrode pairs are recorded from chains of electrodes (F_{P1}–F_3, F_3–C_3, C_3–P_3, and so on) in either parasagittal or coronal positions. Occasionally, bilateral symmetric positions are used (e.g., F_{P1}–F_{P2}, F_3–F_4), but rarely bilateral asymmetric positions.

Bipolar Montages. Bipolar chains have several characteristics of importance. When the EEG is recorded in a bipolar chain, the focus of unusual activity is often recognized by the increase in amplitude of the activity as the recording pairs approach the site, together with a change in the polarity of the activity as seen by channels on opposite sides of the focus. Although this is quite valuable for the encephalographer trying to identify a seizure

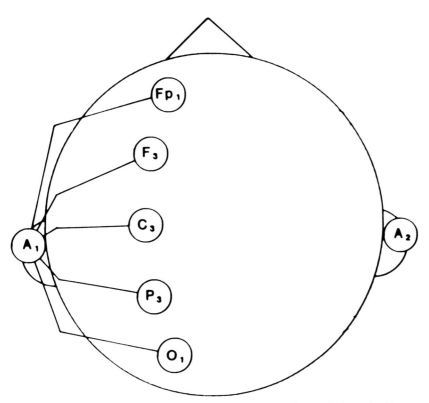

Figure 20–3. A common reference montage is created by recording each channel with one electrode in common. In this example, each of the channels has A_1, the left ear, as one of the two active electrodes. A_2, the ground electrode, is also common to all channels.

focus, it is of little value to the anesthesiologist using processed EEG analysis techniques, because none of the techniques currently in use provides information about wave polarity or phase. A more important characteristic is the tendency for bipolar recordings to emphasize focal effects while minimizing global ones.[7] Thus, with both electrodes over an area of hypoxic slowing, the bipolar recording shows a prominent change, a highly desirable characteristic for a monitor of intraoperative ischemia. Finally, the bipolar recording is physically robust, with only one electrode (the ground electrode) common to all channels. Thus, the loss of electrical contact at any other single electrode does not preclude EEG recording, although this can happen with referential montages.

Referential Montages. Referential montages differ from bipolar montages by the existence of a reference electrode that is used in the recording of all channels of the EEG (or at least all ipsilateral channels) (Fig. 20–3). Normally, one attempts to place the common reference electrode in an area of little EEG activity, thus allowing the electrical activity directly under the other recording electrode to predominate. (This has led to the somewhat erroneous term "unipolar recording.") The ipsilateral ear is commonly used. Occasionally, a quiescent site cannot be found, and an average reference electrode montage may be created by electrically averaging several electrodes in order to provide a new and more stable reference.

Recording Problems

Several problems are common to both common and average reference electrode montages. First, activity occurring near the reference electrode appears on all channels. Thus, when it is used to monitor for ischemia, activity at the reference electrode can give the appearance of adequate perfusion when areas of ischemia are present. Also, artifact derived from the reference electrode can obliterate the entire EEG recording, something that could not occur with a bipolar montage. Even worse, with an average reference electrode, artifact on any one of many channels is added into all channels of the recording, making high-quality recordings more difficult to obtain in an electrically noisy environment such as the operating room.

If the details of electrode positioning, application, and interconnection appear imposing, several approaches can be used to simplify the task, including employing the assistance of a qualified electrophysiologist technician. Although few anesthesia services can justify a full-time technician, it is often possible to utilize one of the hospital technicians to apply electrodes preoperatively, even the night before surgery, which then need only be checked or refilled with conductive jelly. Alternatively, anesthesia personnel can be trained in recording techniques in the neurology clinic by the EEG technologists. The ready availability of a reasonable patient schedule allows the rapid assimilation of the necessary experience. Such an experience does not provide all the skills of an electrophysiologist, but it greatly improves the ease and quality of patient preparation for intraoperative EEG monitoring.

In order to use a commercial EEG monitoring system, one need not comprehend in detail the electronics that it comprises. However, there is little doubt that a general overview of such matters not only satisfies intellectual curiosity but also assists in understanding why certain problems occur and how best to rectify them. For example, it is not intuitively obvious how it is possible to record EEG (at an amplitude of 10–100 μV) from a patient whose ECG has an amplitude of many millivolts and who is exposed to other forms of electrical noise (especially 60 Hz) whose amplitude may be measured in volts. The most important step in this process occurs with equipment in the very earliest stage of amplification of the signal—the differential amplifier.

Differential Amplifiers

Although it is common to speak of a channel of EEG activity as if recorded from a pair of electrodes (e.g., E_1 and E_2), the actual amplification process requires three electrodes. The third electrode, the ground (G), is critical to the differential amplification of the desired signal and the rejection of artifact. The differential amplifier does not amplify a single voltage but actually amplifies only the difference in voltage between two pairs of electrodes. The pairs of electrodes are created by each single active electrode (E_1 and E_2) and the ground (G). Thus, the amplifier actually amplifies the voltage between E_1 and G minus the voltage between E_2 and G. The result is the voltage between E_1 and E_2, which is desired; even more important, any signal common to both E_1-G and E_2-G gets subtracted out (rejected) and not amplified. This process, called common mode rejection, may reduce the amplitude of a common signal like 60-Hz artifact a millionfold (120 db or 99.9999% rejection), provided that the amplifiers are working optimally; this requires that the common signal be of equal amplitude on each differential channel E_1-G and E_2-G.

One of the major factors that causes common mode signal to appear to be of differing amplitude on each channel of the amplifier is a difference in the electrode characteristics, particularly unequal electrode impedances at E_1 and E_2. The amplification process is such that if the impedance at E_1 is much higher than it is at E_2, a common signal (like 60-Hz noise) actually appears to be larger in E_1-G than in E_2-G. Since the common signal is not equal, not all of it is removed, and some common signal (noise) appears as real, amplified signal (EEG).

A similar phenomenon can be responsible for the appearance of ECG signal on the EEG, even though the electrode impedances are not unbalanced or faulty. By placing a ground electrode at a distant site (e.g., the shoulder), the amplitude of ECG signal on each side of the differential amplifier is greatly increased. In addition, volume conduction effects (which occur because of the transmission of a signal from a large volume, the chest, to a smaller one, the head) can change the amplitude of the ECG in the half-channels, so that they do not completely cancel and ECG appears in the EEG. For this reason, it is usually undesirable to put the EEG ground electrode on the torso.

Filters

Another important aspect of EEG monitoring involves the use of filters and the resultant potential for distortion of the EEG. Almost all EEG recording systems are equipped with filters that reduce both high-frequency and low-frequency activity. Filters are described by the frequency at which they reduce the amplitude by 70% (the 3-db point) and the rate at which they reduce activity outside of the band of interest, typically halving the voltage for a doubling of the frequency. One of the frequent uses of high-frequency filters is to reduce 60-Hz artifact. However, a 30-Hz filter only reduces 60-Hz artifact by 50%, and a lower-frequency filter reduces the amplitude of the high-frequency EEG activity often associated with light anesthesia or barbiturates.

At the low-frequency end of the EEG, similar problems exist. Low-frequency filters at 3 Hz are capable of eliminating baseline artifact in the frequency range below 0.5 Hz, but they do so at the expense of low-frequency delta activity (1.5-Hz components are 50% below 3-Hz waves of equal amplitude and 65% below 6-Hz theta activity of equal amplitude, which would be essentially unfiltered). Lower-frequency filters, e.g., 1 Hz, do far less damage to the EEG waveform but are much less effective at reducing low-frequency artifact.

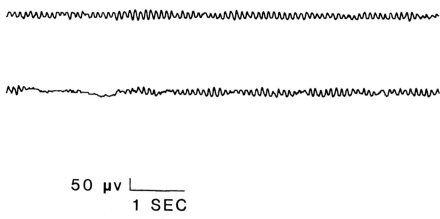

50 µV └─────

1 SEC

Figure 20–4. This electroencephalogram (EEG) exemplifies the rhythm and amplitude patterns characteristic of the alpha rhythm. The frequency is about 10 Hz with an amplitude of 30–40 µV (peak to peak).

CONVENTIONAL MULTICHANNEL EEG

Having amplified and filtered the electrical activity from the scalp, conventional EEG techniques do no further processing. They simply display the signal as a graph of amplitude (i.e., voltage) over time. Depending on the activity being recorded, full-scale deflection of the pen is usually 100–500 µV, and the paper speed is 15–60 mm/second. This process results in patterns of waves that can be associated with specific physiologic states, drug effects, or pathologic conditions.

EEG Patterns

The best known of these patterns is the alpha rhythm (Fig. 20–4), a pattern of activity containing waves of 8–12 Hz, predominating posteriorly, and masked by mental activity, particularly eye opening and attention to stimuli.[8] For any given individual, the frequency of alpha activity is quite stable, although slowing can occur with age.[9] Occasionally, this slowing is of such a degree that the peak of the alpha rhythm falls outside of the normal alpha band (8–12 Hz), and a slow alpha or 7–8-Hz variant alpha is seen.

Not all patients demonstrate baseline alpha rhythms. Various studies estimate the incidence of nonalpha activity to be between 15 and 35%. About half of these nonalpha patterns are low-voltage mixed patterns, with the remainder divided among pure beta (above 12 Hz), theta (4–8 Hz), and mixed and irregular variants. Pure delta activity (below 4 Hz) is not seen in healthy patients under standard recording conditions (awake with eyes closed and without psychotropic drugs).

There are other patterns of activity as well, some of which are closely associated with certain levels of mental status. For example, sleep spindles—fusiform bursts of activity at about 14 Hz—are commonly seen during

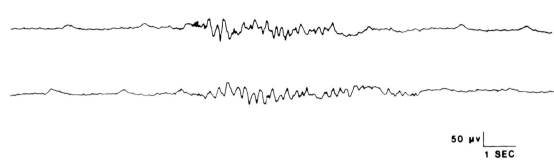

Figure 20–5. This EEG demonstrates the pattern of activity and quiescence characteristic of burst-suppression.

certain stages of natural sleep. Spike and wave activity is classically seen during seizures, at a frequency of about 3 Hz. Isolated spikes of a duration of 0.01–0.08 second can also be seen, as can slightly slower "sharp wave" activity, which is similar in shape but of slightly longer duration (0.08–0.2 second). Burst-suppression (Fig. 20–5) is another pattern of activity commonly observed by the anesthesiologist, who induces it with hypothermia or the administration of barbiturates, isoflurane, or other agents.

Intraoperative EEG Recording

The conventional multichannel strip-chart recording is the gold standard against which all other EEG systems must be compared. However, this standard was set for diagnostic not monitoring purposes, and a number of problems occur in the translocation of this technique (and the equipment) to the operating room. Despite improvements owing to the miniaturization of electronic components, a standard EEG machine is a large, cumbersome device without a home in the crowded operating room. It may not even be possible to put the device where the anesthetist can see both the EEG and the usual monitors and still attend to the administration of an anesthetic. Another disadvantage derives from the use of electrocautery, which not only obliterates the EEG but also produces wild gyrations of the pen and sprays ink over the machine and anything nearby. EEG recording at conventional rates (30 mm/second) utilizes prodigious amounts of paper (360 pages/hour), and simply finding a previous event for comparison may be a heroic task. Lastly, most intraoperative events of interest are not associated with specific, identifiable waveforms; thus, the ability to make such identifications does not add to the usefulness of the technique.

Nonetheless, the ability to examine the unprocessed analog EEG, on either a strip-chart or a video display, is most important when using processed EEG monitors. It may be necessary for EEG interpretation when burst-suppression or seizure activity occurs. Analog display may be useful for artifact identification, including the recognition of electrocardiographic contamination of the signal. Examination of the raw signal is also helpful when trying to eliminate baseline drift and movement artifact. In short, assessment of the analog EEG is a quality-control measure to ensure that the signal being processed accurately reflects cortical electrical activity.

PROCESSED EEG MONITORS

Difficulty in using the strip-chart EEG as a monitor stimulated the development of EEG processing systems for monitoring. Three distinct patterns of processing and data display emerged in the late 1960s and early 1970s: power spectrum analysis, cerebral function monitor, and aperiodic analysis. The first of these, power spectrum analysis,[10] evolved from engineering work in the 1950s and was applied to the EEG as a research tool in the 1960s.[11] Technology had not yet produced microcomputers, so the technique remained an investigational tool for many years. However, during this time, display techniques were developed and enhanced. The second analysis technique, the cerebral function monitor,[12] was developed in England in 1969 for monitoring the EEG after resuscitation, not during anesthesia. The third branch of the EEG analysis tree evolved in 1975 when Demetrescu proposed a technique, called aperiodic analysis, for quantifying the EEG.[13]

Although one may discuss the concept of a monitoring technique and its implementation separately, the two are inseparably linked for the clinician who cannot (and probably should not) develop his or her own system. Unfortunately, technologic change in this area is rapid, and critiques based on specific features may suddenly become obsolete. Accordingly, the discussion that follows tries to emphasize general concerns and theoretic aspects of EEG analysis rather than the presence of specific "front panel" features on each monitor. Since many commercial systems now contain other monitors (e.g., evoked potentials), the ultimate decision to obtain a particular instrument is clearly influenced by other factors.

THE CEREBRAL FUNCTION MONITOR AND CEREBRAL FUNCTION ANALYZING MONITOR

Although the use of power spectrum analysis predated the cerebral function monitor (CFM), the latter was the first device specifically designed and built for monitoring the EEG in the clinical setting. It was designed for the continuous monitoring of one channel of EEG between conventional EEG recordings. The unit incorporated a continuous record of electrode impedance, which functioned to identify both movement artifact and electrode malfunction. Unfortunately, the name of the device suggested that a quantity called cerebral function existed and that this device measured it. In fact, the device measured the peak voltage of a rectified, heavily filtered EEG. The filtration served to de-emphasize low-frequency activity (which tends to be higher in amplitude than high-frequency activity) and emphasize high-frequency activity. As an indicator of EEG activity in patients with decreased brain function, this is a reasonable approach. However, its appropriateness for processing the EEG during general anesthesia is questionable. Nonetheless, extensive work was done with CFM, identifying EEG changes dur-

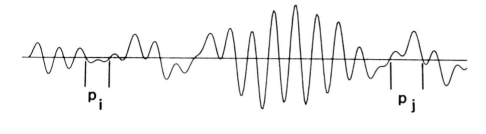

$$F = 1/P$$

Figure 20–6. Zero-crossing analysis determines the period of a wave by measuring the time that the wave is above (or below) the isoelectric line. The frequency of the wave is the inverse of the period.

ing carotid endarterectomy,[14] deliberate hypotension,[15] and cardiopulmonary bypass,[16-18] correlating changes with anesthetic agents,[19-20] and even providing control of anesthetic depth in animals.[21] Despite this success, the inability to examine the behavior of different frequencies within the EEG was a major drawback of this device.

The cerebral function analyzing monitor (CFAM) evolved from the CFM to address this need.[22] The CFAM still filters the EEG before processing, and it generates CFAM units as a logarithmic function of the root-mean-square (RMS) voltage generated by the filter. The output from the filter is further analyzed using a modified zero-crossing technique. This allows the computation of activity in individual frequency bands as a fraction of total activity. Like its predecessor, the CFAM analyzes only a single channel of the EEG, but improvements over CFM include the ability to display portions of unprocessed signal and to transmit digital data about the CFAM analysis to a computer for further analysis.

Technique of Analysis

The underlying analysis technique, zero-crossing analysis, is conceptually straightforward. A signal is analyzed, as shown in Figure 20–6, by determining the amount of time (the period) that the polarity remains the same. By definition, the frequency is the inverse of the period (i.e., frequency = 1/period), so that the frequency is easily calculated. The RMS amplitude is easily computed by electronic means, and the amplitude can then be summed (integrated) into the frequency band indicated by the frequency computation for the wave.

The process of summing the EEG waves into frequency bands evolved from the classic description of wave frequency:

delta waves: $f < 4$ Hz
theta waves: $4 \leq f < 8$ Hz
alpha waves: $8 \leq f \leq 13$ Hz
beta waves: 13 Hz $< f$

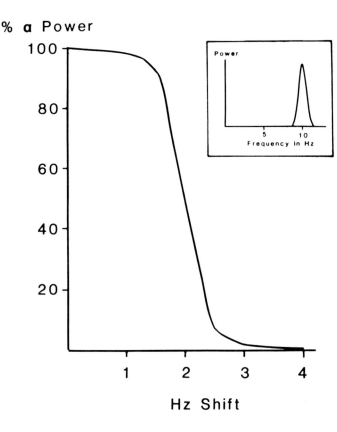

Figure 20–7. Shown here is the percentage of power in the alpha band as a (hypothetic) band of activity (*inset*) is slowed. Almost no change in power is noted during the first 1 Hz of slowing, with very rapid changes in the percentage of power in the alpha band between 1.5 Hz and 2.5 Hz of slowing. Thus, the use of fixed bands makes the uniform slowing appear very sudden and nonuniform.

The CFAM uses slightly different bandwidths, considering activity up to 13 Hz to be alpha, moving the alpha-theta transition to 7.5 Hz, and moving the theta-delta transition to 3.5 Hz. For computer analysis purposes, each band is further subdivided; however, the details are not relevant to this discussion. The appearance that this process imposes on the processed output is, however, most important.

When examining the behavior of the EEG during anesthesia, it is clear that there may be activity that does not fit into the classically defined bands but spreads across bands. Furthermore, as the EEG changes, owing to drug effects or other factors, these bands of activity shift gradually, but the use of arbitrary limits makes the transition appear abrupt (Fig. 20–7). Perhaps more importantly, the process of lumping EEG activity into bands implies that a shift within a band (e.g., from 11 to 8 Hz) is less important than a shift between bands (e.g., 8 to 7 Hz), even though there are no data derived from the analysis of the EEG recorded during anesthesia to suggest this to be true.

Aperiodic Analysis

In 1975, Demetrescu published a single abstract concerning a new EEG analysis technique[13] and began to develop a commercial venture from it (patented in 1982). As a result, it was 1986 before the actual analysis tech-

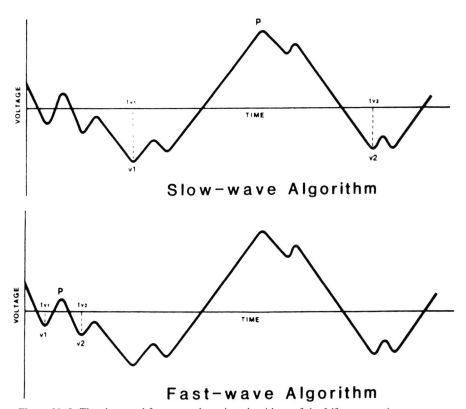

Figure 20–8. The slow- and fast-wave detection algorithms of the Lifescan monitor are exemplified. The slow-wave algorithm identifies negative voltage minima separated by a positive voltage, whereas the fast-wave algorithm identifies minima and maxima without regard to polarity.

nique was published.[23] In the interval, the initial machine was extensively revised and a number of important improvements made; however, the characteristic analysis technique and display format were not changed.

Unlike the CFAM, which uses the polarity to identify the duration of a wave, the aperiodic analysis does so by determining the time of voltage between two voltage minima. Two different algorithms (for slow and fast activity) are used to select voltage minima (Fig. 20–8). The slow-wave algorithm operates on a signal that has been filtered by an 8.2-Hz low-pass filter and selects negative voltage minima that are separated by positive voltage EEG activity. The fast-wave algorithm operates on waveform filtered at 29.4 Hz and determines the period of the wave from successive minima, regardless of polarity of the EEG activity. Having identified the minima, the largest amplitude between them is considered as the peak, and the amplitude for that wave is computed as the average of the voltage difference between the peak voltage and each of the minima.

The Lifescan Monitor

The Lifescan monitor displays the processed EEG (aperiodic analysis) in a unique format. Waves are displayed as vertical spikes (often called telephone poles) on an isometric three-dimensional cathode-ray tube display. The size of the spike indicates the amplitude of the wave; its horizontal position and color are determined by the frequency; and time is displayed on the Z-axis by placing new data in the front and scrolling older data into a more distant–appearing position. Current versions of this device include the ability to monitor evoked potentials, computer communication protocols, and two-channel capability.

Many publications attest to the function of the device as a waveform processor. Both ischemia[24] and anesthetic effects[25-26] have been demonstrated using it. No side-by-side comparisons have been made with any other processing technique, so that it is unclear whether aperiodic analysis truly represents an advantage over zero-crossing or power spectrum techniques. Further confusing the comparison is the unique display, which some observers enjoy and others find difficult to interpret.

Power Spectrum Analysis

Although Blackman and Tukey "wrote the book" on power spectrum analysis in 1958,[10] it was 10 years before these techniques migrated from the engineering world to anesthesia. This is hardly surprising, since a refrigerator-sized computer was required to process even a single channel of EEG data. Real-time analysis, without which monitoring is impossible, was still a gleam in the designers' eyes, realized nearly 5 years later and then only by telephone data transmission.[27] In spite of these difficulties, this period allowed for the development of two alternative display techniques.[28-29] In addition, as computers became smaller and faster, a number of researchers developed their own systems; and this research provided additional understanding for the technique before its clinical use became common.

Method of Analysis

Power spectrum analysis is a general-purpose technique for describing the amplitudes of component waves of a sample of EEG (or any signal that varies with time). It requires that the original signal be digitized and mathematically manipulated through a complex process known as Fourier transformation (Fig. 20–9). This transformation process defines certain characteristics of the resultant power spectra. Failure of the EEG to meet the mathematic assumptions strictly necessary for the application of this transformation has raised questions about its applicability.

In order to perform Fourier transformation, the analog EEG data must be sampled (digitized), a process that defines the highest frequency that can be resolved by the subsequent Fourier analysis. (This frequency is one half the sampling frequency). In fact, if the data are not sampled at a sufficiently high frequency, high-frequency waves appear at lower frequencies, an artifact known as aliasing (Fig. 20–10). (This is true of digitization for all types of analysis, not just power spectrum analysis.)

The process of Fourier transformation converts a collection of data

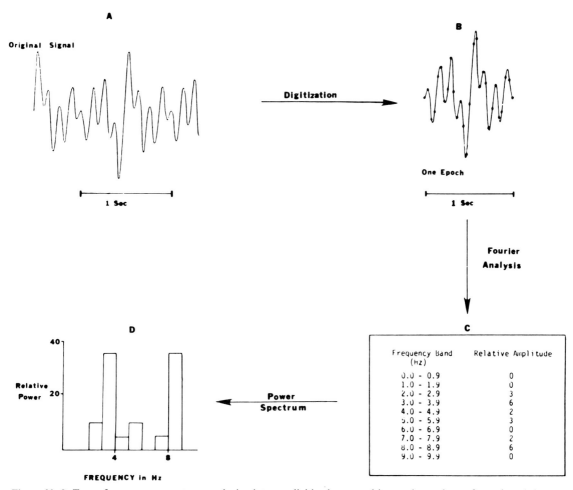

A

Original Signal

1 Sec

Digitization

B

One Epoch

1 Sec

**Fourier
Analysis**

C

Frequency Band (Hz)	Relative Amplitude
0.0 - 0.9	0
1.0 - 1.9	0
2.0 - 2.9	3
3.0 - 3.9	6
4.0 - 4.9	2
5.0 - 5.9	3
6.0 - 6.9	0
7.0 - 7.9	2
8.0 - 8.9	6
9.0 - 9.9	0

**Power
Spectrum**

D

Relative Power

40

20

4   8

FREQUENCY in Hz

Figure 20–9. To perform power spectrum analysis, data are digitized, grouped in epochs, and transformed, and the power spectrum is computed.

points (an epoch) into a series of sine wave components at regularly spaced frequency intervals. For each two data points, one frequency interval can be calculated; thus, if 500 data points are transformed, there are 250 frequency intervals ranging from 0 to the highest frequency that can be resolved by the sampling rate. The relationship between the number of data points and the sampling rate defines both the length of the epoch (epoch length = number of data points/sampling rate) and the frequency resolution of the power spectra (which is simply the inverse of the epoch length in seconds).

One of the major areas of contention about power spectrum analysis is the appropriateness of the application of this technique to the EEG.[30] Strictly speaking, Fourier analysis may be applied to a periodic, stationary signal. The EEG is well known to be nonstationary, although if epochs are not excessively long, stationary behavior may be reasonably well approximated. The EEG is also not, strictly speaking, periodic, since sequential epochs are not identical. These failures to meet the mathematic criteria necessary to

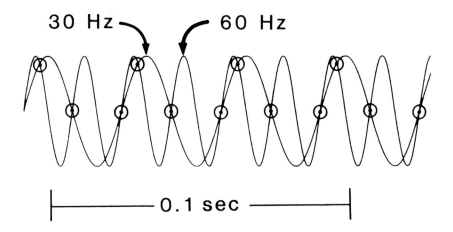

Figure 20–10. Aliasing occurs when a signal is sampled too slowly to be resolved. In this example, a 60-Hz wave is sampled at 90 samples/second; however, a 30-Hz wave can also be drawn through these points. Thus, the 60-Hz wave is made to appear to be 30 Hz, and it appears to be such in all subsequent analyses.

apply power spectrum analysis are often cited by those who favor other analytic approaches; however, they do not, in general, appear to be reasons for not applying power spectrum analysis to the EEG.

These issues become more problematic when the EEG demonstrates burst-suppression activity, because this is clearly nonstationary activity, and analysis with epochs of shorter duration than a complete burst-suppression cycle can be misleading *if taken out of context*. When clinical monitoring is performed, the pattern of burst-suppression activity is easily identified in the graphic display and confirmed by examination of the unprocessed recording.[31] Investigation of the effects of epoch length (and thus spectral resolution) has supported the use of short epochs in all other monitoring situations and recommended the recognition of burst-suppression by its characteristic pattern on the graphic display.[32]

Display

The graphic display of the power spectrum analysis normally takes one of two general forms: a linear graphic or a topographic picture. The linear graphic is almost always utilized for the display of a single epoch of data. Frequency is plotted on the X-axis and amplitude on the Y-axis. Although frequency is a nearly self-explanatory concept, amplitude is not. Strictly speaking, the amplitude of the power spectrum should be plotted in units of intensity − V^2/Hz.[33] This can be converted to actual units of power (watts) if one is willing to assume that the brain behaves as a 1-Ω resistor—hardly a reasonable assumption. The normalization by spectral resolution (Hz) is necessary in order to correct for the reduction in intensity that occurs in each spectral component when the spectral resolution is increased. When

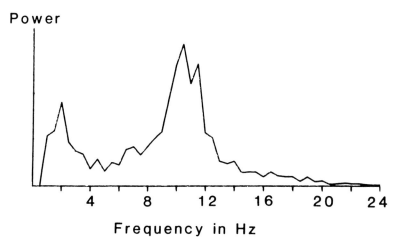

Figure 20–11. Complex Power Spectrum. Although it would be convenient if power spectra yielded narrow, bell-shaped curves, the diffuse bimodal distribution exemplified here is much more typical. Describing this spectrum as a single number must, of necessity, omit much information.

all data are analyzed at the same spectral resolution, the normalization is often omitted, and occasionally, the square root of this unnormalized intensity is plotted as volts.

Even though a graph of intensity and frequency is relatively easy to understand, it may be difficult to describe (Fig. 20–11). Such complexity could be eliminated if the power spectrum could be reduced to one number that could summarize the behavior of the spectrum. From a mathematic standpoint, such a wish is clearly a dream. Even the gaussian distribution, or bell-shaped curve as it is commonly called, requires two numbers, the mean and variance (which describes its width), to describe it. Such logical arguments have failed to deter clinicians, who regularly describe new combinations of spectral frequencies and powers in an attempt to derive the ideal univariate descriptor. At least 27 such descriptors have been proposed,[34] but none has proved useful in all situations.

Spectral Edge Frequency

The spectral edge frequency (SEF)[35] has been one of the most widely used of the univariate descriptors of the EEG power spectrum. This variable is loosely defined as the highest frequency at which there are components in the power spectrum. Although this is not the original description, many have taken this to be the frequency of the ninety-fifth percentile of the power. These differing definitions of SEF account for some of the different results obtained using it. When diffuse slowing of the EEG is a prominent component of the changes under study, the SEF is a useful adjunct for the description of the power spectrum. In this way, hypoxia during carotid endarterectomy has been monitored,[36] the pharmacodynamics of narcotic agents have been differentiated,[37] and questions of acute tolerance to thiopental sodium have been addressed.[38] Other drugs, such as the benzodiazepines,[39] do not produce this slowing, and thus, the SEF has been ineffective in analyzing the EEG effects of these agents.

The reduction of the power spectrum to a single value also simplifies

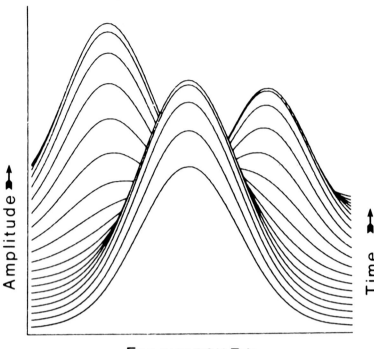

Figure 20–12. The compressed spectral array, a format for power spectral data, places time and amplitude on the same (vertical) axis. New data is placed at the back of the figure and is easily obscured by the preceding information.

the display of these data over time, since a single value is easily graphed as a trend. However, when the entire spectrum is to be displayed over time, the problem becomes more complex, since three-dimensional data must now be compressed into two. Although it is common to do so by shifting the origin both up and to the right, the initial attempts to do this for the EEG power spectrum involved only an upward displacement. The resulting display (Fig. 20–12), known as the compressed spectral array,[28] possesses several disadvantages for monitoring. The primary problem is difficulty in identifying reductions in EEG activity, especially in monitoring activity following artifact, since there is a tendency for low-amplitude data to be hidden by previous activity.

One solution to this problem involved modifying the time axis, so that new data is placed below the old, ensuring the visibility of the most recent data (Fig. 20–13). This format improves the legibility of the data when it is displayed in this fashion, and it is found on commercial equipment utilizing compressed spectral array–type displays.

Density-modulated Spectral Array

The alternative display format, known as the density-modulated spectral array,[29] utilizes a topographic compression of the three-dimensional data into two dimensions. This type of compression requires the color or grayscale encoding of amplitude information, which is then displayed on a graph of time (X-axis) and frequency (Y-axis) (Fig. 20–14). Although it appears

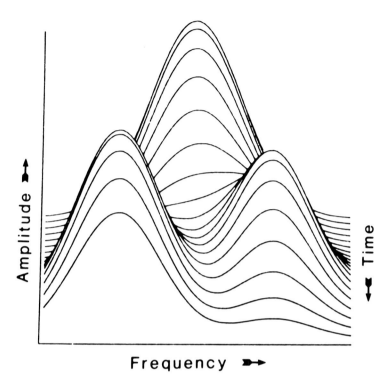

Figure 20–13. This compressed spectral array inverts the time axis (compared with Fig. 20–12). As a result, new data are placed at the front, where changes are more easily discerned.

complex, the process of topographic compression is not only simple but also well known to grade-school children, whose maps often show mountains in various shades of brown, valleys in greens, coastlines in white, and oceans in blue, i.e., altitude data has been encoded in colors. Whether such encoding is performed with colors or shades of gray, the end result is the same. Colors, however, tend to emphasize differences more dramatically. The advantages of this display include a horizontal time axis that is easily scaled to coincide with other physiologic data and elimination of any hiding of data behind "hills."

Differences among Processing Techniques

From a clinician's viewpoint, the differences among analysis techniques are much less significant than the characteristics of the equipment that has been designed to implement these techniques. Qualitatively, all analysis techniques show frequency changes when the EEG slows and amplitude changes when it flattens. Quantitatively, however, these techniques produce different results when applied to the same EEG, and applications that depend on quantitative analysis can be influenced by both analysis technique and the parameters that define it. This has been shown most extensively for power spectrum analysis. The variability from epoch to epoch is reduced by shortening the epoch unless burst-suppression is present.[32] The resolution of high-frequency activity is not influenced by such changes, but it may be

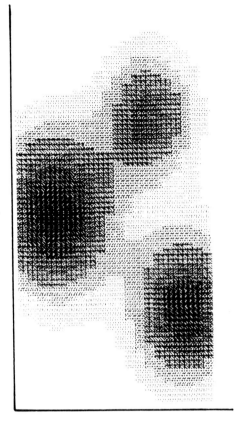

Figure 20–14. Density-modulated spectral array. The data shown in Figs. 20–12 and 20–13 are replotted in the density-modulated format. Darker areas are peaks of greater intensity, and new data are placed at the right margin.

affected when other analysis techniques are used (Fig. 20–15). Most important, different frequency distributions may be observed with different analysis techniques (Fig. 20–16), thus reducing the applicability of data developed with one technique to situations in which another monitoring technique is utilized. This is most unfortunate, since it increases the importance of using a particular monitoring technique, produces apparently conflicting reports of the usefulness of EEG monitoring in particular situations, and impedes research and understanding.

INDICATIONS FOR EEG MONITORING

The appropriate use of the EEG as an intraoperative monitor depends upon three factors. First, the phenomenon must have identifiable EEG correlates that can be recognized by visual inspection or simple analysis of the EEG, whether in processed or analog form. Second, the phenomenon must not be associated with other, more easily identifiable signs that would elimi-

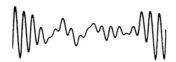

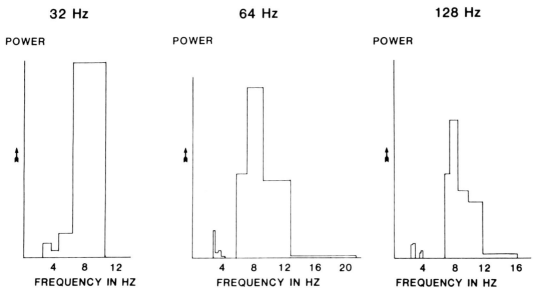

Figure 20–15. Effect of sampling frequency on zero-crossing analysis. Analysis of the 2-second waveform (at top) yields quantitatively different spectra when sampled at 32, 64, and 128 Hz.

nate the need for a more complex monitoring technique like the EEG. Third, the phenomenon should have clinically significant consequences, and therapeutic options should exist that can reduce the magnitude or the severity of these consequences.

Cerebral Ischemia

One of the earliest uses of the EEG was in monitoring for the occurrence of cerebral ischemia during deliberate hypotension[40] and cardiopulmonary bypass.[41] Subsequently, there has been substantial interest in such monitoring for the determination of ischemia during carotid endarterectomy as well.[14, 36, 42–44] In order to complete the picture of ischemia/hypoxia detection, use of the EEG has been proposed as a way to identify hypoxia during routine administration of anesthetics. Although each situation involves monitoring for ischemia (or hypoxia), the applicability of the EEG to each varies greatly.

Ischemia detection by electroencephalographic techniques easily fulfills the first of the criteria established previously. Ischemia produces readily identifiable EEG changes consisting of the loss of high-frequency activity (if present) combined with an increase in low-frequency activity, particularly

ELECTROENCEPHALOGRAPHY

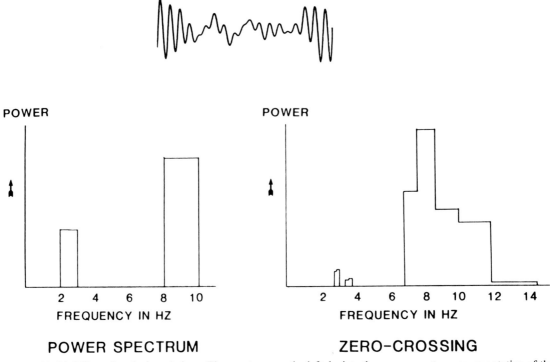

Figure 20–16. Effect of analysis technique. The spectrum on the left depicts the power spectrum representation of the waveform at the top. On the right is a distribution of the waves identified by zero-crossing analysis. Although these are generally similar, there are many quantitative differences.

if such activity was not prominent before the ischemic insult. When the preischemic EEG consists of high-amplitude, low-frequency activity, the early identification of ischemia may be more difficult, but continued inadequate perfusion produces the loss of low-frequency EEG activity, and the amplitude may decrease to nearly an isoelectric level. These changes are gross and easily detected in both analog and processed EEGs (Fig. 20–17).

When considering the presence of other signs of ischemia, it is important to distinguish end-organ ischemia (or hypoxia) from systemic hypoxia. The former is rarely accompanied by other signs and thus fulfills the second requirement for monitoring. As a general-purpose monitor of oxygenation during routine anesthesia, however, the EEG appears ineffective in comparison with the modern pulse oximeter. The pulse oximeter is a simple, robust device, requiring only seconds to apply, that yields qualitative data about systemic hypoxia at the very beginning of arterial desaturation. By comparison, the EEG is more time-consuming to apply, more easily obliterated by artifact, and more difficult to interpret; it yields qualitative (not quantitative) data and is less specific (owing to anesthetic influences) and less sensitive. In awake human volunteers, the EEG does not begin to change until the oxygen saturation of the blood has fallen below 60%,[45] long after the pulse oximeter has warned of the desaturation. Clearly, EEG monitoring is not indicated as a monitor of systemic hypoxia for routine anesthesia care.

The third requirement is for clinical significance and therapeutic op-

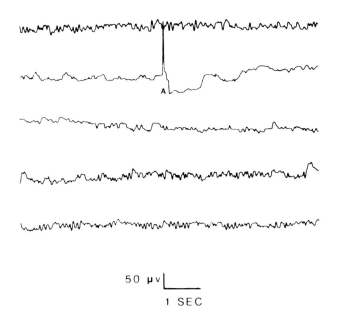

50 μv

1 SEC

Figure 20–17. Cerebral hypoxia. Continuous EEG recorded during a severe ventricular arrhythmia (terminated at A, the artifact due to defibrillation). Diffuse slowing is evident about 4 seconds before this artifact and for about 12 seconds thereafter. The power spectrum display of this data (shown below the raw signal) also depicts the ischemic slowing and recovery. The defibrillation artifact is again prominent.

FREQUENCY IN HZ

— 20

— 10

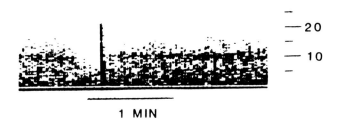

1 MIN

tions, and it is in this area that the indications for hypoxia monitoring begin to weaken. This is not, however, because of the lack of clinical significance of a hypoxic event. Cerebral hypoxia, or ischemia, of sufficient severity to produce EEG changes is no less significant than myocardial ischemia sufficient to change the ECG. It is, by definition, a clinically significant event. Our ability to provide therapeutic options, however, varies markedly. During deliberate hypotension, therapeutic options include increasing the blood pressure. Since many indications for deliberate hypotension are relative (i.e., reducing blood loss during orthopedic surgery), EEG monitoring may provide a margin of safety for these patients. It should be noted, however, that cerebral autoregulation begins to fail at 50–60 mmHg, and an additional 30% reduction in cerebral perfusion is required to produce EEG evidence of ischemia.[46] It is exceedingly rare for these levels of hypotension to be achieved during any procedures except neurosurgery or during cardiopulmonary bypass. Thus, for routine, modest levels of hypotension, cerebral ischemia is so rare that electroencephalographic monitoring is of marginal value.

Cardiovascular Surgery

During cardiopulmonary bypass, neurologic complications are not rare,[47] and hypoperfusion is common. Does this represent an appropriate opportunity for EEG monitoring? It probably does not, because most neurologic complications during bypass are embolic,[48] and there are no specific therapies available to prevent or treat this complication. Furthermore, most cerebral ischemia during bypass occurs during hypoperfusion undertaken to facilitate specific surgical maneuvers (e.g., removing the aortic cross-clamp). Although these maneuvers may produce ischemia, there is no acceptable alternative, and these brief episodes do not appear to pose a threat to the neurologic well-being of the patient.[49] In addition, the high-dose narcotic anesthetics commonly used during cardiac anesthesia and hypothermia during bypass induce profound EEG slowing, similar to changes caused by ischemia. However, the EEG can be used to titrate effects of drugs (barbiturates) during cardiac surgery.[48] Thus, the routine use of EEG monitoring is probably unnecessary for procedures involving extracorporeal circulation.

Only in the case of cerebrovascular surgery (e.g., carotid endarterectomy) are all the requirements for EEG monitoring achieved. Not only does carotid occlusion produce ischemia frequently and without systemic signs, but the placement of a vascular shunt also markedly reduces the severity of ischemia or eliminates it entirely. Perhaps most important, shunting is, itself, associated with surgical morbidity due to emboli and intimal dissection; thus, it is undesirable to shunt except when there is evidence of ischemia. The shunt also complicates surgical access to the vessel, another reason to avoid its unnecessary use. Although this rationale strongly supports the use of EEG monitoring and selective shunting, satisfactory studies comparing selective shunting with alternative techniques have not been performed. Such comparisons may, in fact, be impossible since the incidence of stroke is often reported to be less than 2%, and comparative studies would require thousands of subjects. Since the debate is clearly unsettled,[50] each individual anesthesiologist must decide the appropriateness of these monitoring techniques.

Assessment of Anesthetic Depth

Another commonly proposed indication for EEG monitoring is the assessment of anesthetic depth. This vague term may refer either to anesthesia near the level at which recall for intraoperative events occurs or to much deeper levels of anesthesia necessary to blunt the autonomic response to painful stimulation. Other clinicians use the term to refer to EEG changes produced by anesthetic agents themselves, without surgery, in which the drug concentration represents the evidence of anesthetic depth. Although the EEG may be applicable to each of these areas, in most situations the clinical utility of this technique seems lacking.

If one reviews case reports and series involving intraoperative recall, EEG data is almost uniformly missing. Considering the infrequent occurrence of these events, this is not surprising—such a study would represent a heroic undertaking. It does mean, however, that any usefulness of the EEG must be extrapolated from studies in unstimulated subjects using different and largely irrelevant stimuli. Such extrapolation must be undertaken with caution. The onset of unresponsiveness during anesthetic induction has been shown to correlate with changes in the EEG;[51] however, these changes were specific to the drug under study. Enflurane produces high-frequency activity, whereas the addition of nitrous oxide produces similar unresponsiveness without this high-frequency activity. In other studies, analgesic doses of nitrous oxide by itself have produced high-frequency activity.[52] With isoflurane, the change in responsiveness is associated with the slowing of the alpha rhythm, if it is present. Its absence, usually the result of perioperative anxiety, precludes the use of changes in the alpha rhythm as an indication of unresponsiveness. Since attention to stimuli changes the EEG, one might also expect that attention to surgical stimuli during light anesthesia might also change the EEG. There is evidence that the EEG changes in response to surgical stimulation,[53] particularly in lightly anesthetized patients. However, there is no evidence that this is indicative of awareness or cognitive function.

At greater depths of anesthesia, there is somewhat more evidence that the EEG can be used as a measure of anesthetic depth. This includes both classic studies of EEG changes with large variations in anesthetic concentration[11, 54, 55] and more recent ones that suggest that high-frequency activity in the power spectrum (spectral edge over 14 Hz) is a predictor of inadequate anesthetic depth for intubation, as evidenced by a hypertensive response.[56] Confirmation by other researchers and extension of these findings to other anesthetics and stimuli would be a valuable advance and might even justify more frequent EEG monitoring in those patients (e.g., with aneurysms and severe coronary artery disease) for whom a hypertensive response to intubation is particularly hazardous. However, EEG monitoring only becomes valuable if there are no other signs of anesthetic depth to utilize and if the subject is sufficiently stable to allow adjustment of the anesthetic depth at will. Clearly, the clinical role for the electroencephalographic monitoring of anesthetic depth remains to be defined.

In spite of the problems of applying pure pharmacologic data in the clinical setting, studies of the electroencephalographic effects of drugs continue and often demonstrate close associations between drug dosage and electroencephalographic changes.[57, 58] Thus, EEG effects of fentanyl citrate and alfentanil hydrochloride are grossly similar, but EEG studies explained differences in the clinical behavior of the drugs that were the result of different pharmacodynamics. Similar studies have been performed with other drugs, although certain technical problems have arisen concerning the drug-specific nature of the EEG descriptors.

With the inhalational anesthetics, such pharmacologic data are extensive but older and less applicable to the mixed anesthetic techniques applied clinically. Nonetheless, the EEG changes in a dose-dependent and drug-specific fashion for all the anesthetic agents. With light enflurane, high-frequency activity is more noticeable than with halothane or isoflurane; but at moderate concentrations, the differences are less striking. Isoflurane is the only modern inhalational agent to produce burst-suppression, particularly at clinically useful doses, although this electroencephalographic pattern can also be achieved with the barbiturates. Even though each agent tends to produce a specific EEG pattern, the concept of an "anesthetic signature," which would allow the identification of the anesthetic in use in any particular patient, does not seem achievable, at least not at present. Perhaps this reflects the integration by the brain of many stimuli, not only the anesthetic chemicals administered. If so, each patient must be considered as an individual, not simply as a biologic mass spectrometer that converts drug input into bioelectric output.

Despite these problems and objections, physicians who are comfortable with interpreting the intraoperative EEG often identify changes in anesthetic depth using the EEG before such changes become evident by hemodynamic or somatic signs. In a given anesthetic in a particular patient, changes in anesthetic depth too small to be identified by other means can be evident in the EEG, and the presence of such changes can often predict future clinical developments. The skill to detect such changes is not difficult to develop and might represent a reasonable clinical endeavor for one so inclined; whether it justifies the use of a complex, albeit safe, monitoring modality like the EEG is open to question.

Electroencephalography in the Intensive Care Unit

There are two distinct indications for electroencephalographic recording in the intensive care unit: for diagnosis and for monitoring. The indications for diagnostic recordings include the determination of brain death and the identification of seizures, both postoperatively and during status epilepticus. Such recordings are performed by technicians, using standard multichannel strip-chart recorders, and interpreted by neurologists.

The applicability of processed EEG is less clear. The original CFM was developed to help confirm the diagnosis of brain death, but such monitoring has not become a component of the criteria for brain death. Another application for EEG monitoring is to follow the progress of patients with drug overdoses.[59] Although it is interesting, there is no evidence that this monitoring improves care or modifies therapeutic choices that would be made on a purely clinical basis.

When dealing with victims of head trauma, there may be indications for continuous EEG monitoring. EEG patterns have been compared with the Glasgow coma score as a predictor of outcome, and the EEG performs comparably.[60] In such a situation, the simple clinical evaluation of patients seems preferable to something as complex as continuous EEG monitoring. On the other hand, the depth of barbiturate coma can easily be assessed from burst-suppression activity, and thus, EEG monitoring may allow more rapid adjustment of this therapy than is possible with intermittent determinations of blood barbiturate concentrations. There may also be EEG evidence of "lightening" of coma, which is particularly valuable when neuromuscular-blocking drugs are used to facilitate control of ventilation but patients are not heavily sedated. Evidence of sleep/waking patterns in monitored EEG can also be observed, but it is not clear whether these findings offer sufficient indications to routinely monitor EEG in the neurologic intensive care unit.

SUMMARY

Modern technology has made intraoperative EEG monitoring reliable and practical, provided attention is given to technical detail. There are several different approaches to EEG analysis. No single approach has been shown convincingly to be preferable to others. In general, clinicians select equipment based on such criteria as the number of channels of EEG processed, other monitors incorporated, flexibility, display mode, cost, user interface, length of epoch, and personal taste. The application of EEG monitoring in carotid endarterectomy procedures seems well justified, but for the identification of ischemia in other situations, the benefits are less evident. Although it is useful as a research tool for drug effects, the EEG cannot currently be recommended as a means of assessing anesthetic depth; however, further work has the potential for changing this assessment.

References

1. Gibbs FA, Gibbs EL, Lennox WG: Effect on the electroencephalogram of certain drugs which influence nervous activity. Arch Intern Med 1937; 60:154–166.
2. Peronnet F, Sindon M, Laviron A, et al: Human cortical electrogenesis: Statigraphy and spectral analysis. *In* Petsche H, Brazier MAB (eds): Synchronization of EEG Activity in Epilepsies. New York: Springer-Verlag, 1972; 235–262.
3. Delucchi MR, Garoutte B, Aird RB: The scalp as an electroencephalographic averager. Electroencephalogr Clin Neurophysiol 1962; 14:191–196.
4. Allison T: Calculated and empirical evoked-potential distributions in human recordings. *In* Otta DA (ed): Multidisciplinary Perspectives in Event-related Brain Potential Research. Washington, DC: US Environmental Protection Agency, 1978.
5. Blom JL, Anneveldt M: An electrode cap tested. Electroencephalogr Clin Neurophysiol 1982; 54:591–594.
6. Jasper HH: The ten-twenty electrode system of the International Federation. Electroencephalogr Clin Neurophysiol 1958; 10:371–375.
7. MacGillivray BB: Handbook of EEG and Clinical Neurophysiology, Vol 3–C. Amsterdam: Elsevier, 1974.
8. Chatrian GE, Bergamini L, Dondey M, et al: Report of the Committee on Terminology, Appendix A. Electroencephalogr Clin Neurophysiol 1974; 37:538–548.
9. Pichlmayr I, Lips U, Kunkel H: The Electroencephalogram in Anesthesia. New York: Springer-Verlag, 1984; 37.
10. Blackman RB, Tukey J: The Measurement of Power Spectra. New York: Dover, 1958.
11. Findeiss JC, Kien GA, Huse KOW, Linde HW: Power spectral density of the electroencephalogram during halothane and cyclopropane anesthesia in man. Anesth Analg 1969; 48:1018–1023.

12. Maynard D, Prior PF, Scott DF: A device for continuous monitoring of cerebral activity in resuscitated patients. Br Med J 1969; 4:545–546.

13. Demetrescu TM: The aperiodic character of the electroencephalogram (EEG): New approach to data analysis and condensation. (Abstract.) Physiologist 1975; 18:189.

14. Cucchiara RF, Sharbrough FW, Messick JM, Tinker JH: An electroencephalographic filter-processor as an indicator of cerebral ischemia during carotid endarterectomy. Anesthesiology 1979; 51:77–79.

15. Patel H: Experience with the cerebral function monitor during deliberate hypotension. Br J Anaesth 1981; 53:639–644.

16. Sechzer PH, Ospina J: Cerebral function monitor: Evaluation in anesthesia/critical care. Curr Ther Res 1977; 22:335–347.

17. Kritikou PE, Branthwaite MA: Significance of changes in cerebral electrical activity at onset of cardiopulmonary bypass. Thorax 1977; 32:534–538.

18. Schwartz MS, Colvin MP, Prior PF, et al: The cerebral function monitor. Anaesthesia 1973; 28:611–618.

19. Dubois M, Savege TM, O'Carroll TM, Frank M: General anaesthesia and changes on the cerebral function. Anaesthesia 1978; 33:157–164.

20. Frank M, Savege TM, Leigh M, et al: Comparison of the cerebral function monitor and plasma concentrations of thiopentone and alphaxalone during total IV anaesthesia with repeated bolus doses of thiopentone and althesin. Br J Anaesth 1982; 54:609–616.

21. Prior PF, Maynard DE, Brierley JB: EEG monitoring for the control of anaesthesia produced by the infusion of althesin in primates. Br J Anaesth 1978; 50:993–1000.

22. Sebel PS, Maynard DE, Major E, Frank M: The cerebral function analysing monitor (CFAM). Br J Anaesth 1983; 55:1265–1270.

23. Gregory TK, Pettus DC: An electroencephalographic processing algorithm specifically intended for analysis of cerebral electrical activity. J Clin Monit 1986; 2:190–197.

24. Spackman TN, Faust RJ, Cucchiara RF, et al: A comparison of the Lifescan EEG monitor with EEG and cerebral blood flow for detection of cerebral ischemia. (Abstract.) Anesthesiology 1985; 63:A187.

25. Smith NT, Demetrescu M: The EEG during high-dose fentanyl anesthesia. (Abstract.) Anesthesiology 1980; 53:S7.

26. Demetrescu M, Kavan E, Smith NT: Monitoring the brain condition by advanced EEG. (Abstract.) Anesthesiology 1981; 53:A130.

27. Myers RR, Stockard JJ, Fleming NI, et al: The use of on-line telephonic computer analysis of the EEG in anaesthesia. Br J Anaesth 1973; 45:664–670.

28. Bickford RG, Fleming NI, Billinger TW: Compression of EEG data by isometric power spectral plots. (Abstract.) Electroencephalogr Clin Neurophysiol 1971; 31:632.

29. Fleming RA, Smith NT: Density modulation. A technique for the display of three-variable data in patient monitoring. Anesthesiology 1979; 50:543–546.

30. Brazier MAB, Walter DO (eds): Handbook of Electroencephalography and Clinical Neurophysiology, Volume 5-A. Amsterdam: Elsevier, 1974; 5A33–5A43.

31. Levy WJ: Intraoperative EEG patterns: Implications for EEG monitoring. Anesthesiology 1984; 60:430–434.

32. Levy WJ: Effect of epoch length on power spectrum analysis of the EEG. Anesthesiology 1987; 66:489–495.

33. Walter DO: On units and dimensions for reporting spectral intensities. Electroencephalogr Clin Neurophysiol 1968; 24:486–487.

34. Matteo RS, Orenstein E, Schwartz AE, et al: Effects of low-dose sufentanil on the EEG. Elderly vs young. (Abstract.) Anesthesiology 1986; 65:A553.

35. Rampil IJ, Sasse FJ, Smith NT, et al: Spectral edge frequency—a new correlate of anesthetic depth. (Abstract.) Anesthesiology 1980; 53:S12.

36. Rampil IJ, Holzer JA, Quest DO, et al: Prognostic value of computerized EEG analysis during carotid endarterectomy. Anesth Analg 1983; 62:186–192.

37. Scott JC, Ponganis KV, Stanski DR: EEG quantitation of narcotic effect. The comparative pharmacodynamics of fentanyl and alfentanil. Anesthesiology 1985; 62:234–241.

38. Hudson RJ, Stanski DR, Meathe E, Saidman LJ: Does acute tolerance to thiopental exist? Anesthesiology 1982; 57:A501.

39. Burhrer M, Maitre PO, Ebling WF, Stanski DR: Pharmacological quantitation of midazolam's CNS drug effect in hypnotic doses. (Abstract.) Anesthesiology 1987; 67:A658.

40. Mannheimer WH, Keats AS, Chamberlin JA: Safety in hypotensive anesthesia. Surgery 1963; 54:883–890.

41. Coons RE, Keats AS, Cooley DA: Significance of electroencephalographic changes occurring during cardiopulmonary bypass. Anesthesiology 1959; 20:804–810.

42. Sharbrough FW, Messick JM Jr, Sundt TM: Correlation of continuous electro-encephalograms with cerebral blood flow measurements during carotid endarterectomy. Stroke 1973; 4:674–683.

43. Sundt TM Jr: The ischemic tolerance of neural tissue and the need for monitoring and selective shunting during carotid endarterectomy. Stroke 1983; 14:93–98.

44. Chiappa KH, Burke SR, Young RR: Results of encephalographic monitoring during 367 carotid endarterectomies: Use of a dedicated minicomputer. Stroke 1979; 10:381–388.

45. Cohen PJ, Alexander SC, Smith TC, et al: Effects of hypoxia and normocarbia on cerebral blood flow and metabolism in conscious man. J Appl Physiol 1967; 23:183–189.

46. Finnerty FA Jr, Witkin L, Fazekas JF: Cerebral hemodynamics during cerebral ischemia induced by acute hypotension. J Clin Invest 1954; 33:1227–1232.

47. Slogoff S, Girgis KZ, Keats AS: Etiologic factors in neuropsychiatric complications associated with cardiopulmonary bypass. Anesth Analg 1982; 61:903–911.

48. Nussmeier NA, McDermott JP: Macroembolization. Prevention and outcome modification. *In* Hilberman M (ed): Brain Injury and Protection during Heart Surgery. Boston: Martinus Nijhoff, 1988; 85–106.

49. Levy WJ, Parcella PA: Electroencephalographic evidence of cerebral ischemia during acute extracorporeal hypoperfusion. J Cardiothorac Anesth 1987; 4:300–304.

50. Ferguson GG: Intra-operative monitoring and internal shunts: Are they necessary in carotid endarterectomy? Stroke 1983; 13:287–289.

51. Levy WJ: Power spectrum correlates of changes in consciousness during anesthetic induction with enflurane. Anesthesiology 1986; 64:688–693.

52. Yamamura T, Fukuda M, Takeya H, et al: Fast oscillatory EEG activity induced by analgesic concentrations of nitrous oxide in man. Anesth Analg 1981; 60:283–288.

53. Bimar J, Bellville J: Arousal reactions during anesthesias in man. Anesthesiology 1977; 47:449–454.

54. Martin JT, Faulconer A, Bickford RG: Electroencephalography in anesthesiology. Anesthesiology 1959; 20:359–376.

55. Clark DL, Rosner BS: Neurophysiologic effects of general anesthetics. Anesthesiology 1973; 38:564–582.

56. Rampil IJ, Matteo RS: Changes in EEG spectral edge frequency correlate with

the hemodynamic response to laryngoscopy and intubation. Anesthesiology 1987; 67:139–142.

57. Sebel PS, Bovill JG, Wauquier A, Rog P: Effects of high-dose fentanyl anesthesia on the electroencephalogram. Anesthesiology 1981; 55:203–211.

58. Brandt L, Pokar H: EEG power spectrum analysis during isoflurane anesthesia in man. (Abstract.) Anesthesiology 1984; 61:A340.

59. Myers RR, Stockard JJ: Neurologic and electroencephalographic correlates in glutethimide intoxication. Clin Pharmacol Ther 1975; 17:212–220.

60. Karnaze DS, Marshall LF, Bickford RG: EEG monitoring of clinical coma: The compressed spectral array. Neurology 1982; 32:289–292.

chapter twenty-one

Monitoring the Neuromuscular Junction

STUART C. LAW, M.D.
■ D. RYAN COOK, M.D.

Neuromuscular-blocking agents are administered in nearly three quarters of general anesthetics in order to facilitate endotracheal intubation, control of mechanical ventilation, and surgery.[1] Despite their widespread use, the use of these agents is not without risk.

In 1954 Beecher and Todd conducted a retrospective study of 599,548 patients and showed a 6-fold increased mortality in patients in whom a muscle relaxant had been used.[2] Even though this study has been criticized, it nonetheless pointed out the need for increased diligence when using these agents. Over 25 years have passed since Beecher and Todd's study and Churchill-Davidson and Christie's proposal to use nerve stimulators to monitor neuromuscular blockade.[3] Several studies, however, have shown that neuromuscular blockers are still administered without nerve stimulators and that many patients have significant degrees of neuromuscular block in the immediate postoperative period. Viby-Mogensen and colleagues demonstrated that patients receiving muscle relaxants had a 42% incidence of residual neuromuscular blockade on arrival in the recovery room.[4] Other studies have shown a 21–25% incidence.[5, 6] These studies evaluated patients who received muscle relaxants without monitoring by a nerve stimulator.

Two general problems are encountered each time a muscle relaxant is administered. The proper dose of relaxant and antagonist must be determined, and residual blockade must be evaluated in the operating room and the recovery room. It is impossible to accurately predict the response to a muscle relaxant of a given patient based solely upon pharmacokinetic data. Katz has demonstrated the marked individual variability in response to d-tubocurarine.[7] A dose of 0.1 mg/kg produced no demonstrable blockade in 6% of patients, whereas 7% of the patients developed complete blockade.[7] There may be as much as a 4-fold difference in the serum concentration of a relaxant required to produce a given degree of relaxation in different patients.[8]

In addition to the normal wide variability in response to relaxants, many other factors are known to influence neuromuscular blockade. Temperature, plasma pH, plasma protein concentration, age, and coexisting disease, including renal and hepatic function, affect the response to relaxants. The concomitant administration of a variety of drugs also alters the response to relaxants. Even in a single patient, changing physiologic parameters may alter the dose-response relationship.

Given these arguments, there is no question that administering muscle relaxants based solely upon clinical parameters, without the aid of a peripheral nerve stimulator, is a practice that should be avoided. Use of a peripheral nerve stimulator with visual or tactile evaluation of evoked responses markedly reduces the incidence of residual blockade in the recovery room.[9] This chapter reviews neuromuscular structure/function and describes the techniques of monitoring neuromuscular blockade.

THE NEUROMUSCULAR JUNCTION

Anatomy

The motor unit is composed of a motor neuron and a group of muscle fibers to which it branches. The interface between the nerves and the muscle fibers is called the neuromuscular junction (NMJ). Motor neurons are single cells that extend, uninterrupted, from the ventral horn of the spinal cord to the muscle. After entering the muscle, they branch and send unmyelinated axons to individual muscle fibers. In most muscles, there is only one NMJ. The extraocular muscles of the eye, however, have multiple NMJs and, unlike other muscles, contract in response to depolarizing relaxants. The NMJ is required to amplify the electrical impulse in nerve fibers in order to depolarize the relatively larger muscle fibers.

The NMJ consists of a nerve terminal and a specialized area of the muscle fiber known as the motor end-plate. The nerve terminal is an unmyelinated extension of the axon that has an abundance of mitochondria and 300 Å spheres, called vesicles, which contain acetylcholine (ACh), adenosine triphosphate, calcium, choline, and a variety of lipids and proteins.[10] The motor end-plate is contiguous with the muscle fiber membrane and

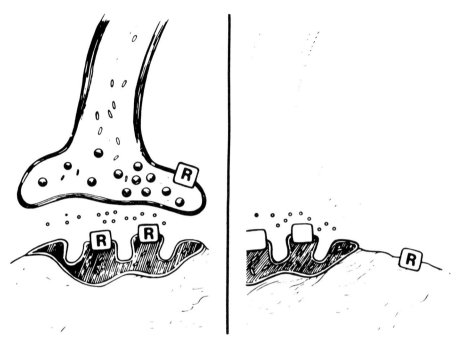

Figure 21–1. *Left*, The anatomy of the normal neuromuscular junction (NMJ) includes the motor nerve containing vesicles of acetylcholine, which diffuse across the junction to activate postjunctional and prejunctional receptors (R). *Right*, The denervated muscular junction with extrajunctional receptors. (From Standaert FG: Donut and holes; molecules and muscle relaxants. Semin Anesth 1984; 4[3]. with permission.)

features extensive infoldings that contain concentrated amounts of acetylcholinesterase.[11] The nerve terminal and motor end-plate are separated by a distance of 500 Å. The motor end-plate is literally paved with ACh receptors at a density of 10,000–20,000/μm (Fig. 21–1).[2,12] Electron micrographs have demonstrated specialized areas of the terminal axon membrane, called active zones, that face invaginations of postsynaptic folds on the outside and feature a twin row of 20–30 synaptic vesicles on the inside. There are 500–1000 zones/terminal (Fig. 21–2).[13]

Physiology

ACh Synthesis, Storage, and Release

Synthesis and Storage

ACh is synthesized in the axon terminal of the motor nerve from acetylcoenzyme A (AcCoA) and choline by the enzyme choline-O-acetyltransferase, which is synthesized in the motor neuron cell body and transported to the nerve terminal (Fig. 21–3). AcCoA is derived from pyruvate, which in turn is a product of glycolysis. Hydrolysis of ACh and dietary intake provide choline, which is actively transported into the cell.[14] Muscle fibers are also known to produce ACh, probably through the enzyme carnitine

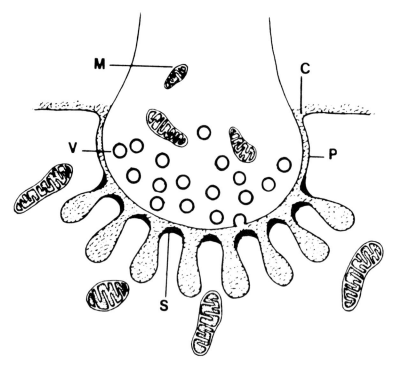

Figure 21–2. Microscopic anatomy of the NMJ showing the twin row of 20–30 synaptic vesicles on the inside of the nerve ending, which face the invaginations of the postsynaptic folds in the "active zones." (M = mitochondria, V = vesicles, P = postjunctional membrane, S = synaptic fold, C = synaptic cleft.) (From Maclean IC: Neuromuscular junction. *In* Johnson EW [ed]: Practical Electromyography, 75. © 1980, the Williams & Wilkins Co., Baltimore.)

acetyltransferase.[15] The rate of ACh synthesis and choline uptake increases with impulse activity of the axon terminal.[16] About 50% of the ACh within the neuron terminal is free in the cytosol, whereas the other 50% is in vesicles.[11] Each vesicle contains approximately 5000–10,000 molecules of ACh.[17]

Release of ACh

The Role of Calcium. Stimulation of a motor neuron causes voltage-responsive ion channels to propagate an action potential down the axon to

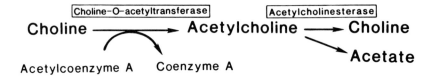

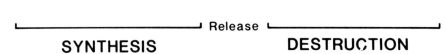

SYNTHESIS   Release   **DESTRUCTION**

Figure 21–3. Acetylcholine is synthesized in the motor nerve terminal from choline and acetylcoenzyme A by the enzyme choline-O-acetyltransferase. It is degraded by acetylcholinesterase to choline and acetate. (From Durant NN: The physiology of neuromuscular transmission. Semin Anesth 1984; 4[3]. with permission.)

the nerve terminal. Nerve terminals, however, lack Na^+ channels and cannot generate an action potential.[18] Depolarization is spread through the nerve terminal by cable conduction and causes voltage-sensitive calcium channels to open. The resulting flux of calcium ions into the terminal initiates ACh release. The released ACh molecules cross the synaptic cleft and bind to ACh receptors. The ACh-bound receptors open channels that allow ionic flux to depolarize the motor end-plate and generate an end-plate potential (EPP). The EPP is conducted to the surrounding membrane where it triggers opening of voltage-sensitive channels and thereby generates a muscle fiber action potential that is transmitted through the T tubule system to initiate contraction. Calcium channels close in response to terminal repolarization induced by an outward potassium current. Thesleff suggests that these voltage-dependent calcium channels may exist exclusively at the active zones.[13]

The mechanism by which calcium promotes the release of ACh at the active zones is not known. It is known, however, that calcium is required for quantal release of ACh. Without Ca^{2+} the nerve terminal can depolarize, but no quantal ACh release occurs.[19] In his review of neuromuscular transmission, Thesleff notes that calcium may act through calmodulin kinase to phosphorylate dephosphosynapsin I, an enzyme that hinders vesicle association with the membrane.[13] Agents that block potassium channels, such as 4-aminopyridine, prolong the influx of calcium and thereby increase calcium-mediated ACh release. Other mediators of ACh release have been identified. Calcium and magnesium ions have opposite actions. Magnesium has been shown to decrease the number of quanta released in response to an action potential.[20]

Quantal Theory. Quantal release implies that ACh is released from the nerve terminals in discrete packets of a uniform size called a quantum. Each quantum contains 5000–10,000 ACh molecules.[21] Spontaneous release of a quantum of ACh produces a postsynaptic voltage potential change called a miniature end-plate potential (MEPP). Neurally evoked ACh release produces an EPP that is actually a summation of many MEPPs. The vesicular hypothesis was developed to incorporate the observance of nerve terminal vesicles into the quantal theory. The central theme of this hypothesis is that ACh is stored in vesicles and is released into the synaptic cleft. Spontaneous discharge of a single vesicle produces a MEPP, whereas the neurally evoked release of many vesicles produces an EPP. The EPP after nerve terminal depolarization consists of a summation of several hundred quanta.[10]

Unfortunately, the actual mechanism for ACh release appears to be more complicated than the vesicle hypothesis suggests. Different types of ACh release have been demonstrated, and some investigators have therefore questioned the validity of the vesicle hypothesis. There now appear to be at least three different mechanisms of ACh release into the synaptic cleft (Table 21–1). There is, at present, debate regarding the validity of the vesicular hypothesis. The evidence for and against this theory is presented in Table 21–2.

Receptor Types

Three populations of nicotinic ACh receptors are involved with neuromuscular transmission. They are classified according to their location as prejunctional, postjunctional, or extrajunctional (see Fig. 21–1).

Table 21–1. DIFFERENT TYPES OF CALCIUM RELEASE

Calcium-mediated quantal release
 Responsible for neurally evoked transmission[10]
 May be a summation of MEPP size discharges, which
  may in turn consist of smaller subunits[10]
Quantal release that is not calcium-mediated
 Consists of events larger than MEPPs referred to as
  giant MEPPs
 Is unaffected by nerve terminal depolarization or by
  presynaptic calcium fluxes*
Nonquantal leakage
 May account for 99% of the ACh in the synaptic cleft
 Does not appear to be involved with the process of
  neurally evoked transmission†

---

* Thesleff S, Molgó J: A new type of transmitter release at the neuromuscular junction. Neuroscience 1983; 9:1–8.

† Katz B, Miledi R: Transmitter leakage from motor nerve endings. Proc R Soc Lond [Biol] 1977; 196:59–72.

Prejunctional Receptors

The prejunctional receptors are located in the membrane of the nerve terminal and modulate ACh mobilization and release. They have different binding characteristics and possibly different channel characteristics than the postjunctional receptors do.[21] Antagonism of this receptor results in diminished ACh release from neurons stimulated at high frequency. These nicotinic receptors increase ACh mobilization to readily releasable stores and provide feedback control during high-frequency stimulation.

Postjunctional Receptors

Postjunctional receptors are packed into the end-plate region at a density of $10,000–20,000/m^2$.[12] The receptor consists of 5 subunits ranging from 40,000 to 65,000 daltons. There are two alpha subunits (45,000 daltons), both of which must be bound by ACh in order to initiate channel opening and the resultant flux of Na^+, K^+, and Ca^{2+} ions.[22]

Extrajunctional Receptors

The extrajunctional receptors are located in the muscle fiber membrane outside of the motor end-plate region. They respond to agonists by allowing ionic flow to occur, as do the other ACh receptors. They are not capable of producing an action potential because their density is insufficient to allow the development of threshold EPP. A deficiency of neural stimulation (as after spinal cord injuries) may initiate the production of these extrajunctional receptors. Although the density of these receptors is low, the absolute numbers may be very high. It is postulated that the receptors bind to agonists

Table 21–2. VALIDITY OF THE VESICLE HYPOTHESIS

Factors in Favor of the Vesicular Hypothesis
  Vesicles contain an amount of ACh that corresponds to a MEPP.
  Rapid-freeze techniques show that depolarization results in the appearance of pits in the membrane that seem to be associated with vesicles.
  The transmembrane potential does not influence the amount of ACh released, which would be expected if ACh was transported through a gate mechanism.
  Osmotically induced changes in the nerve terminal volume and a corresponding decrease in cytosolic ACh concentration does not alter ACh release.

Factors Against
  Newly synthesized ACh is released preferentially by nerve stimulation.[49] Newly synthesized ACh is found in the cytoplasm but not in the vesicles.[10]
  The number of vesicles is not altered by physiologic levels of stimulation, whereas cytoplasmic free ACh is depleted.[10]
  Vesicles contain both ACh and adenosine triphosphate (ATP). The ACh/ATP ratio within vesicles differs from the ratio observed within the synapse after stimulation.[10]
  Stimulation depletes cytoplasmic stores of ACh in the same amount released during depolarization, whereas the vesicular content does not change.*

* Israel M, Lesbats B: Continuous determination by a chemiluminescent method of acetylcholine release and compartmentation in Torpedo electric organ synaptosomes. J Neurochem 1981; 37:1475–1483.

quite avidly and allow for ionic flux, resulting in the well-described increase in potassium after administration of succinylcholine chloride.[23–25]

Impulse Formation

Neurons, muscle fibers, and most other living cells maintain ionic gradients across their membranes. Energy-requiring pump mechanisms transport Na^+ into and K^+ ions out of the cell while producing a voltage gradient of -70 to -90 mV. The K^+ ions are able to slowly leak back out along the concentration gradient and thus leave the inside of the cell negatively charged with respect to the outer membrane.[26] The membrane possesses voltage-gated channels that allow rapid ionic flux to occur if the membrane is depolarized beyond a threshold value.[27] Thus, an electric current sufficient in amplitude to depolarize a motor neuron membrane to more than -50 mV triggers a propagated wave of depolarization. When this impulse reaches the nerve terminal, it must be transmitted across the synaptic cleft to the muscle fiber that it supplies. This is accomplished by the transmitter ACh. Its effect is terminated rapidly as ACh is enzymatically degraded by acetylcholinesterase (see Fig. 21–2).

NEUROMUSCULAR BLOCKERS

Neuromuscular blockers that are in clinical use at present are described as being either depolarizing or nondepolarizing, depending upon their effect on the motor end-plate. A thorough review of the relaxant-receptor interaction has been done by Standaert.[22]

Depolarizing Blockade

Succinylcholine chloride is the most common nondepolarizing relaxant. It is unusual in that it produces two different types of block: phase 1 and phase 2.

Phase 1 Block

During phase 1, succinylcholine chloride binds to ACh receptors, causing membrane ionic channels to open in the same fashion that ACh does. The molecules remain bound to the receptor for an extended period and cause the membrane to remain depolarized and unable to trigger any further muscle action potentials. Characteristics of phase 1 block include: (1) muscle fasciculation prior to onset of block; (2) absence of fade with fast or slow stimulation including train-of-four (TOF) stimulation and tetanus (TOF ratio is 0.6–0.7); (3) absence of post-tetanic facilitation; (4) antagonism by prior administration of a nondepolarizing relaxant; (5) potentiation by other depolarizing agents;[28] and (6) absence of tachyphylaxis.

Phase 2 Block

With prolonged exposure and doses of 2–5 mg/kg, a succinylcholine chloride–induced block assumes the characteristics of a nondepolarizing block and is referred to as phase 2, desensitization, or dual block.[29-32] As phase 2 block develops, fade is seen with both tetanus and TOF stimulation. The TOF ratio decreases to 0.3–0.4.[29] Additional doses of succinylcholine chloride cause tachyphylaxis and even reversal of the block (Fig. 21–4).[33] The mechanism of phase 2 block is presently unknown. Phase 2 block may be more likely to develop in the presence of potent inhalation agents than during nitrous oxide narcotic anesthesia.[34] Characteristics of a phase 2 block include: (1) fade with tetanic or TOF stimulation; (2) post-tetanic facilitation; (3) antagonism with anticholinesterase agents; and (4) diminished response after repeated doses (tachyphylaxis).

Reversal of Phase 2 Block

Phase 2 block, produced by 5 mg/kg succinylcholine chloride given over a period of more than 90 minutes, can be antagonized by neostigmine. The infusion must be stopped 10 minutes prior to the neostigmine in order to

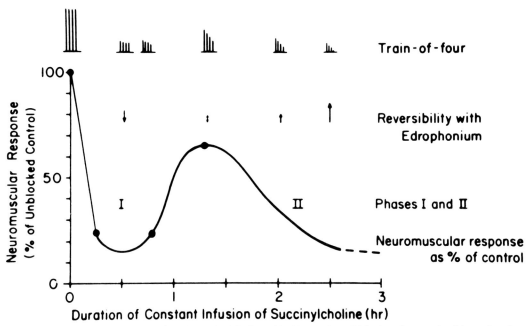

Figure 21–4. During continuous infusion of succinylcholine chloride, a phase 1 block—characterized by reduced neuromuscular response, little fade on train-of-four (TOF), and increased blockade with edrophonium—is seen initially. During phase 2, there is fade on TOF, increasing reversibility of the block by edrophonium, and accumulation of the slowly recovering residual block. (From Lee C: Succinylcholine: Its past, present, and future. Semin Anesth 1984; 4[3]. with permission.)

allow circulating succinylcholine chloride levels to diminish and thus terminate phase 1 block.[35] Furthermore, a 90% block produced by succinylcholine chloride after development of phase 2 can be reversed with neostigmine more rapidly than can a 90% pancuronium bromide–induced block.[36]

Nondepolarizing Blockade

This type of block is produced by d-tubocurarine, pancuronium bromide, metocurine iodide, atracurium besylate, gallamine triethiodide, vecuronium bromide, mivacurium chloride, and pipecuronium bromide. All these agents bind to the alpha subunits of the ACh receptor or physically block the ion channel in the motor end-plate. Some agents cause direct physical blockade of channels. This effect is more common at high concentrations of relaxant in the synaptic cleft. Characteristics of nondepolarizing blockade include: (1) absence of fasciculations; (2) fade with rapid stimulation; (3) post-tetanic facilitation; and (4) antagonism by anticholinesterase drugs.

Receptor Function

Administration of nondepolarizing relaxants diminishes the peak tension developed in response to neural stimulation. Besides this diminution in ten-

---

Table 21–3. EVIDENCE SUPPORTING
PREJUNCTIONAL ETIOLOGY FOR FADE

The motor endplate response to ACh does not change during rapid stimulation that causes fade.[25]
d-Tubocurarine causes progressive decline in ACh release during high-frequency stimulation.[25]
Postjunctional blockers erabutoxin or alpha-bungarotoxin decrease twitch tension without fade of TOF or tetanus.[25]
The onset and recovery of fade and twitch depression have differing pharmacokinetics.[91,92]
Pancuronium bromide, primarily a postjunctional blocker, may not cause much tetanic fade.*

---

* Cashman JN, Jones RM, Vella LM: Fade characteristics and onset times following administration of pancuronium, tubocurarine and a mixture of both agents. Br J Anaesth 1985; 57:488–492; and Stanec A, Baker T: Prejunctional and postjunctional effects of the tubocurarine and pancuronium in man. Br J Anaesth 1984; 56:607–611.

sion, there is also a phenomenon called fade. When tetanic stimulation or stimulation greater than 0.1 Hz is applied to a motor neuron, the developed motor tension progressively decreases. At present, it is thought that these two phenomena, diminished tension and fade, are the result of postjunctional and prejunctional receptor blockade, respectively. There is ample evidence to support this theory (Table 21–3). These observations indicate that depression of twitch and peak tetanic tension differ from fade of TOF or tetanus in that they are the result of ACh receptor antagonists acting at different sites. It is thought, at present, that prejunctional receptor antagonists prevent these receptors from promoting ACh synthesis and mobilization.[25] Postjunctional effects can be measured by single twitch, peak tetanic tension, or by the first twitch in a TOF. Prejunctional effects are evaluated by the T-1/T-4 ratio and by tetanic fade.

EVALUATION OF NEUROMUSCULAR BLOCKADE

Clinical Criteria versus Evoked Responses

Evaluation of neuromuscular blockade is frequently done purely on the basis of clinical impression. Doses of relaxants are selected empirically, and clinical cues such as gross movement and muscle tone are used to determine subsequent muscle relaxant doses. Postoperatively, the evaluation of neuromuscular blockade is based upon observation of various volitional motor responses of the awake patient.

Clinical criteria commonly used to indicate adequate recovery of neuromuscular function are listed in Table 21–4. These criteria represent a variety of ways in which the integrity of NMJ can be evaluated during stress. Such methods are imprecise and nonrigorous, and they cannot be used to

Table 21–4. CLINICAL CRITERIA FOR ADEQUACY OF NEUROMUSCULAR TRANSMISSION

Head lift for 5 seconds[100,103]
Sustained hand grasp[36,103]
Absence of nystagmus/diplopia[100,104]
Coordinated breathing pattern
Wide opening of the eyes[103]
Normal voice
Coordinated swallowing[103,104]
Tongue protrusion[103]
Normal abdominal and sternocleidomastoid tone
Negative inspiratory force of at least -20 to -25 cm H_2O[104]
Vital capacity of 15 cc/kg[103]
Sustained leg lift*
Sustained arm lift (45 seconds)[48]

* Mason LJ, Betts E: Leglift and maximum inspiratory force, clinical signs of neuromuscular blockade reversal in neonates and infants. Anesthesiology 1980; 52:441–442.

evaluate the anesthetized patient. They usually do not compare the postoperative response with a measured preoperative baseline. For example, the majority of patients can perform a head lift far in excess of 5 seconds preoperatively; hence, the ability to do this for only 5 seconds postoperatively does not indicate a return to baseline. Viby-Mogensen and colleagues demonstrated that 28% of patients evaluated in the recovery room were able to sustain a 5-second head lift but still had evidence of residual blockade using TOF.[4] The head lift test was useful only as a gross indicator of residual blockade, since no patient with a TOF ratio <0.40 was able to perform the test.[4]

More recent studies have confirmed these findings.[5, 6] Russell and Serle evaluated hand grip as an indicator of residual blockade.[37] They used a hydraulic hand dynamometer to establish a preanesthetic baseline, and they showed that patients able to sustain head lift for 5 seconds had a mean hand grip strength about 29% of preoperative baseline as compared with hand grip strength of 77% in those patients who had not received muscle relaxants. Half the patients who could perform a 5-second head lift had less than 25% of baseline hand grip strength. This study shows that the lack of sensitivity demonstrated by the usual clinical tests is primarily due to failure to obtain an accurate baseline measurement. Although it is clear that individual bedside tests of neuromuscular function are insensitive, there are no studies evaluating the ability of experienced clinicians using a variety of examinations to detect residual blockade.

Evoked Responses

The most reliable method for evaluating recovery from neuromuscular-blocking agents is to stimulate a peripheral motor nerve and evaluate the

Table 21–5. COMMONLY UTILIZED
PERIPHERAL NERVES

Nerve	Location	Movement Observed
Ulnar	Wrist or elbow	Thumb adduction Fifth digit movement
Posterior tibial	Posterior to the medial malleolus	Plantar flexion of the big toe
Peroneal	Lateral to the neck of the fibula	Foot dorsiflexion
Facial	Near the earlobe where the nerve emerges from the stylomastoid foramen	Orbicularis oculi contraction
Mandibular*	At the condyle and ramus angle	Jaw closure

* Nakatsuka M, Franks P, Keenan R: A method of rapid sequence induction using high-dose narcotics with vecuronium or vecuronium and pancuronium in patients with coronary artery disease. J Cardiothorac Anesth 1988; 2:177–181.

resultant motor response. The first step in the process is accomplished by delivering electrical impulses to a superficial motor nerve. Motor responses to electrical stimuli are determined by: (1) the contractile state of the muscle (electromyogram [EMG] excluded); (2) the functional state of the NMJ; (3) the site of stimulation; (4) electrical stimuli characteristics (duration, intensity, waveform); and (5) pattern of frequency of stimulation (single twitch, tetanus, TOF, post-tetanic).

Site of Stimulation

Although any motor nerve can be stimulated, it is best to use a nerve that is close to the skin surface (readily accessible to the anesthesiologist), and a muscle whose action is easily monitored. Examples of common monitoring sites are shown in Table 21–5. The ulnar nerve–adductor pollicis muscle is a particularly useful nerve-muscle unit, since stimulation over the ulnar nerve can cause thumb movement only by transmission through the nerve and not by direct muscle stimulation (Fig. 21–5; Table 21–6). A second muscle, the flexor pollicis brevis (deep head), is also innervated by the ulnar nerve and is superficial to the adductor pollicis. Visual, tactile, EMG, and in some cases, mechanomyographic (MMG) methods of evaluation may not be able to differentiate the contributions of these two muscles. The adductor pollicis is a deep muscle with the major portion being covered dorsally by the first dorsal interosseous muscle, and its palmar aspect being partially covered by the flexor pollicis brevis and the first lumbrical. Despite frequent reference to the adductor pollicis *brevis* in the literature, there is no such entity. The proper name is adductor pollicis.

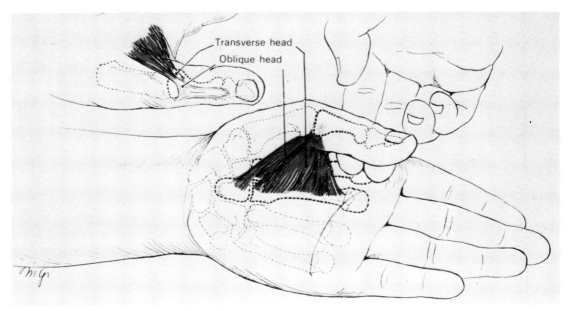

Figure 21–5. The adductor pollicis muscle of the thumb, innervated by the ulnar nerve, is a convenient site to monitor neuromuscular blockade. (From Kendall FP, McCreary ER: Muscle Testing and Function, 61. © 1963, the Williams & Wilkins Co., Baltimore.)

The response to muscle relaxants varies somewhat with the nerve-motor unit being monitored. The facial nerve, for example, is relatively resistant to relaxants and tends to underestimate the degree of relaxation.[38] Caffrey and coworkers[38a] compared thumb twitch with orbicularis oculi twitch using force transducers. During recovery from atracurium block, four facial twitches could be present before the thumb had recovered a single twitch of the TOF. Some researchers have tried to demonstrate the relationship between block seen in peripheral muscle groups and that occurring in the diaphragm. By measuring transdiaphragmatic pressures during bilateral phrenic nerve stimulation Chauvin and coworkers showed that vecuronium bromide–induced block had more rapid onset and offset of blockade in the diaphragm than in the adductor pollicis (1.6 minutes versus 2.5 minutes).[36]

Table 21–6. HAND MUSCLES SUPPLIED BY THE ULNAR NERVE

Abductor digiti minimi
Adductor pollicis
Dorsal and palmar interossei
Flexor digiti minimi
Flexor pollicis brevis (deep head)
Lumbricales 3 and 4
Opponens digiti minimi
Palmaris brevis

Data from Pansky B: Review of Gross Anatomy. New York: Macmillan, 1979.

This may have been secondary to increased blood flow to the diaphragm. Several studies have demonstrated that the diaphragm is only about 50% as sensitive to muscle relaxants as is the adductor pollicis.[38-41]

A common problem when using nerve stimulators is the determination of whether a given motor response is the result of neural stimulation or of direct muscle stimulation. It is also possible to rule out direct muscle stimulation by noting the *presence of fade* with TOF stimulation or with 50-Hz tetanus for 5 seconds. Post-tetanic potentiation, however, can be caused by either direct muscle or neural stimulation.

Characteristics of Electrical Stimuli

Motor responses are evoked by stimulating peripheral nerves with electrical impulses. The physical characteristics of electrical stimuli influence the motor responses that they evoke. As a result, there are standard methods of stimulating peripheral nerves.

Supramaximal

The stimulation current required to trigger an action potential varies among nerves in a given bundle. As stimulation current is increased, the number of nerves reaching the threshold increases until all the nerves are responding (Fig. 21–6). Once the threshold has been reached for a given nerve, it depolarizes and releases ACh at the motor end-plates of all the muscle fibers it supplies. In the absence of neuromuscular blockers, motor end plate depolarization induces these muscle fibers to contract in an all-or-none fashion. In theory, a plateau is reached at which further increments in stimulating current do not produce increased motor response. If all the neurons are being depolarized, any subsequent changes in motor response result from effects at the NMJ or from changes in contractility. It is usual practice to stimulate at *supra*maximum currents, 25–50% greater than that required to elicit maximum response.[42] This ensures that despite alterations in electrode impedance or position, all neurons in the bundle continue to be depolarized.

Duration and Waveform

Pulses greater than 0.2–0.3 m/second that are not square waves may exceed the nerve refractory period, thereby causing repetitive firing.[43, 44]

Patterns of Stimulation

There are four methods in which individual, supramaximal, 0.1–0.2 msec square wave impulses are used clinically: single twitch, TOF, tetanic, and post-tetanic single twitch. It is important to understand the basis for their use and their individual limitations. The comparison of these techniques in clinical practice is discussed in this section.

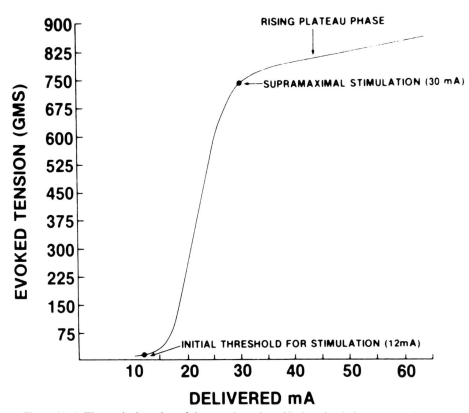

Figure 21-6. The evoked tension of the muscle varies with the stimulating current. As current increases, the number of nerves reaching threshold increases until all are responding. After all nerves have reached threshold, further increases in current fail to increase the motor response (plateau). Supramaximal currents are used to ensure depolarization of all neurons. (From Kopman EA, Lawson D: Milliamperage requirements for supramaximal stimulation of the ulnar nerve with surface electrodes. Anesthesiology 1984; 61:84. With permission.)

Single Twitch

The simplest pattern of stimulation is the single twitch. The degree of relaxation is determined by dividing the measured elicited response (T_1) by the control response (Tc). Recovery from relaxants is sometimes measured by the recovery index or time interval between 25% and 75% recovery.

Frequency. In the presence of relaxants, high-frequency neural stimulation results in a progressive decline in the amount of ACh released from the motor neuron terminals.[45, 46] Normally, no decrement in response is observed below frequencies of 50 Hz, because of the margin of safety afforded by the NMJ.[47, 48] When a nondepolarizing blocking agent is administered, prejunctional effects greatly decrease the amount of ACh released. The motor response to single stimuli exceeding 0.15 Hz (1 twitch/7–10 seconds) declines to a baseline that is less than the initial response and represents an equilibrium between ACh liberation and synthesis.[49, 50] Thus, rapid stimulation rates potentiate the relaxant-induced stress of the NMJ.

Without neuromuscular block, a response that has been conditioned

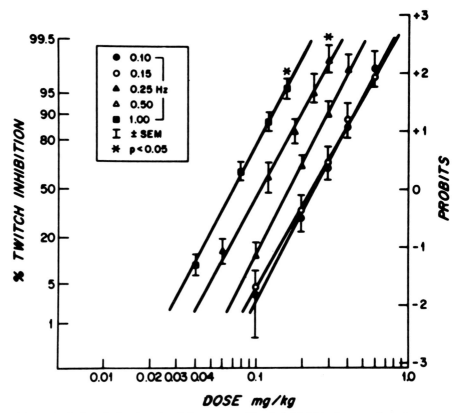

Figure 21–7. Cumulative dose (mg/kg)–response (% twitch inhibition) curves for a d-tubocurarine at different stimulation frequencies (symbols in box). Increase in stimulation frequency shifts the dose-response curve to the left. The dose of d-tubocurarine required to produce 50% or 95% twitch inhibition is increased by stimulation at 1 Hz compared with 0.1 Hz. (From Ali HH, Savarese JJ: Stimulation frequency and dose response to d-tubocurarine in man. Anesthesiology 1980; 52:37. With permission.)

(conditioning means a stimulation occurring in the 10-second interval preceding the measured response) by a preceding response less than 10 seconds earlier has an increased amplitude. In the presence of a nondepolarizing relaxant, however, the second response is reduced.[50] Ali and Savarese have demonstrated that as stimulation frequency is increased, the apparent dose-response curve to d-tubocurarine is shifted to the left.[49] The dose of d-tubocurarine required to produce 50% and 95% depression of the response height (ED_{50} and ED_{95}, respectively) was greater at 0.1 Hz than at 1.0 Hz. A key point is that the dose of d-tubocurarine producing 95% twitch depression at 0.1–0.15 Hz was associated with excellent intubating conditions, whereas at 1.0 Hz there was inadequate relaxation (Fig. 21–7). Single twitch frequency of 0.1–0.15 Hz therefore provides a means of monitoring neuromuscular blockade over a clinically significant range of muscle relaxation.

There are two drawbacks to the single twitch method of stimulation: (1) A baseline prior to administration of relaxants must be established; hence, the technique is not helpful in patients who have already received relaxants; and (2) It is insensitive for the detection of residual blockade.

Table 21–7. COMPARISON OF TOF AND SINGLE STIMULATION TECHNIQUES

Twitch Disappearance	T_1 Depression
Fourth	75%
Third	80%
Second	90%
First	100%

The relationship between the depression of the first mechanical thumb twitch (T_1) of a TOF and the last twitch in the train during d-tubocurarine relaxation. (Data from Lee CM: Train-of-4 quantitation of competitive neuromuscular block. Anesth Analg 1975; 54:649–653.)

TOF

The use of TOF stimuli to monitor neuromuscular block during anesthesia was first introduced by Ali and colleagues in 1970.[51] Conventionally, TOF stimulation consists of four supramaximal, 0.1–0.2 msec, square wave impulses delivered at a rate of 2/second (2 Hz). The TOF method is based on the principle that stimulation at frequencies greater than 0.1–0.15 Hz in the presence of nondepolarizing relaxants causes a rapid decline in the evoked response until a new baseline is reached, usually after the third stimuli. The degree of relaxation determines the response height of the second, third, and fourth stimuli. Blockade can thus be evaluated by comparing the ratio of the fourth response with that of the first response. Since this method uses the first response as the reference point, no preblock baseline needs to be established. There must be at least a 10-second quiescent interval between each TOF, so that the first twitch of each is unconditioned. In each TOF, the three twitches after the first are conditioned. Failure to wait 10 seconds until the next TOF conditions the first response in the train and thus decreases the difference between the first and the last response. As a result, the degree of blockade is underestimated. Stimulation with fewer trains or slower frequencies sacrifices sensitivity, whereas higher-frequency stimulation causes fusion of individual mechanical responses.[51]

The TOF method can be used to monitor both mild and intense relaxation. For monitoring residual blockade, a TOF ratio of 0.7 has been used as a bench mark to indicate a level of relaxation that does not compromise respiration. Surgical degrees of relaxation are monitored by counting the number of twitches present in a TOF. Adequate surgical relaxation is usually indicated by the presence of only one or two twitches in a TOF. Lee compared the first and last twitches in a TOF after administration of d-tubocurarine using a force transducer to measure thumb abduction.[52] He found that there was no change in the single twitch until the TOF ratio was decreased by 20–25%. He also demonstrated the relationship between fade of TOF and the depression of single response at varying levels of block (Table 21–7). Intense neuromuscular block is evaluated by counting the number of twitches present after tetanic stimulation.

The advantages of the TOF method include greater sensitivity than sin-

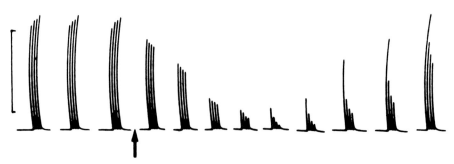

Figure 21-8. The TOF varies during onset and offset of nondepolarizing block. Vecuronium bromide was given (*arrow*) to a cat nerve–tibialis muscle preparation. Fade of the TOF is more marked during recovery of neuromuscular function than with initial twitch depression. (From Bowman WC: Prejunctional and postjunctional cholinoreceptors at the neuromuscular junction. Anesth Analg 1980; 59:940. With permission.)

gle twitch for evaluation of residual blockade, lack of need to establish a baseline response, and performance in awake patients with minimum discomfort. It has also been shown to be useful in monitoring high degrees of blockade and avoids the distortion of neuromuscular transmission that results from tetanic stimulation.

A problem with the method is that the TOF ratio can only be determined by quantitative method such as EMG or MMG. Some patients may have TOF fade despite the absence of fade with 50-Hz tetanus for 5 seconds.[53] It has also been clearly demonstrated that the relationship between TOF ratio and single twitch depression varies with onset and offset of block as well as with relaxant dose, duration of relaxation, and different reversal agents. There is usually significantly more fade present during offset of block compared to onset. This probably reflects differing pharmacokinetic properties at pre- and postjunctional receptors (Fig. 21-8).

Tetanus

Tetanic stimulation consists of single, supramaximal, 0.1–0.2 msec square waves delivered at rates of 20 or more/second. Tetanic stimulation, therefore, is rapid single twitch stimulation taken to the extreme. At a stimulation rate greater than 5 Hz, the mechanical response begins to fuse and fails to return to its original position. Complete fusion occurs at 20–30 Hz.[54] By using EMG techniques, it is possible to observe the muscle response to each stimulation within a tetanic burst. As previously mentioned, rapid stimulation stresses the mechanisms responsible for ACh release. Although there is a margin of safety, sustained rapid stimulation produces fade even in the absence of neuromuscular relaxants (Table 21-8).[55] The range of frequencies used clinically has been 30–200 Hz. Most investigators now feel that tetanus of 50 Hz of 5 seconds' duration should be used. This conclusion is based on the findings by Merton in 1954, demonstrating that with 50 Hz stimulation, the force of contraction is the same as that produced by a maximum effort of an awake patient (Fig. 21-9).[56] Other investigators demonstrated that tetanic pulses of 80 Hz applied during maximum voluntary contraction do

Table 21–8. TETANIC STIMULATION
WITHOUT FADE

Tetanus (Hz)	Duration (seconds)
300	1
150–200	2
80–100	3
70	5
50	10

The maximum duration of tetanic stimulation at various frequencies that can be delivered in the absence of relaxants without developing fade. (Data from Stanec A, Heyduk J, Stanec G, Orkin LR: Tetanic fade and post tetanic tension in the absence of neuromuscular blocking agents in anesthetized man. Anesth Analg 1978; 57:102–107.)

not produce an increase in contractile force or in compound action potential.[57] Waud and Waud showed that with d-tubocurarine, tetanic stimulation is more sensitive than single twitch stimulation for detecting residual blockade. They showed that the sustained response to single twitches required 25% of receptors to be free, whereas sustained 100-Hz tetanus response required 50% receptor availability.[47]

There are two limitations to the use of tetanic stimulation: Tetanus of

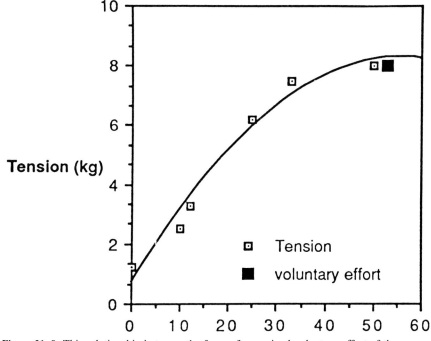

Figure 21–9. This relationship between the force of a maximal voluntary effort of the adductor pollicis and its response to tetanic stimulation at different frequencies demonstrates that at 50 Hz, the tension (force) is identical. (Adapted from Merton PA: Voluntary strength and fatigue. J Physiol [Lond] 1954; 123:553–564.)

Resting thumb tension	Developed twitch tension
g	g ± SE
50	312.8 ± 34.8*
100	371.3 ± 39.0†
200	399.8 ± 37.7
300	410.0 ± 35.6

Figure 21–10. Developed twitch tension varies with the load or counterforce on the muscle (thumb). NMJ function should always be evaluated against a resistance and at baseline conditions before administration of a neuromuscular blocking drug.
* $p < 0.001$ from 100, 200, 300 g.
† $p < 0.05$ from 200, 300 g.
(Reprinted with permission from the International Anesthesia Research Society from Cumulative dose response curves for gallamine: Effect of altered resting thumb tension and mode of stimulation, by Donlon JV, Savarese JJ, Ali HH, Anesthesia and Analgesia, 1979; 58:379).

50 Hz causes considerable discomfort and is, therefore, not well suited for use in awake patients; and tetanic stimulation may condition subsequent stimuli for a period of 6–30 minutes.[50, 58] Repeated administration of tetanic stimuli may demonstrate a false recovery from muscle relaxants.

The typical practice of simply observing the tetanic response against no resistance is not acceptable, since patients can sustain this type of contraction preoperatively for extended period without much effort. Counterforce to thumb movement should be provided in order to compare the force with the estimated baseline force (Fig. 21–10). If supramaximal stimulating current is used with 50-Hz tetanus, the resultant contraction is identical to the patient's maximum voluntary response.

Post-Tetanic Potentiation

Tetanic stimulation enhances the response of a twitch immediately following it. This is called post-tetanic potentiation and may be due to both augmentation of contraction and facilitation of transmission.[59] Augmentation of contraction occurs as a result of increased calcium release within the muscle fiber and is detected in the absence of neuromuscular blocking drugs by all methods of measurement except EMG.[60] Facilitation of transmission occurs only in the presence of nondepolarizing neuromuscular-blocking drugs and is the result of increased ACh synthesis/mobilization that persists after tetanic stimulation. Facilitation is not observed in the absence of neuromuscular blockade, since an excess of ACh is normally released.[61]

The technique of post-tetanic stimulation may be used to demonstrate either nondepolarizing or phase 2 block or the degree of intense neuromuscular blockade.[58, 62, 63] Ridley and Hatch used tetanic stimulation of 50 Hz for 5 seconds followed by single twitch at 1 Hz to evaluate depth of block, a modification of the post-tetanic count method. They noted that a post-tetanic count less than 10 ensured adequate surgical relaxation, whereas a count greater than 15 indicated easy reversibility.[64]

Nerve Stimulators

Requirements

Since current density causes nerve depolarization, peripheral nerve stimulators (PNSs) should deliver a constant current over a range of impedances. Constant voltage stimulators have been shown to provide inadequate stimulation with high impedances that are typical of surface electrodes.[65] The amount of current required to produce supramaximal stimulation varies between patients and is a function of electrode type and position, skin resistance, edema, obesity, and wrist diameter. Pollmaecher and associates demonstrated that, with surface electrodes, maximum stimulation required 38 ± 23 mA, but 6% of patients required greater than 80 mA.[54] Kopman and Lawson showed that 30 mA was adequate to produce supramaximal stimulation using surface electrodes with wrist circumferences less than or equal to 16 cm. They concluded that battery-operated PNSs should deliver no less than 50–60 mA.[66] The requirements for needle electrodes are considerably less. Gravenstein and Paulus reported supramaximal stimulation with 5–8 mA using needle electrodes.[67] A test of six commercially available PNSs showed that none was able to produce either constant current or constant voltage over the range of clinically relevant impedances. The output current in all the PNSs tested declined at resistances above 1 KΩ.[68]

Electrode Placement and Nerve Depolarization

Electrode placement affects the ability to deliver supramaximal stimuli using clinically available PNSs. As electrodes are moved farther apart, the interelectrode impedance increases, and eventually, inadequate stimulating current results. Care must be taken when applying the surface electrodes to seal the outer edges before applying pressure to the central portion. If this is not done, gel can be extruded beyond the electrode, creating a large contact area or possibly forming a direct contact with the other electrode (cathode-anode bridge). This bridging effect can be observed on the ohmmeter as very low impedance (<1–2 KΩ).

An electrode placed over a nerve is called the active electrode and concentrates the current on the nerve. The effect is greatest on the nerve wall closest to the electrode. Nerve depolarization resulting from electrical current takes place under the cathode (black, $-$), whereas hyperpolarization occurs under the anode (red, $+$).[42, 69–71] Berger and coworkers, using needle electrodes, demonstrated submaximum stimulation when the electrodes pacemaker (facial nerve stimulation) and tachycardia in an atrium and ventricle paced, sensed, inhibited, or triggered (DDD) pacemaker (median nerve somatosensory evoked potential) has also been described.[77a]

Needle versus Surface Electrodes for Stimulation

Electrodes can be either needles that are inserted through the skin or surface electrodes placed on the skin. Needle electrodes have lower impedance than surface electrodes do, but they are more invasive and present the possibility for infection and tissue trauma. When needles are used, care must be exercised to avoid penetration of muscle fascia, since this may produce movement artifact. Normally, surface electrodes are satisfactory to provide supramaximal stimulation, and in the case of the EMG, they provide accurate recording of evoked potentials.

The adequacy of surface or needle electrodes can be checked by the use of a variable output stimulator. By incrementally increasing the applied current, one should be able to achieve a maximum response followed by a plateau. The stimulator can then be set at 25–50% above the maximum response (*supra*maximal stimulation). If no plateau is reached, inadequate current is being delivered to the nerve, and the electrodes should be changed or a more powerful stimulator used. In some cases, therefore, surface electrodes produce *sub*maximal stimulation, resulting in overestimation of neuromuscular block. In a study of 50 awake volunteers, surface electrodes resulted in 6% incidence of submaximal stimulation despite the use of a stimulator capable of 80 mA output.[54] Pierce and coworkers showed that reliable supramaximum stimulation could be achieved using either surface or needle electrodes as long as adequate current was provided.[73]

Preparation of the skin prior to placement of surface electrodes markedly decreases the measured impedance. One of the most effective methods is to thoroughly clean the skin with alcohol, abrade lightly with gauze or abrasive paste, and finally, rub a commercial electrolyte gel into the area of contact with a wooden applicator stick. This removes the high-resistance superficial layers of skin as well as any sweat, which is itself a good conductor. This method decreases the impedance by 50% or more. Surface electrodes must not be stored for extended periods of time. Electrodes stored for approximately 2 years demonstrated an impedance increase of over 100%, secondary to drying of the electrolyte gel. After electrode application, impedance decreases over time, with the final value being dependent on the method of skin preparation used (Fig. 21–11).

Complications of Monitoring

There are very few reported complications related to monitoring neuromuscular transmission. Burn injuries have been reported secondary to interaction with an electrocautery and by intermittent stimulation using spherical metal electrodes.[74,75] A case of ulnar nerve palsy resulting from pressure over the ulnar groove by a surface electrode connector and improper arm positioning has been described.[76] Thumb paresthesia lasting 4–14 days has been reported after the use of a particular type of thumb twitch force transducer.[77] Interference from peripheral nerve stimulators, including inhibition of a ventricle paced, ventricle sensed, inhibited (VVI) pacemaker (facial nerve stimulation) and tachycardia in an atrium and ventricle paced, sensed, inhibited, or triggered (DDD) pacemaker (median nerve somatosensory evoked potential) has also been described.[77a]

PNS Testing

Actual testing of stimulator output is rarely done. One can set the stimulator on a low setting and feel the electrodes for a shock. An alternative

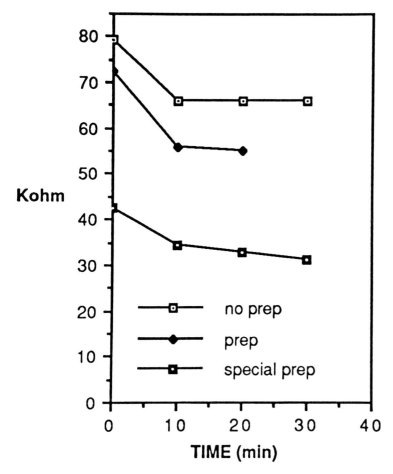

Figure 21–11. A comparison of the impedances of surface electrodes after no skin preparation, skin preparation with alcohol (preparation), and skin preparation with alcohol/abrasion/electrolyte gel (special preparation), as described in text.

to this method is to attach the leads to a neon lamp (type NE-2) available from most electronic parts suppliers.[78]

Quantifying Evoked Responses

Two methods are used at present to assess the motor response resulting from nerve stimulation. The mechanical response, actual movement, can be simply observed or quantified on a graph (MMG). The second method, EMG, measures the compound action potential, which represents the total current created by the action potentials of the contracting muscle fibers.

The simplest method of evaluating mechanical responses is by visual or tactile estimation. These methods are unreliable for the detection of residual blockade. Donati and associates have shown that experienced observers are frequently unable to detect fade on TOF stimulation, even when the ratio was as low as 0.40.[79] Thomas and colleagues noted a case in which force transduction demonstrated significant fade of TOF and tetanus that experienced observers were unable to detect using visual or tactile means.[80] Any visible fade of TOF is associated with a TOF ratio less than 0.7.[50] Viby-

Mogensen and coworkers investigated the correlation between tactile or visual methods and force transduction.[81] They concluded that inability to detect TOF ratio between 0.41–0.70 using visual or tactile means is common. Two years' experience with PNS did not improve performance, feeling or seeing a control response did not improve TOF evaluation, and TOF ratios as low as 0.3–0.4 were sometimes undetectable.[81]

Visual and tactile means are adequate for evaluating more profound block associated with surgical relaxation.[82] MMG is a more precise method of evaluating the motor response, since a transducer provides a quantitative measurement of the motor response.

EMG versus MMG

EMG involves the measurement of the combined action potentials of the contracting motor units. Both EMG and MMG represent ways to quantitate the number of muscle fibers that contract with a given stimulus. Since supramaximum stimuli are used, the motor response is dependent upon the number of motor end-plates that are depolarized beyond threshold. It is important to note that the graded motor response is produced by varying the number of muscle fibers contracting in an all-or-none fashion. In the case of MMG, the measured response is also dependent upon the contractile state of the muscle fibers. For example, a patient given dantrolene sodium has a diminished force tension but an unchanged EMG response. Post-tetanic potentiation in the absence of muscle relaxants is observed on MMG, whereas its presence during EMG is indicative of phase 2 depolarizing block or of nondepolarizing blockade.[60, 61] Another difference between these two methods is that evaluation using MMG measures the response of the entire muscle, whereas the EMG measures the response of only those fibers lying beneath the active electrode.[34] The EMG therefore samples a population of nerve fibers and assumes that this represents the entire muscle. In theory, errors result if needle electrodes are used to record the compound action potential, since a very small population of fibers is sampled. This is probably only a concern when using needles containing active and recording electrodes in the same barrel (bipolar).

Many studies have evaluated the correlation between EMG and MMG. For nondepolarizing agents, the EMG method tends to show less blockade present than does MMG.[61, 83–85] Depolarizing agents produce the opposite results, with EMG overestimating the degree of block.[86] Thus EMG underestimates nondepolarizing blockade and overestimates depolarizing blockade when compared with the gold standard, MMG. The results produced by either of these techniques are highly dependent upon the nerve-muscle unit being monitored. Muscles vary in their response to neuromuscular-blocking drugs. The reasons for this are not clear but may be related to differences in temperature, perfusion, and content of slow- and fast-twitch fibers. An example is the difference observed between the thenar MMG and the hypothenar EMG. Using single twitch, tetanus, and post-tetanic twitch, Katz evaluated hypothenar EMG, thenar EMG, and mechanical thumb twitch. Extrapolation of his data shows that 90% depression of the single mechanical twitch correlated with 82% thenar and 72% hypothenar EMG

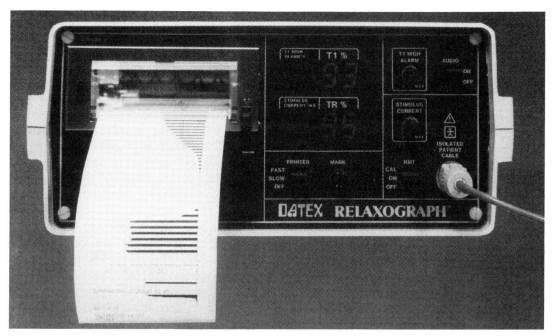

Figure 21–12. A clinical EMG monitor is the Datex Neuromuscular Transmission Monitor Relaxograph. It measures the compound action potential resulting from TOF stimulation. The first twitch is compared with that prior to neuromuscular blockade as well as to the fourth twitch (if present). (From Datex Medical Instrumentation, Tewksbury, MA. With permission.)

depression.[60] These figures agree with Kopman's data, which show that the single thumb twitch MMG was depressed 15% more than was hypothenar EMG.[85] Epstein and Epstein also demonstrated 14% greater depression of the thenar MMG than the hypothenar EMG.[61] These studies indicate that the relationship between thenar and hypothenar EMG is MMG thenar + 0.14% = EMG hypothenar. It may be appropriate to use different criteria for onset and reversal of nondepolarizing blockade based upon the type of monitoring used.

EMG. This technique measures a summation of biphasic action potentials called the compound muscle action potential. The compound action potential is a brief, low-voltage event that must be amplified. This response is a biphasic wave that can be quantified either by amplitude or by integration of the area under the curve. Either technique produces similar results.[86]

An example of a commercially available EMG monitor is the Puritan-Bennett Datex Neuromuscular Transmission Monitor 221 (Puritan-Bennett, Wilmington, MA). (Fig. 21–12). This device produces TOF stimuli and then measures the integrated compound action potential. Individual stimuli are square wave, 0.1-msec duration, and are generated by a fully isolated constant current stimulator. The supramaximal stimulation current level is determined after start-up by giving single twitches at 5 mA increments until no further increase in EMG is produced. The current is then increased by 20% to produce supramaximal stimulation. The maximum stimulation current is 70 mA.

Traditional TOF stimuli are given at 20-second intervals. The compound action potential resulting from each stimulation is amplified, rectified, and then electronically integrated. A stimulation artifact is produced with each twitch. It occurs before, and is independent of, the resultant muscle response. The amplitude of this artifact after each TOF is compared with the initial artifact, and a decrease of 30% or more is presumed to be secondary to an increase in electrode impedance and "ELEC OFF" is noted in the display. The first twitch of the TOF is compared with the prerelaxation baseline and is displayed as a ratio (first twitch/reference). If four twitches are present, the ratio of last twitch/first twitch is displayed. The monitor can be moved with the patient from operating room to postanesthesia recovery area, since the calibration values are retained for 15 minutes after power disconnect. An RS-232 port is provided for computerized data acquisition (see Chapter 11).

EMG Electrodes. The key to successful EMG monitoring is skin preparation and placement of the surface electrodes. A pair of electrodes, called the reference and the active electrodes, monitors the compound action potential. These electrodes convert varying ion currents generated by nerve and muscle activity into varying electric currents in wires that are connected to the amplifier. The optimum location for the active ($-$) electrode of the pair is over the innervation zone of the muscle, usually midway between origin and insertion. Some authors suggest using a strip electrode oriented perpendicular to the muscle belly and positioned over the innervation zone.[87] The reference ($+$) electrode is positioned away from muscles that are innervated by the nerve being stimulated. Some investigators position the reference electrode over the insertion of the muscle, since this ensures that no contracting muscle is under the electrode and, at the same time, places the electrodes parallel to the axis of depolarization, thus maximizing the signal. Kalli compared several electrode placements and demonstrated that positioning the active electrode over the adductor pollicis innervation zone and the reference electrode on the index finger produced the least response variation and drift.[87a]

Pregelled silver–silver chloride surface electrodes work well with adequate skin preparation. Surface electrodes that connect to the EMG leads through a hinged flap work best. This design allows lead movement without transmission to the skin-electrode interface. The optimum interelectrode distance is unknown. Distances larger than 6 cm should probably be avoided, since an increase in impedance requires higher amplification leading to interference from background noise. Needle electrodes of the monopolar type can be used, although surface electrodes are usually adequate.

A ground electrode should be positioned between the stimulating and the ground electrodes in order to decrease stimulation artifact. The ground electrode should be large in order to decrease skin-electrode impedance.[88] The EMG is also dependent upon the location of the stimulating electrodes. The positioning of the stimulating electrodes affects the ability to achieve supramaximal stimulation and alters the shape of the compound action potential. As the stimulating electrodes, specifically the cathode, are moved to a more proximal position, the EMG response demonstrates diminished amplitude and longer duration. This occurs because differential conduction

---

Table 21–9. ADVANTAGES OF EMG
OVER MMG

Less immobilization required
Greater flexibility in muscles monitored
Easier to perform on infants
Individual responses to tetanic train measurable
Measure of neuromuscular refractory period
Enhanced portability

Data from Lee C, Katz RL, Arnold SJL, Glaser B: A new instrument for continuous recording of the evoked compound electromyogram in the clinical setting. Anesth Analg 1977; 56:260–270.

velocity along the motor neurons is magnified by increased distance. This disperses motor unit activation over a larger time span.[88]

Advantages and Disadvantages of EMG. The advantages of EMG over MMG are listed in Table 21–9. Common recording sites are the abductor pollicis (thenar), the abductor digiti minimi (hypothenar), and the first dorsal interosseous muscles of the hand. The hand and electrode leads should be well secured, since movement can produce artifact resembling action potentials. The EMG is a brief event and therefore cannot be recorded on a polygraph. The response can be photographed from an oscilloscope or stored in memory and then displayed on paper. This method avoids some of the problems that are inherent with MMG, including extremity fixation, transducer overload, preload requirement, and twitch angle. Unfortunately, the EMG method has its own assortment of problems. The available EMG monitors are somewhat unreliable, requiring readjustment by the manufacturer during the course of operation. Furthermore, the methodology is not well established, especially in regard to electrode types and placement. The output from two EMG monitors on the same patient may not be identical.

MMG. It is most common to measure the adductor pollicis contraction in response to ulnar nerve stimulation. A force transducer is used to convert the contractile force into electrical current that can be quantified. The motor response is of longer duration than the EMG, therefore the response can be recorded on a strip chart (Fig. 21–13). Accurate measurement requires maintenance of a constant thumb angle and resting tension. A 200–800 gm preload on the muscle is necessary to provide for maximum tension development.[48, 61] Movement during the use of MMG that reduces resting tension from 200 to 50 gm may decrease twitch tension by 20–25%.[89] The transducer should be capable of responding to tensions in the 0–15 kg range, since the maximum force generated by thumb abduction is about 8 kg (see Fig. 21–10).[56] The Grass transducer that is most commonly used is the FT-10, which accurately responds to a maximum of 10 kg. The FT-03 overloads with tensions greater than 2.2 kg and, therefore, is unsuitable for abductor pollicis monitoring in the adult.[61] A force transducer apparatus has been described that can be used in the operating room with output read directly from a standard monitor that accepts transducers with 5 V/mmHg sensitivity.[48, 90]

Both EMG and MMG techniques require significantly more preparation

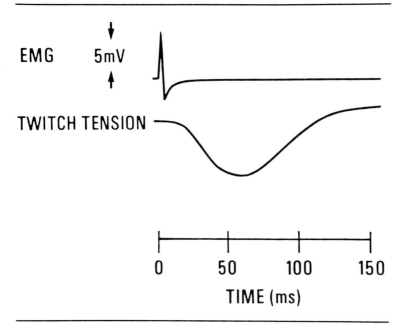

Figure 21–13. The motor response (twitch tension) is longer in duration than the electromyograph and can be recorded on a strip chart. (From Donati F, Bevan JC, Bevan DR: Neuromuscular blocking drugs in anesthesia. Can Anaesth Soc J 1984; 31:326. With permission.)

than does monitoring responses by visual or tactile means. Despite advances in both methods, their primary use continues to be related to research and teaching.

CLINICAL CORRELATIONS

This section demonstrates how the phenomenon of neuromuscular transmission and methods used to monitor it are applied to clinical management. It is difficult to provide a precise "cookbook" approach, since anesthetic depth, type of anesthetic agent used, monitoring site, technique, and patient-determined variables are all interrelated and together determine the response to neuromuscular blockers.

Intubation

When relaxants are utilized to facilitate endotracheal intubation, the goal is to produce a relaxed glottis and a motionless patient. In essence this amounts to relaxation of laryngeal, jaw, abdominal, and intercostal muscles. These muscles are more sensitive to relaxants than the diaphragm is and can be evaluated by monitoring the thumb twitch. One study suggests that jaw relaxation may precede peripheral relaxation.[87] The resistance to the diaphragm to blockade may not be of as much concern during intubation, since its action is on inspiration rather than on the forceful expiration characteristic of "bucking." It is crucial to note that neuromuscular blockers cannot substitute for adequate anesthesia.

Since any movement at all is undesirable, it is most logical to monitor single twitch, peak tetanic response, or the first response of a TOF. These are all measurements of postjunctional effect. Evaluation using TOF ratio during the onset of block may be unreliable, since the TOF ratio at onset varies with the dose. Both atracurium besylate and vecuronium bromide have been shown to exhibit less fade at onset when larger doses are used.[91, 92] Naguib and colleagues demonstrated that for atracurium besylate the priming principle speeds relaxation by an effect at the postjunctional receptor.[93]

In the majority of *adequately anesthetized* patients, 80% depression of the thumb twitch measured by MMG or EMG is adequate for intubation. For those patients in whom coughing may be hazardous, 100% depression is desirable, although total suppression of the peripheral twitch response does not guarantee lack of response to noxious stimuli in the setting of inadequate anesthesia.[94] Abolition of the twitch response can be monitored with PNS combined with visual or tactile evaluation of the elicited response.

Surgical Relaxation

The degree of blockade required during a procedure depends upon the type of anesthetic and the risk associated with spontaneous movement. Abdominal relaxation is difficult to study. Katz used abdominal EMG and noted that the spontaneous abdominal EMG correlated with degree of thumb twitch, anesthetic depth, and mechanical hyperventilation.[95] He noted that 90–95% depression of the single twitch was sufficient to produce adequate abdominal relaxation in most patients. This is probably an overestimation, since he used stimulation rates of 0.3 Hz, which would indicate more profound block than is actually present.[49] He also demonstrated an increase in spontaneous abdominal EMG activity during skin incision that could be prevented by prior infiltration with local anesthetic. This degree of relaxation corresponds to one twitch being present in TOF.[52] During surgical procedures in which patient movement constitutes a hazard, 100% depression is desirable. In this situation, it is imperative to use supramaximal stimulation. With EMG, it is possible to continuously check electrode contact by evaluation of the stimulus artifact. When a PNS is used, the use of needle electrodes increases the likelihood of delivering adequate stimulation current. Intense degrees of blockade can be evaluated by use of the post-tetanic count method.[58, 63, 82] By maintaining at least one post-tetanic twitch, the degree of block can be assessed, the recovery time predicted, and the stimulator's function evaluated.

Reversal of Relaxants

A frequent issue that arises during the clinical use of neuromuscular-blocking drugs is the reversal of intense blockade. Although it is obviously best to avoid this situation by careful monitoring and dosing practices, it is not uncommon to have a patient with >90% block at the end of the case. By using the post-tetanic count method described by Viby-Mogensen and associates, it is possible to predict the recovery time from intense blockade.[58] The post-tetanic count is the number of twitches after a tetanic stimulus of 50 Hz for 5 seconds. The times from appearance of the first post-tetanic twitch to the appearance of the first twitch of the TOF for atracurium besylate, pancuronium bromide, and vecuronium bromide are 9 minutes, 37–38 minutes, and 8.5 minutes, respectively.[58, 62, 63, 82] According to Lee's results, the appearance of the first twitch of the TOF corresponds to 90–99% block.[52] Using neostigmine, a 90% block can be reversed to a TOF ratio <0.7 for atracurium besylate or vecuronium bromide, in less than 10 minutes.[21, 96, 98] Reversal of intense pancuronium or d-tubocurarine block may take up to 30 minutes. Katz used neostigmine, 2.5 mg, in adults and showed that, when the single twitch was depressed by 80% or less by pancuronium bromide, a return to baseline twitch was achieved in 3–14 minutes. When there was greater than 80% depression, reversal took 8–29 minutes.[7, 55] Some authors feel that compared with edrophonium neostigmine provides more rapid and reliable reversal of intense block.[98] Regardless of the relaxant used, reversal of intense block takes longer and is more variable than is reversal of fewer degrees of relaxation. When reversing 90% block, enough time must be allowed for full reversal to occur. The maximum dose of antagonist should be given well ahead of time. Factors affecting reversal, such as acidosis or hypothermia, should be corrected.

Assessment of Recovery from Relaxants

In an ideal world, no patient would have residual blockade after surgery. Since this is not the case, it is necessary to determine what degree of recovery is adequate for the majority of patients to ventilate and clear their airways without assistance. Many patients arrive in the recovery area with significant residual relaxation and survive because 100% strength is not needed for airway control or ventilation in relatively healthy patients.

RESPIRATORY FUNCTION AND RESIDUAL BLOCKADE

A margin of safety separates the minimum degree of relaxation that can be detected from the level of relaxation that causes ventilatory failure. An example is that ventilatory failure may not occur in healthy patients until the TOF ratio is less than 0.45.[5] There are several factors contributing to this margin of safety. In their classic study of receptor occupancy, Waud and Waud demonstrated that patients may have normal inspiratory force and vital capacity even when 75–80% of the ACh receptors are blocked.[47] Another contribution comes from the relative sensitivities of respiratory and nonrespiratory muscle groups to neuromuscular-blocking drugs. Investigators have repeatedly shown that the diaphragm is less sensitive to muscle relaxants than are peripheral muscles.[36, 40, 41, 99, 100] Of the muscles involved in respiration, the abdominal, intercostal, and scalene muscles are more sensitive to these agents than is the diaphragm.[101] As a result, neuromuscular blockade has variable effects on respiratory tests depending upon the muscle group being tested.

In unanesthetized subjects, Foldes and coworkers demonstrated that 77% depression of grip strength induced by d-tubocurarine was associated with only a 12% decrease in vital capacity.[40] More recent research of this type by Gal and Goldberg also examined the relationship between peak inspiratory and peak expiratory force. Using d-tubocurarine to depress hand grip to 3% of control, they demonstrated that vital capacity, peak inspiratory force, and peak expiratory force was 66%, 48%, and 29% of control, respectively.[41] Even when head lift and hand grip are abolished, tidal volume may be preserved, although the ventilatory reserve as measured by maximum ventilatory volume is compromised by pharyngeal and nondiaphragmatic respiratory muscle weakness.[100] These studies clearly show that patients without muscle or respiratory disease are capable of coughing and ventilating despite residual peripheral weakness. It is important to note that patients with partial blockade may have nearly normal tidal volume, vital capacity, and inspiratory force but may be at increased risk of complications resulting from expiratory and pharyngeal muscle weakness (inability to clear and maintain an open airway). Tidal volume is an insensitive indicator of recovery from neuromuscular blockade.

Several investigators compared the response to TOF stimulation with respiratory parameters in order to develop criteria to be applied to anesthetized or uncooperative patients. In 1973, Ali and Kitz noted that after neostigmine reversal, patients with a thumb twitch, MMG TOF ratio of 74 ± 5% had clinical evidence of full recovery.[102] Subsequent studies in awake volunteers and in American Society of Anesthesiologists class 3 and 4 patients demonstrated that recovery to thumb twitch TOF ratio of $\geqq 0.70$ is associated with clinical signs of complete recovery and a return to baseline respiratory parameters, vital capacity 96.5% of control, control peak inspiratory force, and vital capacity of 17 ml/kg.[103–105] The conclusion from these studies is that patients with recovery to TOF ratio $\geqq 0.70$ have coughing and ventilatory capabilities comparable with their baseline values. Jones disagrees with these guidelines and suggests that with atracurium besylate or vecuronium bromide, recovery to thumb twitch TOF $\geqq 0.5$ is adequate.[105] As a result of the relative insensitivity of the hypothenar EMG, Kopman suggested using TOF ratio of $\geqq 0.9$ to indicate adequate reversal when monitoring this particular muscle group.[85]

It is evident that patients without preoperative respiratory compromise can tolerate moderate degrees of residual blockade. There is, however, a subpopulation of patients with severe respiratory compromise who may not tolerate any degree of relaxation. These patients should not have any thenar EMG or MMG fade with TOF stimulation.

Evaluation of Antagonism

Accurate evaluation of the TOF ratio requires quantitative methods such as EMG or MMG.[50, 79, 80] As previously discussed, visual and tactile methods are not accurate for precise evaluation of the TOF ratio or fade with teta-nus.[80] This is a lesser problem with atracurium or vecuronium since only a few minutes separates recovery of TOF ratio 0.4 and 0.7. The clinician lacking this equipment must rely upon the use of precise relaxant doses directed by intraoperative monitoring in order to avoid intense relaxation at the conclusion of surgery, which may be difficult to antagonize. Detection of residual blockade without EMG or MMG is probably best accomplished by careful and rigorous application of a variety of bedside tests. The results of these bedside tests should be compared with an estimated preoperative baseline. There should be no detectable fade with either tetanus (anesthetized patients) or TOF stimulation as measured by tactile or visual means. If tetanus is used, the response should be of the same magnitude as a maximum volitional contraction. Evaluation of residual blockade is greatly facilitated by the availability of quantitative equipment.

The TOF and tetanic methods of stimulation are more sensitive than single twitch, since the TOF may show significant fade when the single twitch has returned to baseline.[53, 106] Tetanic stimulation of 50 Hz for 2 seconds is more sensitive than is TOF for detecting residual block. Kopman and coworkers showed that fade to 2-second 100-Hz tetanus can be present despite a TOF ratio of $\geqq 0.7$.[107] They concluded, however, that since the TOF ratio of 0.7 correlated well with clinical parameters, fade with 100 Hz for 2 seconds should not be used as an index of recovery. Since TOF stimulation is not as painful as tetanic stimulation and does not alter the subsequent response, it is the method of choice for monitoring residual blockade.

References

1. Lunn JN, Mushin WW: Mortality associated with anaesthesia. Nuffield Provincial Hospital Trust 1982:48.
2. Beecher HK, Todd DP: A study of the deaths associated with anesthesia and surgery based on a study of 599,548 anesthesias in ten institutions 1948–1952 inclusive. Ann Surg 1954;140:2–34.
3. Churchill-Davidson HC, Christie TH: The diagnoses of neuromuscular block in man. Br J Anaesth 1959; 31:390–395.
4. Viby-Mogensen J, Jorgenson BC, Ording H: Residual curarization in the recovery room. Anesthesiology 1979; 50:539–541.
5. Beemer GH, Rozental P: Postoperative neuromuscular function. Anaesth Intensive Care 1986; 14:41–45.
6. Lenmarken C, Lofstrom JB: Partial curarisation in the postoperative period. Acta Anesthesiol Scand 1984; 28:260–262.
7. Katz RL: Neuromuscular effects of d-tubocurarine, edrophonium and neostigmine in man. Anesthesiology 1967; 28:327–336.
8. Matteo RS, Spector S, Horowitz PE: Relation of serum d-tubocurarine concentration to neuromuscular blockade in man. Anesthesiology 1974; 41:440–443.
9. Hutton P, Burchett KR, Madden AP: Comparison of recovery after neuromuscular blockade by atracurium or pancuronium. Br J Anaesth 1988; 60:36–42.
10. Dunant Y: On the mechanism of acetylcholine release. *In* Smythies JR, Bradley

RJ (eds): International Review of Neurobiology. Orlando: Academic, 1985; 27:55–92.

11. Durant NN: The physiology of neuromuscular transmission. *In* Katz RL (ed): Muscle Relaxants. Basic and Clinical Aspects. Orlando: Grune & Stratton, 1985; 13–38.

12. Heuser JE, Salpeter SR: Organization of acetylcholine receptors in quick frozen, deep etched and rotary-replicated Torpedo post synaptic membrane. J Cell Biol 1979; 82:150–174.

13. Thesleff S: Different kinds of ACh release from the motor nerve. *In* Smythies JR, Bradley RJ (eds): International Review of Neurobiology. Orlando: Academic, 1986; 59–88.

14. Collier B, Katz HS: Acetylcholine synthesis from recaptured choline by a sympathetic ganglion. J Physiol (Lond) 1970; 206:145–166.

15. Tucek S: The synthesis of acetylcholine in sketetal muscles of the rat. J Physiol (Lond) 1982; 322:53–69.

16. Thesleff S: The mode of neuromuscular block caused by acetylcholine, nicotine, decamethonium and succinylcholine. Acta Physiol Scand 1955; 34:218–231.

17. Kuffler SW, Yoshikami D: The number of transmitter molecules in a quantum: An estimate from iontophoretic application of acetylcholine at the neuromuscular synapse. J Physiol (Lond) 1975; 251:465–482.

18. Brigent JL, Mallart A: Presynaptic currents in mouse motor endings. J Physiol (Lond) 1982; 333:619–636.

19. Katz B: Nerve, Muscles and Synapse. New York: McGraw-Hill, 1966.

20. Hubbard JI, Jones SF, Landau EM: On the mechanisms by which calcium and magnesium affect the release of transmitter by nerve impulses. J Physiol (Lond) 1968; 196:75–86.

21. Standaert FG: Donut and holes: Molecules and muscle relaxants. *In* Katz RL (ed): Muscle Relaxants. Basic and Clinical Aspects. Orlando: Grune & Stratton, 1985; 1–18.

22. Standaert FG: Basic physiology and pharmacology of the neuromuscular junction. *In* Miller RD (ed): Anesthesia. New York: Churchill Livingstone, 1986; 835–870.

23. Tobey RE, Jacobsen PM, Cahil CT, et al: The serum potassium response to muscle relaxants in neural injury. Anesthesiology 1972; 37:332–337.

24. Peper K, Bradley RJ, Dreger K: The acetylcholine receptor at the neuromuscular junction. Physiol Rev 1982; 62:1271–1340.

25. Bowman WC: Prejunctional and postjunctional cholinoreceptors at the neuromuscular junction. Anesth Analg 1980; 59:935–943.

26. Vassalle M: Contribution of the Na^+/K^+ pump to the membrane potential. Experientia 1987; 43:1135–1140.

27. Brown WF: The Physiological and Technical Basis of Electromyography. Boston: Butterworths, 1984; 12–13.

28. Ali HH, Savarese JJ: Monitoring neuromuscular function. Anesthesiology 1976; 45:216–249.

29. Lee C: Dose relationships of phase II, tachyphylaxis and train-of-four fade in suxamethonium-induced dual neuromuscular block in man. Br J Anaesth 1975; 47:841–845.

30. Bevan JC, Donati F, Bevan DR: Prolonged infusion of suxamethonium in infants and children. Br J Anaesth 1986; 58:839–843.

31. Sutherland GA, Bevan JC, Bevan DR: Neuromuscular blockade in infants following intramuscular succinylcholine in two or five percent solution. Can J Anaesth 1980; 30:342–346.

32. Goudsouzian NG, Liu LM: The neuromuscular response of infants to a continuous infusion of succinylcholine. Anesthesiology 1984; 60:97–101.

33. Lee C: Self antagonism: A possible mechanism of tachyphylaxis in suxamethonium-induced neuromuscular block in man. Br J Anaesth 1986; 48:1097–1101.

34. Donati F, Bevan DR: Long-term succinylcholine infusion during isoflurane. Anesthesiology 1983; 58:6–10.

35. Donati F, Bevan DR: Antagonism of phase II succinylcholine block by neostigmine. Anesth Analg 1985; 64:773–776.

36. Chauvin M, Lebrault C, Duvaldestin P: The neuromuscular blocking effect of vecuronium on the human diaphragm. Anesth Analg 1987; 66:117–122.

37. Russell WJ, Serle DG: Hand grip force as an assessment of recovery from neuromuscular block. J Clin Monit 1987; 3:87–89.

38. Stiffel P, Hammeroff SP, Blitt C, Cork RC: Variability in the assessment of neuromuscular blockade. Anesthesiology 1980; 52:436–437.

38a. Caffrey RR, Warren ML, Becker KE: Neuromuscular blockade monitoring comparing the orbicularis oculi and adductor pollicis muscles. Anesthesiology 1986; 65:95–97.

39. Wymore ML, Eisele JH: Differential effects of d-tubocurarine on inspiratory muscles and two peripheral muscle groups in anesthetized man. Anesthesiology 1978; 48:360–362.

40. Foldes FF, Monte AP, Brunn HM, Wolfson B: Studies with muscle relaxants in unanesthetized subjects. Anesthesiology 1961; 22:230–236.

41. Gal TJ, Goldberg SK: Diaphragmatic function in healthy subjects during partial curarization. J Appl Physiol 1980; 48:921–926.

42. Swett JE, Bourassa CM: Electrical stimulation of peripheral nerve. *In* Patterson M, Kesner RP (eds): Electrical Stimulation Research Techniques. New York: Academic, 1981; 244–298.

43. Epstein RA, Jackson SH: Repetitive muscle depolarization from a single indirect stimulation in man. J Appl Physiol 1970; 28:407–410.

44. Epstein RA, Wyte SR, Jackson SH, Sitter S: The electrical response to stimulation by the Block-Aid monitor. Anesthesiology 1969; 30:43–47.

45. Brooks VB, Theis RD: Reduction of quantum content during neuromuscular transmission. J Physiol (Lond) 1962; 162:298–310.

46. Liley AW, North AK: An electrical investigation of the effects of repetitive stimulation on mammalian neuromuscular junction. J Neurophysiol 1953; 16:509–527.

47. Waud BE, Waud DR: The relation between tetanic fade and receptor occlusion in the presence of competitive neuromuscular block. Anesthesiology 1971; 35:456–564.

48. Stanec A, Heyduk J, Stanec G, Orkin LR: Tetanic fade and post tetanic tension in the absence of neuromuscular blocking agents in anesthetized man. Anesth Analg 1978; 57:102–107.

49. Ali HH, Savarese JJ: Stimulation frequency and dose response to d-tubocurarine in man. Anesthesiology 1980; 52:36–39.

50. Lee C, Katz RL: Neuromuscular pharmacology. A clinical update and commentary. Br J Anaesth 1980; 52:173–188.

51. Ali HH, Uting JE, Gray C: Stimulus frequency in the detection of neuromuscular block in humans. Br J Anaesth 1970; 42:967–977.

52. Lee MC: Train-of-4 quantitation of competitive neuromuscular block. Anesth Analg (Cleve) 1975; 54:649–653.

53. Ali HH, Savarese JJ, Lebowitz PN, Ramsey FM: Twitch, tetanus and train-of-four as indices of recovery from nondepolarizing neuromuscular blockade. Anesthesiology 1981; 54:294–297.

54. Pollmaecher JT, Steirt H, Buzello W: A constant current peripheral nerve stimulator (neurostim T4). Br J Anaesth 1986; 58:1443–1446.
55. Katz RL: Clinical neuromuscular pharmacology of pancuronium. Anesthesiology 1971; 34:500–506.
56. Merton PA: Voluntary strength and fatigue. J Physiol (Lond) 1954; 123:553–565.
57. Moritani T, Muro M, Kijima A, et al: Electromechanical changes during electrically induced and maximal voluntary contractions: Surface and intramuscular EMG responses during sustained maximal voluntary contraction. Exp Neurol 1985; 88:484–499.
58. Viby-Mogensen J, Howardy-Hansen P, Chraemmer-Jorgensen B, et al: Posttetanic count (PTC). A new method of evaluating an intense nondepolarizing neuromuscular blockade. Anesthesiology 1981; 55:458–461.
59. Calvey TN: Assessment of neuromuscular blockade by electromyography: A review. J R Soc Med 1984; 77:56–59.
60. Katz RL: Electromyographic and mechanical effects of suxamethonium and tubocurarine on twitch, tetanic and post-tetanic responses. Br J Anaesth 1973; 45:849–859.
61. Epstein RA, Epstein RM: The electromyogram and the mechanical response of indirectly stimulated muscle in anesthetized man following curarization. Anesthesiology 1973; 38:212–223.
62. Muchhal KK, Viby-Mogensen J: Evaluation of intense neuromuscular blockade caused by single bolus vecuronium using posttetanic count (PTC). Anesthesiology 1987; 66:846–849.
63. Bonsu AK, Viby-Mogensen J, Fernando PU, et al: Relationship of post-tetanic count and train-of-four response during intense neuromuscular blockade caused by atracurium. Br J Anaesth 1987; 59:1089–1092.
64. Ridley SA, Hatch DJ: Post-tetanic count and profound neuromuscular blockade with atracurium infusion in paediatric patients. Br J Anaesth 1988; 60:31–35.
65. Capan LM, Satyanarayana T, Patel KP, et al: Assessment of neuromuscular blockade with surface electrodes. Anesth Analg 1981; 60:244–245.
66. Kopman AF, Lawson D: Milliamperage requirements for supramaximal stimulation of the ulnar nerve with surface electrodes. Anesthesiology 1984; 61:83–85.
67. Gravenstein J, Paulus D: Monitoring Practice in Clinical Anesthesia. Philadelphia: JB Lippincott, 1982; 178.
68. Mylrea KC, Hameroff SR, Calkins JM, et al: Evaluation of peripheral nerve stimulators and relationship to possible errors in assessing neuromuscular blockade. Anesthesiology 1984; 60:464–466.
69. Rosenberg H, Greenhow DE: Peripheral nerve stimulator performance: The influence of output polarity and electrode placement. Can J Anaesth 1978; 25:424–426.
70. de Weerd JPC: Instrumentation, electrodes, electrical interference and safety. In Notermans SLH (ed). Current Practice of Electromyography. New York: Elsevier, 1984; 29–56.
71. Ranck JB: Extracellular stimulation. In Patterson M, Kesner R: (eds): Electrical Stimulation Research Techniques. New York: Academic, 1981; 2–36.
72. Berger JJ, Gravenstein JS, Munson ES: Electrode polarity and peripheral nerve stimulation. Anesthesiology 1954; 56:402–404.
73. Pierce PA, Mylrea KC, Watt RC, et al: Effects of pulse duration on neuromuscular blockade monitoring: Implications for supramaximal stimulation. J Clin Monit 1986; 2:169–173.
74. Lippman M, Fields WA: Burns of the skin caused by a peripheral nerve stimulator. Anesthesiology 1974; 40:82–84.

75. Brock-Utne JG, Downing JW: Rectal burn after the use of an anal stainless steel electrode/transducer system for monitoring myoneural junction. Anesth Analg 1984; 63:1139–1144.

76. Gertel M, Shapira SC: Ulnar nerve palsy of unusual etiology. (Letter.) Anesth Analg 1987; 66:1343.

77. Sia RL, Straatman NJ: Thumb paresthesia after neuromuscular twitch monitoring. Anaesthesia 1985; 40:167–169.

77a. Merritt WT, Brinker JA, Beattie C: Pacemaker-mediated tachycardia induced by intraoperative somatosensory evoked potential stimuli. Anesthesiology 1988; 69:766–768.

78. Sarnat JA: A simple device for testing peripheral nerve stimulators. Anesthesiology 1984; 61:624–625.

79. Donati F, Bevan JC, Bevan DR: Neuromuscular blocking drugs in anesthesia. Can Anaesth Soc J 1984; 31:324–336.

80. Thomas PD, Worthley LTG, Russel WJ: How useful is visual and tactile assessment of neuromuscular blockade using a peripheral nerve stimulator? Anaesth Intensive Care 1984; 12:68–69.

81. Viby-Mogensen J, Jensen NH, Engback J, et al: Tactile and visual evaluation of the response to train-of-four nerve stimulation. Anesthesiology 1985; 63:440–443.

82. Howardy-Hansen P, Viby-Mogensen J, Gottschau A, et al: Tactile evaluation of the posttetanic count (PTC). Anesthesiology 1984; 60:372–374.

83. Weber S, Muravchick S: Electrical and mechanical train-of-four responses during depolarizing and nondepolarizing neuromuscular blockade. Anesth Analg 1986; 65:771–776.

84. Astly BA, Katz RL, Payne JP: Electrical and mechanical responses after neuromuscular blockade with vecuronium and subsequent antagonism with neostigmine or edrophonium. Br J Anaesth 1987; 59:983–988.

85. Kopman KF: The relationship of evoked electromyographic and mechanical responses following atracurium in humans. Anesthesiology 1985; 63:208–211.

86. Weber S, Muravchick S: Monitoring technique affects measurement of recovery from succinylcholine. J Clin Monit 1987; 3:1–5.

87. McComas AJ: Neuromuscular Function and Disorders. Woburn, MA: Butterworths, 1977.

87a. Kalli I: Effect of surface electrode positioning on the compound action potential evoked by ulnar nerve stimulation in anesthetized infants and children. Br J Anaesth 1989; 62:188–193.

88. Jabre JF, Hackett ER: EMG Manual. Springfield: CC Thomas, 1983.

89. Donlon JV, Savarese JJ, Ali HH: Cumulative dose response curves for gallamine: Effect of altered resting thumb tension and mode of stimulation. Anesth Analg 1979; 58:379–381.

90. Stanec A: Abductor pollicis monitor. Anesth Analg 1984; 63:1139–1144.

91. Powers SJ, Joknes RM: Relationship between single twitch depression and train-of-four fade: Influence of relaxant dose during onset and spontaneous offset of neuromuscular blockade. Anesth Analg 1987; 66:633–636.

92. Pearce AC, Casson WR, Jones RM: Factors affecting train-of-four fade. Br J Anaesth 1985; 57:602–606.

93. Naguib M, Abdulatif M, Gyasi HK, et al: The pattern of train-of-four fade after atracurium: Influence of different priming doses. Anesth Analg 1987; 66:427–430.

94. Duvaldestin P, Chauvin M: Does diaphragmatic paralysis precede hand paralysis with vecuronium? In response. Anesth Analg 66:1342–1343.

95. Katz RL: Comparison of electrical and mechanical recording of spontaneous and evoked muscle activity. Anesthesiology 1965; 26:204–211.

96. Casson WR, Jones RM: Profound atracurium-induced neuromuscular blockade. A comparison of evoked reversal with edrophonium or neostigmine. Anaesthesia 1986; 41:382–385.

97. Donati F, McCarrol SM, Antazka C, et al: Dose-response curves for edrophonium, neostigmine and pyridostigmine after pancuronium and d-tubocurarine. Anesthesiology 1987; 66:471–476.

98. Kopman A: Recovery times following edrophonium and neostigmine reversal of pancuronium, atracurium and vecuronium steady-state infusions. Anesthesiology 1986; 65:572–578.

99. Maclean IC: Neuromuscular junction. *In* Johnson EW (ed): Practical Electromyography. Baltimore: Williams & Wilkins, 1980; 73–89.

100. Gal TJ, Goldberg SK: Relationship between respiratory muscle strength and vital capacity during partial curarization in awake subjects. Anesthesiology 1981; 54:141–147.

101. DeTroyer A, Bastenier J, Delhez L: Function of respiratory muscles during partial curarization in humans. J Appl Physiol 1980; 49:1049–1056.

102. Ali HH, Kitz RJ: Evaluation of recovery from nondepolarizing neuromuscular block using a digital neuromuscular transmission analyzer: Preliminary report. Anesth Analg 1973; 52:740–745.

103. Brand JB, Cullen DJ, Wilson NE, Ali HH: Spontaneous recovery from nondepolarizing neuromuscular blockade: Correlation between clinical and evoked responses. Anesth Analg 1977; 56:55–58.

104. Ali HH, Wilson RS, Savarese JJ, Kitz RJ: The effect of tubocurarine on indirectly elicited train-of-four muscle response and respiratory measurements in humans. Br J Anaesth 1975; 47:570–574.

105. Jones RM, Pearce AC, Williams JP: Recovery characteristics following antagonism of atracurium with neostigmine or edrophonium. Br J Anaesth 1984; 56:453–457.

106. Gissen AJ, Katz RL: Twitch tetanus and posttetanic potentiation as indices of nerve-muscle block in man. Anesthesiology 1969; 30:481–487.

107. Kopman AF, Epstein RH, Flashburg MH: Use of 100-Hertz tetanus as an index of recovery from pancuronium-induced non-depolarizing neuromuscular blockade. Anesth Analg (Cleve) 1982; 61:439–441.

chapter twenty-two

Evoked Potentials

CAROL L. LAKE, M.D.

Sensory evoked responses or potentials are the obligatory electrical response of the brain, spinal cord, or nerve to sensory, motor, magnetic, electrical, or cognitive stimuli that cause ionic flow. The electroencephalogram (EEG), on the other hand, is the summation of continuous spontaneous electrical activity in the brain. Evoked potentials can be motor, auditory, visual, olfactory, or somatosensory. Examples of sensory stimuli are clicks or tone-bursts near the ear, light flashes or reversed patterns through closed eyelids, and electric shocks to peripheral nerves. Clinically, these electrophysiologic responses to stimulation are used to identify the functional integrity of cranial and peripheral nerves; to monitor function of auditory, brainstem, and peripheral neural pathways during craniotomy or spinal cord surgery; and to determine effects of drugs, therapeutic interventions, or pathophysiologic alterations such as hypoxia or hypotension on neurologic function.[1-14] A major advantage of evoked potentials is that monitoring can occur during altered states of consciousness and neuromuscular blockade. Despite their usefulness in both intensive care unit and operating room, there are numerous problems with evoked potentials, including: the uncertainty of their origins; recording difficulties so that a waveform normal in one laboratory is abnormal elsewhere; failure of all recorded potentials to contain all components of an evoked potential; influences of age, gender, diet, socioeconomic status, state of awareness, and diurnal variation.

HISTORY

Caton, while recording electroencephalographic activity from the cerebral cortex in animals in 1875 with a galvanometer, noted that cerebral

757

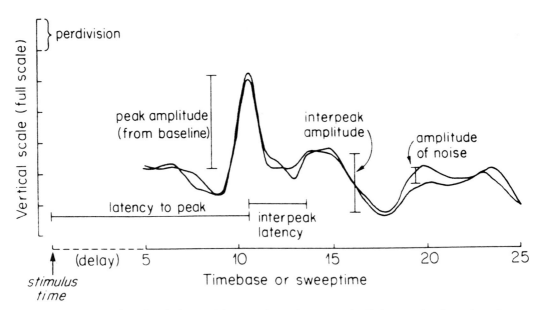

Figure 22–1. A representation of evoked potential nomenclature from two stimuli. See text for discussion. (From Nuwer MR: Evoked Potential Monitoring in the Operating Room. New York: Raven Press, 1986; 28. With permission.)

activity changed in response to visual and somatosensory stimulation.[15, 16] Human cortical evoked potentials were first published by Davis in 1939.[17, 18] Brainstem auditory evoked potentials were initially reported in 1967.[19] Evoked potentials recorded from the eye were described in 1865, but it was not until the response of the visual cortical neurons to complex visual patterns was recognized that clinical pattern-reversal stimulation for visual evoked potentials became practical.

Superimposition of the series of responses after a stimulus was difficult prior to the computer era. Methods used included written graphic displays, cathode ray oscilloscopes, and photographic displays. The initial computer application to evoked potential monitoring was by Brazier, who used the average-responses computer of Clark to retrieve evoked potentials from EEG activity.[20, 21] Present-day digital evoked potential equipment is derived from this system.

COMPONENTS OF THE EVOKED RESPONSE

Four characteristics describe evoked potentials: poststimulus latency of peaks, troughs, and other complexes in the waveform; distance of neural generator from recording electrode; neural origin of evoked response; and mode of sensory stimulation (somatosensory, auditory, visual).

The recorded potential is a plot of voltage against time as is the EEG (see Chapter 20) (Fig. 22–1).[22] Identification of specific peaks in the waveform is by visual recognition, not automatically by maximum deflection within a specific latency, thus precluding computer analysis. The number after each peak is the poststimulus latency.

Latency

Latency, measured in milliseconds, is the time between the occurrence of a peak or complex in the evoked waveform and the stimulus. It can be short (less than 40 msec), intermediate (40–120 msec), or long (120–500 msec).[23] Short latency potentials originate closer to the stimulus site. Examples are cortical evoked potentials recorded from scalp electrodes. Intermediate latency potentials originate in the cerebral cortex and are termed the primary specific complex. Long latency potentials arise in the association areas of the cortex and represent responses to pain or cognition. Intermediate latency visual and somatosensory and short latency auditory and somatosensory potentials are commonly used intraoperatively. Long latency potentials, obliterated by anesthesia and other factors, are of limited interest intraoperatively. Latency is affected by intensity of stimulation and other factors. Latency increases as stimulus intensity decreases. Prolongation of latency is usually abnormal, although latencies are related to patient height (posterior tibial to cortex).[24]

Amplitudes

Amplitudes are measured in microvolts from peak to peak, average zero baseline to peak, or zero point at onset of recording to peak. Commonly, the peak-to-peak method is used. Amplitude is variable but sensitive to abnormalities. At higher stimulus rates, the amplitude of evoked potentials is decreased, particularly after spinal cord injuries.[25] Representation of the polarity of the waves is also undecided, with some investigators displaying positive waves (P) as upright and others with negative (N) peaks up (see Fig. 22–1). Designation of polarity must always be indicated because it is variable among different laboratories. Polarity is also dependent upon the orientation of electrodes.

Central Conduction Time and Velocity

In addition to latency, the central conduction time (CCT) and conduction velocity are usually measured when recording evoked potentials. CCT is the interval or latency between the evoked potential peaks generated in peripheral or cranial nerves, cervical spinal cord, or brainstem and later peaks from the midbrain, thalamic projections, or cortex. Conduction velocity in stimulated peripheral nerve is estimated from the poststimulus latency and the distance between the stimulus site and the recording electrode.

Distances between Neural Generators and Recording Electrodes

The distances between the generator and the electrodes can be near-field or far-field. Near-field evoked potentials are recorded by electrodes adjacent to the origin. Such potentials recorded from the scalp originate from the cerebral cortex, and their amplitude is between 1 and 50 μV. Near-field potentials are also recorded from peripheral nerves from electrodes placed directly on or near them.

Far-field potentials are small signals because they originate far from the recording electrode. Thus, they are little affected by changes in electrode position, but they are smaller than the EEG, requiring averaging of thousands of individual responses in order to extract the signal from the EEG. Far-field potentials have short latencies and are little affected by anesthesia. However, it should be appreciated that potentials described as far-field when recorded from the scalp may be near-field when recorded by invasive electrodes near the nerve. Far-field potentials often include potentials generated by more than one structure, whereas near-field potentials are usually elicited from a localized portion of the nervous system.

Neural Generators

Neural generators can be spinal cord, spinal nerve roots, or cerebral cortical or subcortical regions. Cortical potentials originate in the pyramidal cells. Responses recorded from primary sensory receiving areas were termed primary specific responses by Walter in 1975.[26] Primary specific responses are complex, consistent cortical potentials produced by both meaningful and nonmeaningful stimuli. Secondary specific responses are waves not present in the primary specific complex that arise from regions near the primary sensory areas. Nonspecific responses are recorded from frontal and temporal regions in response to various sensory stimuli. They are enhanced by meaningful stimuli or subject attention. Contingent responses, such as the contingent negative variation, are changes in the surface negative potential of the cerebral cortex dependent upon a relation between a signal and a subject action. About 1 second before voluntary movement or intent to move, cortical responses occur over cortex that are termed antecedent or imaginary responses. Of these cortical responses, only the primary specific response is important to intraoperative monitoring.

MODE OF SENSORY STIMULATION

The primary classification of evoked potentials is by type of stimulation, i.e., sensory (somatosensory, visual, or auditory) and motor.

Somatosensory Evoked Responses

Cortical Potentials

Somatosensory evoked potentials (SSEP) are evaluated by stimulation of either the median or the ulnar nerves of the upper extremity or the common peroneal or the posterior tibial nerves of the lower extremity on the surface or subcutaneously. Potentials are recorded from the scalp, brainstem, spinal cord, or peripheral nerves. Although thermal, mechanical, or magnetic stimuli elicit potentials, electrical stimuli are most commonly used. Electrical current is easily applied, measured, and controlled using pairs of electrodes applied at the site of stimulation. The stimulus intensity, which should be recorded, is usually in the range of 10–15 mA for SSEP. Each extremity is stimulated in turn in order to detect unilateral lesions. Bilateral extremity stimulation gives larger responses and allows comparisons of the differences caused by surgery versus global changes caused by hypothermia, hypotension, or anesthesia.

Typical placements of recording electrodes are called montages. For SSEP a common montage is C3 and C4' (2 cm behind C3 and C4), EP (Erb's point behind the clavicle), CII or C2S (second cervical vertebra), L1 and L3 (lumbar), and IC (iliac crest).[7] See Recording Electrodes.

When stimulating the median nerve and recording at Erb's point (brachial plexus), a nerve action potential is seen. Where the nerves enter the spinal cord, additional potentials, composed of nerve action potentials and excitatory postsynaptic potentials, are generated.[7] At the level of the C2S or other surfaces of the spinal cord, a reproducible pattern consisting of an initial triphasic spike is the response to stimulation. Different investigators use slightly different terminology to describe the subsequent peaks. The negative peak at 9 msec (N_9) is generated in the brachial plexus. Peak N_{11} originates from the spinal roots or dorsal columns, $N_{13,14}$ from spinal cord gray matter or dorsal columns, $N_{14,15}$ from brainstem, thalamus, or both, and N_{20}, P_{20}, N_{30}, P_{25}, and N_{35} from primary somatosensory cortex.[27] Less distinct peaks are generated by stimulation of the lower extremity. This is probably due to temporal dispersion of the neural activity in the long pathway.

Cortical SSEP consist of (1) an early positive wave with a latency of 12–18 msec after the stimulus; (2) an M- or W-shaped deflection or the primary specific complex whose positive trough has a latency of 23–33 msec; (3) a negative wave with a latency of 30–45 msec with two components separated from one another by 10–15 msec. The entire response consists of three positive waves, P_1, P_2, and P_3, and two negative waves, N_1 and N_2. Waves are described by latencies and by amplitudes (distance from P to N) (Fig. 22–2). The short latency sensory potential is subcortical.[28] The initial cortical wave originates from the thalamus or thalamocortical radiation. Recording of the first negative wave is possible over the posterior quadrant of the cerebral hemisphere, whereas the positive potential is centered over the parietal area. The primary specific complex probably originates from the cortex, although the thalamus or thalamocortical radiation may contribute

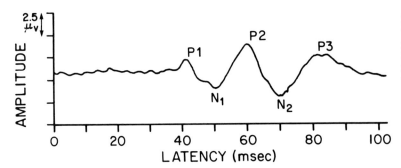

Figure 22–2. A normal SSEP with three positive (P) and two negative (N) peaks. Amplitude is 2.5 μv/division, whereas latency is measured in milliseconds from the stimulus (0).

to P_1. The scalp distribution of SSEP depends upon whether the stimulus is delivered to the tibial or femoral nerve.[29] During somatosensory stimulation, cortical activation closely correlates with regional cerebral blood flow.[30]

Spinal Potentials

Spinal SSEP are elicited by stimulation of the posterior tibial nerve at the knee. They are recorded from electrodes on the surface over the cervical, thoracic, or lumbar cord inserted into interspinous ligaments, spinous processes, dorsal epidural space of the cervical, thoracic, or lumbar spine, or directly on the spinal cord (electrospinogram). The first negative wave in the lumbar region is N_{20}. Immediately after N_{20} is a positive peak and a second negative peak. Two small peaks, the N_{24} and N_{27}, occur in the cervical region.[31] On the scalp, a negative peak at 35 msec and a positive peak at 40 msec are seen.

The amplitude of spinal SSEP, about 0.5–5 μV, is slightly larger than cortical potentials. Electrodes directly on the cord or in the epidural space have the highest amplitudes. Spinous process recordings have the lowest amplitudes and are least adequate for monitoring. Spinal potentials are less affected by electrical interference, blood pressure, or anesthetic depth. However, there is no evidence that they are more sensitive than cortical SSEP.[32] Attenuation of amplitude to 30–50% of control is usually indicative of clinical sequelae.[16]

Direct spinal cord stimulation has been used in Japan, but it is infrequently used in the United States.[33–35] An electrode is placed either directly in the epidural or subarachnoid space during surgery or using the standard percutaneous technique for epidural or continuous spinal anesthesia. Reasons for using direct cord stimulation are that evoked potential amplitudes are large, stable, and simple in pattern with evaluation of both ascending and descending tracts.[33] The response evoked by cord stimulation consists of an initial positive/negative/positive spike wave (from posterolateral spinal cord) followed by a polyphasic portion (from the dorsal column and similar to N and P waves noted by Shimoji and Kano).[33–35] However, the potentials are affected by electrode location, neurologic status, and individual variation. Each patient must serve as his or her own control during direct spinal cord stimulation. Recordings must be made at several levels in order to localize cord injuries. Injured cord is recognized by positivity of the waveform or abrupt degradation of the peak amplitude.[33] However, the exact amount of amplitude degradation that is critical is unclear. Other problems with this technique include stimulation of multiple pathways (producing large amounts of electrical activity at each spinal segment), risk of spinal cord damage, and possibility of overlooking unilateral injury.

Cerebral lesions that destroy or disturb function in the primary sensory cortex, cortical afferent pathways, or thalamic sensory relay nuclei abolish SSEP. However, SSEP are also helpful in the diagnosis of multifocal or diffuse lesions of peripheral nerve, nerve plexuses, brainstem, midbrain, and cortex.[36–43]

Visual Evoked Potentials

Cortical visual evoked potentials (VEP) are evoked by reversal of a checkerboard pattern or light flashes. Flash evoked potentials are stimulated by light-emitting diodes mounted in opaque goggles placed over the patient's closed eyelids, by light-emitting diodes attached to contact lenses, or with strobe lights. Stimulation rates of 1–2/second are used. Intraoperative use of flash evoked potentials has had only limited success. There are substantial problems with the visual stimulators themselves because of the potential for prolonged ocular pressure if the stimulator goggles slip off the bony orbit, corneal damage from contact lenses, skin damage from rigid eye patches, and infringement of strobe light stimulators in the surgical field. Recordings are made from a single electrode on the mid-occipital scalp just above the inion. The reference electrode is placed at the vertex.

VEP consist of five principal waves recorded over the calcarine visual cortex from electrodes on the midline (vertex) of the occipital scalp within 250 msec after a light flash or pattern shift stimulus to the closed eyes. The visual pathway includes the retina, optic nerve, optic chiasm, optic tracts, lateral geniculate nucleus, optic radiation, and occipital visual cortex. Wave I is a large positive wave, occurring after 100 msec. Its latency is greater in the parietal than in the occipital region. Wave II has a similar latency in all cortical areas and an average amplitude of 7.4 μV. Wave III has a similar latency everywhere but greater amplitude in the occipital cortex. Wave IV has a variable latency in the occipital region. The occipital wave V has the lowest amplitude in the occipital region.

Waves I, II, and III are present at birth, but their latency decreases with age, reaching adult values by age 3–4 years. Waves IV and V are barely discernible at birth, and their latencies increase until 2–4 months of age, after which they decrease and remain constant until age 5–6 years when they increase again (Fig. 22–3). As indicated previously, VEP are late potentials with peaks 100–300 msec after the stimulus. Because of this feature, they are more difficult to record and more affected by drugs, temperature, or other factors. The amplitude of VEP decreases with even small degrees of hypothermia. Russ and colleagues noted disappearance of VEP during hypothermic cardiopulmonary bypass at 25°C.[44]

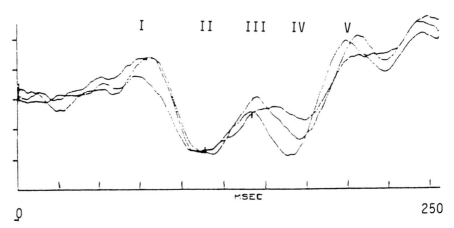

Figure 22–3. A series of VEP demonstrating the characteristic waves as described in the text. (From Nuwer M: Evoked Potential Monitoring in the Operating Room. New York: Raven Press, 1986; 172. With permission.)

Although theoretically VEP should aid in preventing optic nerve injury, false-negatives, false-positives, and absence of a specific pattern of injury have complicated routine intraoperative application.[45–47] VEP elicited by flashes are adversely affected by anesthesia, visual pathway lesions, and cranial surgical manipulation.[48] VEP are, however, employed in surgical procedures for pituitary tumors, anterior cerebral artery aneurysms, or craniopharyngiomas. They are also helpful in nonoperative settings to diagnose retrobulbar dysfunction in multiple sclerosis, hydrocephalus, and epilepsy.[49–51]

Brainstem Auditory Evoked Potentials

Brainstem auditory evoked potentials (BAEP) provide information about the integrity of the auditory pathway and brainstem structures between the midpons and the upper midbrain, but not the cerebral cortex. The auditory pathway is relatively dorsal in the brainstem, so BAEP do not provide useful information about more ventral pathways such as the motor tracts. The neural pathway of BAEP is shown in Table 22–1. Their specific neural generators are controversial but clinically useful. However, most of the components of BAEP are generated in multiple auditory structures.[52]

BAEP are high-frequency waves detected on the scalp within 10 msec of an auditory stimulus such as application of a click or tone to the ear. Intraoperative recordings were initially made by Sohmer and Feinmesser and Jewett and Williston.[19, 53] The entire auditory pathway is evaluated by BAEP, direct recordings of compound action potentials from nerve VIII, and the electrocochleogram. Clinically, they are the easiest potentials to record.

In preparation of intraoperative testing of BAEP, the auditory canals and tympanic membrane are examined and cerumen removed. Either headphones or transducers in molded ear inserts are used to generate stimuli.

Table 22–1. NEURAL GENERATORS OF
BAEP

Wave I Extracranial auditory nerve VIII
Wave II Activation of cochlear nuclei (intracranial nerve
  VIII)
Wave III Cochlear nucleus in pons
Wave IV Superior olive (pons) or lateral lemniscus (mid-
  brain)
Wave V Lateral lemniscus or inferior colliculus (rostral
  midbrain)
Wave VI Thalamus
Wave VII Thalamic or auditory radiation

Compiled from Moller, 1988; Stockard, Rossiter, Neurology 1977; Achor, Starr (I, II), 1980; Starr, Hamilton,
1976.

The same transducers are used for preoperative and intraoperative recordings. The intensity of auditory stimulation is based on the patient's hearing
threshold. The actual stimulus intensity is calibrated in decibels peak equivalent sound pressure level (db pe SPL). Stimuli 60–70 db higher than the
patient's auditory threshold or sensation level (SL) are usually used. The
SL is compared with the hearing level (HL), the mean sensation level of
normal subjects.[5] Time bases of 10 msec are used. A series of 2000 trials
are needed to establish most BAEP (at stimulus rates of 40/second, the entire
series takes less than 1 minute).

Stimulus and recording parameters for BAEP are listed in Friedman and
associates.[7] Usual stimulus parameters are rates of 10–100/second and intensities of 65–76 db, with the actual stimulus being a square wave electrical
pulse of 100 microseconds.[16] Two channels of BAEP should be recorded.
Both ears are stimulated in order to provide the normal control and to differentiate peaks in abnormal waveforms. Moller recommends recording of
the nerve action potential directly from the acoustic nerve during ear surgery.[54] However, electrode movement caused by the surgery produces noise
interference on the recording. Four recording electrodes are placed: both
earlobes, vertex, and a ground on the forehead.

BAEP consist of five to seven waves. Wave I has a latency of 1.6 msec
and is observed with the greatest consistency. It probably results from the
auditory nerve and sometimes has two components: an earlier high amplitude
and a later component present after a wide variety of stimulus intensities
and pitches.[16] Activation of the cochlear nuclei produces wave II, which
has a latency of 2.8 msec. Wave III is due to activity in the superior olive
(pons) and is observed with great consistency with a latency of 3.8 msec.
Waves IV and V, with latencies of 4.8 msec and 5.5 msec, respectively, are
due to activity in the lateral lemniscus and inferior colliculus. Wave VI, with
a latency of 7.1 msec, originates from the medial geniculate (thalamus).
Wave VII, with a latency of 9 msec, originates from the thalamus or auditory
cortical projection. Waves VI and VII are not always evident (Fig. 22–4).
Clinical monitoring uses waves I through V and particularly I, III, and V.

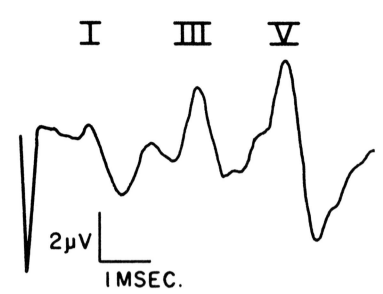

Figure 22–4. A BAEP in a human with normal hearing after 83-decibel stimulation. The horizontal axis is time in msec, whereas the vertical axis is amplitude in microvolts. (From Shaia FT, Albright P: Clinical use of brainstem evoked response audiometry. Virginia Medical 1980; 107:44. With permission.)

Wave I of the BAEP is the same activity recorded as N_1 of the electrocochleogram (the response of the cochlea and auditory nerve to sound). The first component of the electrocochleogram (ECochG) is the cochlear microphonic, resulting from the sensory hair cells of the inner ear. The ECochG is recorded using a needle electrode in the middle ear.

Only lesions of the eighth nerve completely obliterate BAEP. If BAEP are absent, differentiation must be made between peripheral and central neurologic abnormalities. The ECochG distinguishes between the two causes. If the ECochG is absent, peripheral hearing loss is usually present. A normal ECochG and an absent BAEP indicate intracranial abnormality.

The five principal features of the BAEP recommended by the American Electroencephalographic Society to assess the integrity of the auditory pathway are: (1) absence of all waves; (2) absence of waves beyond II or III; (3) increased I–V interpeak interval; (4) decreased V/I amplitude ratio; and (5) interaural I–V interval asymmetry.[33] The interpeak interval has normal values of less than 4.5 msec. Asymmetry between sides should be no more than 0.4 msec. Normal interpeak intervals for I–III and III–V are 2.5 msec, with only 0.4 msec of asymmetry. The V/I amplitude ratio should be 50% to 300%.[16]

BAEP are affected by hearing acuity, temperature, and head size. Monitoring of BAEP is used in surgical procedures of the cerebellopontine angle, floor of the fourth ventricle, or fifth or seventh cranial nerves. Intraoperative BAEP predict postoperative auditory nerve and pathway function by prolongation of latency or loss of waves after waves I or II.[55–57] Asymmetric evoked waveforms occur with unilateral lesions of the auditory pathway or lesions affecting the cross auditory cortical projections.[58, 59] After unilateral or bilateral internal jugular vein ligation, prolongation of the interpeak intervals of waves I–III and III–IV was observed and may detect brainstem compression after head or neck surgery.[60] Auditory evoked responses are also used in infants or in uncooperative subjects to test the integrity of the auditory pathway in the brainstem and hearing.

Motor Evoked Responses

Although motor evoked potentials were described in 1964 by Pagni and associates during internal capsule stimulation, they are still not used extensively.[61] Most direct stimulation of a motor nerve and observation of the resultant muscle contraction have been limited to stimulation of the facial nerve during parotidectomy, the brachial plexus during brachial blocks, or the ulnar nerve to verify neuromuscular blockade. Two techniques for monitoring motor evoked responses are under investigation: (1) Transcranial electrical stimulation and recording of peripheral nerve action potentials; and (2) nervous system stimulation in an electromagnetic field.[62, 63] In recent work, Estrem and coworkers used electrical or magnetic stimulation of the motor cortex to evaluate cranial nerves of the face or tongue.[64, 65] The present state of magnetic stimulation of the brain has been reviewed by Hallett and Cohen.[66]

Multimodality Potentials

Combinations of visual, auditory, and somatosensory evoked potentials are referred to as multimodality evoked potentials. Because the refractory effect of one stimulus on the response to a subsequent stimulus is less if the stimulus is in a different modality, responses to multiple modalities can be recorded simultaneously rather than separately. However, filtering and randomization of stimulus timing may be necessary in order to eliminate distortion of potentials due to interweaving.[67] Multimodality techniques have been used primarily in intensive care units to evaluate outcome after coma or severe head injury. Narayan and colleagues noted that multimodality evoked potentials and intracranial pressure were the best predictors of neurologic outcomes after head injury.[68]

RECORDING TECHNIQUE AND INSTRUMENTATION

Systems for recording evoked potentials can be either created from individual components or purchased complete. Essential components include stimulators; equipment to acquire, amplify, and filter the signals; signal processors; and systems to display, measure, and store evoked waveforms. Systems can be individually configured for specific applications or investigators. Desirable parameters for intraoperative evoked potential recordings are described in Nuwer and Table 22–2.[16] The American Electroencephalographic Society suggested standards for personnel, equipment, and doc-

---

Table 22–2. PARAMETERS FOR EVOKED
POTENTIAL RECORDINGS

---

1. Stimulus current, duration, rate
2. Sites—left or right median or posterior tibial nerve
   (SSEP)
3. Electrodes
       Stimulating type, size, position of cathode
       Recording type, impedance, sites
4. Recording channels
5. Stimulation filters, sweep time, sampling rate
6. Sensitivity
7. Repetitions or trials

---

umentation of electrophysiologic testing in 1984 and 1987.[69, 70] The personnel requirements for evoked potential monitoring include an EEG technologist to apply electrodes, operate the equipment, and troubleshoot the system while an immediately available neurologist, neurosurgeon, or neuroanesthesiologist provides interpretation of the waveforms.

Two, preferably four, and often more channels or comparisons between two electrodes are used for intraoperative monitoring of evoked potentials. Whenever possible, evoked potentials are recorded from both areas at risk and areas not at risk of damage during operative procedures in order to distinguish changes caused by the operative procedure from those produced by anesthesia, temperature, or other global systemic changes.

Stimulating Electrodes

Both invasive and noninvasive techniques can be used. However, invasive techniques are infrequently used in the United States except when the spinal cord, brain, or other structure is open during surgery. Peripheral somatosensory stimuli are delivered as an electrical current through paired electrodes placed about 3 cm apart with the cathode proximal. Although ring electrodes, hand-held balls, and surface electrodes mounted on rigid bars may be used in neurology laboratories, intraoperative stimulation is facilitated by use of subdermal platinum electrodes. Stimuli are delivered through the electrodes at a set rate. Although faster stimulus rates attenuate the amplitude of the evoked potential, they permit more rapid averaging of responses and identification of abnormalities.

Recording Electrodes

For recording of cortical potentials, as with recording of the electroencephalogram, correct position and application of electrodes are essential. Scalp electrodes are positioned according to the International 10–20 system (see Chapter 20), but positions are modified by placing electrodes 2 cm behind positions Cz, C3, and C4 (called Cz′, C3′, and C4′). Another modification is the placement of the electrodes halfway between each of the 10–20 system electrodes.[71] The difference in the signal between a pair of electrodes is amplified and displayed as the evoked potentials. One electrode of the pair is designated as the active electrode, having a stronger signal, but the other or reference electrode is frequently active as well. Reference electrodes are often placed at the mastoid, forehead, mandible, or earlobe.

Preferred electrodes are 1 cm in diameter, silver–silver chloride, applied with collodion, and filled with conducting gel. Electrodes must be securely fastened in order to minimize movement artifacts. Other types are cup, self-adhesive, and needle electrodes. When cup electrodes are used, the gel is placed inside using a blunt-tipped needle, and plastic tape covers the hole to prevent electrode drying. Preparation for self-adhesive electrodes includes rubbing the skin with alcohol followed by rubbing with dry gauze or specially prepared abrasive pads. An easier method of electrode application for anesthesiologists is the use of spiral-needle electrodes (commonly used for fetal scalp monitoring in obstetrics), inserted after mild abrasion of the skin with alcohol and spraying of ethyl chloride in order to minimize discomfort.[72] Careful preparation is necessary to assure low impedances of 1000–3000 ohms. Higher impedances are acceptable only if they are similar bilaterally.

For recordings from sterile surgical fields, platinum needle electrodes are used. Higher impedances are present with such electrodes because of the smaller surface area. Use of needle electrodes requires careful attention to grounding of the electrocautery. An improperly grounded cautery causes more extensive injury, owing to the small surface area of a needle, than does a larger electrode. Silastic or Teflon sheets of electrodes are also used to record from cortical surfaces because of their convenience over individual electrodes.

Signals and Signal Processing

The amplitude of the response evoked by the stimuli is so small that it would usually be indistinguishable from other electrical activity such as the electrocardiogram (ECG) or EEG. Thus, the response must be separated from this background noise. The process of separation involves multiple repetitions of the stimulus, averaging of many responses (signal averaging), and recordings over a specific time after each stimulus. The unprocessed signal is observed in order to suspend recording when excessive noise (such as electrocautery) is present. Four types of filters are used: (1) low filter (filters out low-frequency activity), (2) high filters (filters out high-frequency activity), (3) 60-Hz notch filter (filters out 60-cycle interference from electrical power lines), and (4) smoothing filters.[16] Automatic artifact rejection, based on amplitude criteria, may include certain artifacts not exceeding the limits while excluding physiologic signals.

The variety of signal processing techniques (dual time base, synchronous averaging, asynchronous parallel averaging, and pseudorecursive averaging) are discussed in Nuwer and Moller.[16, 54] Continual monitoring of spontaneous EEG activity allows suspension of evoked potential recordings whenever the signal becomes unduly noisy.

Complex processing of noisy waveforms may produce spurious results because highly processed noise actually resembles evoked potentials but is unrelated to electrophysiologic processes. Common sources of interference on evoked potentials are ECG, EMG, stimulus artifacts, 60-Hz artifacts, and amplifier noise. Such interference is minimized by placing all electrodes and wires as far as possible from sources of mechanical (movement, other patient tubes or cables) or electrical (power cords) artifacts. A detailed discussion of the problem of electromagnetic interference is presented in Moller.[54] Other sources of interference are movement artifacts generated by patient muscle motion such as blinking of eyelids, eye movements, tongue motion, and muscle potentials. Most of these are eliminated by adequate anesthesia and neuromuscular blockade.

Analysis and Storage of Recorded Waveforms

Multiple epochs or sweeps are averaged, converted to an analog waveform, and displayed or measured. Detailed recording parameters for somatosensory, brainstem auditory, and visual (flash) evoked potentials are presented in Friedman and associates and Grundy.[7, 27] Extraneous pharmacologic, physiologic, or other variables possibly affecting the evoked potentials during recording are noted. Evoked potentials can be quantitated by power spectral analysis, correlation analysis, parametric predictive modeling, significance probability mapping, and measurement of wave area.[73-76] Recorded potentials should be reviewed immediately after acquisition, but they may be stored electromagnetically on disks or tape.

When unexpected changes occur in evoked potentials, a thorough search for technical problems should be made before assuming that they result from a pathologic process. Confirmation of stimulation by presence of initial electrophysiologic responses; checking of electrode impedance to evaluate displacement, drying of gel, disconnection, or breaking of leads; evaluation of machine settings for stimulation and recordings; and finally recording of EEG without stimulation all assure that changes in evoked potentials are the result of pathologic and not technical processes.[27] Despite these precautions, false-negatives (stable evoked potentials but postoperative deficits) and false-positives (abnormal evoked potentials without postoperative deficits) occur.[23]

Physiologic Alterations in Evoked Potentials

There is diurnal variation of amplitude, with the greatest amplitude between 6:00 P.M. and 6:00 A.M. in monkeys.[77] In humans, fast frequency potentials appear on the ascending and descending phases of slow negative waves in the awake state, but they are markedly attenuated or disappear during sleep.[78]

Normal values for various types of evoked potentials have been published.[70] Evoked responses may be asymmetric owing to cortical dominance, but they usually do not vary between right and left sides of the body. Evoked potentials vary with both gender and age.[79-82] Maturation of evoked responses has been confirmed in infants.[83] Taylor and Fagan present detailed changes in waveforms associated with maturation.[84] Negative peak latencies of N_9, N_{13}, and N_{14} directly relate to patient age and height. However, the initial negative wave N_{18} and positive wave P_{28} are unrelated to age. CCT decreases during the first decade of life, attaining adult values by 8 years of age.[85]

Published values must be confirmed in the individual laboratory before subsequent recordings are classified as technically inadequate, technically adequate but abnormal, or normal. In intraoperative settings, the patient serves as his or her own control, thus facilitating recording even in the presence of abnormalities.

EFFECTS OF ANESTHETICS, DRUGS, AND PATHOPHYSIOLOGIC CONDITIONS

Anesthesia

Anesthetics minimally affect the early specific evoked responses but greatly affect the later-occurring waves (Fig. 22–5; Table 22–3). Potentials arising in the cerebral cortex are affected by all drugs acting in the central nervous system. VEP are more susceptible to anesthesia than are BAEP.[54, 86] Proper interpretation of changes in evoked potentials during surgical procedures depends upon observation and knowledge of anesthetic effect.[87]

Premedication. Premedicant drugs given more than 60 minutes prior to the procedure are unlikely to significantly affect intraoperative monitoring of SSEP and actually facilitate preoperative analysis by decreasing muscular twitches. However, drugs commonly used for premedication such as diazepam,[88] fentanyl,[89] morphine,[90] and barbiturates all affect evoked potentials. Fentanyl and diazepam given to awake patients minimally affect SSEP. Atropine in clinically used doses does not affect BAEP in animals.[91] In very large doses (40 mg/kg), atropine increases the amplitude of P_1, P_2, and P_3 of the BAEP in rats.[91] The cortical responses are more affected by anesthetics than are the brainstem and spinal cord responses. Nitrous oxide–narcotic–relaxant anesthesia with constant concentrations (less than minimum alveolar concentration [MAC]) of volatile anesthetics maintains the requisite constant depth of anesthesia. Avoidance of bolus administration of narcotics and other intravenous (IV) agents and their administration by infusions minimizes changes in anesthetic depth.[89]

Volatile Anesthetics. In general, the effects of volatile anesthetics such as halothane, enflurane, and isoflurane are greater than those of narcotics and barbiturates in equi-anesthetic concentrations. Concentrations of volatile anesthetics in excess of 0.75% are likely to obliterate cortical SSEP.

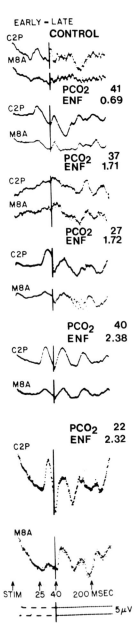

EARLY – LATE

Figure 22–5. Alterations in SSEP waveform associated with enflurane (ENF) anesthesia. The inspired concentration (%) and the arterial PCO_2 at each time are indicated. (From Clark DL, Rosner BS: Neurophysiologic effects of general anesthetics. I. The electroencephalogram and sensory evoked responses in man. Anesthesiology 1973; 38:575. With permission.)

Wolfe and Drummond, Samra and associates, and Peterson and co-workers[92–94] noted that 0.5, 1.0, and 1.5 MAC isoflurane caused dose-related decreases in the amplitude of cortical SSEP. However, subcortical potentials were not significantly affected.[92, 93] Amplitude was more significantly affected than CCT or peak latency.[100] Peterson and coworkers noted that enflurane and halothane produced dose-related reductions in amplitude and prolongation of SSEP latency in humans.[94] Specifically, halothane, up to 0.5%, permitted continuous intraoperative evaluation of SSEP, although

Table 22–3. DRUG EFFECTS ON EVOKED POTENTIALS

Drug	SSER	VER	BAER
Barbiturate	↑ latency[102] →, ↓ amplitude[103,104]	Enhanced early specific activity[105] ↑ latency ⎤ deep ↓ amplitude ⎦ anesthesia	↑ latency, limited effects on amplitude
Etomidate[103,104]	↑ latency N_{20}, P_{23} → latency N_{10}, N_{14} ↑ amplitude N_{20}, P_{23} → amplitude N_{10}	?	No effect
Ketamine[109]	?	?	No effect[109] ↑ latency, decreased amplitude (rats)[110]
Droperidol	↑ latency ↓ amplitude	?	?
Fentanyl	↑ latency[89] ↓ amplitude	Unchanged latency amplitude effects variable	No effect[112]
Sufentanil	→ latency ↓ amplitude	?	?
Propofol[108]	↑ latency sl* ↓ amplitude	?	?
Meperidine	↑ latency ↓ amplitude	?	?
Morphine	↑ latency[89] ↓ amplitude	?	?
Nitrous oxide	↓ amplitude → latency	↓ amplitude ↑ latency	↓ amplitude unchanged latency
Halothane[94,96]	↑ latency ↓ amplitude	↑ latency Amplitude effects variable (increased) Amplitude effects unknown	↑ latency ↓ amplitude
Enflurane[94,96]	↓ specific activity ↑ latency ↓ amplitude	↑ ↓ → latency	↑ latency
Isoflurane[92–94,96]	↑ latency ↓ amplitude	↑ latency ↓ amplitude	↑ latency
Midazolam[103]	sl* ↑ latency → ↓ amplitude	?	?
Diazepam	sl* ↑ latency sl* ↓ amplitude	?	?

* sl = slight.

the latency of P_{53} increased, amplitude of N_{25} and P_{30} decreased, and N_{25}, N_{40}, N_{53}, and N_{71} were occasionally obliterated.[95] Pathak and colleagues, however, noted that subcortical potentials were affected by isoflurane, halothane, and enflurane (increased latency and decreased amplitude), although less than cortical SSEP were.[96] Nitrous oxide decreases the amplitude and increases the latency of SSEP.[97] Halothane, enflurane, and isoflurane produce dose-related increases in latency of BAEP.[98, 99] The findings for halothane and enflurane, however, are controversial.[100]

Induction Agents. Barbiturates enhance evoked potential amplitude before its suppression.[35, 101] Recent studies in unmedicated patients confirm that thiopental causes variability of somatosensory evoked potential amplitude, with a tendency to decrease.[102, 103] A transient increase in the latency of the cortical N_{20} and interwave conduction times of second cervical ver-

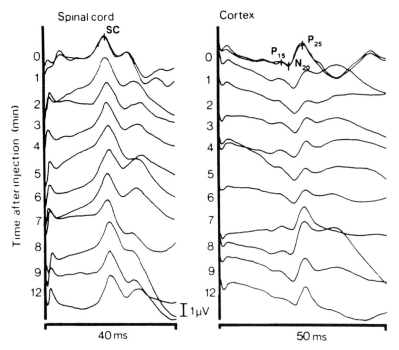

Spinal cord

Cortex

Time after injection (min)

SC

P_{25}

P_{15} N_{20}

40 ms

50 ms

1 μV

Figure 22–6. The effects of thiopental, 4 mg/kg intravenously, on spinal cord (SC) and cortical SSEP in unpremedicated humans are decreased amplitude and increased latency. In the cervical cord response, negative responses are upward, whereas in the cortical response positive responses are upward. See text for discussion on P_{15}, P_{20}, and N_{20}. (From Sloan TB, Kimovec MA, Serpico LC: Effects of thiopentone on median nerve somatosensory evoked potentials. Br J Anaesth 1989; 63:51–55. With permission.)

tebra to sensory cortex primary cortical response waves 15 and 25 is seen (Fig. 22–6).[102, 103] Thiopental does not affect the amplitude of N_{10}, N_{14}, or waves recorded from the scalp.[104] Barbiturates do not depress VEP and may actually enhance early specific activity at occipital sites.[105] In clinical doses, barbiturates have limited or no effect on latencies and amplitudes of BAEP. After large doses, the latency of BAEP waves I, III, and V increases, but amplitude is unchanged.[106]

Etomidate in doses of 0.4 mg/kg changes the evoked waveform by increasing the amplitude of N_{20}–P_{23} and P_{15}–N_{20}, although N_{10} amplitude was unchanged and N_{14} amplitude decreased. Latencies of N_{20} and P_{23} were increased, but N_{10} and N_{14} were unchanged.[103, 104] The increased amplitude seen after etomidate administration may be used to advantage in patients with preexisting neurologic abnormalities reducing evoked responses.[107] However, it may be less desirable to use etomidate for induction of anesthesia because decreases in evoked responses occur as etomidate concentrations decrease.[104]

Propofol, 2.5 mg/kg, causes disappearance of SSEP waves after N_{14} and N_{20}. Latency of potentials increases, and amplitude decreases slightly.[108] Short latency subcortical SSEP are minimally affected by anesthetics such as ketamine and pentobarbital.[109] Church and Gritzke, however, noted increased latency and decreased amplitude of BAEP in rats receiving ketamine 100 mg/kg.[110] Bobbin and associates, however, noted no effect of ketamine on BAEP at the same doses.[109]

Narcotics. Morphine increases the latency of N_1, N_2, and P_2 and decreases the peak-to-peak amplitude of the primary complex (P_2–N_2) of cortical SSEP.[89] However, morphine had no effect on BAEP in monkeys given

3.2 mg/kg intravenously.[111] Fentanyl in normal unpremedicated humans decreased P_{15}–N_{20} amplitude and increased N_{20} and P_{23} latency of SSEP.[89, 104] However, in doses up to 50 μg/kg, it does not affect either the latency or the amplitude of BAEP.[112] Chi and coworkers reported no effect on amplitude of VEP after up to 60 μg/kg of fentanyl.[113] The decrease in amplitude of VEP after fentanyl was variable and may have been caused by pupillary constriction.[113]

Benzodiazepines. Midazolam does not affect the amplitude of SSEP but increases latency.[103] Lorazepam increased the latency and decreased the amplitude of N_1 and P_3 of the auditory evoked response.[114] Diazepam, up to 0.2 mg/kg IV, does not affect BAEP.[115] Scopolamine in doses of 0.1 or 0.32 mg/kg did not change amplitude or latency of BAEP in monkeys.[111]

Local Anesthetics. Application of local anesthetics to peripheral nerves, by blocking sensory input, tends to abolish responses evoked by stimulation of those nerves. Blood levels of lidocaine similar to those achieved during regional anesthesia significantly decreased the amplitude and increased the latency of wave V of the BAEP in humans.[116] BAEP waves I and III were unaffected by lidocaine, indicating its more central effects. Epidural local anesthesia decreases, but does not abolish, SSEP. Intrathecal lidocaine completely abolishes SSEP.[117] Both epidural and subarachnoid bupivacaine anesthesia decrease the amplitude of SSEP from stimulation within the area of neural blockade, but the amplitude reduction is unrelated to sensory or motor blockade.[118, 119]

The optimum anesthetic for evoked potential recordings is a balanced technique of nitrous oxide, narcotic, neuromuscular blockade, and constant concentrations of volatile agents at less than 0.5% if necessary. Because of the effects of anesthesia on evoked potentials, Hogan and coworkers suggest monitoring of early far-field potentials recorded from vertex to neck and lumbar spinal cord potentials during halothane anesthesia.[120] Another approach to monitoring evoked potentials during anesthesia is to use a ratio of the amplitude of the evoked potentials from median and posterior tibial nerves during sequential stimulation, as suggested by Madigan and associates.[121] Subtraction of 1 standard deviation from the mean postdistraction value in 38 patients undergoing scoliosis surgery yielded a critical value for decreased spinal cord conduction. York and colleagues reported no neurologic deficits during scoliosis repair if SSEP were within ±2 standard deviations of the anesthetized control value.[122] Neuromuscular blockers should not be given until the position of stimulating electrodes for SSEP is verified by motor response, although neuromuscular blockade, by eliminating muscle artifacts, actually facilitates recordings.

Drugs

Thyroid hormone increases the early cortical activity related to sensory stimulation.[123] Propranolol has no effect on evoked potentials but eliminates the changes seen with thyroid hormone.[124] Mitchell and coworkers, however, noted no significant changes in VEP before or after therapy for hyperthyroidism.[125] Although ethyl alcohol changes cortical sensory evoked potentials, it minimally affects evoked potentials of subcortical origin.[126]

Drugs used to produce hypotension should be administered in a way that produces a new stable clinical state as rapidly as possible when evoked potentials are being recorded. Although such drugs may produce no intrinsic effect on evoked potentials, alteration of blood pressure has significant effects, which are discussed later in this chapter.

Pathophysiologic Effects

Temperature

Hypothermia increases latency and decreases amplitude. Van Rheineck Leyssius and associates noted that the latency of P_1 of the SSEP increased by 1.15 msec/°C during cooling on cardiopulmonary bypass. Later cortical waves showed even greater increases in latency.[127]

Markand and colleagues studied the effects of cooling on VEP, BAEP, and SSEP.[128] The latency of VEP increased with hypothermia, becoming unrecordable at 23°C during hypothermic cardiopulmonary bypass. Russ and colleagues noted that VEP disappeared at higher temperatures with more rapid rates of cooling (Fig. 22–7).[44] VEP were somewhat more temperature-sensitive than SSEP. BAEP disappeared at temperatures of 20–25°C. SSEP were unrecordable between 20 and 27°C. The configuration of evoked responses can be altered by changes in temperature along the transmission pathway, e.g., exposed extremities, room temperature fluids applied to cord or brain with open dura, or irrigation at cerebellopontine angle.

Hemodilution

Nagao and associates noted changes in VEP and SSEP with hemodilution.[129] At hematocrits of 16–20%, the amplitude of VEP increased. Below 10% hematocrit, amplitude decreased and latency increased, probably because of hypoxia. Similar changes occurred in SSEP.[129]

Oxygen Tension

McPherson and coworkers evaluated the effects of hypoxia on cortical SSEP in dogs.[130] When P_{O_2} decreased to less than 30, there were changes in latency and amplitude, but an evoked response could be recorded at an isoelectric EEG. Grundy and colleagues found marked distortion of somatosensory cortical evoked potentials when other monitors such as ECG, esophageal stethoscope, blood, and skin color failed to detect hypoxia to a P_{O_2} of 41.[131]

Carbon Dioxide Tension

Latencies of cervical and cortical responses to median nerve stimulation decreased significantly during hypocapnia to 20 mmHg.[132] However, Tach-

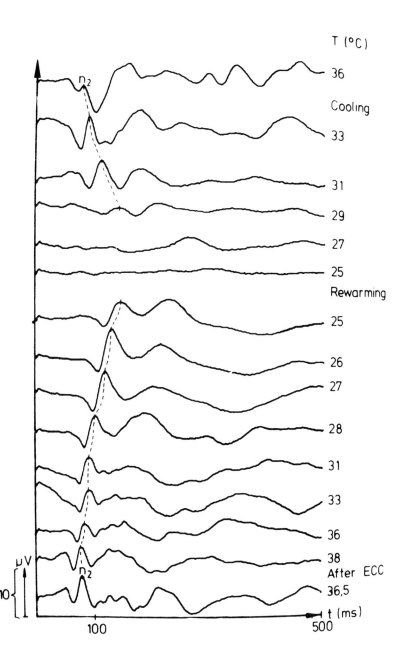

Figure 22–7. The latency of n_2 of the VEP is increased during cooling on extracorporeal circulation. At 25–27°C, the potentials disappear completely but reappear promptly on rewarming. (From Russ W, Kling D, Loesevitz A, Hempelmann G: Effect of hypothermia on visual evoked potentials [VEP] in humans. Anesthesiology 1984; 61:207–210. With permission.)

ibana noted small changes in amplitude.[133] Hypercapnia seems unlikely to affect evoked potentials, but it has not been tested systematically.

Perfusion Pressure

SSEP are preserved to the lower limits of autoregulation. Below mean pressures of about 50 mmHg, SSEP change in response to decreased blood flow.[134–136] However, cortical evoked responses are more sensitive to pressure than are subcortical or spinal evoked responses (Fig. 22–8).[136, 137]

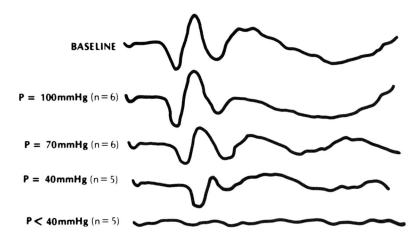

Figure 22–8. In a canine experimental preparation, decreases in perfusion pressure (maintained with left heart–femoral artery bypass) distal to an aortic clamp cause decreased amplitude and prolonged latency in SSEP below 70 mmHg. (From Laschinger JC, Cunningham JN Jr, Baumann FG, et al: Monitoring of somatosensory evoked potentials during surgical procedures on the thoracoabdominal aorta II. J Thorac Cardiovasc Surg 1987; 94:266–270. With permission.)

Ischemia

In the spinal cord, ischemia produces a time-related deterioration and eventual loss of SSEP. In an experimental canine model of thoracic aortic occlusion, Coles and coworkers noted more than 50% diminution in the amplitude of P_1 of the SSEP within 4 minutes of occlusion.[138] Total loss of cortical evoked potentials to sciatic nerve stimulation occurred with loss of P_2 after 12 minutes of occlusion. If reperfusion was initiated at that time, there was no neurologic deficit. If reperfusion was delayed for 15 minutes, significant neurologic deficits were present. The early component, P_1, was most sensitive to ischemia.

Neurologic Injury

The SSEP criteria for acute neurologic injury are unclear. Usually an amplitude reduction of greater than or equal to 50% of the dominant wave is accepted. However, this definition has not been substantiated, and reports of larger alterations without neurologic sequelae exist.[139, 140] In important events there is rapid progression to total or near-total loss of the SSEP. Serious events demonstrate decreased amplitude, increased latency, and changed wave configuration. Reductions in amplitude associated with environmental factors, changes in anesthesia, or gradual reduction are usually inconsequential. Evoked responses can be elicited during isoelectric EEGs. After hypoxic episodes, evoked potentials recover within 5 minutes and are complete within 30 minutes of reoxygenation, significantly before the EEG returns to normal. However, evoked potentials are affected by injuries along their neural pathway.

The status of BAEP wave V is often used to assess injury to the auditory pathway. However, it is not highly specific, since substantial and persistent increases in latency may occur without postoperative hearing loss.[56, 141] Transient loss of the peak intraoperatively with its reappearance later in the procedure is compatible with preservation of hearing postoperatively.

BAEP are useful in the evaluation of comatose patients to separate

Figure 22–9. Cortical SSEP (C_4' − FP_2) and spinal responses (SC_2 − FP_2) in awake state (*A*); after induction of anesthesia (*B*), showing increased latency and decreased amplitude; loss of cortical potentials (*C*) bilaterally when patient with a posterior fossa tumor whose head was flexed, rotated to the left, and placed left side down, causing brainstem ischemia; and restoration of cortical potentials (*D*) after repositioning of head. Responses to stimulation of left median nerve on left and to right median nerve on right side of figure. (From McPherson RW, Szymanski J, Rogers MC: Somatosensory evoked potential changes in position-related brain stem ischemia. Anesthesiology 1984; 61:88–90. With permission.)

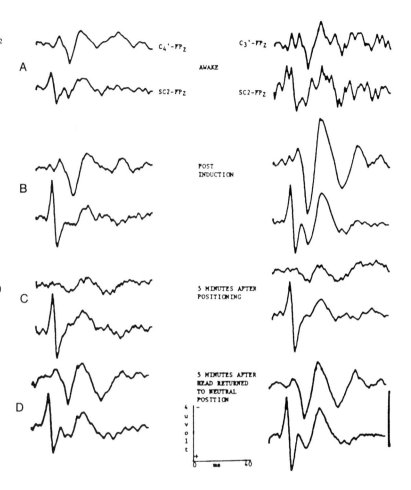

metabolic and toxic encephalopathies from structural lesions of the brainstem, to localize brainstem injury, to assess auditory function, and to clarify prognosis.[16] Wave I of the BAEP or N_1 of the ECochG must be present to evaluate all except the ear itself.

Positioning

Alterations in evoked potentials can result from changes in patient position causing pathologic processes. Normally, changes in position, e.g., sitting to standing, do not change evoked potentials.[23] There should be no differences in latency or amplitude between right and left sides of the body.[23] McPherson and colleagues[142] noted transient loss of cortical SSEP with preserved cervical potentials due to displacement of the brainstem causing ischemia when a patient with a posterior fossa tumor was placed in the parkbench position[143] with the left side down (left arm outstretched) and the head slightly flexed and rotated to the left on a neurosurgical head support. Return of the head to a neutral position restored configuration of the evoked potentials (Fig. 22–9). In a related incident, Mahla and associates noted loss

---

Table 22–4. GRADING OF CHANGES IN EVOKED POTENTIALS

Category I Minimum change (presumably due to anesthesia and temperature changes only)
Category II Transient latency increase, with return toward normal before emergence from anesthesia
Category III Obliteration of the evoked potential, with return toward normal before emergence from anesthesia
Category IV Evoked potential obliteration, without recovery before emergence from anesthesia
Category V Study abandoned for technical reasons
Category VI Absent evoked potential preoperatively and intraoperatively, with associated preoperative neurologic deficits

---

From Grundy BL, Jannetta PJ, Procopio PT, et al: Intraoperative monitoring of brain-stem auditory evoked potentials. J Neurosurg 1982; 57:674–681. With permission.

of both peripheral and cortical SSEP in two patients placed in the park-bench position due to excessive peripheral neural pressure.[144] Repositioning to avoid pressure on the brachial plexus restored the potentials.

Quantitation of Changes in Evoked Potentials

Abnormal waveforms that are not improved by alterations in blood pressure, temperature, position, or technical variables have been categorized by Grundy and coworkers in Table 22–4.[28] Greenberg and colleagues have a useful grading system to evaluate patients with head injury.[145] In their system, grade I is mildly abnormal, grade II is moderately abnormal, grade III is severely abnormal, and grade IV is absent. An example of such a grading system is shown in Figure 22–10.

These alterations result from ischemia,[146] neural path disruption,[147, 148] pressure on spinal cord or cortex,[149–151] and distortion of neural tissue.[151, 152] Additional details of the changes associated with these processes are discussed under specific applications of evoked potential monitoring.

CLINICAL USES OF EVOKED POTENTIALS

One of the major problems with the intraoperative use of evoked potentials has been inappropriate application and interpretation. Because many anesthesiologists lack the time or skill to apply and continuously evaluate the responses during surgery and continuous availability of a neurologist may be equally difficult, intraoperative use of evoked potentials has been limited to centers with the requisite personnel in either neurology or anesthesiology, or both. A reasonable compromise is a registered evoked potential technician who continuously monitors the potentials and consults with neurologists, anesthesiologists, and surgeons when abnormalities are present. Appropriate application of techniques, control of technical difficulties, and skilled interpretation of changes in evoked potentials should minimize false-negative or false-positive results.[153]

Injury grades	Somatosensory evoked potentials	Visual evoked potentials	Auditory evoked potentials

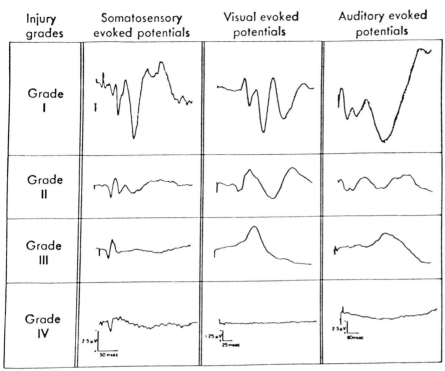

Figure 22–10. Graded responses to injury as demonstrated by sensory evoked potentials. (Reproduced by permission from Cottrell JE, Turndorf H: Anesthesia in Neurosurgery, 2nd ed. St Louis, 1986, The CV Mosby Co.)

Depth of Anesthesia

Evoked responses are affected by depth of anesthesia as described previously. Activating effects on evoked potentials may monitor neurophysiologic effects of anesthesia. Sebel and associates noted insignificant changes in SSEP with tracheal intubation but significant decreases in latency and increases in amplitude with surgical incisions.[154] Their results are corroborated by similar findings from Newton and coworkers using auditory evoked responses.[155] Other studies suggest that the latency of the early cortical wave N_b (less than 44.5 msec) is the best feature to distinguish the "three-wave" auditory evoked response waveform associated with light anesthesia and awareness (indicated by positive responses to Tunstall's isolated forearm test). With addition of increasing concentrations of enflurane, a "two-wave" pattern (latency greater than 44.5 msec) was present.[156] Samra and colleagues were unable to demonstrate a relationship between the long latency auditory evoked potentials and amnesia after lorazepam administration.[114]

Neurosurgery

Cerebral Aneurysmectomy

SSEP have been used extensively in neurosurgical operations, including arteriovenous malformation, intracranial aneurysms, and procedures on the brachial plexus or peripheral nerves. During intracranial surgery, evoked potentials are altered by hypotension, arterial occlusion either directly or from spasm, and brain compression.[157-159] Median nerve stimulation is usually used for evoked potential testing during intracranial vascular surgery. However, for anterior communicating and anterior cerebral artery aneurysms where the areas of the cortex supplying the lower extremity are at risk, posterior tibial nerve stimulation should be used. Kidooka and coworkers noted marked prolongation of the CCT during temporary occlusion of major cerebral arteries or hypotension secondary to aneurysm rupture.[159] In 8 of 20 patients with poor neurologic outcome, the N_{20} peak was obliterated or prolonged by 1.2 msec. Similar findings were made by Ducati and colleagues, who suggested that an intraoperative CCT value of 9 msec was safe when normal values of 6.7 msec were present preoperatively.[160] Such CCTs were present during hypotension to mean arterial pressure of 60 mmHg.[160]

The efficacy of SSEP or BAEP to monitor neurologic damage during cerebral aneurysmectomy was also confirmed by Friedman and associates.[161] In 50 procedures, they noted that prolongation of the CCT, decreased cortical amplitude, or disappearance of the evoked potential was associated with postoperative motor or sensory deficits. However, in patients undergoing basilar aneurysmectomy, such changes in evoked potentials unreliably predicted outcome. Occlusions of basilar aneurysms may not always affect auditory or somatosensory pathways, thus limiting their value as intraoperative monitors.

Posterior Fossa Surgery

Cerebellar retraction, dissection of the eighth cranial nerve, hypotension, and patient positioning may cause BAEP changes. BAEP may be completely obliterated during retraction of the auditory nerve, but function is preserved if changes are reversible in the operating room.[5, 28] Radtke and colleagues note that monitoring of BAEP reduced the incidence of profound postoperative hearing loss from 6.6% to 0% in patients having posterior fossa microvascular surgery for trigeminal neuralgia, hemifacial spasm, or other lesions.[162] However, in Little and coworkers' series of patients undergoing basilar artery aneurysmectomy, four patients had postoperative evidence of brainstem ischemia not predicted by intraoperative monitoring.[163] These events probably occurred in small, unmonitored anatomic areas such as the basilar bifurcation. Changes in BAEP of significance include latency changes of 1 msec and amplitude changes of 50%.[16]

Cortical Localization

Mapping of the cortex by SSEP is less time-consuming than is traditional Penfield electrical stimulation of the cortex to precisely locate sensory and motor cortex.[164] Median nerve stimulation is commonly used, and recording electrodes are applied directly to the brain. Wood and associates used SSEP to localize sensorimotor cortex as maximum SSEP amplitudes are recorded at the hand area of the precentral and postcentral gyri.[165] At the sensory cortex, the SSEP consists of $N_{20}–P_{30}$, whereas at the motor cortex in the precentral gyrus a mirror image (P_{20}, N_{30}) potential is obtained. Reliable identification of the central sulcus depends upon the polarity inversion of the evoked potential.[7]

False-positive changes in evoked potentials occur with accumulation of gas in the cranium beneath cortical electrodes.[166, 167] In both instances, changes in patient position restored evoked potentials to normal, and displacement of intracranial air was verified radiographically.

Brachial Plexus and Peripheral Nerves

Testing of evoked responses is very helpful in determining the functional continuity of the brachial plexus and the necessity for nerve grafting.[10] Preservation of injured, but not transected, nerves is facilitated by electrophysiologic testing in which stimulating and recording electrodes are placed proximal and distal to the lesion, respectively. Nerve injuries are neurapraxic, axonotmetic, or neurotmetic. Neurapraxic lesions are reversible injuries resulting from acute/chronic compression or shear forces, local electrolyte imbalance, or neural ischemia.[7, 16] Nerve action potentials are conducted proximally and distally to, but not through, the lesions. Recovery of the nerve segment occurs in days to weeks but may require neurolysis if chronic compression is present.

In axonotmetic lesions, axons and myelin are lost, but connective tissue elements are preserved and axon regrowth occurs at a rate of 1 mm/day. Nerve action potentials are conducted across the injured area. Neurotmetic lesions involve nerve transection with lack of conduction. Only neurotmetic lesions require resection and nerve anastomosis or grafting.[7]

Orthopedic (Spinal) Surgery

Indications for monitoring SSEP are scoliosis procedures, spinal cord tumors or arteriovenous malformations, and spinal fusions or fracture reduction.

Scoliosis. Although there is a less than 1% incidence of spinal cord damage with spine surgery, procedures such as Luque rodding are more likely to produce injury than those using Harrington rods.[168] Because of this possibility, orthopedic surgeons have relied upon wake-up tests[169] or evoked potentials in order to prevent cord damage. Spinal cord lesions produce changes in amplitude, latency, and form of the evoked response. During spinal cord surgery, the earliest negative peak is evaluated since it is least affected by anesthesia. Figure 22–11 demonstrates the changes in evoked potentials associated with distraction of a Harrington rod. When there is any doubt about the findings from evoked potential testing intraoperatively, a wake-up test is essential. Posterior tibial SSEP are used for surgery involving the thoracic or lumbar spine, whereas median or ulnar stimulation is used to evaluate compression or lesions of the cervical cord. Changes in

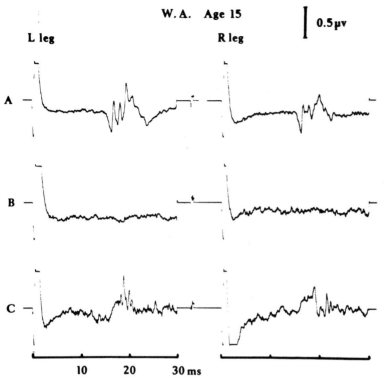

W. A. Age 15

L leg   R leg   0.5 μv

10   20   30 ms

Figure 22–11. During correction of idiopathic scoliosis, normal SSEP from the left and right knees (posterior tibial nerve stimulation) are demonstrated in *A*. In *B*, distraction with the Harrington rod caused bilateral loss of potentials, and loss of function was confirmed with a wake-up test. Twenty minutes after release of distraction, partial restoration of potentials is seen in *C*. (From Jones SA: The value of evoked potentials in surgical monitoring. *In* Cracco RQ, Bodis-Wollner I [eds]: Evoked Potentials. New York: Alan R Liss, 1986; 426. With permission.)

SSEP during anterior cervical spine fusion may also result from carotid arterial compression by retractors in addition to that caused by cord compression. The two processes may be differentiated by preservation of cervical spine responses and absence of cortical potentials.[170]

Spinal Cord Injury. In addition to scoliosis surgery, SSEP are often used during surgery for acute spinal injuries. Fehlings and colleagues noted a correlation among the severity of spinal cord injury, cord blood flow, and both motor and somatosensory evoked potentials in an experimental rat model.[171] As cord injury increased, cord blood flow decreased. SSEP were more sensitive to the degree of injury than were motor evoked potentials. Spielholz and coworkers noted that amplitudes of SSEP increased upon decompression of the spinal cord in 4 of 11 patients undergoing surgical decompression and stabilization of acute cord injuries.[172] However, clinical outcome was unrelated to changes in intraoperative SSEP. Friedman and associates,[7] however, demonstrated the usefulness of SSEP testing in a series of 76 patients undergoing surgical repair of spinal fracture dislocation. Changes in SSEP occurred in two patients; in one, SSEP were lost after passage of the Luque rod but subsequently recovered, and the patient had no postoperative deficit. In the other patient, SSEP from right leg stimulation disappeared during instrumentation whereas left leg SSEP remained normal. The patient subsequently suffered cardiac arrest secondary to myocardial infarction, and on autopsy acute right hematomyelia of the cord confirmed the intraoperative evoked potentials. Meyer and coworkers noted new postoperative deficits in only 0.7% of patients monitored with SSEP during surgical spinal fixation compared with 6.9% in unmonitored patients. They concluded that although subtle alterations might be missed, severe alterations in cord function could be prevented.[173]

Spinal Cord Tumors. Macon and associates,[174] McCallum and Bennett,[175] and McPherson and colleagues[176] have used SSEP during surgical excision of tumors in the spinal canal. In these cases, preoperative absence of evoked potentials precludes monitoring. However, if reproducible waveforms can be obtained, even if they are abnormal, intraoperative monitoring is valuable. Increased stimulus current or stimulus duration and decreased rate of stimulation may facilitate recording of abnormal SSEP. Grundy and coworkers report that monitoring of SSEP during resection of arteriovenous malformations might allow test occlusions of large feeding vessels prior to their sacrifice.[6]

Carotid Artery Surgery

Although the EEG is usually used to monitor cerebral ischemia during carotid endarterectomy, SSEP in response to upper extremity median nerve stimulation has been used for many years.[177] Multichannel EEG is probably preferable since it provides global information, whereas SSEP monitors function in a localized cortical area. However, Moorthy and coworkers confirmed the presence of ischemia on evoked potentials with changes in neurologic status during endarterectomy (Fig. 22–12).[178] In a subsequent report, Markand and associates concluded that SSEP could indicate a need for shunting in patients under general anesthesia when amplitude reduction, latency prolongation, or waveform distortion occurs.[179] Russ and coworkers suggested that a decrease in amplitude of N_{20} and P_{25} or complete loss of SSEP with carotid clamping was 99% specific and 83% sensitive for cerebral ischemia.[180] In cats with unilateral middle cerebral artery occlusion, Steinberg and colleagues noted that recovery of cortical evoked potentials correlated with the severity of cerebral ischemia.[181]

Bilateral comparisons are essential to eliminate the effects of hypotension, anesthesia, or equipment malfunction during evoked potential recording. A comparison of multichannel EEG and SSEP during a large series of carotid endarterectomies has not been performed. Finally, the need for specific monitors of cerebral function during carotid endarterectomy is controversial if regional anesthesia or routine shunting are used.

Cardiac Arrest and Resuscitation

SSEP have recently been used to evaluate the effectiveness of pharmacologic and mechanical methods of cardiopulmonary resuscitation (CPR).[182] Although evoked potentials rapidly disappear during cardiac arrest, effective CPR maintains waves of normal amplitude but slightly prolonged latency. Rapid normalization occurs with restoration of normal circulation (Fig. 22–13).

786

EVOKED POTENTIALS

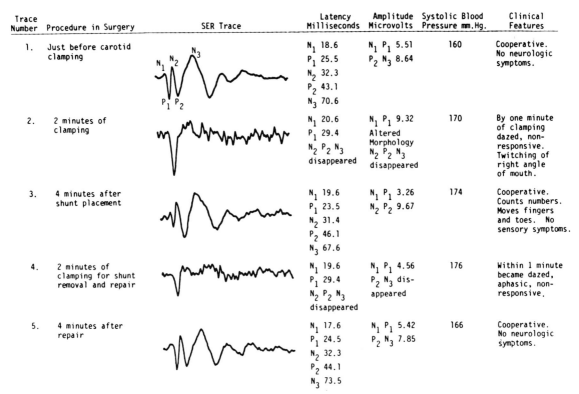

Trace Number	Procedure in Surgery	SER Trace	Latency Milliseconds	Amplitude Microvolts	Systolic Blood Pressure mm.Hg.	Clinical Features
1.	Just before carotid clamping		N_1 18.6 P_1 25.5 N_2 32.3 P_2 43.1 N_3 70.6	$N_1 P_1$ 5.51 $P_2 N_3$ 8.64	160	Cooperative. No neurologic symptoms.
2.	2 minutes of clamping		N_1 20.6 P_1 29.4 $N_2 P_2 N_3$ disappeared	$N_1 P_1$ 9.32 Altered Morphology $N_2 P_2 N_3$ disappeared	170	By one minute of clamping dazed, non-responsive. Twitching of right angle of mouth.
3.	4 minutes after shunt placement		N_1 19.6 P_1 23.5 N_2 31.4 P_2 46.1 N_3 67.6	$N_1 P_1$ 3.26 $N_2 P_2$ 9.67	174	Cooperative. Counts numbers. Moves fingers and toes. No sensory symptoms.
4.	2 minutes of clamping for shunt removal and repair		N_1 19.6 P_1 29.4 $N_2 P_2 N_3$ disappeared	$N_1 P_1$ 4.56 $P_2 N_3$ dis-appeared	176	Within 1 minute became dazed, aphasic, non-responsive.
5.	4 minutes after repair		N_1 17.6 P_1 24.5 N_2 32.3 P_2 44.1 N_3 73.5	$N_1 P_1$ 5.42 $P_2 N_3$ 7.85	166	Cooperative. No neurologic symptoms.

Figure 22–12. Alterations in SSEP associated with neurologic symptoms during clamping of the carotid artery during carotid endarterectomy. During ischemia, N_2, P_2, and N_3 of the evoked response disappeared but immediately returned after shunt placement. (Reprinted with permission from the International Anesthesia Research Society from Somatosensory evoked responses during carotid endarterectomy by Moorthy SS, Markand ON, Dilley RS, et al, Anesthesia and Analgesia, 1982; 61:879.)

Cardiopulmonary Bypass

Cortical visual, brainstem auditory, or somatosensory evoked potentials are used during cardiopulmonary bypass to monitor cerebral perfusion and to detect events such as embolism, hypotension, venous congestion, or mal-positioned cannulae potentially associated with postoperative neurologic dysfunction. However, the associated hypothermia also alters CCT. CCT increases 6.6%/°C as body temperature decreases.[183, 184] The latency of spinal and cortical SSEP increases linearly with hypothermia.[185, 186] All sensory evoked potentials cease at about 20°C.[7]

Coles and coworkers noted that cortical evoked potentials were lost at 18°C in nine infants undergoing profound hypothermia.[187] After rewarming, cortical SSEP recovered within 30 minutes. In the one infant with a prolonged time to recovery of SSEP on rewarming, postoperative seizures occurred. Comparing continuous cardiopulmonary bypass with profound hypothermia and circulatory arrest, Keenan and associates noted less increase in the P_{145} latency during rewarming with continuous bypass than with circulatory arrest.[188]

However, the inability of SSEP to evaluate global cerebral ischemia is demonstrated by two infants in Coles and coworkers' series with postop-

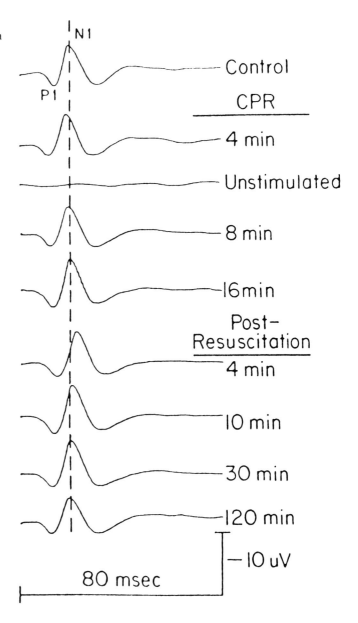

Figure 22–13. SSEP waveforms during cardiac arrest, cardiopulmonary resuscitation (CPR), and after resuscitation in a single experimental animal. The absence of artifact is demonstrated by the "unstimulated" line. Amplitude is measured from P_1 to N_1. The dotted line is a reference for control latency. Latency may be prolonged during resuscitation but rapidly normalizes with restoration of circulation. (From Schleien CL, Koehler RC, Gervais H, et al: Organ blood flow and somatosensory-evoked potentials during and after cardiopulmonary resuscitation with epinephrine or phenylephrine. Circulation 1989; 79:1332–1342. By permission of the American Heart Association, Inc.)

erative cortical blindness. Either multilead EEG or multimodal evoked potentials must be used to assure global evaluation.

Latency for flash evoked potentials increased with hypothermia in rats.[189] BAEP have also been monitored successfully during hypothermic cardiopulmonary bypass.[128]

Aortic Surgery

Surgery on the thoracic or abdominal aorta may result in disruption of critical intercostal or lumbar vessels supplying the spinal cord or ischemia due to decreased spinal cord blood flow during aortic clamping. Spinal cord blood supply includes a single anterior and two posterior spinal arteries. Anterior spinal arteries supply the majority (about $3/4$) of the gray and white matter of the cord. Only the posterior parts of the posterior horns and posterior columns are supplied by the posterior spinal arteries. The small, inconstant circumflex arteries connecting the anterior and posterior spinal arteries are insufficient to sustain circulation to the cord. Radicular arteries, arising from the intercostal and lumbar arteries, provide important supplemental circulation to the anterior spinal arteries. The largest radicular artery, the artery of Adamkiewicz, usually originates in the upper lumbar or lower thoracic region between T-9 and L-2.

SSEP have been used to evaluate spinal cord function during surgical procedures on the aorta in which radicular vessels may be compromised or sacrificed. Neurologic deficits may occur after repair of coarctation, aneurysms of thoracic or abdominal aorta, or resections for aortic occlusive disease. The risk of neurologic injury is less after coarctectomy than after aneurysms because of the presence of collateral circulation. Nevertheless, Dasmahapatra and colleagues noted reversible spinal cord ischemia (decreased interpeak amplitude of N_1–P_1) in 26% of patients undergoing coarctectomy.[189] In these patients, the severity of spinal cord ischemia related to decreased distal aortic pressure.

Laschinger and coworkers noted that interruption of flow to certain vessels caused cord ischemia and that reperfusion resulted in reactive hyperemia.[190] Epidural electrodes were more sensitive than was peripheral nerve stimulation in the detection of cord ischemia secondary to aortic clamping.[191] Preservation of evoked potentials was also pressure-dependent, ceasing below 70 mmHg (see Fig. 22–8). Recent studies also implicate lower distal aortic perfusion pressures resulting from administration of sodium nitroprusside to control proximal hypertension. In canine studies, increased cerebrospinal fluid pressure, decreased distal aortic perfusion pressure, and earlier loss of SSEP associated with nitroprusside administration resulted in postoperative spastic paraplegia.[192]

However, monitoring of sensory evoked potentials does not guarantee that paraplegia will be prevented. SSEP monitor only the posterior and lateral columns of the spinal cord, whereas motor activity is located in the anterior column. Obliteration of SSEP for 15–30 minutes is associated with loss of motor function but sparing or recovery of dorsal column function.[193–195] Monitoring of motor evoked potentials may obviate the false-negative findings occasionally seen during monitoring for spinal cord ischemia.[196] Laschinger and coworkers, using noninvasive peripheral motor evoked potentials monitoring in dogs, noted that ischemic changes occurred from distal to proximal cord as cross-clamp time increased. Reversal of motor evoked potential changes with reperfusion occurred from proximal to distal cord.

Ischemia present on SSEP should be treated by adjustment of distal perfusion pressure, early reversal of ischemia by reimplantation of critical lumbar or intercostal vessels, changes in spinal fluid pressure (cerebrospinal fluid drainage),[197] or administration of pharmacologic adjuncts (calcium blockers, papaverine,[198] free radical scavengers). These modalities should be attempted while false-positive results from central nervous system ischemia, anesthesia, or other causes are eliminated. Grossi and coworkers[191] noted that maintenance of distal mean aortic pressure at 95 mmHg during aortic clamping for 60 minutes prevented ischemic changes on motor evoked potentials. Drainage of cerebrospinal fluid increased spinal cord perfusion pressure during aortic clamping, although it did not affect distal aortic pressure.[192] Finally, a combination of sensory and motor evoked potentials, coupled with monitoring and maintenance of distal aortic perfusion pressure may be required to identify all episodes of spinal cord ischemia during aortic surgery.[190]

Intensive Care Units

CCT is a particularly useful monitor in the postoperative period or after head trauma. During recovery from head trauma, CCT decreases, and its prolongation correlates with the severity of injury. The CCT may be asymmetric in the presence of cerebral injury. Because CCT correlates well with regional cerebral blood flow, it can be used to recognize the onset of ischemia.[199-201] Comas of nontraumatic origin also prolong CCT, as does cerebral hypothermia.[200]

In infants, BAEP correlate well with ultrasonographic abnormalities indicative of brain injury.[202] BAEP are usually normal in comas due to metabolic or toxic causes and may differentiate them from brain injury.

After resuscitation from cardiac arrest, evoked potentials correlate well with outcome.[203-205] If recordings from Erb's point or cervical spine are intact, but no cortical or thalamocortical activity is present, the patient is unlikely to recover beyond a vegetative state. Evoked potentials are also helpful in the assessment of patients with both head and spinal injuries, since evoked potentials do not require patient cooperation.[206]

Despite the expense and complexity of evoked potentials, they are valuable monitors of the central and peripheral nervous system in the perioperative period.[202] Further development of motor evoked potentials, magnetic stimulation, and additional verification of their clinical utility should enhance their use in operating rooms and intensive care units.

References

1. Grundy BL: Monitoring of sensory evoked potentials during neurosurgical operations: Methods and applications. Neurosurgery 1982; 11:556–575.
2. Grundy BL: Electrophysiologic monitoring: Electroencephalography and evoked potentials. *In* Newfield P, Cottrell J (eds): Manual of Neuroanesthesia. Boston: Little Brown, 1983; 28.
3. Bertrand C, Martinez SN, Hardy J, et al: Stereotactic surgery for parkinsonism: Microelectrode recording, stimulation, and oriented sections with a leucotome. Prog Neurol Surg 1973; 5:79–112.
4. Celesia GG: Somatosensory evoked potentials recorded directly from human thalamus and Sm 1 cortical area. Arch Neurol 1979; 36:399–405.

5. Grundy BL, Lina A, Procopio PT, Jannetta PJ: Reversible evoked potential changes with retraction of the eighth cranial nerve. Anesth Analg 1981; 60:835–838.

6. Grundy BL, Nelson PB, Doyle E, Procopio PT: Intraoperative loss of somatosensory evoked potentials predicts loss of spinal cord function. Anesthesiology 1982; 57:321–322.

7. Friedman WA, Theisen GJ, Grundy BL: Electrophysiologic monitoring of the nervous system. *In* Stoelting RK, Barash PG, Gallagher TJ (eds): Advances in Anesthesia 1989; 6:231–290.

8. Haider M, Ganglberger JA, Groll-Knapp E, Schmid H: Averaged cortical and subcortical potentials during stereotactic operations in humans. *In* Speckmann EJ, Caspers H (eds): Origin of Cerebral Field Potentials. Stuttgart: Georg Thieme, 1979; 141–150.

9. Kline DG, Judice DJ: Operative management of selected brachial plexus lesions. J Neurosurg 1983; 58:631–649.

10. Landi A, Copeland SA, Wynn Parry CB, Jones SJ: The role of somatosensory evoked potentials and nerve conduction studies in the surgical management of brachial plexus injuries. J Bone Joint Surg 1980; 62B:492–496.

11. Levy WJ, Grundy BL, Smith NT: Electroencephalography and evoked potentials. *In* Saidman LJ, Smith NT (eds): Monitoring in Anesthesia, 2nd Ed. Boston: Butterworths, 1984.

12. Leuders H, Lesser RP, Hahn J, et al: Cortical somatosensory evoked potentials in response to hand stimulation. J Neurosurg 1983; 58:885–894.

13. Papakostopoulos D, Crow HJ: Direct recording of the somatosensory evoked potentials from the cerebral cortex of man and the differences between precentral and postcentral potentials. *In* Desmedt JE (ed): Clinical Uses of Cerebral, Brainstem, and Spinal Somatosensory Evoked Potentials. Basel: S Karger, 1980; 15–26.

14. Rasmussen T: Cortical resection for medically refractory focal epilepsy: Results, lesions and questions. *In* Rasmussen T, Marino R (eds): Functional Neurosurgery. New York: Raven Press, 1979; 253–269.

15. Caton R: The electric currents of the brain. Br Med J 1875; 2:278.

16. Nuwer MR: Evoked potential monitoring in the operating room. New York: Raven Press, 1986; 5–218.

17. Davis PA: Effects of acoustic stimuli on the waking human brain. J Neurophysiol 1939; 2:494–499.

18. Davis PA: The electrical response of the human brain to auditory stimuli. Am J Physiol 1939; 126:475–476.

19. Sohmer J, Feinmesser M: Cochlear action potentials recorded from the external ear in man. Ann Otol Rhinol Laryngol 1967; 76:427–435.

20. Brazier MAB: Some uses of computers in experimental neurology. Exp Neurol 1960; 2:123–140.

21. Clark WA, Brown RM, Goldstein MG, et al: The average response computer (ARC): A digital device for computing averages and amplitude and time histograms of electrophysiological response. IRE Trans Biomed Electronics 1961; 8:46–51.

22. Anthony PF, Durrett R, Pulec LJ, Hartstone JL: A new parameter in brain stem evoked response: Component wave areas. Laryngoscope 1979; 89: 1569–1578.

23. Grundy BL: Sensory-evoked potentials. *In* Boulton AA, Baker GB, Boisvert DPJ (eds): Imaging and Correlative Physicochemical Techniques. Clifton NJ: Humana Press, 1988.

24. Alonso JA, Hajdu M, Gonzalez EG, et al: Cortical somatosensory evoked

potentials: Effects of positional changes. Arch Phys Med Rehabil 1989; 70: 194–198.

25. Schubert A, Drummond JC, Garfin SR: The influence of stimulus presentation rate on the cortical amplitude and latency of intraoperative somatosensory evoked potential recordings in patients with varying degrees of spinal cord injury. Spine 1987; 12:969–973.

26. Walter WG: Evoked response. *In* Van Leeuwen WS, Lopes da Silva FN, Kamp A (eds): Handbook of Electroencephalography and Clinical Neurophysiology, Vol 8. Evoked Responses. Amsterdam: Elsevier Scientific, 1975; 20–32.

27. Grundy BL: Evoked potential monitoring. *In* Blitt CD (ed): Monitoring in Anesthesia and Critical Care Medicine. New York: Churchill Livingstone, 1985; 345–411.

28. Grundy BL, Jannetta PJ, Procopio PT, et al: Intraoperative monitoring of brainstem auditory evoked potentials. J Neurosurg 1982; 57:674–681.

29. Wang J, Cohen LG, Hallett M: Scalp topography of somatosensory evoked potentials following electrical stimulation of femoral nerve. Electroencephalogr Clin Neurophysiol 1989; 74:112–123.

30. Foit A, Larsen B, Hattori S, et al: Cortical activation during somatosensory stimulation and voluntary movement in man: A regional cerebral blood flow study. Electroencephalogr Clin Neurophysiol 1980; 50:426–436.

31. Leuders H, Dinner DS, Lesser RP, et al: Origin of the far-field subcortical potentials evoked by stimulation of the posterior tibial nerve. Electroencephalogr Clin Neurophysiol 1981; 52:336–344.

32. Tamaki T, Takano H, Nakagawa T: Evoked spinal cord potential elicited by spinal cord stimulation and its use in spinal cord monitoring. *In* Cracco RQ, Bodis-Wollner I (eds): Evoked Potentials. New York: Alan R Liss, 1986; 428–433.

33. Jones SJ: The value of evoked potentials in surgical monitoring. *In* Cracco RQ, Bodis-Wollner I (ed): Evoked Potentials. New York: Alan R Liss, 1986; 421–427.

34. Tamaki T, Tsuji H, Inoue S, et al: The prevention of iatrogenic spinal cord injury utilizing the evoked spinal cord potential. Int Orthop 1981; 4:313–317.

35. Shimoji K, Kano T: Evoked electrospinogram: Interpretation of origin and effects of anesthetics. Int Anesthesiol Clin 1975; 13:171–189.

36. Rowed DW, McLean JAG, Tator CH: Somatosensory evoked potentials in acute spinal cord injury: Prognostic value. Surg Neurol 1980; 9:203–210.

37. Perot PL Jr: The clinical use of somatosensory evoked potentials in spinal cord injury. Clin Neurosurg 1972; 20:367–381.

38. Nash CL Jr, Lorig RA, Schatzinger LA, Brown RH: Spinal cord monitoring during operative treatment of the spine. Clin Orthop 1977; 126:100–105.

39. Engler GL, Spielholz NI, Bernhard WBN, et al: Somatosensory evoked potentials during Harrington instrumentation for scoliosis. J Bone Joint Surg 1978; 60A:528–532.

40. Kondo M: Clinical study of somatosensory evoked potentials (SEPs) in orthopaedic surgery. Int Orthop 1977; 1:9–15.

41. Sundt TM Jr, Sharbrough FW, Piepgras DG, et al: Correlation of cerebral blood flow and electroencephalographic changes during carotid endarterectomy with results of surgery and hemodynamics of cerebral ischemia. Mayo Clin Proc 1981; 56:533–543.

42. Grundy BL, Nash CL, Brown RH: Arterial pressure manipulation alters spinal cord function during correction of scoliosis. Anesthesiology 1981; 54:249–253.

43. Grundy BL, Nash CL, Brown RH: Deliberate hypotension for spinal fusion: Prospective randomized study with evoked potential monitoring. Can Anaesth Soc J 1982; 29:452–462.

44. Russ W, Kling D, Loesevitz A, Hempelmann G: Effect of hypothermia on visual evoked potentials (VEP) in humans. Anesthesiology 1984; 61:207–210.

45. Allen A, Starr A, Nudleman K: Assessment of sensory function in the operating room utilizing cerebral evoked responses: A study of fifty-six surgically anesthetized patients. Clin Neurosurg 1981; 28:457–481.

46. Raudzens PA: Intraoperative monitoring of evoked potentials. Ann NY Acad Sci 1982; 388:308–332.

47. Costa E, Silva ICE, Wang ADJ, Symon L: The application of flash visual evoked potentials during operations on the anterior visual pathways. Neurol Res 1985; 7:11–16.

48. Cedzich C, Schramm J, Mengedoht CF, Fahlbusch R: Factors that limit the use of flash visual evoked potentials for surgical monitoring. Electroencephalogr Clin Neurophysiol 1988; 71:142–145.

49. Chiappa KH: Pattern shift visual, brainstem auditory, and short-latency somatosensory evoked potentials in multiple sclerosis. Neurology 1980; 30: 110–123.

50. De Vlieger M, Sadikoglu S, van Eijndhoven JHM, Atac MS: Visual evoked potentials, auditory evoked potentials and EEG in shunted hydrocephalic children. Neuropediatrics 1981; 12:55–61.

51. Halliday AM, Halliday E: Cerebral somatosensory and visual evoked potentials in different forms of myoclonus. *In* Desmedt JE (ed): Clinical uses of cerebral, brainstem and spinal somatosensory evoked potentials. Basel: S Karger, 1980; 292–310.

52. Moller AR, Jannetta P, Bennett M, Moller MB: Intracranially recorded responses from the human auditory nerve: New insights into the origin of brainstem evoked potentials (BSEPS). Electroencephalogr Clin Neurophysiol 1981; 52:18–27.

53. Jewett DL, Williston JS: Auditory-evoked far fields averaged from the scalp of humans. Brain 1971; 94:681–696.

54. Moller AR: Evoked Potentials in Intraoperative Monitoring. Baltimore: Williams & Wilkins, 1988; 1–205.

55. Raudzens PA, Shetter AG: Intraoperative monitoring of brainstem auditory evoked potentials. J Neurosurg 1982; 57:341–348.

56. Ojemann RG, Levine RA, Montgomery WM, McGaffigan P: Use of intraoperative auditory evoked potentials to preserve hearing in unilateral acoustic neuroma removal. J Neurosurg 1984; 61:938–948.

57. Hardy RW, Kinney SE, Leuders H, Lesser RP: Preservation of cochlear nerve function with the aid of brain stem auditory evoked potentials. Neurosurgery 1982; 11:16–19.

58. Hashimoto I, Ishiyama Y, Tozuka G: Bilaterally recorded brain stem auditory evoked responses: Their asymmetric abnormalities and lesions of the brain stem. Arch Neurol 1979; 36:161–167.

59. Oh SJ, Kuba T, Soyer A, et al: Lateralization of brainstem lesions by brainstem auditory evoked potentials. Neurology 1981; 31:14–18.

60. Yung MW, Soliman AM: Changes in the brainstem evoked responses following jugular vein ligation. J Laryngol Otol 1988; 102:861–864.

61. Pagni CA, Ettorre G, Infuso L, Marossero F: EMG responses to capsular stimulation in the human. Experientia 1964; 20:691–692.

62. Levy WJ, York DH, McCaffrey M, Tanzer F: Motor evoked potentials from transcranial stimulation of the motor cortex in humans. Neurosurgery 1984; 15:287–302.

63. Barker AT, Jalinous R, Freeston L: Noninvasive magnetic stimulation of human motor cortex. (Letter.) Lancet 1985; 1:1106–1107.

64. Estrem SA, Haghighi S, Levy WJ, et al: Motor-evoked potentials of facial musculature in dogs. Laryngoscope 1988; 98:1012–1015.
65. Estrem SA, Haghighi S, Levy WJ, et al: Motor-evoked potentials of tongue musculature in dogs. Laryngoscope 1988; 98:628–631.
66. Hallett M, Cohen LG: Magnetism: A new method for stimulation of nerve and brain. JAMA 1989; 262:538–541.
67. Plourde G, Picton T, Kellett A: Interweaving and overlapping of evoked potentials. Electroencephalog Clin Neurophysiol 1988; 71:405–414.
68. Narayan RK, Greenberg RP, Miller JD, et al: Improved confidence of outcome prediction in severe head injury: A comparative analysis of the clinical examination, multi-modality evoked potentials, CT scanning and intracranial pressure. J Neurosurg 1981; 54:751–762.
69. American Electroencephalographic Society: Guidelines for intraoperative monitoring of evoked potentials. J Clin Neurophysiol 1987; 4:397–416.
70. Chatrian GE (ed): American Electroencephalographic Society guidelines for clinical evoked potential studies. J Clin Neurophysiol 1984; 1:3–53.
71. Chatrian GE, Lettich E, Nelson PL: Ten percent electrode system for topographic studies of spontaneous evoked EEG activities. Am J EEG Technol 1985; 25:83–92.
72. Dubin S, Martin D: Spiral needle electrodes for evoked potential monitoring. (Letter.) Anesthesiology 1988; 69:282.
73. Boston JR: Spectra of auditory brainstem responses and spontaneous EEG. IEEE Trans Biomed Eng 1981; 28:334–341.
74. Duffy FH, Bartels PH, Burchfiel JL: Significance probability mapping, an aid in the topographic analysis of brain electrical activity. Electroencephalogr Clin Neurophysiol 1981; 51:455–462.
75. Steeger GH: A new reliability test for the correlation analysis of cortical evoked responses using a maximum-likelihood detector. Scand Audiol [Suppl] 1980; 11:15–23.
76. Wong PKH, Bickford RG: Brainstem auditory evoked potentials: The use of noise estimate. Electroencephalogr Clin Neurophysiol 1980; 50:25–34.
77. Dowman R, Wolpaw JR: Diurnal rhythms in primate spinal reflexes and accompanying cortical somatosensory evoked potentials. Electroencephalogr Clin Neurophysiol 1989; 72:69–80.
78. Yamada T, Kameyama S, Fuchigami Y, et al: Changes of short latency somatosensory evoked potential in sleep. Electroencephalogr Clin Neurophysiol 1988; 70:126–136.
79. Desmedt JE, Cheron G: Somatosensory evoked potentials to finger stimulation in healthy octogenarians and in young adults: Wave forms, scalp topography and transit times of parietal and frontal components. Electroencephalogr Clin Neurophysiol 1980; 50:404–425.
80. Desmedt JE: Clinical uses of cerebral, brainstem and spinal somatosensory evoked potentials. Basel: S Karger, 1980; 146–161.
81. Stockard JJ, Hughes JF, Sharbrough FW: Visually evoked potentials to electronic pattern reversal. Latency variations with gender, age and technical factors. Am J EEG Technol 1979; 19:171–204.
82. Stockard JJ, Rossiter VS: Clinical and pathologic correlates of brainstem auditory evoked response abnormalities. Neurology 1977; 27:316–325.
83. Chin KC, Taylor MJ, Menzies R, Whyte H: Development of visual evoked potentials in neonates. A study using light emitting diode goggles. Arch Dis Child 1985; 60:1166–1168.
84. Taylor MJ, Fagan ER: SEPs to median nerve stimulation: Normative data for paediatrics. Electroencephalogr Clin Neurophysiol 1988; 71:323–330.

85. Whittle IR, Johnston IH, Besser M: Short latency somatosensory-evoked potentials in children. Part I. Normative data. Surg Neurol 1987; 27:9–18.
86. Koht A: Anesthesia and evoked potentials: Overview. Int J Clin Monit Comput 1988; 5:167–173.
87. Veilleux M, Daube JR, Cucchiara RF: Monitoring of cortical evoked potentials during surgical procedures on the cervical spine. Mayo Clin Proc 1987; 62: 256–264.
88. Loughnan BL, Sebel PS, Thomas D, et al: Evoked potentials following diazepam or fentanyl. Anaesthesia 1987; 42:195–198.
89. Pathak KS, Brown RH, Cascorbi HF, Nash CL: Effects of fentanyl and morphine on intraoperative somatosensory cortical-evoked potentials. Anesth Analg 1984; 63:833–837.
90. Maruyama Y, Shimoji K, Shimizu H, et al: Effects of morphine on human spinal cord and peripheral nervous activities. Pain 1980; 8:63–73.
91. Church MW, Gritzke R: Dose-dependent effects of atropine sulfate on the brainstem and cortical auditory evoked potentials in the rat. Brain Res 1988; 456:224–234.
92. Wolfe DE, Drummond JC: Differential effects of isoflurane/nitrous oxide on posterior tibial somatosensory evoked responses of cortical and subcortical origin. Anesth Analg 1988; 67:852–859.
93. Samra SK, Vanderzant CW, Domer CW, Sackellares JC: Differential effects of isoflurane on human median nerve somatosensory evoked potentials. Anesthesiology 1987; 66:29–35.
94. Peterson DO, Drummond JC, Todd MM: Effects of halothane, enflurane, isoflurane and nitrous oxide on somatosensory evoked potentials in humans. Anesthesiology 1986; 65:35–40.
95. Salzman SK, Beckman AL, Marks HG, et al: Effects of halothane on intraoperative scalp-recorded somatosensory evoked potentials to posterior tibial nerve stimulation in man. Electroencephalogr Clin Neurophysiol 1986; 65: 36–45.
96. Pathak KS, Amaddio MD, Scoles PV, et al: Effects of halothane, enflurane, and isoflurane in nitrous oxide on multilevel somatosensory evoked potentials. Anesthesiology 1989; 70:207–212.
97. McPherson RW, Mahla M, Johnson R, Traystman RJ: Effects of enflurane, isoflurane, and nitrous oxide on somatosensory evoked potentials during fentanyl anesthesia. Anesthesiology 1985; 62:626–633.
98. Thornton C, Heneghan CPH, James MFM, et al: Effects of halothane or enflurane with controlled ventilation on auditory evoked potentials. Br J Anaesth 1984; 56:315–323.
99. Mainninen PH, Lam AM, Nicholas JF: The effects of isoflurane and isoflurane-nitrous oxide anesthesia on brainstem auditory evoked potentials in humans. Anesth Analg 1985; 64:43–47.
100. Duncan PG, Sanders RA, McCullough DW: Preservation of auditory-evoked brainstem responses in anesthetized children. Can Anaesth Soc J 1979; 26: 492–495.
101. Shaw NA, Cant BR: The effect of pentobarbital on central somatosensory conduction time in the rat. Electroencephalogr Clin Neurophysiol 1981; 51: 674–677.
102. Sloan TB, Kimovec MA, Serpico LC: Effects of thiopentone on median nerve somatosensory evoked potentials. Br J Anaesth 1989; 63:51–55.
103. Koht A, Schutz W, Schmidt G, et al: Effects of etomidate, midazolam, and thiopental on median nerve somatosensory evoked potentials and the additive effects of fentanyl and nitrous oxide. Anesth Analg 1988; 67:435–441.

104. McPherson RW, Sell B, Traystman RJ: Effects of thiopental, fentanyl and etomidate on upper extremity somatosensory evoked potentials in humans. Anesthesiology 1986; 65:584–589.

105. Domino EF, Corssen G, Sweet RB: Effects of various general anesthetics on the visually evoked response in man. Anesth Analg 1963; 42:735–747.

106. Drummond JC, Todd MM, U HS: The effect of high dose sodium thiopental on brainstem auditory and median nerve somatosensory evoked responses in humans. Anesthesiology 1985; 63:249–254.

107. Sloan TB, Ronai AK, Toleikis JR, Koht A: Improvement of intraoperative somatosensory evoked potentials by etomidate. Anesth Analg 1988; 67: 582–585.

108. Scheepstra GL, DeLange JJ, Booij LDHJ, Ros HH: Median nerve evoked potentials during propofol anesthesia. Br J Anesth 1989; 62:92–94.

109. Bobbin RP, May JG, Lemoine RL: Effects of pentobarbital and ketamine on brainstem auditory potentials. Latency and amplitude intensity functions after intraperitoneal administration. Arch Otolaryngol 1979; 105:467–470.

110. Church MW, Gritzke R: Effect of ketamine anesthesia on the rat brain-stem auditory evoked potential as a function of dose and stimulus intensity. Electroencephalogr Clin Neurophysiol 1987; 67:570–583.

111. Samra SK, Krutak-Krol H, Pohorecki R, Domino EF: Scopolamine, morphine, and brainstem auditory evoked potentials in awake monkeys. Anesthesiology 1985; 62:437–441.

112. Samra SK, Lilly DJ, Rush NL, Kirsh MM: Fentanyl anesthesia and human brain stem auditory evoked potentials. Anesthesiology 1984; 61:261–265.

113. Chi OZ, McCoy CL, Field C: Effects of fentanyl anesthesia on visual evoked potentials in humans. Anesthesiology 1987; 67:827–830.

114. Samra SK, Bradshaw EG, Pandit SK, et al: The relation between lorazepam-induced auditory amnesia and auditory evoked potentials. Anesth Analg 1988; 67:526–533.

115. Doring WH, Daub D: Acoustically evoked responses under sedation with diazepam. Arch Otorhinolaryngol 1980; 227:522–525.

116. Ruth RA, Gal TJ, DiFazio CA, Moscicki JC: Brain-stem auditory-evoked potentials during lidocaine infusion in humans. Arch Otolaryngol 1985; 111: 799–802.

117. Chabal C, Jacobson L, Little J: Effects of intrathecal fentanyl and lidocaine on somatosensory-evoked potentials, the H-reflex, and clinical responses. Anesth Analg 1988; 67:509–513.

118. Lund C, Selmar P, Hansen OB, Kehlet H: Effect of intrathecal bupivacaine on somatosensory evoked potentials following dermatomal stimulation. Anesth Analg 1987; 66:809–813.

119. Lund C, Selmar P, Hansen OB, et al: Effect of epidural bupivacaine on somatosensory evoked potentials after dermatomal stimulation. Anesth Analg 1987; 66:34–38.

120. Hogan K, Gravenstein M, Sasse F: Effects of halothane dose and stimulus rate on canine spinal, far-field and near-field somatosensory evoked potentials. Electroencephalogr Clin Neurophysiol 1988; 69:277–286.

121. Madigan RR, Linton AE, Wallace SL, et al: A new technique to improve cortical-evoked potentials in spinal cord monitoring. A ratio method of analysis. Spine 1987; 12:330–335.

122. York DH, Chabot RJ, Gaines RW: Response variability of somatosensory evoked potentials during scoliosis surgery. Spine 1987; 12:864–876.

123. Short MJ, Wilson WP, Gills JP: Thyroid hormone and brain function. IV. Effect of triiodothyronine on visual evoked potentials and electroretinogram in man. Electroencephalogr Clin Neurophysiol 1968; 25:123–127.

124. Straumanis JJ, Shagass C: Electrophysiological effects of triiodothyronine and propranolol. Psychopharmacologia (Berlin) 1976; 46:283–288.
125. Mitchell KW, Wood CM, Howe JW: Pattern visual evoked potentials in hyperthyroidism. Br J Ophthalmol 1988; 72:534–537.
126. Erwin CW, Linnoila M: Effect of ethyl alcohol on visual evoked potentials. Alcoholism 1981; 5:49–55.
127. Van Rheineck Leyssius AT, Kalkman CJ, Bovill JG: Influence of moderate hypothermia on posterior tibial nerve somatosensory evoked potentials. Anesth Analg 1986; 65:475–480.
128. Markand ON, Warren CH, Moorthy SS, et al: Monitoring of multimodality evoked potentials during open heart surgery under hypothermia. Electroencephalogr Clin Neurophysiol 1984; 59:432–440.
129. Nagao S, Roccaforte P, Moody RA: The effects of isovolemic hemodilution and reinfusion of packed erythrocytes on somatosensory and visual evoked potentials. J Surg Res 1978; 25:530–537.
130. McPherson RW, Zeger S, Traystman RJ: Relationship of somatosensory evoked potentials and cerebral oxygen consumption during hypoxic hypoxia in dogs. Stroke 1986; 17:30–36.
131. Grundy BL, Heros RC, Tung AS, Doyle E: Intraoperative hypoxia detected by evoked potential monitoring. Anesth Analg 1981; 60:437–439.
132. Schubert A, Drummond JC: The effect of acute hypocapnia on human median nerve somatosensory evoked responses. Anesth Analg 1986; 65:240–244.
133. Tachibana N: Somatosensory evoked potentials and analgesia in man. Int Anesthesiol Clin 1975; 13:191–213.
134. Branston NM, Ladds A, Symon L, Wang AD: Comparison of the effects of ischaemia on early components of the somatosensory evoked potentials in brainstem, thalamus, and cerebral cortex. J Cereb Blood Flow Metab 1984; 4:68–81.
135. Kobrine AI, Evans EE, Rizzoli HV: Relative vulnerability of the brain and spinal cord to ischemia. J Neurol Sci 1980; 45:65–72.
136. Sato M, Pawlik G, Umbach C, Heiss WD: Comparative studies of regional CNS blood flow and evoked potentials in the cat. Stroke 1984; 15:97–101.
137. Kobrine AI, Doyle TF, Rizzoli HV: Spinal cord blood flow as affected by changes in systemic arterial blood pressure. J Neurosurg 1976; 44:12–15.
138. Coles JG, Wilson GJ, Sima AF, et al: Intraoperative detection of spinal cord ischemia using somatosensory cortical evoked potentials during thoracic aortic occlusion. Ann Thorac Surg 1982; 34:299–306.
139. LaMont RL, Wasson SL, Green MA: Spinal cord monitoring during spinal surgery using somatosensory spinal evoked potentials. J Pediatr Orthop 1983; 3:31–36.
140. Whittle IR, Johnston IH, Besser M: Recording of spinal somatosensory evoked potentials for intraoperative spinal cord monitoring. J Neurosurg 1986; 64:601–612.
141. Friedman WA, Kaplan BJ, Gravenstein D, Rhoton AL: Intraoperative brainstem auditory evoked potentials during posterior fossa microvascular decompression. J Neurosurg 1985; 62:552–557.
142. McPherson RW, Szymanski J, Rodgers MC: Somatosensory evoked potential changes in position-related brain stem ischemia. Anesthesiology 1984; 61:88–90.
143. Gilbert RGB, Bindle AF, Galdino A: The park bench position. *In* Anesthesia for Neurosurgery. Boston: Little, Brown, 1966; 119–151.
144. Mahla M, Long DM, McKennett J, et al: Detection of brachial plexus dysfunction by somatosensory evoked potential monitoring—A report of two cases. Anesthesiology 1984; 60:248–252.

145. Greenberg RP, Newlon PG, Hyatt MS, et al: Prognostic implications of early multimodality evoked potentials in severely head-injured patients. A prospective study. J Neurosurg 1981; 55:227–236.
146. Astrup J, Symon L, Branston NM, et al: Cortical evoked potential and extracellular K^+ and H^+ at critical levels of brain ischemia. Stroke 1977; 8:51–57.
147. Crockard HA, Brown FD, Trimble J, Mullan JF: Somatosensory evoked potentials, cerebral blood flow and metabolism following cerebral missile trauma in monkeys. Surg Neurol 1977; 7:281–287.
148. Cracco RQ, Evans B: Spinal evoked potential in the cat: Effects of asphyxia, strychnine, cord section and compression. Electroencephalogr Clin Neurophysiol 1978; 44:187–201.
149. Bennett MH, Albin MS, Bunegin L, et al: Evoked potentials during brain retraction in dogs. Stroke 1977; 8:487–492.
150. Kobrine AI, Evans DE, Rizzoli HV: Correlation of spinal cord blood flow, sensory evoked response and spinal cord function in subacute experimental spinal cord compression. Adv Neurol 1978; 20:389–394.
151. Croft TJ, Brodkey JS, Nulsen FE: Reversible spinal cord trauma: A model for electrical monitoring of spinal cord function. J Neurosurg 1972; 36:402–406.
152. Dolan EJ, Transfeldt EE, Tator CH, et al: The effect of spinal distraction on regional spinal cord blood flow in cats. J Neurosurg 1980; 53:756–764.
153. Grundy BL, Villani RM: Evoked Potentials. New York: Springer Verlag, 1988; 1–144.
154. Sebel PS, Withington PS, Rutherfoord CF, Markham K: The effect of tracheal intubation and surgical stimulation on median nerve somatosensory evoked potentials during anesthesia. Anaesthesia 1988; 43:857–860.
155. Newton DEF, Thornton C, Creaegh-Barry P, Doré CJ: Early cortical auditory evoked response in anaesthesia: Comparison of the effects of nitrous oxide and isoflurane. Br J Anaesth 1989; 62:61–65.
156. Thornton C, Barrowcliffe MP, Konieczko KM, et al: The auditory evoked response as an indicator of awareness. Br J Anaesth 1989; 63:113–115.
157. Hargadine JR, Snyder E: Brainstem and somatosensory evoked potentials: Application in the operating room and intensive care unit. Bull Los Angeles Neurol Soc 1982; 47:62–75.
158. Symon L, Wang AD, Costa e Silva IE, Gentili F: Perioperative use of somatosensory evoked potentials in aneurysm surgery. J Neurosurg 1984; 70: 269–275.
159. Kidooka M, Nakasu Y, Watanabe K, et al: Monitoring of somatosensory-evoked potentials during aneurysm surgery. Surg Neurol 1987; 27:69–76.
160. Ducati A, Landi A, Cenzato M, et al: Monitoring of brain function by means of evoked potentials in cerebral aneurysm surgery. Acta Neurochir [Suppl] (Wien) 1988; 42:8–13.
161. Friedman WA, Kaplan BJ, Day AL, et al: Evoked potential monitoring during aneurysm operation: Observations after 50 cases. Neurosurgery 1987; 20: 678–687.
162. Radtke RA, Erwin CW, Wilkins RH: Intraoperative brainstem auditory evoked potentials: Significant decrease in postoperative morbidity. Neurology 1989; 39:187–191.
163. Little JR, Lesser RP, Lueders H: Electrophysiological monitoring during basilar aneurysm operation. Neurosurgery 1987; 20:421–427.
164. Penfield W, Jasper HH: Epilepsy and the functional anatomy of the human brain. Boston: Little Brown, 1954.
165. Wood CC, Spencer DD, Allison T, et al: Localization of human sensorimotor cortex during surgery by cortical surface recording of somatosensory evoked potentials. J Neurosurg 1988; 68:99–111.

166. McPherson RW, Toung TJK, Johnson RM, et al: Intracranial subdural gas: A cause of false-positive change of intraoperative somatosensory evoked potential. Anesthesiology 1985; 62:816–819.

167. Schubert A, Zornow MH, Drummond JC, Luerrsen TG: Loss of cortical evoked responses due to intracranial gas during posterior fossa craniectomy in the seated position. Anesth Analg 1986; 65:203–206.

168. MacEwen GD, Bunnell WP, Sriram K: Acute neurological complications in the treatment of scoliosis: A report of the Scoliosis Research Society. J Bone Joint Surg 1975; 57A:404–408.

169. Sudhir KG, Smith RM, Hall JE, Hansen DD: Intraoperative awakening for early recognition of possible neurologic sequelae during Harrington rod spinal fusion. Anesth Analg 1976; 55:526–528.

170. Sloan TB, Ronai AK, Koht A: Reversible loss of somatosensory evoked potentials during anterior cervical spinal fusion. Anesth Analg 1986; 65:96–99.

171. Fehlings MG, Tator CH, Linden RD: The relationships among the severity of spinal cord injury, motor and somatosensory evoked potentials and spinal cord blood flow. Electroencephalogr Clin Neurophysiol 1989; 74:241–259.

172. Spielholz NI, Benjamin MV, Engler GL, Ransohoff J: SSEP during decompression and stabilization of the spine. Spine 1979; 4:500–505.

173. Meyer PR, Cotler HB, Gireesan GT: Operative neurological complications resulting from thoracic and lumbar spinal internal fixation. Clin Orthop 1988; 237:125–131.

174. Macon JB, Poletti CE, Sweet WH, et al: Conducted somatosensory evoked potentials during spinal surgery. J Neurosurg 1982; 57:354–359.

175. McCallum JE, Bennett MH: Electrophysiologic monitoring of spinal cord function during intraspinal surgery. Surg Forum 1975; 26:469–471.

176. McPherson RW, North RB, Udvarhelyi GB, Rosenbaum AE: Migrating disc complicating spinal decompression in an achondroplastic dwarf: Intraoperative demonstration of spinal cord compression by somatosensory evoked potentials. Anesthesiology 1984; 61:764–767.

177. Jacobs LA, Brinkman SD, Morrell RM, et al: Long-latency somatosensory evoked potentials during carotid endarterectomy. Am Surg 1983; 49:338–344.

178. Moorthy SS, Markand ON, Dilley RS, et al: Somatosensory-evoked responses during carotid endarterectomy. Anesth Analg 1982; 61:879–883.

179. Markand ON, Dilley RS, Moorthy SS, et al: Monitoring of somatosensory evoked responses during carotid endarterectomy. Arch Neurol 1984; 41: 375–378.

180. Russ W, Fraedrich G, Hehrlein FW, et al: Intraoperative somatosensory evoked potentials as a prognostic factor of neurologic state after carotid endarterectomy. Thorac Cardiovasc Surg 1985; 33:392–396.

181. Steinberg GK, Gelb AW, Lam AM, et al: Correlation between somatosensory evoked potentials and neuronal ischemic changes following middle cerebral artery occlusion. Stroke 1986; 17:1193–1197.

182. Schleien CL, Koehler RC, Gervais H, et al: Organ blood flow and somatosensory-evoked potentials during and after cardiopulmonary resuscitation with epinephrine or phenylephrine. Circulation 1989; 79:1332–1342.

183. Hume AL, Durkin MA: Central and spinal somatosensory conduction times during hypothermic cardiopulmonary bypass and some observations on the effects of fentanyl and isoflurane anesthesia. Electroencephalogr Clin Neurophysiol 1986; 65:46–58.

184. Kopf GS, Hume Al, Durkin MA, et al: Measurement of central somatosensory conduction time in patients undergoing cardiopulmonary bypass. An index of neurologic function Am J Surg 1985; 149:445–448.

185. Dolman J, Silvay G, Zappulla R, et al: The effect of temperature, mean arterial pressure, and cardiopulmonary bypass flows on somatosensory evoked potential latency in man. Thorac Cardiovasc Surg 1986; 34:217–222.

186. Gollehon D, Kahanovitz N, Happel LT: Temperature effects on feline cortical and spinal evoked potentials. Spine 1983; 8:443–446.

187. Coles JG, Taylor MJ, Pearce MJ, et al: Cerebral monitoring of somatosensory evoked potentials during profoundly hypothermic circulatory arrest. Circulation 1984; 70 (Suppl 1):I96–102.

188. Keenan NK, Taylor MJ, Coles JG, et al: The use of VEPs for CNS monitoring during continuous cardiopulmonary bypass and circulatory arrest. Electroencephalogr Clin Neurophysiol 1987; 68:241–246.

189. Dasmahapatra HK, Coles JG, Taylor MJ, et al: Identification of risk factors for spinal cord ischemia by the use of monitoring of somatosensory evoked potentials during coarctation repair. Circulation 1987; 76 (Suppl 3):III14–18.

190. Laschinger JC, Izumoto H, Kouchoukos NT: Evolving concepts in prevention of spinal cord injury during operations on the descending thoracic and thoracoabdominal aorta. Ann Thorac Surg 1987; 44:667–674.

191. Grossi EA, Laschinger JC, Krieger KH, et al: Epidural-evoked potentials: A more specific indicator of spinal cord ischemia. J Surg Res 1988; 44:224–228.

192. Marini CP, Grubbs PE, Toporoff B, et al: Effect of sodium nitroprusside on spinal cord perfusion and paraplegia during aortic cross-clamping. Ann Thorac Surg 1989; 47:379–383.

193. Kaplan BJ, Friedman WA, Gravenstein N, et al: Effects of aortic occlusion on regional spinal cord blood flow and somatosensory evoked potentials in sheep. Neurosurgery 1987; 21:668–675.

194. Laschinger JC, Cunningham JN, Cooper MM, et al: Monitoring of somatosensory evoked potentials during surgical procedures on the thoracoabdominal aorta. Parts I, II, III, IV. J Thorac Cardiovasc Surg 1987; 94:260–285.

195. Friedman WA, Grundy BL: Monitoring of sensory evoked potentials is highly reliable and helpful in the operating room. J Clin Monit 1987; 3:38–45.

196. Laschinger JC, Owen J, Rosenbloom M, et al: Direct noninvasive monitoring of spinal cord motor function during thoracic aortic occlusion: Use of motor evoked potentials. J Vasc Surg 1988; 7:161–171.

197. Grubbs PE, Marini C, Toporoff B, et al: Somatosensory evoked potentials and spinal cord perfusion pressure are significant predictors of postoperative neurologic dysfunction. Surgery 1988; 104:216–223.

198. Svensson LG, Stewart RW, Cosgrove DM, et al: Intrathecal papaverine for the prevention of paraplegia after operation on the thoracic or thoracoabdominal aorta. J Thorac Cardiovasc Surg 1988; 96:823–829.

199. Okada Y, Shima T, Yamamoto M, Uozumi T: Regional cerebral blood flow, sensory evoked potentials, and intracranial pressure in dogs with MCA occlusion by embolization or trapping. J Neurosurg 1983; 58:500–507.

200. Cracco RQ, Bodis-Wollner I (eds): Evoked Potentials: Frontiers of Clinical Neuroscience. Vol 3. New York: Alan R Liss, 1986.

201. Hargadine JR, Branston NM, Symon L: Central conduction time in primate brain ischemia—a study in baboons. Stroke 1980; 11:637–642.

202. Karmel BZ, Gardner JM, Zappulla RA, et al: Brainstem auditory evoked responses as indicators of early brain insult. Electroencephalog Clin Neurophysiol 1988; 71:429–442.

203. Goldie WD, Chiappa KH, Young RR, Brooks EB: Brainstem auditory and short-latency somatosensory evoked responses in brain death. Neurology 1981; 31:248–256.

204. Hume AL, Cant BR: Central somatosensory conduction after head injury. Ann Neurol 1981; 10:411–419.

205. Hume AL, Cant BR, Shaw NA: Central somatosensory conduction time in comatose patients. Ann Neurol 1979; 5:370–384.
206. Grundy BL, Friedman W: Electrophysiological evaluation of the patient with acute spinal cord injury. Crit Care Clin 1987; 3:519–548.
207. Achor LJ, Starr A: Auditory brainstem responses in the cat. I. Intracranial and extracranial recordings. Electroencephalogr Clin Neurophysiol 1980; 48:154–173.
208. Achor LJ, Starr A: Auditory brainstem responses in the cat. II. Effects of lesions. Electroencephalogr Clin Neurophysiol 1980; 48:174–190.
209. Starr A, Hamilton AE: Correlation between confirmed sites of neurological lesions and abnormalities of far-field auditory brainstem responses. Electroencephalogr Clin Neurophysiol 1976; 41:595–608.

Index

Note: Page numbers in *italics* refer to illustrations; page numbers followed by (t) refer to tables.

801

pH (*Continued*)
  low. See *Acidity.*
  of buffer systems, 598–599, *601*
  of open systems, 601
Pheochromocytoma, hyperthermia due to, 524
Phlebotomy, preoperative, 565
Phonocardiography, in fetal heart rate monitoring, 398
  systolic time intervals and, 243–244
Photoluminescence quenching, 290–291, *290, 291*
Photometry, flame, 616–617
Pickwickian syndrome, respiratory acidosis due to, 609–610, 609(t)
Piezoelectric detectors, for anesthetic gas monitoring, 491
Piezoelectric microphones, 119
Pipecuronium bromide, 727
Placenta, in normal pregnancy, 366–367
  in preeclampsia, 366–367
  oxygenation of, 396–397
Plaques, atherosclerotic, due to catheter-caused injury, 104
Plasmin, epsilon aminocaproic acid's effect on, 545
  in anticoagulation, *540*, 541
Plasminogen, direct tissue activator of, 541
  epsilon aminocaproic acid's effect on, 545
  in anticoagulation, *540*, 541
Plasminogen activator therapy, for myocardial infarction, 561
Platelet(s), 536–538, *536*
  factor 4 level of, 556
  function of, Sonoclot analyzer monitoring of, 561
  heparin and, 542
  in liver transplant surgery, 564
  in preeclampsia, 365–366
  integrity of, and thromboelastography, 560
Plethysmography, 125
  body, for functional residual lung capacity, 325
    for respiratory resistance, 323, *324*
  inductance, for ventilation flow rate, 328
Plotters, graphics, for computer output, 421
Pneumocephalus, tension, 596–597, 597(t)
Pneumoencephalography, 668
Pneumonia, hypoxia due to, 593
Pneumotachography, 328
Pneumothorax, central venous catheterization and, 164
  risk of, during venous catheterization, 166
  tension, 596–597, 597(t)
Poisoning, carbon monoxide, 597(t)
Polarographic analyzer, for oxygen analysis, 284–285
Polio, bulbar, respiratory acidosis due to, 609(t)
Portacaval shunt, 152
Portex Cardioesophagoscope, 30, *30*
Positioning, of patient, during surgery, 13
Positive end-expiratory pressure, 174
  cardiac effects of, 596
  ideal levels of, 595, 595(t)
  in central venous pressure monitoring, 169

Positive end-expiratory pressure (*Continued*)
  preload and, 212–213
  right ventricular function changes with, 271
  to improve pulmonary compliance, 596
  to prevent high oxygen tension, 596
  to raise airway pressure, 594
  vascular pressure and, 174
Post-tetanic facilitation, 727, 738
Post-tetanic potentiation, 738–742
Posture, effects of, on electrocardiography, 38
Potassium, flame photometry of, 616–617
  increase of, due to succinylcholine chloride administration, 725
  ion-selection membrane for, 619
  levels of, effect of hemolysis on, *635*
    hyperventilation and, *74*
    venous, 598
  measurement of, 633-*635,634*
  physiologic role of, 635–636
Potentials, evoked. See *Evoked potential(s).*
Potentiation, post-tetanic, 738
Potentiometry, direct, 619–620
Power spectrum analysis, 698–699, *710*
  complex, *705*
  compressed spectral array of, *706*
  density-modulated spectral array of, 706–707, *708*
  display of, 704
  high frequency activity in, 713
  method of, 702–704
  spectral edge frequency of, 705–706, *706, 707*
Preeclampsia, 354, 357(t)
  angiotensin sensitivity in, 362–363
  arterial pressure in, monitoring of, 371
  blood volume in, 358–359
  cardiac index in, 359, 359(t)
  central nervous system function in, 365
  central venous pressure in, monitoring of, 370
  defined, 357–358
  epidural analgesia and, 366
    cardiovascular physiology of, 367–368, *367*, 369(t)
    hemodynamic response to, *368*
  fluid therapy for, 359–362
  general anesthesia during, 368, *370*
  hemodynamic data of, 359(t)
  hemodynamic responses in, *360*
  hemostasis in, 365–367
  hypertension in, 357
    therapy for, 363–364
  hypovolemia in, 361
  intervillous blood flow in, 369(t)
  neonatal Apgar scores and, 369(t)
  oliguria in, 361, *361*
  patients with, monitoring of, 368, 370–372
  placenta in, 366–367
  pulmonary artery pressure in, monitoring of, 370–371
  renal physiology of, 364
  uterine blood vessels in, 362–363
  vascular reactivity in, 362–363
  vasodilator therapy for, 359–362, *360*